Complications of PEDIATRIC SURGERY

Prevention and Management

by KENNETH J. WELCH, M.D., F.A.C.S.

Associate Clinical Professor of Surgery,
Harvard Medical School,
Senior Associate in Surgery,
Children's Hospital Medical Center,
Boston, Massachusetts

1982

W. B. SAUNDERS COMPANY
PHILADELPHIA/LONDON/TORONTO/MEXICO CITY/RIO DE JANEIRO/SYDNEY/TOKYO

W. B. Saunders Company: West Washington Square
Philadelphia, PA 19105

1 St. Anne's Road
Eastbourne, East Sussex BN21 3UN, England

1 Goldthorne Avenue
Toronto, Ontario M8Z 5T9, Canada

Apartado 26370 — Cedro 512
Mexico 4, D.F., Mexico

Rua Coronel Cabrita, 8
Sao Cristovao Caixa Postal 21176
Rio de Janeiro, Brazil

9 Waltham Street
Artarmon, N.S.W. 2064, Australia

Ichibancho, Central Bldg., 22-1 Ichibancho
Chiyoda-Ku, Tokyo 102, Japan

Library of Congress Cataloging in Publication Data

Main entry under title:

Complications of pediatric surgery.

1. Children — Surgery — Complications and sequelae.
   I. Welch, Kenneth J. [DNLM: 1. Surgery — In infancy
   and childhood.   2. Postoperative complications. WO
   925 C737]

RD137.C59   617'.9801   80–54852

ISBN 0–7216–9169–2   AACR2

Complications of Pediatric Surgery   ISBN   0-7216-9169-2

Last digit is the print number: 9   8   7   6   5   4   3   2   1

CONTRIBUTORS

HARRY APPLEBAUM, M.D.
Formerly Chief Resident in Pediatric Surgery, St. Christopher's Hospital for Children, Philadelphia, Pennsylvania; Surgeon, Division of Pediatric Surgery, Henry Ford Hospital, Detroit, Michigan
The Neck

KEITH W. ASHCRAFT, M.D.
Clinical Professor of Surgery, University of Missouri at Kansas City School of Medicine; Chief, Section of Urology, The Children's Mercy Hospital, Kansas City, Missouri
Esophagus

A. BARRY BELMAN, M.D., M.S.
Professor of Urology and Child Health and Development, George Washington University School for Health Sciences; Chairman, Department of Pediatric Urology, Children's Hospital National Medical Center, Washington, D.C.
The Male External Genitalia

CLIFFORD D. BENSON, M.D., F.A.C.S., F.A.A.P.
Professor of Clinical Surgery, Wayne State University School of Medicine; Emeritus Surgeon in Chief, Children's Hospital of Michigan; Senior Surgeon, Harper-Grace Hospital, Detroit, Michigan
Stomach and Duodenum

RICHARD E. BLACK, M.D.
Fellow in Pediatric Surgery, College of Medicine, University of Cincinnati; Fellow in Pediatric Surgery, Children's Hospital Medical Center, Cincinnati, Ohio
Colon and Rectum

J. R. CASSADY, M.D.
Associate Professor of Radiation Therapy, Harvard Medical School; Staff, Joint Center for Radiation Therapy, Children's Hospital Medical Center, Beth Israel Hospital, Brigham and Women's Hospital, New England Deaconess Hospital, Sidney Farber Cancer Center, Boston, Massachusetts
Radiation Therapy

ARNOLD G. CORAN, M.D.
Head, Section of Pediatric Surgery, and Professor of Surgery, University of Michigan Medical School, Ann Arbor; Chief of Pediatric Surgical Services, Mott Children's Hospital, University of Michigan Medical Center, Ann Arbor; Chief of Pediatric Surgical Services, Wayne County General Hospital, Wayne, Michigan
Malnutrition and Wound Healing

CONTRIBUTORS

J. S. CRAWFORD, M.D., C.M.

Professor of Ophthalmology, University of Toronto Department of Medicine; Formerly Ophthalmologist in Chief, The Hospital for Sick Children, Toronto, Ontario, Canada

Eyes and Lids

SAMUEL L. CRESSON, M.D.

Clinical Professor of Surgery, Temple University Medical School; Senior Surgeon, St. Christopher's Hospital for Children, Philadelphia, Pennsylvania

The Neck

REUBEN S. DUBOIS, M.B., B.S.

Associate Professor of Pediatrics, Wayne State University School of Medicine; Chief, Division of Pediatric Gastroenterology, Children's Hospital of Michigan, Detroit, Michigan

Small Intestine

ANGELO J. ERAKLIS, M.D.

Associate Clinical Professor of Surgery, Harvard Medical School; Associate Surgeon and Director of Surgical Clinics, Children's Hospital Medical Center, Boston, Massachusetts

Spleen and Portal Circulation

PHILIP R. EXELBY, M.D.

Professor in Surgery, Cornell University Medical College; Chief, Pediatric Surgical Service; Attending Surgeon, Department of Surgery, Memorial Sloan-Kettering Cancer Center, New York, New York

Solid Neoplasms

ROBERT M. FILLER, M.D.

Professor of Surgery, University of Toronto; Surgeon in Chief, The Hospital for Sick Children, Toronto, Ontario, Canada

Pancreas

ERIC W. FONKALSRUD, M.D.

Professor and Chief of Pediatric Surgery, University of California at Los Angeles School of Medicine, Los Angeles, California

The Adrenals

DONALD P. GOLDSTEIN, M.D.

Assistant Clinical Professor of Obstetrics and Gynecology, Harvard Medical School; Gynecologist in Chief, Children's Hospital Medical Center; Gynecologist, Brigham and Women's Hospital, Boston, Massachusetts

The Female Genital Tract

WARREN E. GRUPE, M.D.

Associate Professor of Pediatrics, Children's Hospital Medical Center, Harvard Medical School; Chief of Pediatric Nephrology and Senior Associate in Medicine, Children's Hospital Medical Center, Boston, Massachusetts

Acute Renal Insufficiency

J. ALEX HALLER JR., M.D.

Robert Garrett Professor of Pediatric Surgery, The Johns Hopkins Hospital, Baltimore, Maryland

Arteries and Veins

WILLIAM E. HARMON, M.D.

Instructor in Pediatrics, Harvard Medical School; Director, Dialysis Unit, and Assistant in Medicine, Children's Hospital Medical Center, Boston, Massachusetts

Acute Renal Insufficiency

GERALD B. HEALY, M.D.

Associate Professor of Otolaryngology, Harvard Medical School and Boston University School of Medicine; Otolaryngologist in Chief, Children's Hospital Medical Center, Boston, Massachusetts

Salivary Glands, Larynx, and Oropharynx

W. HARDY HENDREN, M.D.

Professor of Surgery, Harvard Medical School; Chief of Pediatric Surgery, Massachusetts General Hospital, Boston, Massachusetts

Kidneys and Ureters

DONALD W. HIGHT, M.D.

Assistant Professor of Surgery, Wayne State University School of Medicine; Director of Pediatric Surgical Education, Children's Hospital of Michigan; Associate Pediatric Surgeon, and Co-Director of Emergency Ambulatory Services, Children's Hospital of Michigan, Detroit, Michigan

Stomach and Duodenum

THOMAS M. HOLDER, M.D.

Clinical Professor of Surgery, University of Missouri at Kansas City School of Medicine; Chief, Thoracic and Cardiovascular Surgery, The Children's Mercy Hospital, Kansas City, Missouri

Esophagus

NORMAN JAFFE, M.D.

Professor of Pediatrics, University of Texas System Cancer Center; Division Chief, Division of Solid Tumors, Pediatrics Department, M. D. Anderson Hospital and Tumor Institute, Houston, Texas

Cancer Chemotherapy

WILLIAM E. KAPLAN, M.D.

Assistant Professor of Urology, Northwestern University Medical School; Director of Neurologic Urology and Associate in Urology, Children's Memorial Hospital, Chicago, Illinois

The Male External Genitalia

SHERWYN V. KEVY, M.D.

Associate Professor of Pediatrics, Harvard Medical School; Director of Transfusion Service, Children's Hospital Medical Center, Boston, Massachusetts

Hemorrhagic Disorders and Transfusion Therapy

SAMUEL H. KIM, M.D.

Assistant Professor of Surgery, Harvard Medical School; Associate Surgeon, Massachusetts General Hospital, Boston, Massachusetts

Endoscopy

LOWELL R. KING, M.D.

Professor of Urology and Surgery, Northwestern University Medical School; Attending Urologist, Children's Memorial Hospital and Northwestern Memorial Hospital, Chicago, Illinois

Bladder and Urethra

RAPHAEL H. LEVEY, M.D.

Associate Professor of Surgery, Harvard Medical School; Associate in Surgery, Children's Hospital Medical Center, Boston, Massachusetts

Surgical Treatment of End-Stage Renal Disease

JOHN R. LILLY, M.D.

Professor of Surgery and Acting Chairman, Department of Surgery; Chief of Pediatric Surgery, University of Colorado School of Medicine; Staff, University Hospital, Denver, Colorado

Liver, Gallbladder, and Extrahepatic Bile Ducts

LESTER W. MARTIN, M.D.

Professor of Surgery and Pediatrics, College of Medicine, University of Cincinnati; Director of Pediatric Surgery, Children's Hospital Medical Center, Cincinnati, Ohio

Colon and Rectum

TREVOR J. I. McGILL, M.D.

Assistant Professor of Otolaryngology, Harvard Medical School; Associate Chief in Otolaryngology, Children's Hospital Medical Center; Associate in Otolaryngology, Massachusetts Eye and Ear Infirmary, Boston, Massachusetts

Salivary Glands, Larynx, and Oropharynx

JOHN B. MULLIKEN, M.D.

Assistant Professor of Surgery, Harvard Medical School; Associate in Surgery, Children's Hospital Medical Center and Brigham and Women's Hospital, Boston, Massachusetts

Soft Tissues

JOSEPH E. MURRAY, M.D.

Professor of Surgery, Harvard Medical School; Senior Associate in Surgery, Children's Hospital Medical Center and Brigham and Women's Hospital, Boston, Massachusetts

Soft Tissues

JAMES A. O'NEILL, JR., M.D.

Professor of Pediatric Surgery, University of Pennsylvania School of Medicine; Surgeon in Chief, Children's Hospital of Philadelphia, Pennsylvania

Burns

H. BIEMANN OTHERSEN, JR., M.D.

Professor of Surgery and Pediatrics, Medical University of South Carolina; Chief, Division of Pediatric Surgery, Medical University Hospital, Charleston, South Carolina

Trachea, Lungs, and Pleural Cavity

ARVIN I. PHILIPPART, M.D.

Associate Professor of Surgery, Wayne State University School of Medicine; Chief of General Surgery, Children's Hospital of Michigan, Detroit, Michigan

Small Intestine

BRADLEY M. RODGERS, M.D.

Professor of Surgery and Pediatrics, University of Virginia School of Medicine; Chief, Division of Pediatric Surgery, University of Virginia Hospital, Charlottesville, Virginia

Peritoneal Cavity

Marc I. Rowe, M.D.

Professor, Department of Surgery, University of Pittsburgh School of Medicine; Chief of Surgery, Children's Hospital of Pittsburgh, and Staff, Presbyterian Hospital, Pittsburgh, Pennsylvania

Shock and Resuscitation

C. D. Smith, M.D.

Assistant Professor of Surgery and Pediatrics, Medical University of South Carolina; Attending Pediatric Surgeon, Medical University Hospital; University Affiliate, Roper Hospital and St. Francis Hospital, Charleston, South Carolina

Abdominal Parietes

Robert M. Smith, M.D.

Consultant in Anesthesia, Children's Hospital Medical Center, Boston, Massachusetts

Anesthesia

Thomas E. Starzl, M.D., Ph.D.

Professor of Surgery, University of Pittsburgh Health Center, Pittsburgh, Pennsylvania

Liver, Gallbladder, and Extrahepatic Bile Ducts

H. Harlan Stone, M.D.

Professor of Surgery, Emory University School of Medicine; Chief of the Pediatric Surgical, Burn, and Trauma Services, Grady Memorial Hospital; Director, Surgical Bacteriology Laboratory, Emory University School of Medicine, Atlanta, Georgia

Surgical Infections and Antibiotics

Kenneth J. Welch, M.D.

Associate Clinical Professor of Surgery, Harvard Medical School; Senior Associate in Surgery, Children's Hospital Medical Center, Boston, Massachusetts

Thoracic Parietes

Ken R. Winston, M.D.

Assistant Professor of Surgery, Harvard Medical School; Senior Associate in Neurosurgery, Children's Hospital Medical Center, Boston, Massachusetts

Central Nervous System

PREFACE

American pediatric surgery has evolved largely over the past thirty-five years. Currently more than four hundred surgeons devote their entire time to the surgical care of children. This work follows the publication of textbooks and standard reference works in the field, the Journal of Pediatric Surgery, formation of the American Pediatric Surgical Association and the formal recognition of pediatric surgery as a specialty through the awarding of a certificate of proficiency to qualified examinees under the aegis of the American Board of Surgery. This volume logically follows and joins the W. B. Saunders series beginning with the classic work of Artz and Hardy, *Complications in Surgery.*

The goal of this text is to provide surgeons in all specialties who operate upon children with authoritative and detailed advice on the prevention and management of complications that will inevitably occur during the operation or the postoperative period. It is the ultimate surgical postgraduate course and we should all take it. Complications often occur elsewhere. Patients are then referred to a specialized institution for subsequent care and management. Little is learned from this convenient process. One can lecture about staying out of trouble, the zenith of surgical luck or skill, yet as the scope of surgery widens, as new procedures evolve and the surgical tour de force becomes common, major complications will occur at a predictable rate. Having avoided traditional traps and pitfalls, next most important is realistic acceptance that an error has occurred. Delay or unwilling recognition of a complication sets the stage for rapid deterioration of the patient. Corrective surgery may be required when the patient's resources are low. Any unsolved problem will result in complications at least as bad as anticipated.

The surgical audit conducted by most university teaching services is more than a requirement. It is a statement of responsibility to our patients, a fountain of new surgical information, and the most instructive conference of the week. Surgical errors include: error in diagnosis (ED), error in judgment (EJ), error in technique (ET), and error in management (EM). The late I. S. Ravdin added trying to play God (TPG). Such a conference, painful on occasion, has been held weekly from 1967 to 1981 at Children's Hospital Medical Center under the stewardship of Dr. Judah Folkman. Collected complications provided a data base for a full table of contents. Thirty four chapters were assigned to recognized authorities representing 21 major pediatric surgical departments in the United States and Canada. Analysis of similar complications at other institutions revealed a remarkably high correlation as to the type of complication, rate of occurrence, and result of treatment.

I wish to express my gratitude to my secretary, Suzanne Danais, for preparation of manuscripts, for assuming day to day editorial responsibilities, and for good natured but vigorous pursuit of tardy contributors. I would like to thank all members of the W. B. Saunders staff, particularly Lisette Bralow, Associate Medical Editor, and Grace Gulezian, Production Manager. Both made my editorial duties pleasant and instructive. Finally I would like to thank the contributors who took time from their surgical practices and their families to prepare manuscripts for this important work. We hope it will diminish suffering and expedite recovery in our little patients who require surgical treatment.

Kenneth J. Welch, M.D.

CONTENTS

GENERAL | 1

ANESTHESIA

Robert M. Smith, M.D.

Complications of the perioperative period of pediatric surgery start with those related to anesthesia. Table 1–1 suggests many but by no means all of the complications of pediatric anesthesia. To emphasize the more important rather than the more exotic, complications have been coded to indicate their relative incidence and severity. Severity is judged on the bases of mortality (or duration of nonfatal effect), degree of injury, physical suffering of the patient, emotional distress of the patient and parents, and social and financial effect on patient, family, and community. The following discussion will concern early recognition of the more important complications, as well as their treatment and prevention. References are given for details of pathophysiology that are beyond the scope of this chapter.

FATAL COMPLICATIONS

Many discussions entitled "Complications" touch on a variety of mishaps but avoid consideration of the most serious, namely death. Although it is an unpleasant note upon which to open, it seems proper to face the most important problem first.

Because of difficulties in determining the true cause of operative deaths, few reliable data relate to pediatric anesthesia.[38, 43] The report of Beecher and Todd[6] in 1954 supported the current estimate of one death per 1500 anesthetics for adults.[13] It was generally believed at that time that children were "poorer anesthetic risks,"[73] with an expected death rate of approximately one per 1000 anesthetics. Although inclusive studies were not made, many articles mentioned anesthetic deaths in children,[10, 18, 22] frequently caused by posttonsillectomy bleeding problems,[2, 32, 49] hyperpyrexia and

seizures during appendectomy,[70] and aspiration of vomitus during reduction of Colles' fractures in healthy children.[66] For many years the Anesthesia Study Commission instituted by Ruth in 1945[32, 54, 58] did much to point out such errors. For the next 20 years the term "cardiac arrest" was used to designate but not explain deaths that occurred during more extensive surgery. These deaths were undoubtedly caused by blood loss, increasing hypoxia, or airway obstruction of a more subtle nature that went unnoticed until arrest occurred.[47, 62, 66, 72]

Figures now available show that anesthetic mortality for both adults and children is far less than it was 25 years ago. Fatal anesthetic complications are to be neither expected nor excused in patients of any age. Although surgical mortality is relatively high in the perinatal period, such deaths are due chiefly to prematurity and to serious congenital defects rather than to anesthetic or surgical complications or preventable errors. The records of five anesthetic deaths among 89,000 patients, one anesthetic death among 29,000 patients, and one anesthetic death among 50,000 patients (from Boston,[64] Salt Lake City,[24] and Philadelphia,[19] respectively) document the success attained in pediatric hospitals.

Because the incidence of anesthetic mortality is so low, generalizations about its causes have relatively little significance. At present, anesthetic deaths in healthy children should be, and are, an extreme rarity when special equipment and skillful anesthesiologists are available. Fatal complications of anesthesia do occur, however, as noted in news items and legal reports. In some instances they may be traced to inadequate anesthetic skills, but they more frequently result from a lack of overall facilities for supportive care and observation.[14, 15]

TABLE 1–1 ANESTHETIC COMPLICATIONS LISTED IN REFERENCE TO BODY SYSTEMS AND CODED FOR SEVERITY AND INCIDENCE*

Central Nervous System
Death (A-4)
Temporary fear, anxiety, terror (C-1)
Behavior disorders (C-3)
Hypoxic damage
Mental retardation (B-4)
Dementia (A-4)
Spasticity (B-4)
  Blindness (B-4)
Peripheral nerve injury (C-4)

Thermic Disorders
Hypothermia, shivering (D-1)
Nonmalignant hyperthermia (D-4)
Malignant hyperthermia (A-4)

Respiratory System
Hypoxia, hypercarbia (B, C-3)
Hypocarbia (C-3)
Respiratory obstruction
  Anatomic, tongue, secretions (D-1)
  Pathologic, inflammation, tumor (C-3)
  Spasm, aspiration, hiccoughs (B-2)
  Atelectasis, pulmonary edema (B-2)
  Pneumothorax, pneumomediastinum (B-3)
Respiratory depression
  Drug overdose, sensitivity, abnormal response (C-3)

Complications of Endotracheal Intubation
Endobronchial intubation (C-3)
Physiologic trauma, hypoxia (C-3)
Blocked, kinked tube (C-3)
Extubation spasm (C-2)
Postintubation tracheitis (C-3)
Subglottic stenosis (B-4)

Cardiovascular System
Tachycardia (D-2)
Bradycardia (C-3)
Asystole (cardiac arrest) (A, B-3)
Arrhythmias (D-1)
Hypertension (C-1)
Hypotension (C-2)
Pulmonary hypertension (C-3)
Shock (B-3)
Cardiac failure (B-3)
Volume overload (B-3)
Volume depletion (C-2)

Gastrointestinal System
Nausea, vomiting (D-2)
Gastric distention (D-2)
Intestinal ileus (C-3)
Gastric rupture (B-4)
Esophageal and rectal trauma (C-3)

Hepatorenal System
Hepatotoxicity (B-4)
Acute renal failure (B-3)

Iatrogenic Complications
Drug overdosage, toxicity, sensitivity, interaction (B, C-3)
Anesthetic pollution, explosion
Monitoring complications
  Vascular damage, burns, hypothermia, electrical injury (B-4)
Transfusion reactions
Damage to skin, eyes (C-3)
Oxygen toxicity (B-4)
Retrolental fibroplasia (B-4)

Equipment Failure
Separation of breathing apparatus (B-3)
Faulty endotracheal tube cuffs

---

*__Code__ *Severity:* A = fatal or catastrophic; B = major; C = moderate; D = minor. *Incidence:* 1 = 1/10 cases; 2 = 1/100 cases; 3 = 1/1000 cases; 4 = < 1/1000 cases.

NONFATAL COMPLICATIONS

Because of the high incidence of nonfatal complications, much can be learned from close inspection of the many clinical settings in which complications occur and from studies of their causes and management.

Special Diagnostic Features

Most complications appear gradually and may be corrected if recognized in their early stages. Knowing when to expect them and how to detect them is essential. When dealing with young patients, one may anticipate special complications in relation to their physical status, their age, the phase of operation, the type of operation, and the pathologic condition involved.[28, 73]

PHYSICAL STATUS

The American Society of Anesthesiologists has established the following system for classifying the physical status of patients:

Class 1. The patient has no organic, physiologic, biochemical, or psychiatric disturbance. The pathologic process for which the operation is to be performed is localized and does not entail a systemic disturbance.

Class 2. The patient has a mild to moderate disturbance caused either by the condition to be treated surgically or by other pathologic processes. Neonates and octogenarians are included in this class, even when no discernible systemic disease is present (unless they are sick enough to be classified as Class 3, 4, or 5).

Class 3. The patient has a severe systemic disturbance or disease from whatever cause, although it may not be possible to define the degree of disability with finality.

Class 4. The patient has a severe systemic disorder that is already life-threatening and not always correctable by the operative procedure.

Class 5. The patient is moribund and has little chance of survival but is submitted to operation in desperation.

EMERGENCY OPERATION

A patient in any one of the classes listed above who undergoes an emergency opera-tion is considered to be in poorer physical condition. The letter *E* is placed beside the numeric classification.[20, 59]

AGE

The age of the child has much to do with the type and incidence of anesthetic complications. *School-age children* are more likely to receive accidental injuries and hence present the problem of aspiration of undigested stomach contents. They also are more subject to various types of intraoperative fever. Airway problems are bothersome in all pediatric age groups, but *the small child* is affected more than others owing to greater susceptibility to infection and tracheal irritation.[53] Emotional stress is maximal in this age group.[46, 64] These young children are old enough to be frightened but not old enough to understand. It is difficult to determine which phase of the operative experience is most distressing for the child, but needles, induction of anesthesia, and separation from parents are known to cause much grief. Extensive operations followed by the discomforts of intensive care add to the misery of the patient.[74]

Emotional stresses of *neonates* are unknown, but these patients experience a variety of ventilatory problems and have a marked tendency toward hypothermia,[67] hypotension, hypoglycemia,[31] infection, metabolic acidosis, cerebral hemorrhage,[25] and fluid overload.[64] Neonates have varied responses to antibiotics, muscle relaxants, and other drugs.[31, 64] Premature infants are subject to greater complications, the worst of which is combined susceptibility to the respiratory distress syndrome (RDS), which demands high oxygen concentrations, and to retrolental fibroplasia, which may lead to blindness after exposure to increased oxygen levels.[8, 40]

It is reasonable to look for early appearance of complications in children who are in critical condition before the operation is begun.[28, 73]

PHASE OF OPERATION

Certain complications are apt to occur during particular phases of the operation.

Before the procedure, children may become terrified unless they are skillfully managed.[46] Unexpected drug reactions and interactions may appear in this stage, causing excitement, depression, hypotension, or nausea.[15] Induction of anesthesia, a critical challenge that must be met in every operation, presents a real danger of causing respiratory spasm, "induction arrest," hypotension, aspiration, and problems associated with starting intravenous infusions. Endotracheal intubation, marking the end of induction, is a source of numerous problems in normal children and is even more so in the presence of pathologic conditions of the airway.[9, 26, 68]

Many complications may occur intraoperatively. The airway is always a source of danger, the patient's temperature may fall gradually or rise suddenly,[35, 71] cardiac reflexes may be provoked, or blood loss may be misjudged.[16, 44] As reported by Cooper and associates,[14] equipment failure and personal fatigue add considerably to complications during maintenance of anesthesia. The recovery period is known to be associated with vocal cord spasm,[3] aspiration, excitement, shivering, and pain[17, 67] and may be followed by shock, vomiting, croup, or more serious complications such as emotional disturbances, subglottic stenosis,[26, 68] or permanent brain damage.

TYPE OF OPERATION AND LESION

With young patients as well as old, emergency operations increase the danger of errors and complications resulting from haste; inadequate control of dehydration, shock, and hypothermia; and faulty preparation of equipment.[14, 48] Certain precautions always should be taken. Suction must be ready for treatment of the full stomach, tourniquets should not be used on black patients until tests have been made for hemoglobin S,[44] and the child with a ruptured liver should not be operated on until preparations have been made for dealing with sudden exsanguination. Many pre-existing diseases and physiologic defects affect the patient's response to anesthesia. For example, myasthenia gravis renders patients more sensitive to curariform agents so that normal dosages produce prolonged paralysis. Children with neuromuscular disorders have such variable responses to muscle-relaxing agents that it is best to avoid these drugs if possible.[7, 31, 64] Children with dysautonomia are particularly difficult to manage; they have lost temperature control, are unable to swallow secretions, and have poor ventilatory exchange.[42, 64] We have had the greatest success with light, easily controlled anesthesia, preferably endotracheal halothane. Pheochromocytoma, if unsuspected, may cause deep hypotension on induction, followed by bursts of hypertension during the operation. These may be prevented by establishing normal blood volume preoperatively and controlling arterial pressure with phentolamine methanesulfonate (Regitine) and halothane.[55]

COMPLICATIONS OF THE CENTRAL NERVOUS SYSTEM

The most severe complications of operations involving the central nervous system are death and permanent brain damage, usually caused by prolonged or severe hypoxia. It has been thought that the brain cannot tolerate more than 3 minutes of total hypoxia without sustaining some degree of damage. There is evidence, however, that this may vary with body temperature at the time of arrest. Clinical application of this concept has been effective in treating hypoxic patients by means of hypothermia (33°C) and high-dosage barbiturates (serum pentobarbital, 2.5 to 4 mg/dl). Other effects of hypoxic episodes are seizures, various types of psychotic disorders, and temporary or permanent blindness.[36]

Otherwise normal children without hypoxia may become emotionally disturbed after hospitalization. This is best prevented by careful preoperative evaluation, rapport between physician, patient, and parent, and building of mutual confidence.[37, 46, 64] Intelligent use of premedication is important. Postoperative follow-up is of much greater value than is commonly realized, and it can do much to re-establish understanding and confidence that may have been shaken by the surgical procedure. This assumes even greater importance if the child must return for another operation.

THERMAL COMPLICATIONS

Owing to the high incidence of hypothermia in smaller patients and the rare but dangerous hyperthermia in older children, careful intraoperative monitoring of body temperature is now standard practice.[56, 57, 65, 69]

Unintentional Hypothermia

Infants naturally tend to become hypothermic during the operative period.[17, 67] Preventive measures include transportation of infants in heated bassinets,[34] warming of operating rooms to 25°C, and use of infrared heating lamps during preparation for surgery.[31, 65] Although circulating-water mattresses are of some value,[30] it is more helpful to cover the limbs with sheet-wadding and the heads of hairless infants with stockinette caps. Internal warming by means of warmed, humidified gases and avoidance of cold infusions and rinsing fluids are of particular importance. Cooling below 35°C is to be avoided, chiefly to prevent postoperative depression in infants[35, 56] and shivering in older children.

Nonmalignant Hyperthermia

Intraoperative elevation of temperature is definitely abnormal. Common causes include overheating by environmental lighting, room temperature, or excessive use of heating devices; carbon dioxide retention; dehydration; exacerbation of underlying infection (especially during appendectomy and genitourinary procedures[52]); and transfusion reaction.[61] Any rise in temperature should be an indication for appropriate action, beginning with reversal of all warming measures and including hyperventilation and hydration. A further rise in temperature calls for application of icepacks to axillae and groin, gastric irrigation with iced saline solution, irrigation of the chest or peritoneal cavities, and further definitive measures.

Malignant Hyperthermia

This extremely rare complication (one in 15,000 to 50,000 anesthetics) has attracted much attention because of its rapid onset, high mortality (60 to 70 per cent), and as yet uncertain pathophysiology.[1, 11] Premonitory signs, including tachyarrhythmias, rigidity, and mottling of the skin, may precede the sudden temperature elevation. The identification of metabolic acidosis confirms the diagnosis. Treatment includes termination of the operation and of anesthetization, external and internal cooling, maximal hyperventilation, and intravenous administration of cold fluids, procainamide, and dantrolene (1 to 2 mg/kg).[39]

Patients suspected of being at increased risk of developing this syndrome thus far have been managed successfully with fentanyl and droperidol (Innovar) and similar combinations of narcotic and sedative.

RESPIRATORY COMPLICATIONS

The extensive variety of complications involving the respiratory system, their high incidence, and their severity make these the greatest problems in pediatric anesthesia. Most complications lead to hypoxia, through either depression or obstruction of respiration. Hypocarbia and oxygen toxicity are caused by excessive ventilation or oxygenation.

Depression of respiration may occur preoperatively as a result of overmedication, hypothermia, disease of the central nervous system, prematurity, diaphragmatic hernia, or other pathologic entities. The presence of any of these conditions makes ventilation more difficult. Treatment consists of establishing an effective airway, warming the patient, and assisting respiration with oxygen if indicated. Proceed with anesthesia and full control of ventilation as soon as possible. If there is any possibility of hypoxic damage, the operation should be halted and all efforts directed toward reversal of depression.

Intraoperative ventilatory depression should be easy to correct but may go unnoticed during spontaneous respiration, particularly if the surgeon's hands are resting on the infant's chest or abdomen. Even worse is the depression that may occur when a child's lung is retracted for long periods during intrathoracic procedures. The patient's position on the operating table may be hazardous, especially when the child is prone, in the lateral kidney position, or, in connection with repair of an imperforate anus, supine with legs flexed and strapped to the abdomen.[64] Arterial or transcutaneous measurement of oxygen concentration may be useful, but for detection of ventilatory complications there is no substitute for continuous stethoscopic auscultation of actual breath sounds.

Immediate postoperative respiratory depression may be caused by prematurity, intracranial hemorrhage,[25] cold,[35] splinting, general debility, overdosage of drugs, or failure of relaxant reversal due to acidosis, hypothermia, deficient acetylcholinesterase, or underlying neuromuscular diseases.[7] Warmth and specific reversal agents are used as indicated. Reintubation and mechanical ventilation are undertaken if blood gas determinations, rising heart rate, and other signs suggest a need for them.[57, 69]

Pneumothorax may occur as a minor complication after repair of pectus excavatum, as a major complication after cardiac surgery, and as a lethal complication after repair of diaphragmatic hernia. Atelectasis should be ruled out in any small infant with cardiorespiratory difficulty; if present, it should be treated aggressively with chest percussion, position change, and aspiration followed by inflation as indicated.

There are more causes of *respiratory obstruction* than of respiratory depression. Causative factors include the large tongue of the child, tendency to nasal breathing, increased secretions, upper respiratory tract infections, gagging on induction, and airway spasm, which may be serious enough to cause severe bradycardia. Pathologic processes such as hypertrophied tonsils and adenoids, choanal atresia, tumors of mouth and neck, papillomas of vocal cords, and inhaled foreign bodies may add to airway obstruction, while asthma, cystic fibrosis, and bronchospasm may interfere with pulmonary function. Pierre Robin syndrome, Hurler's syndrome, epiglottitis, and Apert's syndrome are a few of the more challenging problems that face the pediatric anesthesiologist.[64]

When an obstructive lesion is known to be present in the airway, it is usually advisable to avoid muscle-relaxant drugs and ketamine. Halothane is generally accepted to be the agent of choice and is frequently used without nitrous oxide. Induction with repeated small amounts of morphine has definite value. The availability of an effective antagonist (naloxone) adds to the safety of morphine.

Aspiration of vomitus during induction or maintenance of anesthesia has become relatively rare since the use of ether was discontinued, but some danger remains during the awakening period if children have large amounts of undigested food in their stomachs. It is a standard rule to intubate such children and to leave the endotracheal tube in place until the child is truly awake.

Bronchospasm is actually a rare complication. Difficulty in ventilation is more often due to light anesthesia or upper airway obstruction. True bronchospasm generally responds to continued halothane anesthesia.

Vocal cord spasm on tracheal extubation, on the contrary, is all too common and not easily controlled. Prevention by intravenous administration of lidocaine (1 mg/kg) is currently advised.[3] Obstruction by secretions, pulmonary edema, or passage of the endotracheal tube into the right main bronchus is most easily detected by constant stethoscopic monitoring. Correction consists of clearing the airway and removing the cause. Pulmonary edema may be a sign of fluid overload, cardiac failure, or prolonged forceful retraction of a lung. Moderate positive ventilatory pressure helps to control the fluid transudate.

As mentioned previously, endotracheal intubation has many potential complications.[9, 26, 45, 68] Deciduous teeth are easily displaced. (Anesthesiologists are not held responsible if the tooth is recovered.) Passage of the tube into the right main bronchus is a common error that should be corrected promptly. Other complications varying from an unsightly pressure ulceration of the external naris[4, 27, 45, 53] to perforation of the esophagus are evidence that passage of an endotracheal tube, although a lifesaving maneuver, still demands precise technique and, after fixation, constant vigilance. Most intraoperative complications should be correctable, but postoperative respiratory complications are more difficult to correct. One example is severe respiratory obstruction and collapse after repair of cleft lip in small infants. For this and other procedures involving the mouth, it is helpful to have the surgeon place a mattress traction suture in the tongue, providing an effective means of opening the airway and stimulating respiration in a single maneuver.[64]

The incidence of postoperative tracheitis has been considerably reduced since the elimination of impurities in the materials from which endotracheal tubes are manufactured and the demonstration of the danger of tightly fitting endotracheal tubes.[45] Evidence of tracheal irritation usually appears within an hour after operation, if it is to appear, and usually starts with a croupy cough, followed in more severe cases by sternal retraction and stridor. Therapy with dexamethasone (1 to 6 mg intravenously) and a mist tent is usually effective. Inhalation of racemic epinephrine may be added.[41] In rare instances it may be necessary to reintubate the trachea for a few hours. The worst complication of endotracheal intubation at present is subglottic stenosis, which is likely to occur after prolonged intubation of neonates supported by ventilators. Although subglottic stenosis is truly a major complication, it is usually not life-threatening and appears to be amenable to corrective surgery.[26, 53, 68]

CARDIOVASCULAR COMPLICATIONS

Important changes in cardiac rate, rhythm, and hemodynamics occur much less frequently than respiratory complications, but several potentially lethal irregularities may appear. Moderate tachycardia is beneficial to cardiac output in young patients. The child with a heart rate of less than 120 beats per minute while anesthetized probably needs an additional 0.2 mg of atropine. Bradycardia is dangerous and should not be tolerated, since it usually denotes a strong vagal response, deep anesthesia, or acute hypoxia. Rapid oxygenation, elimination of anesthetic, and cessation of surgical stimulation followed by administration of atropine usually resolve the bradycardia. Small infants show an increased vagal response to halothane anesthesia, and use of atropine (0.15 to 0.2 mg) is advisable on induction, preferably with the onset of analgesia.[64]

Arrhythmias occurring in anesthetized children seldom are dangerous. They usually are caused by surgical manipulation and should cease when the manipulation is stopped. Unless blood pressure is reduced by the arrhythmia, it probably is not necessary to attempt correction by use of cardiac depressant drugs.

Hypotension not attended by bradycardia occurring on induction of anesthesia with halothane is suggestive of hypovolemia and indicates a need for fluid replacement, preferably as a colloid.

Cardiac Asystole (Cardiac Arrest)

Sudden asystole may occur with stimuli such as traction on the peritoneum or on ocular musculature. More frequently, asystole results from airway obstruction, hypoxia, blood loss, anesthetic overdosage, or overinfusion of fluids. Most instances are due to errors of commission or to inadequate observation.[10, 15, 60, 62, 66]

Successful treatment of asystole depends first upon its immediate recognition through continuous monitoring with the simple precordial stethoscope. Prompt team action attempts simultaneously to determine the cause and to start treatment. Surgeons remove constricting packs and instruments and begin cardiac massage (with aortic compression, if possible), while the anesthesiologist and assistants actively ventilate the child's lungs with oxygen, replace fluid deficits, and give atropine for full vagal suppression. Calcium, epinephrine, isoproterenol, or other cardiotonic agents are used as indicated (Table 1–2). Sodium bicarbonate, once used indiscriminately, should be used only when definitely indicated, and then in moderation (1 to 3 mg/kg, stat dose), repeated only as suggested by blood gas determinations. Children rarely experience

TABLE 1–2 MEDICATIONS FOR CARDIAC RESUSCITATION

Drug	Concentration	Dose	Route	Interval
Atropine	0.04 mg/ml	Neonate 0.15 mg Infant 0.2 mg Child 0.4 mg	Intravenous or intramuscular	20 min, or as needed
Calcium chloride and calcium gluconate	10 per cent, 1000 mg in 10-ml ampule	20 mg/kg (chloride), 60 mg/kg (gluconate)	Intravenous or intracardiac	10 min, or as indicated by serum Ca^{++}
Epinephrine	1 ml, 1:1000	Dilute to 10 ml and give 0.1 ml/kg	Intravenous or intracardiac	5–10 min
Isoproterenol (Isuprel)	0.2 mg/ml, 1:5000	1 mg in 250 ml $D_5W = 4$ μg/ml Give 0.1–0.5 μg/kg/min (titrate for effect)	Intravenous	Constant

From Smith, R. M.: Anesthesia for Infants and Children, 4th edition. St. Louis, C. V. Mosby Co., 1980.

ventricular fibrillation in such situations, but a cardiac defibrillator should be immediately available.[19]

GASTROINTESTINAL AND HEPATORENAL COMPLICATIONS

The occasional child who is nauseated before operation usually is overanxious, whereas postoperative vomiting is frequently caused by sensitivity to narcotics or is related to the operative procedure, particularly after ophthalmic surgery. Droperidol (0.1 mg/kg) is the best preventive agent, and trimethobenzamide (Tigan, 100 mg/kg) is most effective for treatment, in addition to elimination of the narcotic. Gastric distention seen before, during, or after operation may be treated by nasogastric suction or sump. Emergency gastrostomy may be indicated for infants with tracheoesophageal fistula.

Complications due to either liver or kidney malfunction are rarely seen in pediatric surgical patients. The neonatal kidney has limited function and tolerates overload poorly, but acute renal failure is uncommon and is seen chiefly in late stages of low cardiac output failure.

Jaundice is encountered in many neonates and young children, and halothane, with its multihalogenated molecular structure, is frequently blamed. The existence of halogen hepatitis has never been definitely proved, and children have been involved relatively infrequently. A study of more than one million halothane anesthetics in children provided only five cases in which halothane seemed the major cause of hepatic failure.[64] Halothane is generally considered safe for use in children in nearly any circumstance. It seems reasonable, however, to choose other agents for operations lasting more than 6 to 8 hours, for children who have serious illnesses and complicated metabolic disturbances, and for patients who are likely to institute legal action.

COMPLICATIONS DUE TO DRUG OVERDOSAGE, SENSITIVITY, TOXICITY, AND INTERACTION

Simple overdosage of narcotics and sedatives may cause respiratory depression, and excessive amounts of muscle relaxants may result in prolonged immobilization. Both should be effectively handled without harming the child. Excessive concentrations of halothane may cause severe myocardial depression, particularly in small, hypovolemic infants. Standard precautions should avert this danger.

Several agents given by surgeons intraoperatively carry considerable danger. Sodium bicarbonate, as previously mentioned, may induce cerebral hemorrhage in infants who have a high serum osmolality.[23, 25] Epinephrine, used either alone for hemostasis or with local anesthetic agents, often exceeds standard safety limits. This danger can be averted if surgeons use dilute solutions of 1:200,000 or 1:400,000, which would serve most purposes, rather than use more concentrated preparations. The dosage of procaine and lidocaine should be limited to 10 mg/kg and 5 mg/kg, respectively.[21, 51]

The reaction of infants to many drugs is distinctly different from that of older patients and may differ widely among infants of the same age.[31, 64] These factors lead to many undesirable responses and complications. Sensitivity to drugs also exists but is less troublesome. Atropine often causes a facial flush without other effects and does not present a problem. Barbiturates may cause excitement in some children. If they produce such a reaction, these drugs should be avoided in subsequent operations. The excitement is seldom remembered by the patient, however, and leaves no psychic imprint. Patients with porphyria have defective barbiturate metabolism, making them subject to prolongation of sedative effect.

A variety of complications are associated with the use of ketamine and succinylcholine.[31] Ketamine causes elevation of both intraocular and intracranial pressures and may be followed by disturbing hallucinations. Succinylcholine also raises intraocular pressure. In addition, it is one of the outstanding precipitating factors in malignant hyperthermia. It can initiate potentially lethal elevation of serum potassium when administered to patients with severe burns and other types of major trauma.[33, 50] Seizures may be evoked by moderately deep enflurane anesthesia, particularly in children.

One of the most severe and perplexing complications associated with pediatric anesthesia is retrolental fibroplasia, caused by high concentrations of oxygen.[8, 40] This complication is closely associated with low birth weight and prematurity, but it has been impossible to establish limits within which oxygen may be administered safely. The defect has been found in some subjects who had never breathed anything but room air.

IATROGENIC COMPLICATIONS AND COMPLICATIONS OF MIXED ORIGIN

It is not to be assumed that all complications are caused by errors or mismanagement. Excessive effect of a drug may be caused by a patient's unsuspected sensitivity to a standard dose of the drug. Nausea, excessive bleeding, or airway obstruction may occur in spite of expert anesthetic care. In a variety of situations, however, errors of omission or commission, currently termed "anesthetic mishaps," are undeniably at fault.[14, 48, 70] Among these must be included anesthetic explosions (now fortunately eliminated), errors in calculation of drug dosages, actual injury of patients by heating or electrical devices, and tissue damage caused by iodine or pressure injury. Numerous complications related to endotracheal intubation have been mentioned, as has vascular injury due to arterial cannulation, which is occasionally used without clear indication and may result in infection, thrombosis, or loss of tissue.[5] Inadequate or faulty apparatus, resulting in use of the wrong anesthetic gases, ventilator failure, or separation of the endotracheal tube from the oxygen source, belong in the category of iatrogenic and consequently preventable complications. The most common equipment errors are poor choice of airways and use of masks that are too small for the child, reducing rather than increasing ventilatory exchange. The reasons underlying iatrogenic complications have been studied recently by Cooper et al.,[14] who found that fatigue during long operations is a significant factor. For optimal care of patients, they advise relief of anesthesiologists at reasonable intervals.

References

1. Aldrete, J. A., and Vritt, B. A., eds.: Malignant Hyperthermia. Second International Symposium. New York, Grune & Stratton, 1978.
2. Alexander, D. W., Graff, T. D., and Kelley, E.: Factors in tonsillectomy mortality. Arch. Otolaryngol. 82:409, 1965.
3. Baraka, A.: Intravenous lidocaine controls extubation spasm in children. Anesth. Analg. (Cleve.) 57:506, 1978.
4. Baxter, R. J., Johnson, J. D., Goetzman, B. W., and Hackel, A.: Cosmetic nasal deformities complicating prolonged nasotracheal intubation in

critically ill newborn infants. Pediatrics 55:884, 1975.

5. Bedford, R. F., and Wollman, H.: Complications of percutaneous radial artery cannulation: An objective prospective study. Anesthesiology 38:228, 1973.

6. Beecher, H. K., and Todd, D. P.: A study of the deaths associated with anesthesia and surgery based on a study of 599,548 anesthesias in ten institutions 1948–1952, inclusive. Ann. Surg. 140:2, 1954.

7. Bennett, E. J., Dalal, F. Y., and Schmidt, G. B.: Amyotonia congenita. Mid. East J. Anaesthesiol. 4(2):111, 1974.

8. Betts, E. K., and Downes, J. J., Jr.: Retrolental fibroplasia and oxygen administration during anesthesia. Anesthesiology 47:518, 1977.

9. Blanc, V. F., and Tremblay, N. A. G.: The complications of tracheal intubation: A new classification with a review of the literature. Anesth. Analg. (Cleve.) 53:202, 1974.

10. Boba, A.: Death in the Operating Room. Springfield, Ill., Charles C Thomas, Publisher, 1965.

11. Britt, B. A., and Kalow, W.: Malignant hyperthermia: A statistical review. Can. Anaesth. Soc. J. 17:293, 1970.

12. Carney, F. M. Y., and Van Dyke, R. A.: Halothane hepatitis: A critical review. Anesth. Analg. (Cleve.) 51:135, 1972.

13. Clifton, B. S., and Hotten, W. I. T.: Deaths associated with anaesthesia. Br. J. Anaesth. 35:250, 1963.

14. Cooper, J. B., Newbower, R. S., Long, C. D., et al.: Preventable anesthetic mishaps: A study of human factors. Anesthesiology 49:399, 1978.

15. Cooperman, L. H., and Orkin, F. K., eds.: Complications in Anesthesiology. Philadelphia, J. B. Lippincott Co., 1979.

16. Davenport, H. T., and Barr, M. N.: Blood loss during pediatric operations. Can. Med. Assoc. J. 89:1309, 1963.

17. Dawkins, M. J. R., and Scopes, J. W.: Nonshivering thermogenesis in the human newborn infant. Nature 206:201, 1965.

18. Dornette, W. H. L., and Orth, O. S.: Death in the operating room. Anesth. Analg. (Cleve.) 35:545, 1956.

19. Downes, J. J., Jr., and Raphaely, R. C.: Anesthesia and intensive care. *In* Ravitch, M. M., Welch, K. J., Benson, C. D., et al. (eds.), Pediatric Surgery, 3rd edition. Chicago, Year Book Medical Publishers, 1979.

20. Dripps, R. D., Lamont, A., and Eckenhoff, J. F.: The role of anesthesia in surgical mortality. JAMA 178:261, 1961.

21. Eather, K.: Regional anesthesia for infants and children. Int. Anesthesiol. Clin. 13:19, 1975.

22. Edwards, G., Morton, H. J. V., Pask, F. A., and Wylie, W. D.: Deaths associated with anaesthesia; a report on 1000 cases. Anaesthesia 11:194, 1956.

23. Eidelman, A. I., and Hobbs, J. F.: Bicarbonate therapy revisited. A study in therapeutic revisionism. Am. J. Dis. Child. 132:847, 1978.

24. Elwyn, R. A.: Perioperative pediatric mortality. A five year study. Salt Lake City, Postgraduate

Anesthesia Symposium on Pediatric Anesthesia, 1978.

25. Finberg, L.: Dangers to infants caused by changes in osmolal concentrations. Pediatrics 40:1031, 1967.

26. Fishman, N. H.: Post-intubation tracheal stenosis. Ann. Thorac. Surg. 8:47, 1969.

27. Fox, E. J., Sklar, G. S., Hill, C. H., et al.: Complications related to the pressor response to endotracheal intubation. Anesthesiology 47:524, 1977.

28. Goldstein, A., Jr., and Keats, A. S.: The risk of anesthesia. Anesthesiology 33:130, 1970.

29. Gordon, T., Larson, C. P., Jr., and Prestwich, R.: Unexpected cardiac arrest during anesthesia and surgery: An environmental study. JAMA 236:2758, 1976.

30. Goudsouzian, N. G., Morris, R. H., and Ryan, J. F.: The effects of a warming blanket on the maintenance of body temperatures in anesthetized infants and children. Anesthesiology 39:351, 1973.

31. Goudsouzian, N. G., and Ryan, J. F.: Recent advances in pediatric anesthesia. Pediatr. Clin. North Am. 23:345, 1976.

32. Graff, T. D., Phillips, O. C., Benson, D. W., and Kelly, E.: Baltimore Anesthesia Study Committee. Factors in pediatric anesthesia mortality. Anesth. Analg. (Cleve.) 43:407, 1964.

33. Gronert, G. A., Lambert, E. H., and Theye, R. A.: The response of denervated muscle to succinylcholine. Anesthesiology 40:268, 1974.

34. Hackel, A.: A medical transport system for the neonate. Anesthesiology 43:258, 1975.

35. Hackett, P. R., and Crosby, R. M. N.: Some effects of inadvertent hypothermia in infant neurosurgery. Anesthesiology 21:356, 1960.

36. Hagerdal, M., Welsh, F. A., Keyhah, M., and Harp, J. R.: The protective effects of a combination of hypothermia and barbiturates in cerebral hypoxia. Crit. Care Med. 6(2):110, 1978.

37. Haller, G. A.: The Hospitalized Child and His Family. Baltimore, Johns Hopkins University Press, 1967.

38. Hamilton, W. K.: Unexpected death during anesthesia. Wherein lies the cause? Anesthesiology 50:381, 1979.

39. Harrison, G. G.: Control of the malignant hyperpyrexic syndrome in MHS swine by dantrolene sodium. Br. J. Anaesth. 47:62, 1975.

40. James, L. S., and Lanman, J. T., eds.: History of oxygen therapy and retrolental fibroplasia. Pediatrics 57 (Suppl., Part 2), April 1976.

41. Jordan, W. S., Graves, C. L., and Elwyn, R. A.: New therapy for postintubation laryngeal edema and tracheitis in children. JAMA 212:585, 1970.

42. Kadis, L. B., Diaz, P. M., and Lack, J. A.: Neurological disorders. *In* Katz, J., and Kadis, L. B. (eds.): Anesthesia and Uncommon Diseases: Pathophysiologic and Clinical Correlations. Philadelphia, W. B. Saunders Co., 1973.

43. Keats, A. S.: What do we know about anesthetic mortality? Anesthesiology 50:387, 1979.

44. Kevy, S. V.: Surgical implications of hematologic disorders. *In* Ravitch, M. M., Welch, K. J.,

Benson, C. D., et al. (eds.): Pediatric Surgery, 3rd edition. Chicago, Year Book Medical Publishers, 1979.

45. Koka, B. V., Jeon, I. S., Andre, J. M., et al.: Postintubation croup in children. Anesth. Analg. (Cleve.) 56:501, 1977.

46. Korsch, B. M.: The child in the operating room. Anesthesiology 43:251, 1975.

47. Kristoffersen, M. B., Rattenborg, C. C., and Holaday, D. A.: Asphyxial death; the roles of acute anoxia, hypercarbia and acidosis. Anesthesiology 28:488, 1967.

48. Marmer, K. J.: Iatrogenesis in anesthesiology. Anesth. Analg. (Cleve.) 48:612, 1969.

49. Martin, G. E.: Complications following removal of tonsils. J. Laryngol. Otol. 37:80, 1922.

50. McCaughey, T. J.: Hazards of anaesthesia for the burned child. Can. Anaesth. Soc. J. 9:220, 1962.

51. Melman, E., Penuelas, J., and Marrufo, J.: Regional anesthesia in children. Anesth. Analg. 54:387, 1975.

52. Modell, J. H.: Septicemia as a cause of immediate postoperative hyperthermia. Anesthesiology 27:329, 1966.

53. Otherson, H. B., Jr.: Intubation injuries of the trachea in children: Management and prevention. Ann. Surg. 189:601, 1979.

54. Phillips, O. C., Frazier, T. M., Graff, T. D., et al.: The Baltimore Anesthesia Study Committee. Review of 1024 postoperative deaths. JAMA 174:2015, 1960.

55. Pratilas, V., and Pratila, M. G.: Anaesthetic management of phaeochromocytoma. Can. Anaesth. Soc. J. 26:253, 1979.

56. Roe, C. F.: Temperature regulation and energy metabolism in surgical patients. Prog. Surg. 12:96, 1973.

57. Rowe, M. I.: Physiologic monitoring. *In* Gans, S. L., ed.: Surgical Pediatrics. New York, Grune & Stratton, 1973.

58. Ruth, H. S.: Anesthesia study commissions. JAMA 127:514, 1945.

59. Saklad, M.: Grading patients for surgical procedures. Anesthesiology 2:281, 1941.

60. Schoonmaker, G. W.: Axioms on cardiac arrest. Hosp. Med. 14(10):6, 1978.

61. Schweizer, O., Howland, W. S., Ryan, G., and Goldminer, P. L.: Hyperpyrexia in the operative and immediate postoperative period. Anesth. Analg. (Cleve.) 50:906, 1971.

62. Singer, J. J.: Cardiac arrests in children. J. Am. Coll. Emerg. Physicians 6(5):198, 1971.

63. Smith, R. M.: Some reasons for the high mortality in pediatric anesthesia. N.Y. State J. Med. 56:2212, 1956.

64. Smith, R. M.: Anesthesia for Infants and Children, 4th edition. St. Louis, C. V. Mosby Co., 1980.

65. Smith, R. M.: Anesthesia and monitoring. *In* Holder, T. M., and Ashcraft, K. W. (eds.): Pediatric Surgery. Philadelphia, W. B. Saunders Co., 1980.

66. Snyder, W. H., Snyder, M. H., and Chaffin, L.: Cardiac arrest in infants and children; report of 66 original cases. Arch. Surg. 66:714, 1953.

67. Stern, L.: Physiology of the newborn infant. III. Thermoregulation. Res. Pediatr. Surg. 12:23, 1978.

68. Steward, D. J.: Post-intubation stenosis. Can. Anaesth. Soc. J. 17:388, 1970.

69. Talbert, J. L.: Intraoperative and postoperative monitoring in infants. Surg. Clin. North Am. 50:787, 1970.

70. Utting, J. E., Gray, T. C., and Shelley, F. C.: Human misadventures in anaesthesia. Can. Anaesth. Soc. J. 26:472, 1979.

71. Waltermath, C. L.: The febrile patient: Pathologic physiology and anesthetic management. Anesth. Analg. (Cleve.) 48:795, 1969.

72. Waters, R. M., and Gillespie, N. A.: Death in the operating room. Anesthesiology 5:113, 1944.

73. Wilson, R. D., Traber, D. L., Priano, L. L., and Evans, B. L.: Anesthetic management of the poor-risk pediatric patient. South. Med. J. 62:767, 1969.

74. Wilson, W. E.: Preoperative anxiety and anesthesia: their relation. Anesth. Analg. (Cleve.) 48:605, 1969.

SHOCK AND RESUSCITATION

Marc I. Rowe, M.D.

It is rare to scrutinize a general surgical journal without finding at least one article dealing with the clinical or experimental aspects of shock in the adult. In contrast, there is a scarcity of such information in the pediatric medical and surgical literature. Nevertheless, review of experience on any pediatric surgical service reveals that shock is common in newborns, infants, and children. The lack of emphasis on shock in the pediatric age group probably stems from the fact that infants do not present with the "classic" signs of shock. Only recently has physiologic monitoring of sick babies and children been practiced. Shock research has used the adult experimental subject almost exclusively.

There are many similarities between shock in the adult and shock in children. The types and cellular effects of shock appear to be the same in both age groups; hypovolemia and invasive infection are the most common causes. No matter what the age the final common pathway to irreversibility and death is the same — progressive cellular dysfunction and injury. Emphasis on the injured cell as the central feature in shock resulted from intensive research in the late 1960's and the 1970's.* Evidence accumulated that as a result of inadequate perfusion, cellular hypoxia, and, in some cases, direct attack on cell structure, disruption of mitochondria and lysosomes occurs, and molecular and enzymatic processes are disabled. The metabolic consequences of these events are cell death, organ failure, and, eventually, death of the organism. The major difference between shock in the pediatric patient and that in the adult does not

appear to be the type of shock or the critical target — the cell — but rather the difference in physiologic and pathologic response by patients of different ages and levels of maturation.

PATHOPHYSIOLOGY OF SHOCK

Hypovolemic Shock

Hemorrhage in the newborn infant leading to acute hypovolemic shock is usually the result of injury to the umbilical vasculature or rupture of the liver at birth. In childhood, blood loss results from blunt trauma to solid intra-abdominal viscera. Nonhemorrhagic acute hypovolemic shock is usually the result of fulminating diarrhea or extensive burns. Chronic hypovolemia develops more slowly over hours or even days, often without significant external losses. Large quantities of water and electrolytes are sequestered in the "third space." Peritonitis and intestinal obstructions are common examples.

The physiologic adjustment to acute reduction of blood volume is preservation of blood flow to the vital organs. As blood volume decreases, venous return to the heart is reduced, ventricular output falls, and with a decreased stroke volume there is a drop in arterial blood pressure. The carotid and aortic baroreceptors are the main sensors of a fall in blood pressure. The detection of a pressure drop stimulates the secretion of catecholamines from the adrenal medulla and sympathetic nerve endings. Plasma epinephrine and norepinephrine levels rise and parallel the loss of blood volume. The effects of catecholamines in-

---

*See References 8, 9, 14, 32, 35, 46, 92, 109, 120, 125, and 136.

"

clude arterial vasoconstriction and an increase in heart rate and myocardial contractility. Intense vasoconstriction of the arterioles of the gastrointestinal tract, kidneys, muscles, and skin allows blood flow to be redirected to vital organs such as the heart and the brain. The generalized vasoconstriction reduces capillary hydrostatic pressure, and eventually serum oncotic pressure exceeds capillary pressure. Fluid then moves from the interstitial space into the intravascular space (transcapillary refill), increasing blood volume. Blood volume is further increased as a result of intense constriction of the venous system. Since almost 80 per cent of the blood resides in the venous system, reduction in the venous bed produces a sizable "autotransfusion." The vasoconstrictive response is particularly intense in the renal vasculature. The kidney accommodates as much as 25 per cent of the cardiac output. As renal blood flow is reduced, more blood can be shunted to vital organs. There is also a reduction in glomerular filtration and sodium excretion. Urine concentration increases and oliguria develops.

How effective these "autoregulatory" responses are is determined by the severity and duration of the hemorrhage, the characteristics of the patient, and the promptness and effectiveness of treatment. With severe or progressive hemorrhage, or in patients with inadequate reserves, the initial homeostatic responses are insufficient to allow adequate blood flow to tissues. The patient is now in a low flow state. The degree of tissue perfusion failure determines the inadequacy of oxygen delivery to the cells. The magnitude of oxygen deprivation, in turn, determines the extent of cellular dysfunction and ischemic injury. As perfusion decreases and cellular hypoxia increases, a lack of oxygen forces the cells to shift to anaerobic glycolysis to produce energy. The anaerobic environment, by blocking oxidation of pyruvate from glucose, allows the build-up of lactic acid. As intracellular hydrogen ions accumulate, they pass into the interstitial fluid and then into the blood, resulting in metabolic acidemia. Anaerobic combustion of carbohydrates is inefficient and produces minimal amounts of energy.[23, 111] The intracellular sodium-potassium pump requires energy to perform and maintains a low intracellular sodium level by pumping sodium out of the cell against a gradient. The energy shortage leads to pump failure, resulting in a loss of potassium from the cell and the movement of sodium and water from the interstitial space into the cell. Interstitial fluid volume is reduced, and intracellular water and sodium increase. Thus, the effects of hemorrhage on total body fluids are (1) a reduction in blood volume, (2) a severe reduction in interstitial fluid volume as a result of a combination of transcapillary refill and the movement of water from the interstitial space into the cell, and (3) an increase in intracellular fluid volume. With continued low flow and cellular hypoxia, cell damage progresses. As mitochondria and lysosomes are injured and cell membranes are disrupted, cell death occurs. Death of significant numbers of cells leads to organ failure, irreversibility, and death of the patient.*

Chronic hypovolemia leads more slowly, but just as unerringly, to a reduction in tissue perfusion, cellular damage, and eventually cell death. The gradual development of shock that occurs in late intestinal obstruction is an example. Fluid is lost externally as a result of vomiting and internally into the bowel lumen, intestinal wall, and peritoneal cavity. Since the loss is gradual, blood volume is maintained at the expense of the functional interstitial space by transcapillary refill. Eventually compensation is inadequate, and blood volume and tissue perfusion decrease. Cellular hypoxia develops and the sodium pump is affected. Sodium and water then move into the cell, and the functional interstitial space is further reduced. The results are a large volume of fluid sequestered in the nonfunctional interstitial space, a severe functional interstitial deficit, and a moderate decrease in blood volume.

Effective treatment of acute and chronic hypovolemia is relatively simple initially. Continued loss of fluid must be prevented, and hypovolemia and interstitial fluid deficits must be corrected. If this is accomplished promptly, serious cellular damage can be averted and the patient can be rapid-

---

*See References 21, 30, 31, 43, 52, 66, 72, 93, 131–135, and 154.

ly and successfully resuscitated. If fluid losses continue, or if deficits are not adequately replaced, tissue perfusion becomes progressively inadequate. As cellular damage increases, treatment becomes more complex and survival less likely.

Gram-Negative Septic Shock

Septic shock in the pediatric patient is more frequently caused by gram-negative than gram-positive bacteria. Infants and children with reduced or altered host defenses are particularly vulnerable. The source of infection in gram-negative sepsis is usually the urinary tract, intestines, meninges, peritoneum, or lung. Contaminated intravascular lines are sources of infection in all age groups.

Gram-negative shock has a more complex pathophysiology than hypovolemic shock, but the end result is the same — progressive cellular damage leading to cell death and eventually death of the organism. A large body of information[6, 15, 28, 50, 82] has accumulated that suggests that many of the changes seen in patients with septic shock are the result of a violent struggle between the body's defense mechanisms and bacteria and bacterial byproducts rather than direct action of the infective agent on the cell. The process appears to have a primarily immunologic basis, leading to the release of substances that have a profound effect on blood vessels and cells (Fig. 2–1).

Host defense plays an essential role in the pathophysiology of gram-negative shock. As bacteria enter the body, two basic mechanisms, one humoral and the other cellular, are activated to eliminate the invaders. Humoral defenses involve antibodies — immunoglobulins produced by plasma cells. When a microorganism enters the body, it is recognized as a foreign antigen and is bound to a specific immunoglobulin. The resulting complex activates the effector arm of the humoral defense mechanism — the classic complement system. The cascade of reactions begins with C1, the first protein in the sequence, and ends with C9. The latter half of the sequence is a membrane attack phase. The resulting complement products insert themselves into the bacterial cell membrane, causing lysis and death. During the chain reaction of the complement sys-

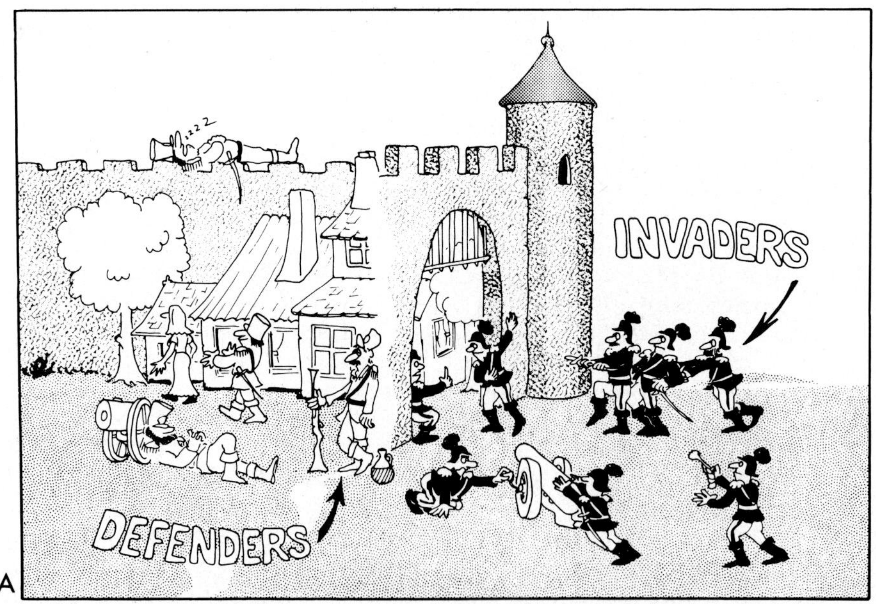

Figure 2–1   Parable of the mechanism of cellular damage in gram-negative shock. The cast of characters: *The Invaders* (bacteria and their byproducts); *The Defenders* (host defense, white blood cells, platelets, complement, reticuloendothelial system, and immunoglobulins); *The City and Civilian Population* (the body, its cells, and its blood vessels). *Scene A,* The invaders approach the city; the defenders allow them to enter unchallenged.

tem, biologically active peptides are broken off and released into the circulation.

Phagocytosis and intracellular killing of bacteria is the second and most important method of combating acute bacterial infection. The principal phagocytic cell is the polymorphonuclear leukocyte. The white blood cell is attracted to the site of the bacterial invasion by elements of the complement system, particularly C3 and C5, in a process known as chemotaxis. Leukocytes next must recognize bacteria and ingest them. These processes are facilitated by opsonization — the binding of immuno-

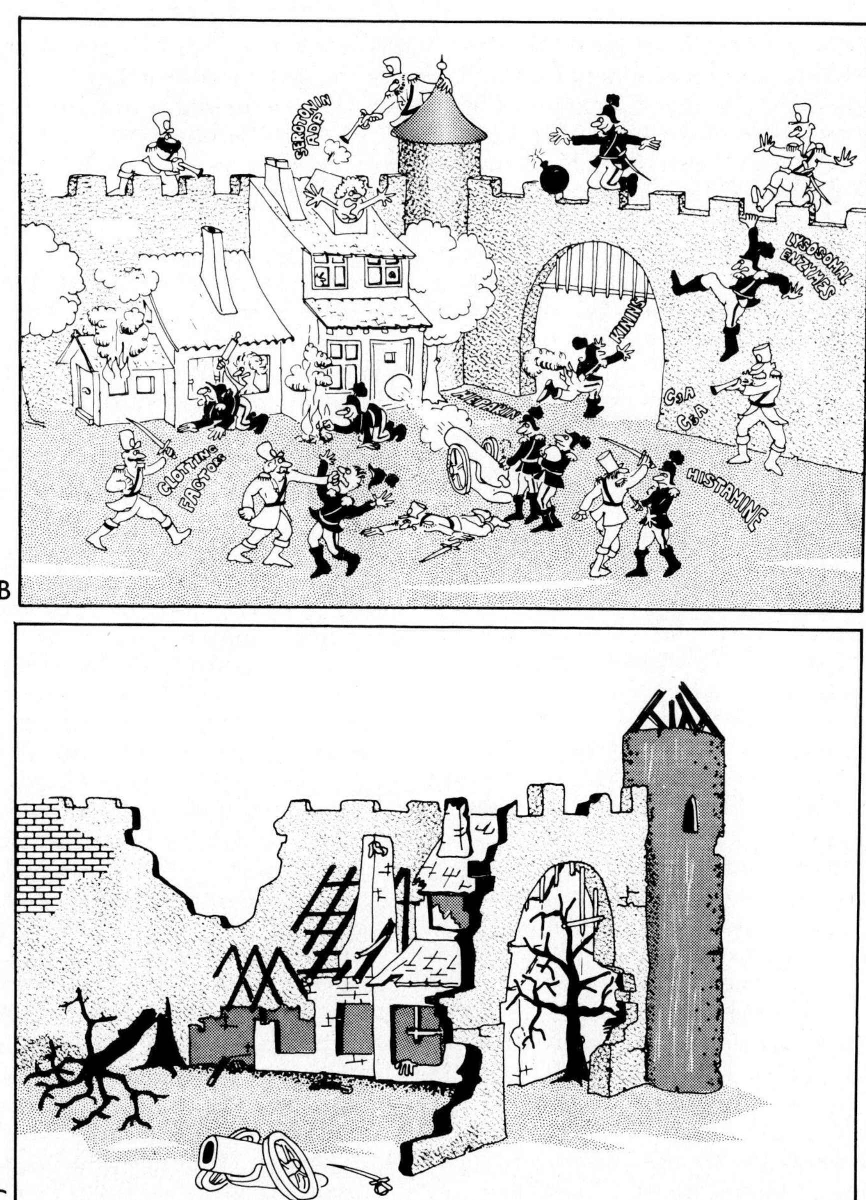

Figure 2–1 *Continued   Scene B,* The defenders take on the invaders in a violent clash within the city. Much of the city and its population are damaged as a result. *Scene C,* The battle may be "won," but the city and its population are irreparably damaged and unable to function properly.

globulins or complement particles to the microorganisms. It appears that the alternate or properdin complement pathway rather than the classic pathway is the principal mechanism for the production of opsonins. Once the microorganisms are prepared for phagocytosis by opsonization, they are ingested by leukocytes. Intracellular killing of the bacteria then occurs as a result of a complex energy-consuming process.[2, 67, 68, 94]

As bacteria are killed, endotoxin, a lipopolysaccharide derived from the cell membrane, accumulates in the circulation. Endotoxin contains at least three antigens. The body eliminates endotoxin by combining it with antibodies, white blood cells, and platelets. These reactions also require activation of the complement system. The bound endotoxin is then phagocytosed by the reticuloendothelial (RE) system, the major site of endotoxin detoxification. In order to effectively phagocytose bound endotoxin, the RE system must contain an opsonizing substance, alpha$_2$-glycoprotein. As the RE system becomes overwhelmed, increasing amounts of endotoxin accumulate in the system.[122] Endotoxin contributes to the overall effects of gram-negative sepsis by causing direct damage to the cells and also by initiating adverse immunologic reactions.

Both the alternate and classic complement pathways are maximally activated by the clash between invading bacteria and the patient's defense mechanisms. Active complement particles are released into the circulation and travel throughout the body, affecting cells and blood vessels. Two complement proteins, C3a and C5a, trigger the release of histamines and heparin.[75] Stimulation of the complement system leads to activation of the kinin and coagulation systems, with release of vasoactive and clotting substances.[6, 28] Platelet aggregation and destruction occurs in the presence of complement and endotoxin and leads to the release of serotonin, adenosine diphosphate (ADP), prostaglandins E$_2$ and F$_2$, and histamine. With the rupture of lysosomal membranes, proteolytic enzymes injurious to the cell are released into the circulation.[4]

Although endotoxin and proteolytic enzymes may cause direct cellular injury, inadequate perfusion, as in hypovolemic shock, is even more damaging to the cell. Low flow results from (1) obstruction and rerouting of the microcirculatory flow,[29, 54, 116, 162] (2) reduction of circulating blood volume,[95] and (3) reduction of cardiac output.[57, 81, 105, 160] Microcirculatory changes are profound in gram-negative shock. With platelet aggregation and destruction, platelet fragments are swept into the microvasculature, producing widespread blockade. Increased platelet adhesiveness results in the adherence of platelets to small blood vessels, reducing flow. Other platelet substances initiate further aggregation, vasoconstriction, vasodilatation, and capillary leak. Several investigators believe that widespread vascular plugging, particularly of the pulmonary microvasculature, results from a complement-granulocyte interaction that produces white blood cell thrombi and emboli. As the coagulation system is activated, diffuse disseminated intravascular coagulation may occur. Vasoactive compounds released by the kinin and complement systems cause arterial vasoconstriction and opening of arteriovenous shunts. Obstruction, constriction injury, and shunting in the microvasculature reduce blood flow to individual cells, causing progressive cellular hypoxia.

Stasis and pooling of blood in the capillary bed leads to reduction of the circulating blood volume. Vasoactive substances cause pooling of blood in the venous system. Proteolytic enzymes and histamine increase capillary membrane permeability. Water, electrolytes, and proteins leak from the capillaries into the nonfunctional interstitial space. As high protein edema develops, blood volume falls. As cellular hypoxia increases, the sodium pump becomes less effective, as in hypovolemic shock; fluid and sodium move intracellularly, and interstitial fluid volume falls.

Myocardial dysfunction develops progressively as the shock state worsens, owing partly to decreased venous return. The principal explanation for the failure of cardiac function appears to be inadequate coronary perfusion and inadequate delivery of oxygen and cellular substrates to the cardiac musculature. A circulating myocardial depressant factor has been postulated but never confirmed. As cardiac output falls, so does tissue perfusion, and cellular damage is accelerated.

To treat a patient suffering from septic shock effectively, the invading bacteria must be controlled or eliminated, tissue perfusion must be restored, and the violence of the host-invader collision must be moderated.

PEDIATRIC PHYSIOLOGY

A host of factors make treatment of shock in the pediatric surgical patient a complex and difficult task. Four important factors are the red blood cells, hyperviscosity, blood volume, and the catecholamine system.

The Red Blood Cells

The production of red blood cells begins at 2 weeks' gestation within the yolk sac blood vessels of the embryo. These cells immediately begin to deliver oxygen to the tissues. By 8 weeks, production shifts to the liver sinusoids, spleen, and lymph nodes, reaching a peak by 5 months and then falling off. Bone marrow production begins during this period. The concentration of hemoglobin in the blood nearly doubles during the course of gestation; it is 9 gm/dl at 10 weeks, 10 gm/dl at 12 weeks, 14 gm/dl at 24 weeks, and 14 to 16.5 gm/dl at term. Hematocrit rises from 33 per cent to 51 per cent over the same period.

Four factors determine the hemoglobin concentration of the infant at birth: (1) the site of blood sampling, (2) fluid shifts, (3) gestational age, and (4) pathologic factors. Owing to sluggish capillary flow and movement of fluid into the interstitial space, hemoglobin concentration in the capillary blood is 2 gm/dl higher than in venous samples; hematocrit is 6 per cent higher. This difference disappears at 2 weeks of age. The same shift of fluid also accounts for the increase in red blood cell volume. The increase is most marked if clamping of the umbilical cord is delayed. The preterm infant tends to have a lower hemoglobin level and the postmature infant a much higher level, to the point of polycythemia. Transfusions between twins and fetal-maternal transfusions can also affect hemoglobin levels.

Hemoglobin levels below 14.5 gm/dl in the full-term infant suggest anemia. In premature babies, the fall in hemoglobin levels after 6 weeks is greater than in the full-term infant. At 2 to 3 months, a hemoglobin level of 9 gm/dl and a 28 per cent hematocrit are found. By 6 months, there is a further rise in hemoglobin in both the full-term and the preterm baby. This rise continues until adolescence, when male and female values diverge. In girls 14 to 18 years of age the hematocrit is 41 per cent. In boys, hematocrit rises to 43 per cent at age 14 years and to 47 per cent by 18 years.[26, 33, 100]

Certain characteristics of neonatal red blood cells may affect susceptibility to and tolerance of shock. Of these, one of the most important is the presence of fetal hemoglobin.[99, 101] Ninety to 95 per cent of hemoglobin produced by the fetus is fetal hemoglobin (HbF); the remainder is adult hemoglobin (HbA). About 75 per cent of the total hemoglobin concentration is HbF at birth; this declines to 20 per cent by 4 months and to 2 per cent by 1 year. The function of hemoglobin is to combine reversibly with oxygen, allowing red blood cells to extract oxygen from the lungs and deliver it to the tissues. This function is determined principally by the affinity of hemoglobin for oxygen. There is a marked difference in oxygen affinity between red blood cells containing HbF and those containing HbA. The affinity of hemoglobin for oxygen can best be depicted by the oxygen dissociation curve. Oxygen saturation of blood is plotted against the partial pressure of oxygen. The P_{O2} at which hemoglobin is 50 per cent saturated is designated P_{50}. The P_{50} of adult hemoglobin is 27 mm Hg. When the P_{O2} of arterial blood falls to 27 mm Hg in the adult, 50 per cent of the oxygen has been released to the tissues. With fetal hemoglobin, the curve shifts to the left. The P_{50} is 20 mm Hg, that is, 7 mm Hg less than in the adult. The fetal blood can thus be 50 per cent saturated or release 50 per cent of its O_2 at a P_{O2} level that is 7 mm Hg less than adult blood.

These characteristics of fetal hemoglobin are well suited for oxygen exchange in the low-oxygen environment of the fetus. The high oxygen affinity favors extraction of oxygen from the maternal vessels (P_{O2} 100 mm Hg) into the fetal vessels (P_{O2} 30 mm Hg). The increased affinity also makes it possible for oxygen delivery to take place at extremely low P_{O2} levels found in the peripheral vessels of the fetus. At a P_{O2} of 15 mm Hg, for example, almost 50 per cent of the oxygen can still be released to the tissues. Although the higher oxygen affinity of fetal blood suits the intrauterine low-oxygen environment, it fails to meet the needs of the neonate, whose P_{O_2} is higher and in whom oxygen release is less efficient. By 3 months of age the curve has shifted from left to right, toward its adult position, because of the decreasing production of HbF and its replacement with HbA.

The leftward shift of the oxygen dissociation curve in the neonate is due to the predominance of fetal hemoglobin in the baby's circulation and the low concentration of 2,3-diphosphoglycerate (2,3-DPG) in HbF. A potent modifier of hemoglobin function, 2,3-DPG decreases the affinity of hemoglobin for oxygen by competing for the binding sites on the hemoglobin molecule. The more 2,3-DPG present in hemoglobin, the lesser the oxygen affinity. Fetal hemoglobin has less 2,3-DPG than does adult hemoglobin because HbF binds 2,3-DPG poorly, and the actual concentration of 2,3-DPG is lower in the neonate than in the adult.

Polycythemia and Hyperviscosity

Any factor that contributes to inadequate tissue blood flow during shock adds significantly to the progressive development of cell injury and death. High blood viscosity is common in the newborn infant; it markedly decreases peripheral blood flow and tissue perfusion. Viscosity is a measure of the internal friction resulting when a layer of fluid is made to move in relation to another layer. Measurements are made at different shear rates and the results recorded as shear force measured in poises. The major determinants of blood viscosity are hematocrit, protein concentration, pH, and temperature. Red blood cell rigidity contributes to a lesser extent.[36, 83, 88] Not only can hyperviscosity intensify the effects of shock, but it

can, itself, be a major source of morbidity and mortality. The hyperviscosity syndrome includes poor feeding, lethargy, seizures, cyanosis, respiratory distress, and congestive heart failure. Hyperviscosity can cause thrombosis of peripheral blood vessels, renal vein thrombosis, brain damage, and necrotizing enterocolitis.

Polycythemia of the newborn has been defined as a venous hematocrit of 65 per cent or more. It occurs in 3 to 4 per cent of the newborn population. Hyperviscosity is diagnosed if the whole blood viscosity is greater than two standard deviations above the mean as defined by Gross et al.[48] It is usually associated with a hematocrit of over 65 per cent but may occasionally be found in blood with hematocrits as low as 60 per cent. The two major causes of neonatal polycythemia and hyperviscosity are (1) intrauterine or intranatal transfusions, such as placental and twin-to-twin transfusions, and (2) intrauterine hypoxia. Dehydration with hemo-concentration intensifies hyperviscosity. Polycythemia and hyperviscosity are more common in small-for-gestational-age infants and babies suffering from Down's syndrome and gastroschisis.

Babies with symptoms of hyperviscosity who have hematocrits above 65 per cent should be treated.[11, 12, 47, 48, 53, 148, 161, 163] We believe that patients without symptoms of hyperviscosity who have hematocrits above 60 per cent and who are in a low flow state as a result of hypovolemia or sepsis should also have their hematocrits lowered. The hematocrits of newborn patients requiring major surgery should be reduced to 55 per cent or less. If hypovolemia is present, a significant decrease in hematocrit can be accomplished by the infusion of red cell–free fluids. In normovolemic patients a partial exchange transfusion using fresh frozen plasma must be performed. The formula shown at the bottom of this page may be used (assume blood volume is 100 ml/kg).

$$\text{volume of exchange (ml)} = \frac{\text{blood volume} \times (\text{observed hematocrit} - \text{desired hematocrit})}{\text{observed hematocrit}}$$

Blood Volume

Total blood, plasma, and red blood cell volumes are all at their highest point at birth. After 6 hours, plasma shifts out of the circulation and total blood volume remains high, primarily because of elevated red blood cell volume. Infants who have had placental transfusions and all small-for-gestational-age babies have a red blood cell volume higher than their plasma volume. Plasma volume is greater than red blood cell volume in preterm and full-term infants. Premature infants have a larger blood volume than full-term infants.

The time of clamping the umbilical cord leads to the presence or absence of placental transfusion, which has a marked effect on the total blood volume and the red blood cell volume. In one study, the average blood volume during the first hours of life averaged 71.7 ml/kg in infants whose cords were clamped immediately and 86.9 ml/kg in babies who had delayed clamping and thus received a placental transfusion. The difference between these two groups is in red blood cell rather than plasma volume. After a few months of age, no difference in blood volume can be measured as a function of early or late cord clamping. The average full-term infant has a blood volume of 85 ml/kg, whereas the blood volume of premature infants averages 90 ml/kg. Volume increases in the preterm infant to 105 ml/kg during the first days of life. In both preterm and full-term infants, blood volume decreases during the first few months. Average blood volume falls to 75 to 77 ml/kg, similar to that in older children and adults.[44, 90, 97, 138, 146, 155]

Catecholamines

Hypovolemia and infection stimulate the secretion of catecholamines from the adrenal medulla and sympathetic nerve endings. These hormones increase cardiac contractility and rate, dilate and constrict blood vessels, and release energy, responses that are essential for the organism to cope successfully with stress. The development of the catecholamine system begins by the seventh week of gestation. The sympathetic trunk ganglia made up of neuroblasts derived from the neural crest are linked by nerve cords to form the sympathetic trunks and plexus. The neuroblasts then migrate down through the adrenal cortex and congregate at its center to form the medulla. They mature to polyhedral chromaffin cells. Cells also migrate to various sites along the aorta and into skin and form chromaffin masses. The largest of these are the paired periaortic organs of Zuckerkandl. In the fetus and the newborn, the adrenal medulla is primitive; it does not take on adult form until the age of 1 year. Most chromaffin tissue in the fetus is found in the extraadrenal masses, particularly the organ of Zuckerkandl. This organ achieves its maximum at term and then atrophies over a 2- or 3-year period.[41, 150]

The biosynthesis of catecholamines begins with tyrosine, which is hydroxylized to dopa in the chromaffin cells of the adrenal medulla and sympathetic nerve endings. Dopa is decarboxylized to dopamine, which is the first active catecholamine formed. Dopamine is metabolized to norepinephrine in the nerve endings and medulla. The conversion of norepinephrine to epinephrine occurs only in the adrenal medulla. The adrenal gland contains a mixture of epinephrine and norepinephrine in a ratio of 4:1. Once formed, the hormones are stored in granules. Secretions from the medulla and sympathetic nerves are predominantly norepinephrine in a ratio of 5:1 to epinephrine. Both hormones are rapidly metabolized. Two to 5 per cent of norepinephrine and epinephrine is secreted by the kidneys unchanged. Twenty per cent appears in the urine as metanephrine and normetanephrine. Vanillylmandelic acid makes up 30 to 50 per cent of the excreted catecholamines.

Catecholamines are believed to exert their physiologic effect on target tissues by being bound to receptor sites on the cell membrane. In response to receptor occupancy, adenylate cyclase is stimulated and adenosine monophosphate (AMP) forms from adenosine triphosphate (ATP). AMP is then released into the cell and alters cell function. The receptor sites have been divided on the basis of agonists that activate the receptor and antagonists that block them. The alpha receptors respond to norepinephrine and result in vasoconstriction, particularly of the blood vessels of the muscles and skin. These sites are blocked by phenoxybenzamine. The beta receptors classically respond to epinephrine and, to a lesser extent, norepinephrine. When stimulated they increase heart rate (chronotropic) and myocardial contractility (inotropic) and cause vasodilatation. The beta receptors are blocked by propranolol. Beta effects have been further subdivided into β_1 and β_2. The cardiac effects are due to β_1 and the dilatation of blood vessels to β_2. Beta receptors are responsible for the profound alterations in intermediate metabolism produced by catecholamines, particularly epinephrine. These alterations include the mobilization of glucose from glycogen stores, the new synthesis of glucose from carbohydrate and noncarbohydrate sources, and the formation and release of free fatty acids from triglyceride stores in adipose tissues. Since dopamine has vasoactive effects that are quantitatively different from those of norepinephrine and epinephrine, a specific dopaminergic receptor site has been postulated. These sites are principally in the lung, brain, intestine, and kidney.[5, 148, 160, 166]

Studies of catecholamine secretion in the pediatric patient are incomplete. Many suggest that secretion of catecholamines is lowest at birth and reaches adult levels by 10 years of age. The levels of norepinephrine, epinephrine, and dopamine in neonates vary according to gestational age. The preterm infant has lower levels than the full-term infant until the fifteenth day of life. A recent extensive study of urine catecholamine metabolites in newborn infants, children, and adults suggests that the maturation process of the sympatheticoadrenal system is relatively slow and is not achieved until the fifth year of life.[34] Another study of plasma catecholamine concentrations in newborns and infants up to 48 hours of age reveals that norepinephrine concentration is much higher than epinephrine concentration.[38] The levels of epinephrine and norepinephrine, extremely high right after birth, fell rapidly within 3 hours and then more slowly over a 12-hour period. It appears that the catecholamine system in newborn and young patients can be stimulated to secrete hormones in concentrations ap-

proaching those of the adult. This suggests that in the usual stressful situations, the sympatheticoadrenal system is adequate to meet the needs of the pediatric patient.

MONITORING

Considering the array of factors that affect the pediatric patient in shock, there is no "standard" pediatric patient who can be managed by set formulas or rules of thumb. Each patient is unique and constantly changing. A system that permits flexibility and individualization must be designed. Techniques must be available to evaluate the physiologic and pathophysiologic state of the patient. Analysis of the data thus provided allows a tentative therapeutic plan to be formulated. The plan is then put into operation for a specific period of time. During that period, the responses of the patient to therapy are constantly monitored, and adjustments are made. A revised plan is then made. Once the new plan is in operation, monitoring and readjustments continue to meet the changing needs of the patient. This feedback system is dynamic and can be likened to a therapeutic chess game between physician and patient.

Serial Measurements of Body Weight

Changes in body weight are a sensitive indicator of the volume of external fluid losses and the adequacy of fluid replacement. Roughly, a loss or gain of 1 gm of body weight can be equated to a loss or gain of 1 ml of water. There can be a significant loss of fluid from the circulation without a decrease in body weight if the fluid is sequestered in the "third space." Patients should be weighed naked and dressings either removed or weighed. The weight of nasogastric and other tubes can be determined by weighing similar tubes.

Urine Output

The kidney is a well-perfused organ with an arterial blood supply that reacts to a reduction in blood flow by prompt and vigorous vasoconstriction in excess of that found in other areas of the body. The kidney receives as much as one quarter of the cardiac output each minute and therefore has the capacity to make large adjustments during periods of low flow. Renal function can be temporarily sacrificed in favor of more vital needs of the body, and blood is thus shunted to vital organs.[19] An individual, regardless of age, will excrete adequate amounts of urine when renal blood flow is ample and scant urine when renal blood flow decreases. Serial measurements of urine output can serve as a valuable indirect guide to tissue blood flow. The full-term newborn infant usually has a urine flow rate of about 25 ml/kg/24 hr; the low-birth-weight infant, 50 to 100 ml/kg/24 hr; and the child, 600 to 700 ml/M²/24 hr, or about 55 ml of urine/100 calories metabolized.[62, 118, 137] In patients already in shock, it is helpful to insert an indwelling bladder catheter and measure half-hourly or hourly urine output.

Arterial Blood Pressure

Arterial blood pressure determinations are often neglected in the small patient but are extremely helpful in assessing the circulatory system in shock. Blood pressure is a product of cardiac output and peripheral resistance (BP = CO × PR). The most direct and accurate method of assessing blood pressure is by an arterial catheter, which is inserted percutaneously or by a cutdown into a peripheral artery or through the umbilical artery into the aorta. Pressure is measured by an electronic strain gauge transducer. Pressure waves are displayed on an oscilloscope and recorded. Electronic devices allow systolic, diastolic, and mean pressures to be digitally displayed and high and low alarms set.

The umbilical artery is readily available during the first week of life. The lumen is easily exposed in the freshly cut umbilical stump. The catheter can then be advanced into the aorta until the tip rests just above the bifurcation of the iliac arteries or at the level of the diaphragm. Septicemia and major vascular thrombosis are the two most serious complications of umbilical catheterization. Low pressure readings may be obtained if the catheter is inadvertently advanced into the ductus arteriosus. When arterial oxygen tensions are also being measured through the catheter, confusing readings may result if the catheter is advanced into the ductus or if there are right-to-left or left-to-right shunts.

The temporal artery is a potential cannulation site because of its accessibility and expendability. Because of its superficial position, it can be entered either by a cutdown or percutaneously. Recently there have been several reports of cerebrovascular accidents and one report of blindness following the use of this vessel as a catheter site. In the past, this has been our "first choice" site for arterial cannulation in the infant. We have performed more than 1000 cannulations and have now found evidence of central nervous system damage by either CAT scan or neurological changes in several patients. We now prefer to use the radial or posterior tibial artery. Radial artery catheterization may rarely result in gangrene of the fingers or even the hand owing to an incomplete palmar arch or to absence or thrombosis of the ulnar artery. Ulnar artery patency can be determined by the Doppler apparatus.

The manometer and inflatable cuff method of measuring blood pressure generally gives accurate readings in large healthy babies, children, and teenagers. The measurements are profoundly affected by the severe vasoconstriction that takes place during deep shock and by technical difficulties of using cuffs on tiny infants. To avoid the dangers of vascular cannulation and the problems presented by the manometric method, Doppler and infrasound devices have become popular. These techniques use ultrasound transducers to sense either arterial wall motion or low-frequency vibrations (infrasounds) in blood vessels. Both methods accurately measure systolic pressure in infants and children.[108, 127] There have been no extensive studies of the use of such apparatus on patients in shock.

Regardless of whether the manometer, Doppler, or infrasound method is utilized, a potential source of error is the choice of inflatable cuff size. The largest cuff that will snugly fit the patient's arm or leg should be used. A table of suggested cuff sizes for different age groups has been published.[18]

In patients of any age, persistent hypotension suggests inadequate perfusion, and its continuation will result in progressive organ failure. One must know the normal blood pressure for patients of different ages, sexes, weights, and levels of maturity. It is best to refer to published tables.[18, 20, 77] Preterm newborn infants have a systolic blood pressure that ranges between 35 and 56 mm Hg. Full-term, full-size infants often have a blood pressure of 75/50; by 1 to 6 months, readings reach 80/46, and by 2 years, 100/82.

Base Excess/Deficit and Blood Lactate Measurements

Tissue hypoxia develops when there is inadequate tissue perfusion. For cellular metabolic activity to continue, anaerobic biochemical pathways must be utilized. Lactate and hydrogen ions are end products of these pathways. Nonvolatile lactic acid is then formed in the blood. Increased concentration of lactic acid results in metabolic acidosis. With effective treatment of shock, tissue perfusion improves, aerobic metabolism is re-established, lactic acid production decreases, and accumulated lactate ions are metabolized to water and carbon dioxide, primarily in the liver.[76] Hydrogen ions are excreted by the kidney. Monitoring of the metabolic portion of acid-base balance or of the blood lactate level is therefore a clinically useful method of indirectly measuring tissue perfusion.

The metabolic or nonrespiratory portion of acid-base balance can be most simply estimated by calculating the base excess/deficit. This calculation is made from pH, P_{CO2}, and hematocrit. Ideally, these measurements should be made on arterial blood, but there is only a minor discrepancy between base excess calculated from arterial blood and base excess calculated from venous or capillary blood. Base deficit is reported as milliequivalents per liter of base above or below the normal buffer-base range. A patient with metabolic acidosis has a minus base excess, which is often referred to as a base deficit. During therapy of shock, if base excess becomes more minus or base deficit increases, there is continued poor tissue perfusion. If base deficit decreases and approaches zero during treatment,

there is strong evidence that tissue blood flow and cellular oxygenation are improving. The value of this monitoring system as a guide to adequacy of tissue blood flow is destroyed if buffers are administered.

Weil and Afifi[159] have used arterial blood lactate levels to indicate the severity of shock and to predict survival. Used alone, they are as accurate as calculations of excess lactate or the lactate-pyruvate ratio.

Central Venous Pressure

Right atrial pressure and right ventricular filling pressure can be measured with a catheter advanced into the superior vena cava or right atrium. In most instances, left atrial pressure and the filling pressure of the left ventricle are similar and provide a rough estimate of the adequacy of blood volume in relation to ventricular function. Although right and left atrial pressures are usually similar, there are important exceptions. When pulmonary disease, overwhelming sepsis, or cardiac lesions are present, there may be a wide discrepancy between left and right atrial pressures. In these cases, central venous pressure measurements will not reflect adequacy of blood volume in relation to left ventricular function.[10, 107]

Central venous pressure monitoring is simple, rapid, and inexpensive. High readings may be obtained when the catheter tip is not in a central position. Proper placement must be checked by roentgenogram. Central venous pressure measured by a water manometer may be inaccurate. The manometer can respond only to one or two variations per second, which may reflect only the maximal pressure rather than the mean central venous pressure. This "lag" error can be eliminated by using an electronic strain gauge transducer, which has a rapid response time. High central venous pressure readings are commonly encountered with respiratory distress or positive pressure ventilation. Markedly elevated pressure also occurs when a catheter is placed in the inferior vena cava of a patient with increased intra-abdominal pressure from intestinal obstruction or ascites. The most effective way of utilizing central venous pressure is by obtaining serial readings and following the response of central venous pressure to therapy.

In infants the central venous catheter is usually placed by a cutdown in the antebrachial or jugular vein and passed into the superior vena cava or the right atrium. Placement through a percutaneous puncture of the subclavian vein has been performed successfully and safely on very small newborn babies.

The Swan-Ganz Catheter

Placement of the Swan-Ganz catheter has become routine during the management of critically ill adult patients. Central venous, pulmonary artery, and pulmonary wedge pressures and cardiac output can be measured repeatedly with the use of this multichannel catheter. The standard balloon catheter has three lumens and is supplied in diameters of 5 to 8 French. It is possible to monitor all three functions in larger babies and children. Because there are no triple-lumen catheters smaller than 5 French, it is impossible to measure pulmonary artery pressure and cardiac output with a single catheter in the small baby. Number 4 French double-lumen balloon-tip catheters are available to measure pulmonary artery and pulmonary wedge pressures in the small infant. A 4 French balloon-tip thermistor catheter can be purchased, to measure cardiac output without the pressure.

The Swan-Ganz catheter can be placed percutaneously or by a cutdown through the subclavian, jugular, cephalic, or femoral vein. In small infants, many physicians prefer to pass the catheter through the saphenous vein into the femoral vein to the inferior vena cava and then to float the catheter into the pulmonary artery. The catheter is advanced under continuous electrocardiographic and pressure monitoring. The electrocardiogram reveals any cardiac arrhythmia that develops during inflation of the balloon, and pressure tracings indicate the position of the catheter. The catheter is advanced with the balloon deflated until right atrial waves are noted on the oscilloscope. The balloon is inflated and allowed to be carried into the right ventricle and then into the pulmonary artery. The balloon is then deflated and the catheter advanced gently as far as it will go. With reinflation of the balloon, characteristic pulmonary wedge pressure tracings should be seen. A portable chest x-ray film is taken for final confirmation of the position of the catheter.

Pressure Monitoring. When the tip of the Swan-Ganz catheter is in the distal pulmonary artery and the balloon is inflated, the resulting pressure is generally an accurate reflection of the left atrial pressure and left ventricular filling pressure. There is a relationship between left ventricular filling pressure and the ability of the left ventricle to perform work. A low pulmonary wedge pressure suggests that blood volume must be expanded for cardiac output to be adequate and for blood flow to improve. A high or normal pulmonary wedge pressure in the face of continued signs of shock suggests that there is adequate blood volume and left ventricular filling pressure, but inadequate myocardial function.

In a study of 13 preterm and full-term infants who had pulmonary artery pressure monitoring, unsuspected congenital heart disease was frequently diagnosed, and changes in wedge pressure helped guide pharmacologic therapy and fluid replacement.[152] A mixed group of 19 patients, ranging in age from 2 days to 19 years, required bedside pulmonary artery catheterization. There were three complications, none fatal.[104]

Cardiac Output

Recent development of thermodilution[27, 84] for estimating cardiac output and incorporation of a thermistor in the Swan-Ganz catheter has made determination of cardiac output a practical clinical tool. Only a single vein need be cannulated, no blood withdrawal is necessary, and only a small quantity of a physiologic injectate is required. The method offers the added advantages of internal electrical calibration, minimal recirculation of the injectate, and the possibility of performing repeated measurements within a short time interval. The principle of detecting blood flow by the thermodilution technique is similar to that of other indicator dilution techniques as described by the Stewart-Hamilton formula. Temperature rather than color serves as the indicator. Cardiac output is determined by injecting a known amount of the indicator, cold saline solution, into the blood at a specific point and measuring the temperature change of the blood at a point downstream. The small 5 French triple-lumen catheter has been successfully used in children and in several babies less than 1 year of age. A bolus of cold saline is injected into the right atrium and sensed by the thermistor in the pulmonary artery. The resulting indicator dilution curve can be displayed on an oscilloscope and printed out. A computer calculates the area under the thermodilution curve and the resultant cardiac output.

There are serious drawbacks to use of the standard Swan-Ganz catheter for cardiac output measurements in the neonatal surgical patient. First, there are the technical problems of constructing a catheter with three lumens that will still allow flow of fluid and remain unobstructed by blood clot. The second problem is the transitional circulation of the newborn. Conditions such as hypoxia and shock result in pulmonary vasoconstriction, dilation of the ductus arteriosus, and development of right-to-left shunts. In the preterm infant, fluid overloading during resuscitation may result in large left-to-right shunts across the ductus. When the saline indicator is injected into the right atrium in the standard manner and there is a left-to-right shunt across the ductus, the flow of blood into the pulmonary artery will warm the indicator and produce an inaccurate curve. With a right-to-left shunt, the indicator will be lost across the ductus to the left side of the heart. In either case, the calculation of cardiac output by the computer will be in error. We have concluded that if a ductus arteriosus shunt is present, injection and sensing on the right side of the heart will not give satisfactory clinical information.

The Swan-Ganz catheter is an extremely valuable addition to the armamentarium of the pediatric surgeon caring for the infant or child in shock, despite its failure to measure cardiac output in the newborn infant with a persistent shunt. Pulmonary wedge pressure alone or pulmonary wedge pressure with cardiac output gives a clear estimate of cardiac function. However, placement of the Swan-Ganz catheter and its position in the distal pulmonary artery have been associated with serious and, at times, fatal complications. We believe that the catheter should be used only in selected patients. Our indications are as follows: (1) when coexisting cardiac disease is present; (2) when shock is associated with respiratory failure, and mechanical ventilation with high positive end-expiratory pressure is required; (3) when there is renal failure; and (4) when adequate fluid replacement and therapy of sepsis do not improve the patient's condition, and a cardiogenic shock component must be ruled out.

Transcutaneous Oxygen Monitoring

The transcutaneous oxygen monitor estimates arterial oxygen tension (Pa_{O_2}) by measuring oxygen tension on the skin surface (TcP_{O_2}). It allows continuous noninvasive monitoring of the low flow state. This device is effective because one of the hallmarks of shock is an intense compensatory peripheral vasoconstriction. Vessels of the skin are the first to undergo this marked constrictor response because of the predominance of alpha-adrenergic receptors. As skin blood flow decreases, regardless of Pa_{O_2}, TcP_{O_2} will fall.

The transcutaneous oxygen device was developed to monitor the hypoxic infant. It functions on the principle that oxygen readily diffuses from the dermal vessels to the skin surface, where it can be measured.[69] Under normal conditions, the amount of oxygen released is equal to the amount consumed by the skin cells; the result is a TcP_{O_2} of zero. With maximum dilatation of the skin vasculature by heating, blood flow increases and a large amount of oxygen diffuses from the arterialized capillaries to the skin surface. The partial pressure of oxygen that reaches the skin surface then approaches that of arterial oxygen tension and is measured by an oxygen electrode. The two essential features of the apparatus are (1) a heating coil to warm the skin and (2) an oxygen sensor to measure oxygen escaping to the skin surface.

A large number of clinical and experimental studies have shown that the correlation between Pa_{O_2} and TcP_{O_2} under normal conditions is very close $(R > 0.9)$.[39, 111, 149] In sick infants who are in the low flow state, the difference between the two measurements is often large. In a study in our laboratory using piglets subjected to a 35 per cent hemorrhage, the relation between the low flow state and transcutaneous oxygen was further qualified.[117] Under controlled conditions, TcP_{O_2} closely reflected Pa_{O_2}. With hemorrhage, however, a marked difference developed between Pa_{O_2} and TcP_{O_2}. TcP_{O_2} fell more rapidly and to a greater extent than the pulse rate, blood pressure, cardiac output, or base deficit. TcP_{O_2} also appeared to be an earlier and more sensitive indicator of the adequacy of resuscitation. We believe that transcutaneous oxygen measurements can be used as a method of monitoring low flow states if TcP_{O_2} readings are interpreted in relation to Pa_{O_2} determinations. When a transcutaneous oxygen monitor is used, Pa_{O_2} and TcP_{O_2} should be measured simultaneously. A close correlation between the two measurements suggests adequate tissue perfusion. If TcP_{O_2} falls during the course of transcutaneous monitoring, Pa_{O_2} should be measured again. A low Pa_{O_2} indicates hypoxia. If Pa_{O_2} has not changed significantly, inadequate tissue perfusion is suggested. A persistent low TcP_{O_2} in spite of resuscitation of the low flow state suggests that treatment is inadequate.

THERAPY

Successful management of shock is based on prevention and, failing that, recognition of the shock state during its earliest stages. Prevention requires appreciation of subtle signs of hypovolemia or infection before there is a significant decrease in tissue perfusion or beginning cellular damage. Treatment is simple and effective at this stage. Later treatment is complex and usually ineffective (Fig. 2–2).

Treatment of Hypovolemic Shock

The treatment of hypovolemic shock can best be discussed by arbitrarily separating the condition into two forms; acute hypovolemia (rapid loss of body fluid, classically blood) and chronic hypovolemia (gradual loss of fluid over hours or even days). Examples of the second form include intestinal obstruction, most diarrheas, and chemical peritonitis. It is important to recognize that the chronic form is often accompanied by infection, which complicates management. Nevertheless, the basic principle in all forms of hypovolemic shock is correction of the

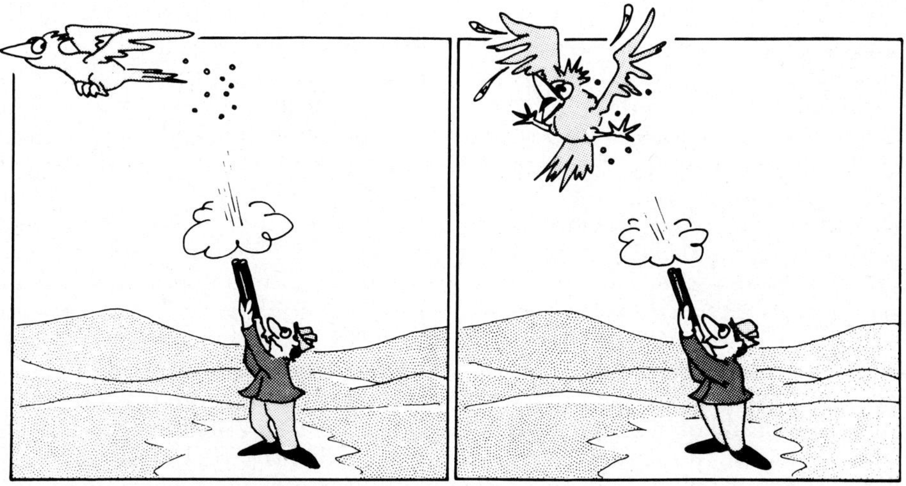

Figure 2–2 The principle of "leading" the patient in the treatment of shock. The hunter must aim ahead rather than directly at a rapidly flying bird. Similarly, the physician must "lead" the patient in treating shock. He must recognize the early signs of shock and begin therapy before advanced cellular damage results.

blood volume, and, in almost all cases, of the accompanying interstitial fluid deficit.

We treat the patient in hemorrhagic shock, regardless of age, with a rapid intravenous infusion of 5 per cent dextrose in lactated Ringer's solution. A volume of 12 to 15 ml/kg is run in over a 15- to 20-minute period. In small infants, the infusion is delivered by a hand-held syringe. Simultaneously, a blood sample is sent for typing and cross matching. Infusion of Ringer's lactate solution usually results in a rise in arterial blood pressure. The extremities become warm and color improves. Pulse rate falls in children, but it increases in newborn infants since babies often respond to acute volume depletion with bradycardia. Observation of the patient and measurement of pulse rate and blood pressure is all that is required initially. With severe or continued hemorrhage, other monitoring techniques become necessary.

If the single intravenous infusion of lactated Ringer's solution results in stabilization, hemorrhage has been minimal and is not continuing. Only transient improvement in vital signs, however, suggests that bleeding is continuing. The initial infusion of lactated Ringer's solution allows time for accurate typing and cross matching of whole blood. Blood transfusion can then be given safely. In the case of extreme blood loss when lactated Ringer's solution has only minimal effect, there is not adequate time for typing and cross matching. Type-specific whole blood can usually be made available in 10 to 15 minutes and then infused immediately. There are occasional patients with exsanguinating hemorrhage in whom crystalloid infusion has no effect. Type O negative blood with low titer of A must be given immediately and the patient rushed to the operating room.

A patient whose vital signs stabilize with only an infusion of Ringer's lactate solution may present later with a severe anemia that requires packed cell transfusion. If there is continued or massive hemorrhage, Ringer's lactate never replaces blood. We agree with Shires that "the treatment of hemorrhagic shock continues to be adequate replacement of whole blood, because this is the fluid that has been lost."[131] Ringer's lactate infusion is used initially in hemorrhage, because it (1) is very effective in determining the extent of bleeding; (2) reduces the quantity of blood

necessary to treat hemorrhage; (3) gives time for adequate typing and cross matching of blood; and (4) replaces interstitial fluid deficit and partially replaces blood volume. For most large hemorrhages, a ratio of 4:1 crystalloid solution to blood corrects the blood volume and interstitial fluid deficits, yet does not leave the patient with significant anemia.[131]

Chronic hypovolemia does not present with signs of low perfusion as does acute hypovolemia. Vital signs are usually only minimally altered. There may be signs of dehydration, such as loose skin, sunken fontanel, or dry mucous membranes. As in acute hypovolemia, blood volume and functional interstitial fluid volume are reduced. However, the "nonfunctional" interstitial space, the so-called third space, is markedly increased. Besides this internal loss in the tissues, large volumes of fluid are lost by evaporation from the skin surface, vomiting, gastrointestinal drainage, and fecal discharge. The extent of the volume deficit may be misjudged and replaced therapy underestimated because of the absence of signs of frank shock and the hidden losses into the tissue. The true extent of the volume deficit may not become apparent until the patient undergoes anesthesia, when vasodilatation and a small degree of hypoxia may precipitate severe circulatory collapse. Since serum sodium, potassium, and chloride values are only slightly reduced or normal, the degree of electrolyte losses may not be appreciated. Solutions containing low concentrations of electrolytes, such as pediatric maintenance solutions or 5 per cent dextrose in water, may be mistakenly given to correct the volume deficit. The serum then becomes markedly hypotonic and hyponatremic with danger of water intoxication.

The degree of volume depletion can be assessed simply and rapidly by serial measurements of hematocrit, urine specific gravity or osmolality, urine output, total protein measured by the refractometer, and serum blood urea nitrogen. The hematocrit and serum total protein are high because of the large water loss in proportion to red blood cell and protein loss. As blood volume decreases the urine becomes more concentrated, urine output falls, and blood urea nitrogen rises.

Hypertonic dehydration is much more

common in hypovolemic infants than in adults and presents a grave risk during resuscitation. Babies tend to become hypertonic for several reasons. Most of the fluid lost, such as vomitus, diarrhea, and peritoneal and bowel fluid, is dilute in relation to serum. Body surface area is large, allowing for increased transepithelial water loss. Metabolic activity is greater, leading to increased utilization of water of metabolism. The neonatal kidney has reduced concentrating ability and lower renal sodium excretion than that of the adult. A serum sodium value of 150 mEq/l or higher or a serum osmolality greater than 300 mOsm/kg is consistent with hypertonicity. Patients with hypertonic dehydration are in grave danger of brain damage if solutions low in electrolytes are infused. A rapid drop in serum osmolality causes cerebral edema and hemorrhage. Because it is impossible to determine by physical examination whether a patient is hypertonic, it is essential that serum sodium and serum osmolality be accurately measured. The initial resuscitation fluid should have a serum sodium concentration of at least 75 mEq/l. If hypertonic dehydration is found, it must be corrected slowly over 24 to 48 hours using sodium-containing solutions and titrating the concentration by serial measurements of serum sodium or serum osmolality. If an emergency operation is necessary, the hypovolemia is corrected but the patient is operated on while still in "electrolyte imbalance." Restoration of normal tonicity continues during the postoperative period.

Our usual resuscitation fluid for older infants and children with chronic hypovolemia is 5 per cent dextrose in Ringer's lactate or normal saline solution. For newborn infants we use 5 per cent dextrose in half-strength Ringer's lactate because of the neonate's reduced ability to handle excess sodium chloride. If hypovolemia is severe, an initial bolus of 10 ml/kg is infused over 15 to 30 minutes. This is followed by an infusion of 5 per cent dextrose in Ringer's lactate or half-strength normal saline solution, depending on the age, at double maintenance fluid volumes. Potassium is not added until urine flow is established. The actual speed and volume of the infusion are gauged by monitorng urine output, specific gravity, central venous pressure, or, when indicated, pulmonary wedge pressure.

In full-term infants and children, moderate leeway is allowed in choosing the volume of fluid to deliver. Overinfusion is usually well tolerated by the lungs, cardiovascular system, and kidneys. This is not the case for the preterm infant, in whom overinfusion may rapidly lead to abrupt expansion of blood volume, opening up of the ductus arteriosus, shunting of blood from right to left across the ductus, and development of right heart failure and pulmonary edema. Resuscitation of the hypovolemic preterm infant requires precise management while monitoring serial urine output, urine specific gravity or osmolality, central venous pressure, transcutaneous oxygen levels, blood gas determinations, and body weights. Resuscitation proceeds at a slower pace. If we err in our estimate of fluid replacement, it is better to err on the low rather than the high side.

Most of the conditions that lead to chronic hypovolemia are associated with bacterial infection. Failure of the patient's condition to improve after volume resuscitation suggests that there is ongoing sepsis requiring vigorous treatment.

A common pitfall in the management of the patient with chronic hypovolemic shock occurs during the postoperative period. Preoperatively, large volumes of fluid are given rapidly to correct deficits and replace continuing losses caused by the untreated disorder. This vigorous therapy is usually continued intraoperatively by the anesthesiologist. After operation, the patient has changed. His physiology has been altered by anesthesia and operative trauma, fluid and electrolyte deficits have been corrected and often overcorrected, and pathologic lesions have been treated either partially or completely. Rapid infusion of high volumes of electrolyte-containing fluids at this stage may lead to circulatory overload. Immediately after operation, the patient must be reassessed and a tentative new therapeutic program outlined. This plan is then instituted for a specific period of time — in seriously ill patients for 2 hours, in relatively stable patients for 6 to 8 hours. At the end of these periods, the tentative program is adjusted to meet the needs of the patient. In this way, treatment is tailored to the constantly changing condition of the infant or child. Postoperative assessment includes calculation of intake and output, monitoring of pulse rate and blood pressure, measurement of urine output and osmolality or specific gravity, and serial determinations of serum osmolality, total protein and electrolytes, blood urea nitrogen, blood hematocrit, blood sugar, and body weight. When shock was profound or continues after operation, serial measurements of central venous pressure or pulmonary wedge pressure and constant monitoring of arterial Pa_{O2}, pH, P_{CO2} and transcutaneous oxygen are helpful.

Treatment of Septic Shock

The treatment of septic shock involves control of infection and restoration of adequate tissue perfusion; treatment of infection is the cornerstone. A combination of antibiotics providing wide-spectrum coverage is administered intravenously in high doses from the beginning of resuscitation. The choice of antibiotics is guided by the clinical presentation of the patient, the primary pathologic condition, and the physician's knowledge of the hospital's pathogens and antibiotic sensitivities. In full-term infants and children without advanced septic shock, we usually employ a combination of gentamicin sulfate and oxacillin. Clindamycin is added to combat anaerobic infections if there has been fecal soiling. For preterm debilitated full-term infants, we use the antibiotic or antibiotics most effective against the current resistant strains of gram-negative organisms in our hospital. We have made this decision because of the fulminating and rapidly fatal course of the compromised patient treated inadequately for infection. In three such patients the peritoneal and blood cultures grew gentamicin sulfate–resistant *Klebsiella aerobacter* that was sensitive to amikacin sulfate, a drug whose use we have been trying to limit. We are now convinced, as are others,[153] that in compromised patients with serious gram-negative infections, one must use the most effective antibiotic available while the opportunity for treatment still exists.

The source of infection should be rapidly identified and, if possible, controlled. Infected intravascular cannulas must be removed. Superficial abscesses of the skin or infected surgical wounds that can be drained without general anesthesia should be incised and drained promptly. When infection is due to perforation of the intestine or necrotic bowel, a vigorous attempt should be made to improve the patient's cardiovascular status before operation is performed. On occasion the grave risk of operating on a patient in shock must be accepted and surgery performed to prevent further seeding of the body with viable bacteria and bacterial byproducts. Elimination of infection is ultimately determined by the effectiveness of the host's defenses. Prematurity, "stress," trauma, operation, anesthesia, certain drugs, starvation, and infection reduce the humoral and cellular defenses against infection. In an attempt to provide additional host defense, blood and blood byproducts have been used.

The administration of fresh frozen plasma and fresh whole blood transfusions will increase elements of the classic and alternate complement pathways and increase the level of circulating immunoglobulins to bind bacteria and serve as opsonins for white blood cells and other phagocytes.[3, 130] Fresh whole blood transfusions have been effective in treating severe group-B streptococcal sepsis of the newborn. The transfused blood rich in opsonic antibodies for streptococci was given in volumes greater than 40 per cent of the blood volume.

Exchange transfusions of fresh whole blood provide complement and immunoglobulins in addition to viable white blood cells. Removing old blood and infusing donor blood may have the added benefit of removing circulating infectious components such as live bacteria, vasoactive substances, platelet and white blood cell aggregates, and endotoxin.[1, 102, 153, 156, 165] Exchange transfusions are also useful when disseminated intravascular coagulation occurs during the course of septic shock. They appear to be more effective than heparin because of the removal of fibrin split-products and the replacement of depleted clotting factors.[49]

The successful use of unmatched granulocytic transfusions in the treatment of neonatal sepsis has recently been reported.[55, 79, 80] In the past, it was believed that white blood cell transfusions were effective only if the donor cells matched those of the recipient. However, Laurenti et al.[79] found increased survival in infants with serious gram-negative infection who were treated with unmatched leukocyte transfusions. Mortality was reduced from 72 per cent to 10 per cent; there were no significant side effects.

Saba and coworkers[16, 17, 98, 122, 124] note that the RE system plays an essential role in removing bacterial byproducts, particularly endotoxin, from the circulation during infection. An alpha$_2$ opsonic glycoprotein must be present in the plasma for the cells of the RE system to act as phagocytes. The concentration of glycoprotein is reduced by trauma and infection. Cryoprecipitated plasma contains a high concentration of the opsonic glycoprotein and may be used in the treatment of infected patients. They report a reduction in septic complications in burn patients. Reduced levels of opsonic glycoprotein were restored by infusion of cryoprecipitated plasma.

We currently resuscitate septic preterm and stressed infants with blood, fresh frozen plasma, and electrolyte-containing solutions. If infection continues unabated, we then give one or more exchange transfusions of fresh whole blood. Exchange transfusion must not be used as a last resort and delayed until the patient is moribund.

The chronic hypovolemia of gram-negative sepsis is treated with blood or plasma as part of the initial resuscitation regimen. These colloid-containing fluids are used not for their oncotic effect but rather because they contain immunologic factors that need to be replaced because of the patient's compromised host defense. The efficacy of crystalloid versus colloid-containing solutions in resuscitation of the patient in shock is still controversial. Two solutions most commonly compared are Ringer's lactate solution and 5 per cent albumin in normal saline solution or plasma. Colloid-containing fluids have the advantage of increasing colloid oncotic pressure. According to Starling's hypothesis,[145] this increase favors absorption of interstitial fluid through the capillary membrane into the vascular compartment and reduces capillary filtration of water out of the vessel. The net result is an increase in the blood volume over and above the increase produced by the addition of the colloid-containing infused fluid. Since the presence of oncotically active molecules in the circula-

tion tends to hold the infused fluid in the circulation, tissue edema is prevented and extravascular fluid mobilized, reducing edema already present. In contrast, the administration of large volumes of protein-free electrolyte solutions dilutes plasma proteins and reduces colloid oncotic pressure. Capillary filtration increases and capillary refill decreases. Blood volume increases only slightly, and theoretically, as more and more fluid diffuses from the vascular space, tissue edema will develop. Several authors[70, 71, 139-142] emphasize that diffusion of fluid into the lung parenchyma is particularly hazardous and may contribute to the development of shock lung.

In septic shock, Starling's hypothesis may not be valid in all areas of the body owing to the damaged capillary membrane.[61-63, 91, 96, 113, 114] Without a properly functioning membrane, protein molecules may leak through the injured capillaries into the tissues. The increased colloid in the interstitium may alter the oncotic gradient and paradoxically increase fluid loss. The non-functional interstitial fluid space will increase as protein and fluid accumulate in the area of injury. Since generalized capillary damage occurs only in late shock, in many areas — particularly muscle and spleen — the capillary membrane will still be intact. In these areas, venous refill will take place and fluid will be drawn from the interstitium, decreasing functional interstitial fluid volume and increasing blood volume. In most forms of shock a significant functional interstitital fluid deficit already exists; the oncotic action of a colloid-containing solution might intensify this deficit.

With all the conflicting data, it is difficult to champion one form of fluid therapy over the other. Our conclusions are as follows:

1. Milliliter for milliliter, a colloid-containing solution will increase blood volume to a much greater extent than a crystalloid solution.

2. Electrolyte solutions are effective in correcting the interstitial fluid deficit, whereas colloid-containing solutions may actually intensify the deficit.

3. Colloid-containing solutions, in spite of increasing colloid oncotic pressure, are no more effective in preventing the pulmonary impairment that develops during

shock than are protein-free electrolyte solutions.

4. In the presence of capillary damage, colloids can leak into the area of tissue injury in large quantities.

5. Blood viscosity is reduced more by infusion of colloid solutions than by infusion of electrolyte solutions.

6. Crystalloids can improve cardiac output and pulmonary wedge pressure to the same extent as colloids, but only if a much greater volume is infused.

7. It is impossible to make generalizations from a review of the literature, first because the amount of colloid administered varies from study to study; doses range from 0.2 gm/kg to 10 gm/kg and have been delivered as a bolus, infused over several hours or over a 24-hour period; second, crystalloid versus colloid effectiveness has been investigated in a host of pathologic conditions: hemorrhagic shock, septic shock, adult respiratory distress syndrome, peritonitis, pancreatitis, major surgery, trauma, intestinal obstruction, and burns. One cannot assume that the pathophysiology of each of these conditions is the same and that the colloids or crystalloids will act similarly in each condition.

8. A large amount of albumin is required to elevate colloid oncotic pressure significantly. In young animals and infants a bolus of 1.5 gm/kg of albumin causes an immediate marked elevation of colloid oncotic pressure lasting about 20 minutes and then leveling off to a moderate elevation. Elevated colloid oncotic pressure can also be produced by infusing 2.5 per cent albumin in electrolyte solution, 2.5 to 3 gm/kg/24 hr.

Our approach at present is to continue to use colloid-containing solutions sparingly. We prefer electrolyte solutions for initial resuscitation because of their safety, availability, cheapness, and effectiveness. During the early phases of shock when capillary leak, interstitial fluid deficit, and poor cellular function occur, colloid solutions may be counterproductive. However, faced with gram-negative septic shock in the infant, solutions such as blood and fresh frozen plasma have the added advantage of buttressing host defenses. When large volumes of colloid-free electrolyte solutions have been used for resuscitation, total protein utilization must be measured by refracto-

TABLE 2–1   REFRACTOMETER TOTAL PROTEIN

Age of Patient	Total Protein (mg/dl)
Term newborn	6.25
Premature newborn	5.04
One to 11 months	6.11
One to 12 years	7.02
Adults, 24 to 40 years	7.45

meter. If there is a persistently low total serum protein level (Table 2–1) and edema is present, we raise the level by a 24-hour infusion of 2½ per cent albumin.

After the initial period of rapid fluid resuscitation, total fluid requirement is evaluated. A rise in arterial central venous and pulmonary wedge pressures, an increase in urine output, a slowing pulse in the older infant and child, an increase in pulse rate in the neonate, a decrease in metabolic acidosis, and a rise in cardiac output suggest that the fluid deficit has been corrected and that the circulatory system is functioning effectively. Occasionally, central venous and pulmonary wedge pressures increase but arterial hypotension persists and there is continued oliguria and metabolic acidosis. These findings suggest that fluid resuscitation is "adequate" but shock persists because of cardiac failure. Cardiac output measurements are particularly helpful in confirming this diagnosis. Continued delivery of large volumes of intravenous fluid will increase the burden on the failing myocardium. The rate of intravenous infusion is decreased, and therapy is directed toward improving cardiac function.

Dopamine[37, 40, 74, 78, 112, 115] is presently our drug of first choice because it increases myocardial contractility, redistributes blood flow to central viscera, and can be titrated to obtain different pharmacologic effects. This agent has alpha and beta effects midway between those of isopropanol and epinephrine. An infusion of 1.5 μg/kg/min increases cardiac output, renal blood flow, and urine output. With larger doses, up to 30 μg, there is a further increase in cardiac output and, presumably, renal blood flow. At higher doses, peripheral vasoconstriction occurs owing to an adrenergic effect. For infants and children, a solution of dopamine (0.8 μg/ml) mixed in 5 per cent dextrose in water is prepared. The infusion is adjusted to run at a rate of 1 to 3 μg/kg/min. The dose is gradually increased if urine output and hemodynamic function do not improve. Methylprednisolone is given intravenously for its reported inotropic effect.

If we accept the concept that the cell is the critical target in shock, and cellular injury and death result from immunologic damage and inadequate delivery and utilization of essential nutrients, treatment must include agents that moderate violent host-invader reactions and act as cellular stabilizers and energizers. Animal and clinical investigations suggest that a water-soluble cortisone compound such as methylprednisolone, given in doses well above physiologic levels, may be such an agent.[51, 73, 85-87, 103, 129, 144, 151] Methylprednisolone reduces the interaction between white blood cells, endotoxin, and complement and between platelets, endotoxin, and complement. These reactions lead to the release of proteolytic and vasoactive compounds. Large doses of corticosteroids may also protect by stabilizing the cellular and lysosomal membranes. Several studies have demonstrated that corticosteroids stimulate hepatic cell gluconeogenesis and support carbohydrate metabolism.[7, 13, 45, 59, 65, 128] They may indirectly enhance cellular metabolism by improving the hemodynamic status of the shocked patient. Sambhi and coworkers[126] reported increased cardiac output in corticosteroid-treated patients in shock, while Hinshaw et al.[58] observed increased coronary blood flow in experimental endotoxin shock. Steroids in large doses decrease peripheral resistance and improve circulatory flow.[22, 60, 106, 157] Recently, Hinshaw and coworkers[56] pointed out that combined steroid and antibiotic therapy increased survival of primates suffering from experimental septic shock. They combined intravenous gentamicin sulfate with continuous infusion of methylprednisolone sulfate in a dose of 75 mg/kg/12 hr.

Several new agents are currently being studied. Prostaglandin E appears to act as a cellular stabilizer and prolongs survival in canine shock.[42, 89, 143] Cells in shock have an increased glucose requirement. This is usually satisfied by intravenous administration of a combination of glucose, potassium, and insulin.[119] An even more direct source of cellular energy is ATP. Chaudry and Baue and coworkers[8, 14, 23, 24] have shown that ATP-Mg complex and ATP-Mg glucose combinations are effective in increasing survival in experimental shock. ATP normally does not enter cells, but it freely invades the cell in shock. These new approaches in cellular support indicate the future direction of shock therapy.

References

1. Adamkin, D. H.: New uses for exchange transfusion. Pediatr. Clin. North Am. 24:599, 1977.
2. Alexander, J. W.: The role of host defense mechanisms in surgical infections. Surg. Clin. North Am. 60:107, 1980.
3. Alexander, J. W., McClellan, M. A., Ogle, C. K., and Ogle, J. D.: Consumptive opsinopathy: Possible pathogenesis in lethal and opportunistic infections. Ann. Surg. 184:672, 1976.
4. Alho, A.: Lysosomal functions in circulatory shock. Ann. Chir. Gynaecol. Fenn. 60:159, 1971.
5. Alho, A., Jaattela, A., Lahdensuu, M., et al.: Catecholamines in shock. Ann. Clin. Res. 9:157, 1977.
6. Altar, S. M.A., Tingey, H. B., McLaughlin, J. S., and Cowley, R. A.: Bradykinin in human shock. Surg. Forum 18:46, 1967.
7. Archer, L. T.: Hypoglycemia in conscious dogs in live Escherichia coli septicemia: A chronic study. Circ. Shock 3:93, 1976.
8. Baue, A. E.: Worth, M. A., and Sayeed, M. M.: Alterations in magnesium and sodium plus potassium activated adenosine triphosphate and Krebs cycle in hemorrhagic shock. Surg. Forum 21:8 1970.
9. Bell, M. L., Herman, A. H., Egdahl, R. H., et al.: Role of lysosomal disruption in the development of refractory shock. Surg. Forum 21:10, 1970.
10. Berglund, E.: Balance of left and right ventricular output: Relation between left and right atrial pressures. Am. J. Physiol. 178:381, 1954.
11. Bergqvist, G.: Viscosity of the blood in the newborn infant. Acta Paediatr. Scand. 63:858, 1974.
12. Bergqvist, G., and Zetterström, R.: Submaximal blood flow and blood viscosity in newborn infants. Acta Paediatr. Scand. 64:253, 1975.
13. Berry, L. J.:Metabolic effects of bacterial endotoxins. In Kadis, S., Weinbaum, G., and Ajl, S. J. (eds.): Microbial Toxins. New York, Academic Press, 1971, p. 165.
14. Blackwood, J. M., Hsieh, J., Fewel, F., Rush, B. F., Jr.: Tissue metabolites in endotoxin and hemorrhagic shock: A comparison. Arch. Surg. 107:181, 1973.
15. Blaisdell, F. W., Linn, R. C., and Stallone, R. J.:

The mechanism of pulmonary damage following traumatic shock. Surg. Gynecol. Obstet. 130:15, 1970.

16. Blumenstock, F. A., Saba, T. M., Weber, P., and Laffin, R.: Biochemical and immunological characterization of human opsonic α_2SB glycoprotein: Its identity with cold-insoluble globulin. J. Biol. Chem. 253:4287, 1978.

17. Blumenstock, F., Weber, P., Saba, T. M., and Laffin, R.: Electroimmunoassay of alpha-2-opsonic protein during reticuloendothelial blockade. Am. J. Physiol. 232(3):R80, 1977.

18. Blumenthal, S., Chairman, and National Heart, Lung and Blood Institute's Task Force on Blood Pressure Control in Children: Report of the Task Force on Blood Pressure Control in Children. Pediatrics 59(suppl): 797, 1977.

19. Brown, C. B.: Shock and the kidney: Pathophysiology and pharmacological support. Intens. Care Med. 3:1, 1977.

20. Bucci, G., Scalamandre, A., Savignoni, P. G., et al.: The systemic systolic blood pressure of newborns with low weight: A multiple regression analysis. Acta Paediatr. Scand. 229(Suppl.):1, 1972.

21. Campion, D. S., Lynch, L. J., Rector, F. C., Carter, N., and Shires, G. T.: The effect of hemorrhagic shock on transmembrane potential. Surgery 66:1051, 1969.

22. Cavanagh, D., Rao, P. S., Sutton, D., et al.: Pathophysiology of endotoxin shock in the primate. Am. J. Obstet. Gynecol. 108:705, 1970.

23. Chaudry, I. H., Sayeed, M. M., and Baue, A. E.: Effect of adenosine triphosphate–magnesium chloride administration in shock. Surgery 75:220, 1974.

24. Chaudry, I. H., Sayeed, M. M., and Baue, A. E.: Evidence for enhanced uptake of adenosine triphosphate by muscle of animals in shock. Surgery 77:833, 1975.

25. Chaudry, I. H., Sayeed, M. M., and Baue, A. E.: Alterations in high-energy phosphates in hemorrhagic shock as related to tissue and organ function. Surgery 79:666, 1976.

26. Chessells, J. M.: Blood formation in infancy. Arch. Dis. Child. 54:831, 1979.

27. Colgan, F. J., and Stewart, S.: An assessment of cardiac output by thermodilution in infants and children following cardiac surgery. Crit. Care Med. 5:220, 1977.

28. Colman, R. W., O'Donnell, T. F., Talamo, R. C., and Clowes, G. H. A., Jr.: Bradykinin formation in sepsis: Relation to hepatic dysfunction and hypotension. Clin. Res. 21:596, 1973.

29. Craddock, P. R., Hammerschmidt, D. E., White, J. G., et al.: Complement (C5a)-induced granulocyte aggregation in vitro: A possible mechanism of complement-mediated leukostasis and leukopenia. J. Clin. Invest. 60:261, 1977.

30. Cunningham, J. N., Jr., Shires, G. T., and Wagner, Y.: Cellular transport defects in hemorrhagic shock. Surgery 60:215, 1971.

31. Cunningham, J. N., Jr., Shires, G. T., and Wagner, Y.: Changes in intracellular sodium and potassium content of red blood cells in trauma and shock. Am. J. Surg. 122:650, 1971.

32. Cunningham, J. N., Wagner, Y., and Shires, G. T.: Changes in intracellular sodium content of red blood cells in hemorrhagic shock. Surg. Forum 21:38, 1970.

33. Dallman, P. R.: Blood and blood-forming tissues. *In* Rudolph, A. M. (ed): Pediatrics. New York, Appleton-Century-Crofts, 1977, pp. 1109–1114.

34. Dalmaz, Y., Peyrin, L., Sann, L., and Dutruge, J.: Age-related changes in catecholamine metabolites of human urine from birth to adulthood. J. Neural. Transm. 46:153, 1979.

35. DePalma, R. C., Harano, Y., Robinson, A. V., and Holden, W. D.: Structure and function of hepatic mitochondria in hemorrhage and endotoxemia. Surg. Forum 21:3, 1970.

36. Dormandy, J. A.: Clinical significance of blood viscosity. Ann. R. Coll. Surg. Engl. 47:211, 1970.

37. Driscoll, D. J., Gillette, P. C., and McNamara, D. G.: The use of dopamine in children. J. Pediatr. 92:309, 1978.

38. Eliot, R. J., Lam, R., Leake, R. D., et al.: Plasma catecholamine concentrations in infants at birth and during the first 48 hours of life. J. Pediatr. 96:311, 1980.

39. Fenner, A., Müller, R., Busse, H. G., et al.: Transcutaneous determination of arterial oxygen tension. Pediatrics 55:224, 1975.

40. Fiddler, G. I., Chatrath, R., Williams, G. J., et al.: Dopamine infusion for the treatment of myocardial dysfunction associated with a persistent transitional circulation. Arch. Dis. Child. 55:194, 1980.

41. Fisher, D. A.: Endocrine physiology II. Part 1: Catecholamines in the fetus and newborn. *In* Smith, C. A., and Nelson, N. M. (eds.): The Physiology of the Newborn Infant, 4th edition. Springfield, Ill., Charles C Thomas, Publisher, 1976, pp. 614–623.

42. Fletcher, J. R., and Ramwell, P. W.: The effects of prostacyclin (PGI$_2$) on endotoxin shock and endotoxin-induced platelet aggregation in dogs. Circ. Shock 7:299, 1980.

43. Fulton, R. Y.: Adsorption of sodium and water by collagen during hemorrhagic shock. Am. Surg. 172:861, 1970.

44. Gairdner, D., Marks, J., Roscoe, J. D., et al.: The fluid shift from the vascular compartment immediately after birth. Arch. Dis. Child. 33:489, 1958.

45. Galis, J. U., Rappaport, E. S., Gerber, L., et al.: A primate model for prolonged endotoxin shock. Lab. Invest. 38:511, 1978.

46. George, B. C., Ryan, N. T., Ullrick, W. C., and Egdahl, R. H.: Persisting structural abnormalities in liver, kidney and muscle tissues following hemorrhagic shock. Arch. Surg. 113:289, 1978.

47. Bergqvist, G., and Zetterström, R.: Blood viscosity and peripheral circulation in newborn infants. Acta Paediatr. Scand. 63:865, 1974.

48. Gross, G. P., Hathaway, W. E., and McGauhey, H. R.: Hyperviscosity in the neonate. J. Pediatr. 82:1004, 1973.

49. Gross, S., and Melhorn, D. K.: Exchange transfu-

sion with citrated whole blood for disseminated intravascular coagulation. J. Pediatr. 78:415, 1971.

50. Guenter, C. A., Ciorica, R., and Hinshaw, L.: Cardiorespiratory and metabolic responses to live E. coli and endotoxin in the monkey. J. Appl. Physiol. 26:780, 1969.

51. Gunnar, R. M.: Clinical experience with corticoids in shock. Internal medicine. *In* Schumer, W., and Nyhus, L. M. (eds.): Corticosteroids in the Treatment of Shock. Urbana, University of Illinois Press, 1970.

52. Hagberg, S., Haljamas, H., and Rockert, H.: Shock reactions in skeletal muscle. III. The electrolyte content of tissue fluid and blood plasma before and after induced hemorrhagic shock. Ann. Surg. 168:243, 1961.

53. Hakanson, D. O., and Oh, W.: Hyperviscosity in the small-for-gestational age infant. Biol. Neonate 37:109, 1980.

54. Hammerschmidt, D. E., White, J. G., Craddock, P. R., and Jacob, H. S.: Corticosteroids inhibit complement-induced granulocyte aggregation: A possible mechanism for their efficacy in shock states. J. Clin. Invest. 63:798, 1979.

55. Hill, H. R.: Phagocyte transfusion — ultimate therapy of neonatal disease? J. Pediatr. 98:59, 1981.

56. Hinshaw, L. B., Archer, L. T., Beller-Todd, B. K., et al.: Survival of primates in LD_{100} septic shock following steroid/antibiotic therapy. J. Surg. Res. 28:151, 1980.

57. Hinshaw, L. B., Archer, L. T., Black, M. R., et al.: Myocardial function in shock. Am. J. Physiol. 226:357, 1974.

58. Hinshaw, L. B., Archer, L. T., Black, M. R., and Greenfield, L. J.: Effects of methylprednisolone sodium succinate on myocardial performance, hemodynamics and metabolism in normal and failing hearts. *In* Glenn, T. M. (ed.): Steroids and Shock. Baltimore, University Park Press, 1974, p. 253.

59. Hinshaw, L. B., Peyton, M. D., Archer, L. T., et al.: Prevention of death in endotoxin shock by glucose administration. Surg. Gynecol. Obstet. 139:851, 1974.

60. Hinshaw, L. B., Solomon, L. A., Freeny, P. C., and Reins, D. A.: Endotoxin shock: Hemodynamic and survival effects of methylprednisolone. Arch. Surg. 94:61, 1967.

61. Holcroft, J. W., and Trunkey, D. D.: Pulmonary extravasation of albumin during and after hemorrhagic shock in baboons. J. Surg. Res. 18:91, 1975.

62. Holcroft, J. W., Trunkey, D. D., and Carpenter, M. A.: Sepsis in the baboon: Factors affecting resuscitation and pulmonary edema in animals resuscitated with Ringer's lactate versus Plasmanate. J. Trauma 17:600, 1977.

63. Holcroft, J. W., Trunkey, D. D., and Carpenter, M. A.: Extravasation of albumin in tissues of normal and septic baboons and sheep. J. Surg. Res. 26:341, 1979.

64. Holliday, M. A., and Segar, W. E.: Parenteral Fluid Therapy. Indianapolis, Indiana University Medical Center, 1956.

65. Holtzman, S., Schuler, J. J., Earnest, W., et al.: Carbohydrate metabolism during endotoxemia. Circ. Shock 1:99, 1974.

66. Horovitz, J. H., Carrico, C. J., and Shires, G. T.: The pulmonary response to major injury. Arch. Surg. 108:349, 1974.

67. Howard, R. J.: Host defense against infection. Part I. Curr. Probl. Surg. 17:266, 1980.

68. Howard, R. J.: Host defense against infection. Part II. Curr. Probl. Surg. 17:318, 1980.

69. Huch, A., and Huch, R.: Transcutaneous, noninvasive monitoring of P_{O_2}. Hosp. Pract. 11:43, 1976.

70. Hutchin, P., Terzi, R. G. G., Hollandsworth, L. C., et al.: The influence of intravenous fluid administration on postoperative urinary water and electrolyte secretion in thoracic surgical patients. Ann. Surg. 170:813, 1969.

71. Hutchin, P., Terzi, R. G. G., Hollandsworth, L. C., et al.: Pulmonary congestion following infusion of large fluid loads in thoracic surgical patients. Ann. Surg. 8:339, 1969.

72. Illner, H., and Shires, G. T.: The effect of hemorrhagic shock on potassium transport in skeletal muscles. Surg. Gynecol. Obstet. 150:17, 1980.

73. Janoff, A., Weissman, G., Zweifach, B. W., and Thomas, L.: Pathogenesis of experimental shock. IV. Studies on lysosomes in normal and tolerant animals subjected to lethal trauma and endotoxemia. J. Exp. Med. 116:451, 1962.

74. Jardin, F., Gurdjian, F., Desfonds, P., and Margairaz, A.: Effect of dopamine on intrapulmonary shunt fraction and oxygen transport in severe sepsis with circulatory and respiratory failure. Crit. Care Med. 7:273, 1979.

75. Johnston, R. B., Jr., and Stroud, R. M.: Complement and host defense against infection. J. Pediatr. 90:169, 1977.

76. Kappy, M. S., and Morrow, G., III: Pediatrics for the clinician. A diagnostic approach to metabolic acidosis in children. Pediatrics 65:351, 1980.

77. Kitterman, J. A., Phibbs, R. H., and Tooley, W. H.: Aortic blood pressure in normal newborn infants during the first 12 hours of life. Pediatrics 44:959, 1969.

78. Kleiber, M.: The Fire of Life: An Introduction to Animal Energetics. New York, John Wiley & Sons, 1961.

79. Laurenti, F., Ferro, R., Isacchi, G. et al.: Polymorphonuclear leukocyte transfusion for the treatment of sepsis in the newborn infant. J. Pediatr. 98:118, 1981.

80. Laurenti, F., LaGreca, G., Ferro, R., and Bucci, G.: Transfusion of polymorphonuclear neutrophils in a premature infant with Klebsiella sepsis (letter). Lancet 2:111, 1978.

81. Lefer, A. M.: Role of a myocardial depressant factor in the pathogenesis of circulatory shock. Fed. Proc. 29(Pt. 2):1836, 1970.

82. Lefer, A. M.: Blood-borne humoral factors in the pathophysiology of circulatory shock. Circ. Res. 32:129, 1973.

83. LeVeen, H. H., Ip, M., Ahmed, N., et al.: Lowering blood viscosity to overcome vascular resistance. Surg. Gynecol. Obstet. 150:139, 1980.

84. Levett, J. M., and Replogle, R. L.: Current research review. Thermodilution cardiac output: A critical analysis and review of the literature. J. Surg. Res. 27:392, 1979.

85. Levitan, H., Kendrick, A., and Kass, E. H.: Effect of route of administration on protective action of corticosterone and cortisol against endotoxin. Proc. Soc. Exp. Biol. Med. 93:306, 1956.

86. Lillehei, R. C., Longerbeam, J. K., Boch, J. H., and Manax, W.: The nature of irreversible shock: Experimental and clinical observations. Ann. Surg. 160:682, 1964.

87. Lillehei, R. C., and MacLean, L. C.: Physiological approach to successful treatment of endotoxic shock in experimental animals. Arch. Surg. 78:464, 1959.

88. Litwin, M. S., Chapman, K., and Stoliar, J. B.: Blood viscosity in the normal man. Surgery 67:342, 1970.

89. Machiedo, G. W., Brown, C. S., and Rush, B. J., Jr.: Prostaglandin E_1 as a therapeutic agent in hemorrhagic shock. Surg. Forum 24:12, 1973.

90. Maclaurin, J. C.: Changes in body water distribution during the first two weeks of life. Arch. Dis. Child. 41:286, 1966.

91. Marty, A. T.: Hyperoncotic albumin therapy. Surg. Gynecol. Obstet. 139:105, 1974.

92. Mela, L., Bacalze, L. V., White, R., and Miller, L. D.: Shock induced alterations in mitochondrial energy-linked functions. Surg. Forum 21:6, 1970.

93. Middleton, E. S., Matthews, R., and Shires, G. T.: Radiosulphate as a measure of the extracellular fluid in acute hemorrhagic shock. Ann. Surg. 170:174, 1969.

94. Miller, M. E.: Host Defenses in the Human Neonate. New York, Grune & Stratton, 1978.

95. Moore, F. D., Olesen, K. H., McMurrey, J. D., et al.: The Body Cell Mass and Its Supporting Environment. Philadelphia, W. B. Saunders Co., 1963.

96. Moss, G. S., Das Gupta, T. K., Newson, B., et al.: The effect of saline solution resuscitation on pulmonary sodium and water distribution. Surg. Gynecol. Obstet. 136:934, 1973.

97. Nelson, N. M.: Respiration and circulation after birth. *In* Smith, C. A., and Nelson, N. M., (eds): The Physiology of the Newborn Infant, 4th edition. Springfield, Ill., Charles C Thomas, Publisher, 1976, pp. 154–159.

98. Niehaus, G. D., Schumacker, P. R., and Saba, T. M.: Reticuloendothelial clearance of blood-borne particulates. Relevance to experimental lung microembolization and vascular injury. Ann. Surg. 191:479, 1980.

99. Oski, F. A.: Hematological problems. *In* Avery, G. B. (ed.): Neonatology. Philadelphia, J. B. Lippincott Co., 1975, pp. 401–422.

100. Pearson, H. A.: The blood — red blood cells. *In* Smith, C. A., and Nelson, N. M. (eds.): The Physiology of the Newborn Infant, 4th edition. Springfield, Ill., Charles C Thomas, Publisher, 1976, pp. 246–272.

101. Pearson, H. A.: The blood — fetal hemoglobins. *In* Smith, C. A., and Nelson, N. M. (eds.): The Physiology of the Newborn Infant. 4th edition. Springfield, Ill., Charles C Thomas, Publisher, 1976, pp. 272–284.

102. Pelet, B.: Exchange transfusion in newborn infants: Effects on granulocyte function. Arch. Dis. Child. 54:687, 1979.

103. Pierce, C. H., Briggs, B. T., and Gutelius, J. R.: Methylprednisolone and phenoxybenzamine in experimental cardiovascular dynamics and platelet function. *In* Forscher, B. K., Lillehei, R. C., and Stubbs, S. S. (eds.): Shock in Low Flow States. Amsterdam, Excerpta Medica, 1972.

104. Pollack, M. M., Reed, T. P., Holbrook, P. R., and Fields, A. I.: Bedside pulmonary artery catheterization in pediatrics. J. Pediatr. 96:274, 1980.

105. Postel, J., and Schloerb, P. R.: Cardiac depression in bacteremia. Ann. Surg. 186:74, 1977.

106. Rao, P. S., and Cavanagh, D.: Endotoxin shock in the subhuman primate. Arch. Surg. 102:486, 1971.

107. Rapaport, E., and Scheinman, M.: Rationale and limitations of hemodynamic measurements in patients with acute myocardial infarction. Mod. Concepts Cardiovasc. Dis. 38:55, 1969.

108. Reder, R. F., Dimich, I., Cohen, M. L., and Steinfeld, L.: Evaluating indirect blood pressure measurement techniques: A comparison of three systems in infants and children. Pediatrics 62:326, 1978.

109. Reed, P. C., Erve, P. R., DasGupta, T. K., and Shumer W.: Endotoxemic effect of E. coli on cardiac and skeletal muscle mitochondria. Surg. Forum 21:13, 1970.

110. Rodman, G. H.: Pathophysiology of shock. Part I: Cellular phenomena. Weekly Anesthesiology Update 2(Lesson 20):1, 1979.

111. Rooth, G.: Transcutaneous oxygen tension measurements in newborn infants. Pediatrics 55:232, 1975.

112. Rowe, M. I.: The role of arterial serum osmolality measurements in the management of the neonatal surgical patient. Surg. Gynecol. Obstet. 133:93, 1971.

113. Rowe, M. I., and Arango, A.: The choice of intravenous fluid in shock resuscitation. Ped. Clin. North Am. 22:269, 1975.

114. Rowe, M. I., and Arango, A.: Colloid versus crystalloid resuscitation in experimental bowel obstruction. J. Pediatr. Surg. 11:635, 1976.

115. Rowe, M. I., Lankau, C., and Newmark, S.: Clinical evaluation of methods to monitor colloid oncotic pressure in the surgical treatment of children. Surg. Gynecol. Obstet. 139:889, 1974.

116. Rowe, M. I., Marchildon, M. B., Arango, A, Malinin, T., and Gans, M. A.: The mechanisms of thrombocytopenia in experimental gram-negative septicemia. Surgery, 84:127, 1978.

117. Rowe, M. I., and Weinberg, G.: Transcutaneous oxygen monitoring in shock and resuscitation. J. Pediatr. Surg. 14:773, 1979.

118. Roy, R. N., and Sinclair, J. C.: Hydration of the low birth weight infant. Clin. Perinatol. 2:393, 1975.

119. Ryan, N. T., and Clowes, G. H. A.: Metabolic effects of glucose-insulin-potassium infusion during experimental intraperitoneal sepsis. Circ. Shock 3:309, 1976.

120. Ryan, N. George, B. C., Harlow, C. L., et al.: Endocrine activation and altered muscle metabolism after hemorrhagic shock. Am. J. Physiol. 233:439, 1977.

121. Saba, T. M.: Physiology and physiopathology of the reticuloendothelial system. Arch. Intern. Med. 126:1031, 1970.

122. Saba, T. M.: Prevention of liver reticuloendothelial system host defense failure after surgery by intravenous opsonic glycoprotein therapy. Ann. Surg. 188:142, 1978.

123. Saba, T. M., and DiLuzio, N. R.: Reticuloendothelial blockade and recovery as a function of opsonic activity. Am. J. Physiol. 216:197, 1969.

124. Saba, T. M., and Scovill, W. A.: Effect of surgical trauma on host defense. Surg. Ann. 7:71, 1975.

125. Sachs, E., Fewel, J., Hsieh, J., and Rush, B.: Electrolyte and enzyme gradients in plasma, lymph and interstitial fluids during shock. Surg. Forum 21:38, 1970.

126. Sambhi, M. P., Weil, M. H., and Udhoji, U. H.: Acute pharmacodynamic effects of glucocorticoids: Cardiac output and related hemodynamic changes in normal subjects and patients in shock. Circulation 31:523, 1965.

127. Savage, J. M., Dillon, M. J., and Taylor, J. F. N.: Clinical evaluation and comparison of the Intrasonde, Arteriosonde, and mercury sphygmomanometer in measurement of blood pressure in children. Arch. Dis. Child. 54:184, 1979.

128. Schuler, J. J., Erve, P. R., and Schumer, W.: Glucocorticoid effect on hepatic carbohydrate metabolism in the endotoxin-shocked monkey. Ann. Surg. 183:345, 1976.

129. Schumer, W.: Steroids in the treatment of clinical septic shock. Ann. Surg. 183:345, 1976.

130. Shigeoka, A. O., Hall, R. T., and Hill, H. R.: Blood-transfusion in group-B streptococcal sepsis. Lancet 1:636, 1978.

131. Shires, G. T.: Pathophysiology and fluid replacement in hypovolemic shock. Ann. Clin. Res. 9:144, 1977.

132. Shires, G. T., Brown, F. T., Canizaro, P. C., and Sommerville, N.: Distributional changes in extracellular fluid during acute hemorrhagic shock. Surg. Forum 11:115, 1960.

133. Shires, G. T., and Carrico, C. J.: Current status of the shock problem. Curr. Probl. Surg., March 1966, p. 3.

134. Shires, G. T., Carrico, C. J., and Canizaro, P. C.: Shock. Philadelphia, W. B. Saunders Co., 1973.

135. Shires, G. T., Coln, D., Carrico, C. J., and Lightfoot, S.: Fluid therapy in hemorrhagic shock. Arch. Surg. 88:688, 1964.

136. Schumer, W.: Localization of the energy pathway block in shock. Surgery 64:55, 1978.

137. Sinclair, J. C., Driscoll, J. M., Heird, W. C., and Winters, R. W.: Supportive management of the sick neonate. Pediatr. Clin. North Am. 17:863, 1970.

138. Sisson, T. R. C., and Whalen, L. E.: The blood volume of infants. III. Alterations in the first hours after birth. J. Pediatr. 56:43, 1960.

139. Skillman, J. J., Bushnell, L. S., and Hedley-Whyte, J.: Peritonitis and respiratory failure after abdominal operations. Ann. Surg. 170:122, 1969.

140. Skillman, J. J., and Feldman, J. B.: Serum oncotic pressure and protein changes after hemorrhage in man. Proc. Soc. Exp. Biol. Med. 137:1293, 1971.

141. Skillman, J. J., Parikh, B. M., and Tanenbaum, B. J. L.: Pulmonary arteriovenous admixture — improvement with albumin and diuretics. Am. J. Surg. 119:440, 1970.

142. Skillman, J. J., and Tanenbaum, B. J.: Unrecognized losses of albumin, plasma and red cells during abdominal vascular operations. Curr. Top. Surg. Res. 2:523, 1970.

143. Slotman, G. J., Machiedo, G. W., Tesoriero, R., and Rush, B. F., Jr.: Effects of prostaglandin E_1 and steroid combinations in the treatment of hemorrhagic shock. *In* Lefer, A. M., et al. (eds.): Advances in Shock Research. Vol. 1, Papers from 1st Annual Conference on Shock, Arlie, Virginia, June 1978. New York, A. R. Liss, 1979.

144. Somani, P., and Arora, R. B.: Effect of hydrocortisone on capillary membrane permeability changes induced by Eschis carinatus (saw-scaled viper) venom in the rat. J. Pharm. Pharmacol. 14:535, 1962.

145. Starling, E. H.: Production and absorption of lymph. In Schafer, E. A. (ed.): Textbook of Physiology. New York, Macmillan Co., 1898, p. 296.

146. Steele, M. W.: Plasma volume changes in the neonate. Am. J. Dis. Child. 103:10, 1962.

147. Steer, M. L.: Adrenergic receptors. Clin. Endocrinol. Metabol. 6:577, 1977.

148. Stevens, K., and Wirth, F. H.: Incidence of neonatal hyperviscosity at sea level. J. Pediatr. 97:118, 1980.

149. Swänstrom, S., Villa Elisaga, I., Cardona, L. et al.: Transcutaneous PO_2 measurements in seriously ill newborn infants. Arch. Dis. Child. 50:913, 1975.

150. Teller, W. M.: Growth and development of the adrenal medulla. *In* Davis, J. A., and Dobbing, J. (eds.): Scientific Foundations of Paediatrics. Philadelphia, W. B. Saunders Co., 1974, pp. 498–502.

151. Thomas, C. S., and Brockman, S. K.: The role of adrenal corticosteroid therapy in Escherichia coli endotoxin shock. Surg. Gynecol. Obstet. 126:61, 1968.

152. Todres, I. D., Crone, R. K., Rogers, M. C., and Shannon, D. C.: Swan-Ganz catheterization in the critically ill newborn. Crit. Care Med. 7:330, 1979.

153. Tollner, U., Pohlandt, F., Heinze, F., and Henrichs, I.: Treatment of septicaemia in the newborn infant: Choice of initial antimicrobial drugs and the role of exchange transfusion. Acta Paediatr. Scand. 66:605, 1977.

154. Trunkey, D. D., Illner, H. M. D., Wagner, I. Y., and Shires, G. T.: The effect of hemorrhagic shock on intracellular muscle action potential in the primate. Surgery 74:241, 1973.

155. Usher, R., Shephard, M., and Lind, J.: Blood volume of the newborn infant and placental transfusion. Acta Paediatr. 52:497, 1963.

156. Vain, N. E., Mazlumian, J. R., Swarner, O. W., and Cha, C. C.: Role of exchange transfusion in the treatment of severe septicemia. Pediatrics 66:693, 1980.

157. Vaughn, D. T., Kirschbaum, T., Bersentes, T., and Assali, N. S.: Effects of corticosteroid hormones on regional circulation in endotoxin shock. Proc. Soc. Exp. Biol. Med. 124:760, 1967.

158. Voorhess, M. L.: Disorders of the adrenal medulla and multiple endocrine adenomatoses. Pediatr. Clin. North Am. 26:209, 1979.

159. Weil, M. H., and Afifi, A.: Experimental and clinical studies on lactate and pyruvate as indicators of the severity of acute circulatory failure (shock). Circulation 41:989, 1970.

160. Weisul, J. P., O'Donnell, T. F., Stone, M. A., and Clowes, G. H. A.: Myocardial performance in clinical septic shock. J. Surg. Res. 18:357, 1975.

161. Wesenberg, R. L., Rumack, C. M., Lubchenco, L. O., et al.: Thick blood syndrome. Radiology 125:181, 1977.

163. Wilson, J. W.: Treatment or prevention of pulmonary cellular damage with pharmacologic doses of corticosteroids. Surg. Gynecol. Obstet. 134:675, 1972.

163. Wirth, F. H., Goldberg, K. E., and Lubchenco, L. O.: Neonatal hyperviscosity. I. Incidence. Pediatrics 63:833, 1979.

164. Xanthou, M., Nicolopoulos, D., Gizas, A., and Matsaniotus, N.: The response of leukocytes in the peripheral blood during and following exchange transfusion in the newborn. Pediatrics 57:570, 1973.

165. Young, J. B., Landsberg, L.: Catecholamines and intermediary metabolism. Clin. Endocrinol. Metabol. 6:599, 1977.

HEMORRHAGIC DISORDERS AND TRANSFUSION THERAPY

Sherwin V. Kevy, M.D.

This chapter will, it is hoped, provide an overview of and approach to the most common hematologic and transfusion complications encountered before, during, and after surgery. With the advent of specific component therapy, one must understand the causes and mechanisms of hemorrhage in order to treat the patient rationally. Transfusion is indicated during and after surgery to provide adequate cardiac output and blood flow to tissues and to improve oxygen-carrying capacity, minimizing the risk of tissue hypoxia.

HEMOSTASIS

Primary Hemostasis

It is important to distinguish between hemostasis and coagulation. Defects in either produce different clinical pictures. The formation of the hemostatic plug occurs as a result of the interaction of platelets and the damaged blood vessel wall. Coagulation produces a fibrin mesh that adds structure and stability to the platelet plug.

Vasoconstriction occurs immediately after damage to or severance of a blood vessel. Circulating platelets are exposed to collagen, to which they adhere. Changes occur within the platelet, causing the release of several intrinsic substances, one of which is adenosine diphosphate. This substance causes platelets to aggregate and results in the formation of a platelet plug. Additional platelet release factors aid in the constriction and retraction of the blood vessel around the platelet plug. Primary hemosta-

sis is now complete and bleeding ceases. If the patient does not have a normal coagulation mechanism, the plug is unstable and rebleeding occurs. This can often be distinguished clinically. The patient with a platelet abnormality has a persistent ooze, whereas the patient with a coagulation defect will usually rebleed during the latter stages of surgery or in the postoperative period.

Platelet Function Tests

The template bleeding time (TBT) is the most sensitive and reliable method for evaluating platelet function. A sterile, disposable TBT device is now available, which has resulted in precise duplicate bleeding time determinations.* Because of the complex primary hemostatic mechanism, numerous patient-related factors may affect the bleeding time. It is important for surgeons to know the normal laboratory range. The TBT becomes prolonged at platelet counts of 75,000/mm³, but significant prolongation occurs only at levels of 30,000/mm³ or less. Spontaneous hemorrhage is rare with counts above 30,000/mm³. Experience has shown that major surgical procedures can be carried out without platelet support in the rate of 30,000 to 50,000/mm³.[11] Further dilutional thrombocytopenia is very likely to occur in the event that the child has to be massively transfused.

---

*Simplate, General Diagnostics, Morris Plains, New Jersey.

The role of platelets in the control of hemorrhage is related not only to their number but also, more importantly, to their stickiness or ability to aggregate. This can be measured in vitro after the addition of various substances to the patient's platelet-rich plasma. There are several congenital abnormalities of platelet release and several drugs that inhibit normal aggregometry patterns. A prolonged bleeding time and a normal platelet count are sufficient to implicate abnormal function, and appropriate treatment should be provided unless the patient has a history of a bleeding diathesis.

Acquired Disorders of Platelet Function

An enormous volume of literature has accumulated during the past 5 years relating defective platelet function to various drugs and disease states. Aspirin, the most commonly used drug in pediatrics, has a marked effect on platelet function. This takes the form of an abnormal TBT for up to 5 days and abnormal aggregometry for up to 7 days following the ingestion of a single aspirin tablet. As shown in Table 3–1, a large number of drugs can cause functional in vitro platelet abnormalities. Buchanan and Handin evaluated antiplatelet drugs and their effect on hemostasis in 30 normal subjects and in 18 patients with severe hemophilia;[29] only aspirin had a significant in vivo effect on hemostasis.

We have encountered 10 instances of significant postoperative bleeding due to functional platelet abnormalities during the past 3 years. Eight were due to aspirin and two to massive doses of semisynthetic penicillin. On the basis of these findings, it is strongly recommended that the question of aspirin ingestion be included in every "surgical history." Elective surgery should be delayed for 5 to 7 days following aspirin intake. If this delay is not possible, a TBT must be performed on patients with a history of intake of any antiplatelet drug prior to surgery. In the event that the TBT is prolonged, one to four units of platelets should be administered preoperatively, depending upon the size of the child.

Many acquired and unrelated clinical conditions are associated with alterations in

TABLE 3–1   DRUGS THAT INTERFERE WITH PLATELET FUNCTION AFTER INGESTION

Antibiotics

Penicillin G	Methicillin
Ampicillin	Carbenicillin (large doses)

Aspirin and Aspirin-containing Compounds

Anacin	Edrisal
Alka-Seltzer	Excedrin
Bufferin	Percodan
Midol	

Antihistamines

Contained in most common cold and hay fever remedies, including

Actifed	Dimetane
Allerest	Novahistine
Benadryl	Ornade
Coricidin	Phenergan

Glyceryl Guaiacolate

Contained in many cough syrups, including
Robitussin
Trind

Phenothiazines

Thorazine
Chlorpromazine

Nitrofurantoin

Nonsteroid, Anti-inflammatory Agents

Phenylbutazone (Butazolidin)
Sulfinpyrazone and related compounds
(Azulfidine)
Indomethacin (Indocin)

Miscellaneous

Dipyridamole (Persantine, colchicine)

platelet function. There is frequently a decrease in platelet factor III and abnormal aggregation studies in patients with uremia. Many uremic patients bleed severely at the time of renal biopsy. These defects are corrected with dialysis and respond to the administration of platelet concentrates.[26]

Idiopathic Thrombocytopenic Purpura

Idiopathic thrombocytopenic purpura (ITP) may occur at any age but is most common between the ages of 2 and 6 years. In contrast to ITP in adults, which occurs in a 4:1 female-to-male ratio, ITP occurs with equal frequency in boys and girls. At least 80 to 85 per cent of patients with ITP will have complete and permanent recovery without any specific treatment. Of the patients who recover spontaneously, slightly more than half do so within 1 month after onset, and 85 per cent recover within 4 months. An additional 5 to 10 per cent will recover within 1 year.[17, 18]

When considering splenectomy one must take into consideration the natural history of ITP in childhood. Persistence of thrombocytopenia for 1 year is indicative of chronic ITP, and spontaneous recovery is rare. Splenectomy is the treatment of choice for chronic ITP: More than 70 per cent of patients recover completely; those who do not recover completely exhibit significant improvement in their bleeding tendency. The peak platelet count is usually seen within 2 weeks following splenectomy. An excellent prognostic sign is a platelet count of greater than $500,000/mm^3$ within 1 week after splenectomy.

Platelet therapy is virtually useless and unwarranted in patients with this disease except in the very rare instance of central nervous system hemorrhage or in adolescence when emergency splenectomy is necessary. Adolescents have a clinical course similar to that of adults.[28]

Of the 29 children who have undergone splenectomy for chronic ITP during the past 15 years, only two have required platelet transfusion during surgery or in the immediate postoperative period. Platelets, if required, should be administered following clamping of the splenic pedicle or by constant infusion when emergency splenectomy is required.

There is an immune disorder of childhood (Wiskott-Aldrich syndrome) that is characterized by thrombocytopenia, eczema, and recurrent infections. Splenectomy in these patients does not modify the course of the thrombocytopenia but does make death by infection a virtual certainty. During a 30-year span we have not had a single patient who required splenectomy for ITP who also had overwhelming infection.[9, 10]

Anaphylactoid Purpura
(Nonthrombocytopenic Purpura, Schönlein-Henoch Purpura)

This syndrome is due to a systemic vasculitis and is characterized by abdominal pain, periarticular swelling, nephritis, and a skin rash. Most cases occur in children less than 7 years of age. The rash is pathognomonic. Initially it is urticarial but there soon develop central red areas that eventually become hemorrhagic, almost exclusively involving the legs, buttocks, and perineal areas. Abdominal colic is severe and usually is associated with gastrointestinal bleeding of varying degree. Intussusception, usually ileoileal in nature, can occur during the abdominal phase of the disease.[1]

Intravenous administration of corticosteroids in high doses leads to dramatic improvement of the abdominal and joint symptoms. In my experience, none of the children so treated has ever developed intussusception. However, corticosteroids do not alter the course of the disease, as evidenced by continuing appearance and disappearance of the skin rash. Care should be taken to taper the steroid therapy gradually.

COAGULATION

Physiology of Coagulation

Coagulation abnormalities tend to produce terror in the heart of even the boldest surgeon. However, investigation of a bleeding diathesis becomes a straightforward diagnostic exercise once the basic elements of clot formation are understood. Hemostasis depends on three variables: (1) the state of the vasculature, (2) the quantity and functional capability of the platelets, and (3) activation of the coagulation factors in plasma.

The current schema of blood coagulation is presented diagrammatically in Figure 3–1. There are two basic mechanisms for generating coagulation. One is initiated when blood contacts tissue, as in the case of an injury, and is called the *extrinsic clotting mechanism.* The other is activated in plasma by exposure to a foreign surface and is known as the *intrinsic clotting mechanism.*

As shown in Figure 3–1, the intrinsic clotting mechanism is initiated when factor XII (Hageman factor) becomes activated and acquires enzymatic activity following interaction of normal plasma with an abnormal surface. This allows it to interact with factor XI (plasma thromboplastin antecedent), and a sequential series of cascading

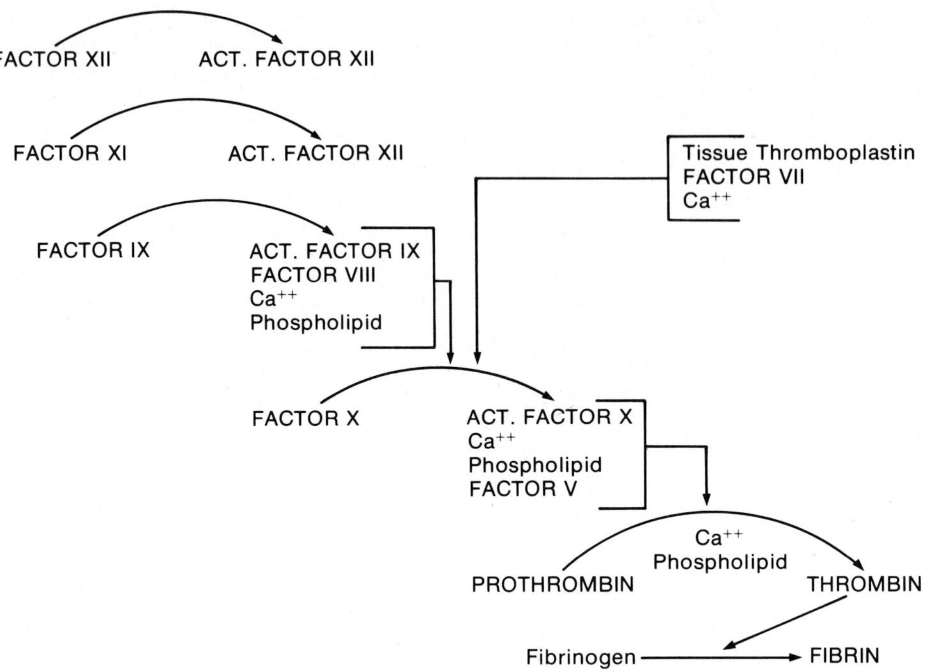

Figure 3–1   The generation of fibrin during blood coagulation.

reactions occurs. Activated factor XI interacts with factor IX (Christmas factor) in the presence of calcium. Ultimately, there is formed a complex composed of activated factor IX, factor VIII, phospholipid, and calcium. This, in turn, activates factor X (Stuart factor), which reacts with factor V (proaccelerin) to catalyze the conversion of prothrombin to thrombin.

In the event that tissues are injured, a shortcut is taken: Thromboplastic material is released from the cells, activating the extrinsic clotting mechanism. As shown in Figure 3–1, a complex forms with factor VII (serum prothrombin conversion accelerator), calcium, and phospholipid to react with activated factor X and ultimately catalyze the conversion of prothrombin to thrombin.

PREOPERATIVE EVALUATION OF COAGULATION AND HEMOSTATIC DISORDERS

A bleeding disorder should be suspected when the child's history reveals (1) unexpected or unexplained bleeding associated with a surgical procedure, (2) bleeding that persists for more than 2 hours after dental extraction, (3) bleeding that begins several hours after dental extraction or suturing of a laceration, (4) the presence of petechiae or ecchymoses larger than 5 cm in diameter, or (5) a family history of a bleeding disorder. Characteristically, bleeding due to a capillary or platelet defect is superficial, begins immediately after trauma, and is effectively stopped by local pressure. Clotting abnormalities should be suspected with such findings as large hematoma, bleeding into joints, delay in onset after trauma, rebleeding after surgery, and only temporary stoppage by local pressure. Four relatively simple tests will confirm or exclude the existence of a bleeding disorder and indicate the area that needs further evaluation. They are the prothrombin time (PT), activated partial thromboplastin time (PTT), platelet count, and template bleeding time (TBT).

The PT is abnormal in persons with virtually all acquired coagulation defects. It is a measure of the overall efficiency of the extrinsic pathway. Thus, an abnormal PT is indicative of a deficiency of factors that enter into the coagulation scheme at the

TABLE 3–2 LABORATORY ABNORMALITIES OF COMMONLY OBSERVED COAGULATION DISORDERS

Defect	Red Blood Cells	Prothrombin Time (PT)	Partial Thrombo-plastin Time (PTT)	Bleeding Time	Platelets	Fibrin Split Products	Euglobulin Lysis Time
Liver disease	Targeting	Prolonged	Normal	Normal	Normal or decreased	Normal or increased	Normal
Hemophilia (factor VIII)	Normal	Normal	Prolonged	Normal	Normal	Normal	Normal
Christmas disease (factor IX)	Normal	Normal	Prolonged	Normal	Normal	Normal	Normal
von Willebrand's disease	Normal	Normal	Prolonged	Prolonged	Normal	Normal	Normal
Thrombocytopenia	Normal	Normal	Normal	Prolonged	Markedly decreased	Normal	Normal
Functional abnormalities of platelets (aspirin)	Normal	Normal	Normal	Prolonged	Normal	Normal	Normal
Intravascular coagulation	Fragmented	Prolonged	Prolonged	Normal or prolonged	Decreased	Increased	Normal
Primary fibrinolysis	Normal	Normal or prolonged	Normal or prolonged	Normal	Normal	Normal	Abnormal

level of factor X or later (see Figure 3–1). The PTT, on the other hand, is a sensitive assessment of the intrinsic pathway and is abnormal when any coagulation factor is below 30 per cent of its normal value. For example, a mildly hemophilic patient with a factor VIII level of 8 per cent will bleed postoperatively and have a normal whole blood clotting time and a prolonged PTT. Both of these tests must be performed in parallel, using normal plasma as a control. The standard for each laboratory must be known so that the significance of any deviation from normal may be evaluated. The TBT is the most sensitive test, not only for the quantitative aspect of platelets but for their functional capability as well. Kits are available with calibrated templates that will enable the technician to perform this test with acceptable reproducibility. Table 3–2 summarizes the results of the laboratory abnormalities in hemostatic disorders encountered most frequently by surgeons.

Hemophilia

Hemophilia, or factor VIII deficiency, is the most common of the congenital coagulation defects. The baseline factor VIII level within the individual patient's plasma is constant and determines the severity of the disease. A severely hemophilic patient will have a baseline level of less than 0.5 per cent. These children, except during the first year of life, have a history of spontaneous bleeding into the joints and soft tissues and excessive bleeding into the joints. Moderately to mildly affected patients have baseline levels that vary between 2 and 15 per cent. These children may remain undiagnosed until a laceration occurs or surgery is performed.

Surgical procedures can be performed with relative ease even in patients with severe hemophilia. However, this does require accurate measurement of clotting factors. Before contemplating elective surgery, the patient must be evaluated for the presence of an inhibitor to factor VIII. This occurs in 6 to 10 per cent of patients with hemophilia and negates the use of factor VII concentrate in the usual manner.

As shown in Table 3–3, factor VIII must be at the 50 per cent level to ensure proper hemostasis. This can be achieved easily even in the tiniest infant by using commercially available concentrates. The initial or priming dose calculated to achieve a factor VIII level of 100 per cent should be administered at least 30 minutes prior to surgery. Since factor VIII has a half-life of 12 hours, half of the initial dose is administered every 12 hours for 7 to 10 days to ensure good wound healing. Emergency surgery must frequently be performed on known hemophilic patients when complete laboratory services are not available. In such cases the PTT should be obtained prior to and one-half hour following the infusion of sufficient factor VIII concentrate to raise the child's level by 100 per cent. If the postinfusion PTT is brought to normal, significant inhibitors can be excluded and the blood level is certain to be greater than 50 per cent of normal. If blood loss and replacement is equivalent to or greater than 15 per cent of the patient's estimated blood volume, we administer one quarter of the initial dose during the immediate postoperative period.[14]

Commercial concentrates frequently contain significant titers of isoagglutinins. It is not unusual, therefore, for children of group A, B, or AB to experience a slight fall in hematocrit level without evidence of bleeding, starting on the sixth postoperative day. This is due to the hemolytic effect of the isoagglutinins.

Detailed management of the child with inhibitors is beyond the scope of this chapter. They have undergone surgery successfully with the combined use of massive doses of factor VIII concentrate, intensive plasma exchange, and activated prothrombin complex concentrates.[3, 21]

Christmas Disease (Factor IX, Plasma Thromboplastin Component Deficiency)

Factor IX deficiency is identical to hemophilia in symptoms, mode of inheritance, and the varying degrees of severity. The preoperative and postoperative management of the patient is similar to that of the hemophilic patient. As shown in Table 3–3, factor IX has a half-life of 24 hours, which allows the physician to administer either factor IX concentrate or plasma only once a day. It is our usual practice to administer factor IX concentrate for the first 4 postop-

TABLE 3–3 THERAPY OF COMMONLY OBSERVED COAGULATION DISORDERS

Defect	Preparation to Use	Half-Life (hours)	Level After Transfusion of 1 Unit/kg	Minimal Hemostatic Level for Surgery (% Normal)	General Comments
Hemophilia (factor VIII, AHF)	Commercial AHF concentrate, Unitage stated on label	8–12	2%	50%	Therapy must be given every 12 hours for 7–10 days
Christmas disease (factor IX, PTC)	Factor IX concentrate, Unitage stated on label	24	1–1½%	30%	Concentrate administered daily up to the post-operative day. Thereafter, plasma administered in a dose of 3 ml/kg body weight for 3–4 days
	Fresh frozen or bank plasma	24			
von Willebrand's disease	Cryoprecipitate or fresh frozen plasma	24–48	3%	50%	Administration of 2 bags of cryoprecipitate/10 kg body weight will achieve this level; daily therapy for 7–10 days
Factor V globulin	Fresh frozen plasma, fresh plasma	36	1½%	15–25% needed for therapy	Administer in dose of 5–10 ml/kg body weight once daily
Liver disease, low levels of factors VII and X	Plasma or commercial factor IX concentrate	36–72	1%	15–25%	Concentrate should not be used if fibrin split products are detected
Thrombocytopenia	Platelet concentrates stored at 22°C	72	100,000/mm³ (1 unit of platelets/5 kg)	30,000–50,000/mm³	

erative days and then switch to plasma, since the necessary hemostatic levels are not as high as those required for hemophilia.

von Willebrand's Disease

This is an autosomal dominant–inherited disorder characterized by a low factor VIII (antihemophilic factor) level in the plasma, prolongation of the bleeding time, and impaired platelet aggregation, platelet adhesiveness, or both. The typical clinical history is one of a mild bleeding tendency characterized by frequent epistaxis, easy bruising, and prolonged bleeding after lacerations and dental extractions. The severity of the disease varies from one affected patient to another and, unlike hemophilia, even within the same kindred.

When normal plasma, stored plasma, or plasma fractions rich in factor VIII are administered to patients with von Willebrand's disease, factor VIII activity exceeds the level predicted from the amount administered and persists longer than it would in a patient with true hemophilia. The apparent induction of synthesis of factor VIII in vivo makes this condition relatively easy to treat but can make the diagnosis virtually impossible to prove in the bleeding surgical patient when a transfusion has been given. In some patients, factor VIII concentrate will rise to almost normal levels without transfusion when the patient is stressed by infection, activity, or hemorrhage. However, platelet aggregometry and the bleeding time remain abnormal. The patient may then have to be treated as would one with von Willebrand's disease, with the condition ultimately confirmed or refuted when a basal state is reached. If the diagnosis has been established preoperatively, therapy can be started 6 to 8 hours prior to operation, as indicated in Table 3–3. The prolonged bleeding time, even though only transiently corrected by factor VIII therapy, should not present problems in the postoperative period.[15, 22]

Disseminated Intravascular Coagulation

Disseminated intravascular coagulation (DIC) is an acquired coagulation disorder resulting from widespread activation of the clotting mechanism that literally converts plasma to serum within the circulation. In the majority of instances, DIC appears to be initiated by entry of thromboplastic substances into the circulation. Another group of cases results from damage to the endothelium of vessels, with exposure of collagen and subsequent activation of factor XII (Hageman factor; see Figure 3–1). A number of conditions are known to be associated with DIC. Among them are (1) gramnegative sepsis, (2) anoxia, (3) tissue ischemia following injury or shock, and (4) acidosis. Platelets are also destroyed or consumed in giant cavernous hemangiomas by accelerated coagulation.

The diagnosis of DIC should be suspected in a patient having one of the underlying conditions who develops an acute deficiency of clotting factors. The laboratory findings depend on the stage of the disorder. Very early in the course, slight to modest thrombocytopenia develops (75,000 to 150,000/mm^3). Fibrinogen levels, which ordinarily are increased to three times normal in the presence of infection or inflammation, are normal or low normal, indicating increased fibrinogen destruction. As the disorder progresses, factors V and VIII are destroyed. The PTT and PT become prolonged, the platelet count drops to very low levels, red blood cells appear fragmented (microangiopathic changes), and fibrin split products usually are detectable in the circulation. The clinical picture in the later stages of the disorder is characterized by mucosal bleeding, generalized ecchymosis, and oozing from venipuncture and wound sites. Treatment should be withheld until it is determined that the disorder is progressive or until clinical manifestations are present.

Treatment should be directed toward amelioration of the condition that precipitated the episode of DIC. The use of heparin in doses of 50 to 75 units/kg intravenously is recommended by many hematologists. However, there are no controlled studies of its efficacy in the human. Replacement of clotting factors with fresh plasma (fresh frozen plasma) and platelet transfusions may be given once the patient is heparinized. Fibrinolysis is always a sequel to DIC and is the mechanism for removal of fibrin from the microcirculation.

FIBRINOLYSIS

In fibrinolytic syndromes, plasminogen, the precursor of a fibrinolytic enzyme, is converted to its active form, plasmin, which has among its substrates fibrin, fibrinogen, and several clotting factors (V, VIII, and IX). A hemorrhagic diathesis due to primary fibrinolysis is extremely rare in pediatric surgery. It nearly always occurs as an aftermath of intravascular coagulation. There are, however, very rare instances in which primary fibrinolysis does occur in children: (1) operative correction of scoliosis, (2) extracorporeal circulation, and (3) operative repair of craniosynostosis. In such instances, the platelet count is normal unless there is evidence of dilutional thrombocytopenia. The euglobulin lysis time, a rapidly and easily performed test, will be less than 45 minutes, and the thrombin time will be prolonged. Epsilon-aminocaproic acid (EACA) should be administered only when one can determine that fibrinolysis is primary. EACA is contraindicated in defibrination.

Liver Disease

Liver disease is probably the most common cause of acquired hemostatic abnormalities. Moderate to severe hepatic insufficiency will result in low plasma levels of clotting factors, since the liver is the site of synthesis of the vitamin K–dependent clotting factors, factor V and fibrinogen. In addition, severe liver disease is often associated with hypersplenism and thrombocytopenia as well as intravascular coagulation.[23, 27] With biliary tract obstruction, lipid absorption is impaired and vitamin K–dependent factors will be low. A prolonged prothrombin time is the most consistent abnormality observed in patients with severe parenchymal hepatic disease.

The use of commercially available concentrates of prothrombin complex in patients unable to synthesize the vitamin K–dependent factors is a rational approach to ensuring adequate hemostasis. They should not be used, however, in patients with laboratory evidence of DIC. The safest replacement therapy for patients with DIC is a modified plasma exchange with fresh frozen plasma using a continuous-flow cell separator.

MASSIVE TRANSFUSION

Unlike in adults, massive blood loss and subsequent transfusion in children most frequently occur in the operating room. A massive transfusion for the pediatric patient is defined as the rapid infusion of blood approaching or exceeding 30 per cent of the patient's own blood volume in a short period of time. A review of 139,751 transfusions during an 11-year period at the Children's Hospital Medical Center in Boston revealed that 15.83 per cent were in this category.

The circumstances surrounding massive transfusion usually do not lend themselves to sufficient data collection to evaluate the efficacy of the approach taken. One is therefore left with anecdotal information that must be correlated with the available data to develop a practical approach for treating future patients. In such patients, initial volume support is more important than replacement of red blood cells. Maintenance or normalization of the child's blood pressure and tissue perfusion can minimize the possible deleterious effects of massive transfusion.

For the patient seen in the emergency room, we utilize the following massive transfusion aphorisms:

1. A hemoglobin decrease within 3 to 6 hours after an injury suggests blood loss greater than 20 per cent of the patient's blood volume.

2. If the hemorrhage is equivalent to 30 per cent or more of the patient's blood volume, the systolic blood pressure determinations shown in Table 3–4 should be expected.

TABLE 3–4 SYSTOLIC BLOOD PRESSURE IN PATIENTS WHO HAVE LOST 30 PER CENT OR MORE OF BLOOD VOLUME

Age	Systolic Pressure
0 to 4 years	<65 mm Hg
5 to 8 years	<75 mm Hg
9 to 12 years	<85 mm Hg
13 to 16 years	<90 mm Hg

Hemoglobin Function

There is little doubt that stored blood is cold, acidotic, and hyperkalemic. This is especially true of blood collected in citrate-phosphate-dextrose anticoagulant fortified with adenine (CPD-A-1), which can be stored for as long as 35 days. The pertinent biochemical values of blood collected in the two most commonly used preservative solutions in relation to the duration of storage are shown in Table 3–5. As will be mentioned in subsequent paragraphs, hyperkalemia is neither a real nor a theoretical problem in most children. The end product of massive transfusion is alkalosis and hypokalemia even in the patient with decreased renal function.

Current methods for storing blood are associated with a loss of 2,3-diphosphoglyceric acid (2,3-DPG), which is most pronounced in adenine-fortified blood (Table 3–5). This increases the affinity of hemoglobin for oxygen so that the red blood cell becomes less efficient in delivering oxygen to the tissues at physiologic gas tensions. Clinical studies supporting this concept were performed in anemic patients, whereas most of the negative studies were in patients who had normal or above-normal hematocrit levels.[4] In an attempt to evaluate these clinically important variables, animal studies were undertaken by Collins and Stechenberg.[5] Animals were bled and then transfused with either fresh or old blood at one of three hematocrit ranges. Considering the age of storage as the variable, there were no differences in survival between animals given fresh blood and those given old blood at near-normal hematocrit levels; at moderate levels of anemia there was a suggestion of better survival with fresh blood. At less than half-normal hematocrit levels, fresh blood was clearly superior to old blood in promoting survival. The results imply that concurrent anemia and replacement with depleted red blood cells may expose the subject to increased risk.

Following the report of Lemieux et al. that skeletal muscle pH is a reliable index of both arterial pH and tissue perfusion,[30] the probe was miniaturized so that it could be easily applied to the surface muscles of an infant. We have used this technique in more than 30 children who predictably were to be massively transfused owing to the nature of the proposed surgical procedure. A detailed analysis of one patient, who was transfused with an equivalent of two blood volumes of whole blood preserved in CPD and was studied in this manner, is shown in Figure 3–2. The first unit of transfused blood was stored for 21 days. This was followed by a unit of blood stored for only 1 day and a freshly collected unit of blood. This replacement, equivalent to 90 per cent of the patient's blood volume, occurred within the first 2 hours of the surgical procedure. As noted in the figure, units of blood low in DPG were then administered (19 to 21 days of storage). There was then a slight rise in the patient's lactate level, with maintenance

TABLE 3–5 COMPARISON OF BIOCHEMICAL VALUES OF CITRATE-PHOSPHATE-DEXTROSE (CPD) BLOOD AND CITRATE-PHOSPHATE-DEXTROSE-ADENINE (CPD-A-1) BLOOD STORED AT 0 TO 4°C*

	Days Stored					
	0	*7*	*14*	*21*	*28*	*35*
pH						
CPD	7.20	6.79	6.73	6.71		
CPD-A-1	7.21	6.78	6.73	6.72	6.69	6.57
Potassium (mEq/l)						
CPD	4.0	10.0	21.0	30.0		
CPD-A-1	4.2	9.8	20.5	29.7	31.2	33.5
Diphosphoglyceric acid (μmol/gm Hgb)						
CPD	13.2	14.1	9.8	3.2		
CPD-A-1	13.6	13.85	8.9	2.85	2.1	1.12
Adenosine triphosphate (μmol/gm Hgb)						
CPD	4.1	3.9	3.7	3.1		
CPD-A-1	4.21	3.98	3.85	3.61	3.27	2.56

*Findings represent average values obtained by analysis of 20 units.

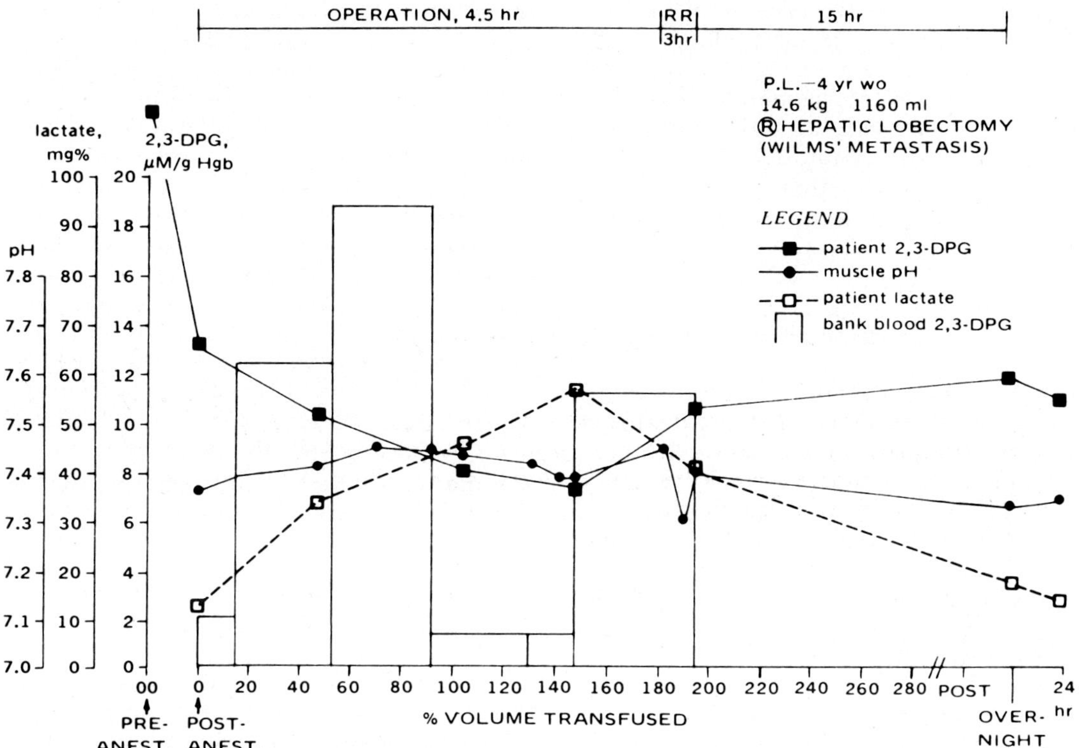

Figure 3–2 A patient transfused with an equivalent of two blood volumes. The alternating of DPG-poor and DPG-rich blood resulted in the maintenance of homeostasis.

of muscle pH. The administration of blood stored less than 1 week then resulted in a normalization of this trend. At no time was there a fall in the patient's blood pressure.

This had led us to the practice of rotating blood of varying age throughout the course of surgery as well as using a blood warmer for massive transfusion. Utilization of blood in this manner has virtually eliminated what those of us involved in blood banking have called the "Transfusion Syndrome." This refers to situations associated with massive transfusion during which time there is a persistent fall in blood pressure despite what is estimated to be adequate replacement. There is increasing evidence that the position of the oxyhemoglobin dissociation curve plays an important, if not critical, role in the function of the heart.[7]

Alkalosis and Hypokalemia

As shown in Table 3–5, the potassium level in CPD and CPD-adenine blood averages 30.2 mEq/l and 33.5 mEq/l, respectively, during the final week of storage. Although the concentration of potassium is relatively high for an infant, the actual potassium content of each unit of blood is approximately 30 per cent of the liter load. This must be taken into account when rapidly transfusing an infant. There is ample evidence to indicate the synergistic effect between high potassium and low-ionized calcium.[25] However, studies in both animals and adults support the rule that infusion rates of less than 1.5 ml/kg/min are safe despite some depression of ionized calcium.

The potassium level of the recipient following massive transfusion has a direct relation to the alkalosis that results from the metabolism of citrate to bicarbonate. Each unit of blood has a citrate content of 7.6 mmole, which generates 22.8 mEq of bicarbonate.[25] The hypokalemia that occurs as a result of this conversion is due to the movement of potassium from the extracellular fluid into the cells and the movement of hydrogen ions from the cells in an attempt to lower the pH of the extracellular fluid. This appears to be true in children and adults except for the neonate, whose metabolism is decreased. It is, therefore, our practice never to administer whole blood older than 5 days to these patients or to combine red blood cells up to 2 weeks of age with fresh frozen plasma.

Hemostasis

Every surgeon who has cared for patients undergoing rapid and massive transfusion in the operating room has observed a breakdown in hemostasis characterized by diffuse oozing. It is well known that multiple-factor coagulation abnormalities can cause bleeding at higher factor levels than is observed when only one factor is abnormal. In addition, higher levels of coagulation factors and platelet counts are essential for hemostasis during surgery and the postoperative period compared with the lower levels needed to prevent spontaneous hemorrhage.

Recent evidence favors occurrence of DIC and not transfusion washout as being responsible for most diffuse bleeding.[13, 14, 20] It is undoubtedly the result of the underlying condition necessitating surgery, of poor tissue perfusion, or of both. Most, if not all, instances leading to massive transfusion in children, such as burns, massive bleeding in patients with leukemia, contaminated wounds and sepsis, and metastatic malignancy with pulmonary and hepatic metastases, are conditions predisposing to intravascular coagulation. A review of 200 consecutive instances excluding open heart surgery during which children were massively transfused in the operating room revealed only three cases of dilutional thrombocytopenia.

The surgeon's main concern, and rightly so, is the management of the patient. We approach the problem as follows:

1. Review the patient's history to determine whether the underlying disease might predispose the patient to bleeding or whether there is a suggestive history of a congenital coagulation defect.

2. The nature of the bleeding problem must be defined, e.g., diffuse oozing suggests an abnormality of hemostasis, whereas massive bleeding from an operative site suggests a localized surgical lesion.

3. The following laboratory tests are performed: platelet count, prothrombin time, activated partial thromboplastin time, fibrin split products, and bleeding time. The latter test is extremely important in pediatric surgery, since so many prescribed and over-the-counter medications contain salicylates or other compounds that produce a qualitative platelet defect. Experience indicates that in a majority of instances, therapy cannot be delayed. Initial therapy is begun with the administration of fresh frozen plasma in a dose of 11 ml/kg body weight. Platelets are administered if the platelet count is below 80,000/mm³ or if the bleeding time is greater than normal for our hospital (3.0 to 8.0 minutes).

TRANSFUSION REACTIONS

Fortunately, untoward reactions to blood transfusion are not as common in pediatric patients as in adults. Statistics from our own hospital during a 19-year period reveal that 2.31 per cent (5358) of 231,967 transfusions were associated with some form of reaction. Of these, 2238 (41.76 per cent) were febrile and nonhemolytic in nature; 3120 (58.23 per cent) were allergic; and two were delayed hemolytic reactions. During this same period, 1.08 per cent of all children and 5.85 per cent of multitransfused children experienced febrile reactions, and 0.83 per cent of all children had allergic reactions. The latter were unrelated to the number of transfusions the children had received.

Immediate reactions vary in importance and severity, but the safest procedure is to stop the transfusion and investigate the cause. The intravenous line should be kept open with a very slow saline drip to facilitate the administration of any therapeutic agent that may be indicated. The transfusion should not be resumed unless there is evidence that it is unrelated to the clinical symptoms. Urticaria and other minor symptoms have occasionally been reported to be the first manifestation of a severe reaction in the adult. This has not been our experience in children.

Procedures to be followed if a transfusion reaction is suspected are available in the hospital blood bank. A brief description and the accepted method of therapy of the commonly observed reactions are detailed below.

Allergic Reactions

Allergic reactions are relatively frequent but seldom serious. They are characterized by urticaria, pruritus, diffuse rash, and occasionally facial and periorbital edema. After they develop, parenteral antihistamine should be administered. Steroids, epinephrine, or both are the treatment of choice if laryngospasm is present. In known reactors, antihistamines may be given orally or parenterally prior to transfusion, but they should never be injected into the unit of blood.

Plasma Reactions

Plasma protein reactions have been identified in patients with antibodies to immunoglobulin A. These reactions are severe and striking. They resemble anaphylaxis, with flushing, abdominal pain, diarrhea, chills, and fever. These patients can be transfused with blood washed by a continuous-flow process or blood that has been previously frozen.

Febrile (Nonhemolytic) Reactions

This type of reaction has an incidence of only 0.08 per cent in children who have not been previously transfused and of 5.85 per cent in multitransfused recipients. The signs and symptoms may vary from mild chilliness and slight temperature elevation to severe chills and higher fever. There may also be myalgia, flushing, nausea, and vomiting. This reaction often cannot be distinguished from hemolytic reaction except that neither hemoglobinemia nor hemoglobinuria is observed. Febrile reactions have been attributed to bacterial pyrogens, plasma sensitivity, citrate sensitivity, circulatory overload, and white blood cell antibodies, which have been confirmed by clinical and laboratory findings. Children who experience multiple febrile reactions should receive white cell–poor blood, either as frozen-deglycerolized red blood cells or as red blood cells prepared by means of a Leukopak or Immugard filter. In our experience the former is preferred, because the incidence of febrile reactions in chronically transfused patients can be reduced by 98.6 per cent.

Acute Hemolytic Reactions

This is a clinical catastrophe that still strikes all too frequently. Some hemolytic reactions are unavoidable, e.g., when antibody levels in the recipient are below the sensitivity of the compatibility tests. Most reactions, however, involve error, usually of a clerical nature when the patient is given the wrong unit of blood during a hectic situation in the operating room or the emergency room. This can result in ABO incompatibility, which has an estimated mortality of 10 to 25 per cent.

A hemolytic transfusion reaction can be defined as the occurrence of clinical and laboratory signs of red blood cell destruction following transfusion. Antibodies that are hemolytic in vitro characteristically bring about intravascular destruction, with consequent rupture of red blood cells within the blood stream and liberation of hemoglobin. Those antibodies that are nonhemolytic in vitro bring about destruction that is predominantly extravascular, but the process is characteristically accompanied by some degree of hemoglobinemia.

The administration of group-incompatible blood or contaminated blood is usually associated with the onset of symptoms before much blood has been introduced. If the transfusion is stopped immediately, serious harm may not result. The symptoms observed include restlessness, anxiety, flushing of the face, precordial oppression and pain, an increase in pulse and respiratory rate, generalized tingling sensations, and pain in the back and thighs. Nausea and vomiting may occur, followed by cyanosis; shock with cold, clammy skin; coma; and a failing pulse. A chill, followed by a rise of temperature to 105°F or higher and possibly delirium, may ensue. In the operating room the only signs of a hemolytic reaction may be generalized diffuse oozing due to intravascular coagulation. When a transfusion reaction is suspected owing to the presence of what may be hemoglobinuria, the plasma must be examined immediately. If the plasma is clear, the reddish-brown urine undoubtedly is indicative of myoglobinuria, a not-infrequent occurrence during surgery.

The postulate that acute renal failure following incompatible transfusion is due to obstruction of the renal tubules by hemoglobin casts was first proposed in 1925. Since then it has had widespread support.[16] The evidence is based solely on morphologic examination of the kidney by either biopsy or postmortem examination. The most convincing evidence that hemoglobin deposition in the renal tubules is not the mechanism of renal failure is based upon the work of Schmidt and Holland.[24] They infused incompatible, hemoglobin-free, red blood cell stroma into two patients. Both patients developed renal complications: one had transient functional impairment; the other, acute tubular necrosis.

The management of such reactions is governed by the patient's condition. Since shock may be an important factor in the development of renal shutdown, hypovolemia must be prevented. Infusion of mannitol has been recommended as a means of maintaining renal blood flow and glomerular filtration. If intravascular coagulation is present, the judicious use of heparin is warranted, followed by coagulation factor replacement with fresh frozen plasma and platelet concentrate. Alkalinization of the urine has always been a time-honored method of therapy based upon animal studies that demonstrated that precipitation of heme pigments in the kidney is favored by an acid reaction. This procedure is of little value once the kidneys have been injured, since renal ischemia rather than pigment precipitation is the etiologic factor in renal failure. The vasomotor disturbances can best be alleviated by alpha-adrenergic blocking agents.[8] Diuretic agents, such as furosemide and ethacrynic acid, can be used for their possible renal vasodilator effects. Although mannitol, furosemide, and ethacrynic acid may be used empirically, none has proved capable of preventing acute tubular necrosis, which is managed as one would manage renal failure resulting from other causes.

Delayed Hemolytic Reactions

Most delayed transfusion reactions are subclinical, the only noticeable signs being a mild transient hyperbilirubinemia, a fall in hematocrit level, and a positive direct Coombs test. If, however, the patient was massively transfused, the reaction may be dramatic. Hemoglobinemia, hemoglobinuria, fever, hyperbilirubinemia, and renal failure have been reported.

Delayed hemolytic reactions classically occur 3 to 10 days following the transfusion of what was apparently compatible blood. Although the recipient was sensitized to red blood cell antigens by previous transfusions, the antibody levels were too low to be detected by existing techniques. Following transfusion, an anamnestic response is initiated and the transfused unit or units are destroyed. We have successfully treated one such massively transfused patient with red blood cell pheresis utilizing a continuous-flow cell separator.

Posttransfusion Purpura

This rare complication of blood transfusion has been observed three times during the past 10 years. Patients present with severe purpura and diffuse bleeding in a clinical setting, which frequently predisposes them to disseminated intravascular coagulation. The latter condition can be ruled out by normal red blood cell morphology, normal prothrombin time, and normal partial thromboplastin time.

Although the disease is self-limited, the bleeding severity and the fact that it can persist for up to 6 weeks may demand therapy. Steroids and platelet transfusions are of no value. The latter may cause a severe reaction. Intensive plasma exchange with a continuous-flow cell separator has, in our hands, been the therapy of choice and has produced immediate amelioration of the condition.

References

1. Allen, D. M., and Diamond, L. K.: Anaphylactoid purpura in children (Schoenlein-Henoch syndrome). Am. J. Dis. Child. 99:147, 1960.
2. Barcenas, C. G., Fuller, T. J., and Knochel, J. P.:

Metabolic alkalosis after massive blood transfusion: Correction by hemodialysis. JAMA 236:953, 1976.

3. Buchanan, G. R., and Kevy, S. V.: Use of prothrombin complex concentration in hemophiliacs with inhibitors: Clinical and laboratory studies. Pediatrics 62:767, 1978.

4. Collins, J. A.: Massive transfusion: What is current and important? Massive Transfusion, American Association of Blood Banks, 1978.

5. Collins, J. A., and Stechenberg, L.: The effects of the concentration and function of hemoglobin on the survival of rats after hemorrhage. Surgery 79:41, 1979.

6. Colman, R. W., and Robboy, S. J.: Disseminated intravascular coagulation (DIC): An approach. Am. J. Med. 52:679, 1972.

7. Dennis, R. C., Hechtman, H. B., Berger, R. L., et al.: Transfusion of DPG enriched red blood cells to improve cardiac function. Surgery 78:17, 1978.

8. Emmanuel, D. S., and Katz, A. I.: Acute renal failure in obstetric shock: Current view on pathogenesis and management. Am. J. Obstet. Gynecol. 117:145, 1973.

9. Eraklis, A. J., Kevy, S. V., Diamond, L. K., and Gross, R. E.: The hazard of overwhelming infection after splenectomy in childhood. N. Engl. J. Med. 276:1225, 1967.

10. Eraklis, A. J., and Filler, R. M.: Splenectomy in childhood: A review of 1413 cases. J. Pediatr. Surg. 7:382, 1972.

11. Harker, L. A., and Slichter, S. J.: The bleeding time as a screening test for evaluation of platelet function. N. Engl. J. Med. 287:155, 1972.

12. Heene, P. L.: Disseminated intravascular coagulation: Evaluation of therapeutic approaches. Semin. Thromb. Hemostasis, 3:291, 1977.

13. Herman, C. M., Moquin, R. B., and Horwitz, D. L.: Coagulation changes of hemorrhagic shock in baboons. Ann. Surg. 93:941, 1966.

14. Hilgartner, M., ed.: Hemophilia in children. Littleton, Mass., Publishing Sciences Group, Inc., 1976.

15. Hoyer, L. W.: Von Willebrand's disease. *In* Spaet, T. (ed.): Progress in Hemostasis and Thrombosis. Vol. 3. New York, Grune & Stratton, 1976, pp. 231–288.

16. Jaenike, J. R.: The renal lesion associated with hemoglobinemia: A study of the pathogenesis of the excretory defect. J. Clin. Invest. 46:378, 1967.

17. Lusher, J. M., and Zuelzer, W. W.: Idiopathic thrombocytopenic purpura in childhood. J. Pediatr. 168:971, 1966.

18. McClure, P. D.: Idiopathic thrombocytopenic purpura in children: Diagnosis and management. Pediatrics 55:68, 1975.

19. McNamara, J. J., Burran, E. L., Stremple, J. F., et al.: Coagulopathy after major injury. Ann. Surg. 176:243, 1977.

20. Miller, R. D., Robbins, T. O., Tong, M. J., et al.: Coagulation defects associated with massive blood transfusions. Ann. Surg. 174:794, 1971.

21. Penner, J. A., and Kelly, P. E.: Management of patients with factor VIII or IX inhibitors. Semin. Thromb. Hemostasis 1:386, 1975.

22. Ratnoff, O. D., and Bennet, B.: Clues to the pathogenesis of bleeding in von Willebrand's disease: Diagnostic criteria. N. Engl. J. Med. 289:1182, 1973.

23. Roberts, H. R., and Coderbaum, A. I.: The liver and blood coagulation: Physiology and pathology. Gastroenterology 63:297, 1972.

24. Schmidt, P. J., and Holland, P. V.: Pathogenesis of the acute renal failure associated with incompatible transfusion. Lancet 2:1169, 1967.

25. Smith, N. T., and Corbascio, A. N.: The interaction of potassium and calcium on the isolated guinea pig atrium. Fed. Proc. 23:326, 1964.

26. Stewart, J. H., and Castaldi, P. A.: Uraemic bleeding: A reversible platelet defect corrected by dialysis. Q. J. Med. 36:409, 1967.

27. Straub, P. W.: Diffuse intravascular coagulation in liver disease. Semin. Thromb. Hemostasis 4:15, 1977.

28. Zerella, J. T., Martin, L. W., and Lampkin, B. C.: Emergency splenectomy for idiopathic thrombocytopenic purpura in children. J. Pediatr. Surg. 13:243, 1978.

29. Buchanan, G. R., and Handin, R. I.: Effects of antiplatelet drugs in hemostasis in normal subjects and in patients with severe hemophilia. Abstr. Am. Soc. Hematology, December, 1976.

30. Lemieux, M. D., Smith, R. N., Couch, D. P., and Macey, A. M.: Effects of acetones and alkalones in surface skeletal muscle hydrogen ion activity. Surg. Gynecol. Obstet. 128:533, 1969.

ACUTE RENAL INSUFFICIENCY

Warren E. Grupe, M.D.
William E. Harmon, M.D.

Acute renal failure is an uncommon complication of surgery in infants and children.[19] Nevertheless, the appearance of a child with an unexplained and sudden change in renal function presents a challenging problem in diagnosis and management. Acute renal failure can be defined as sudden and rapid deterioration or cessation of renal function sufficient to prevent normal homeostasis but with the potential for reversal. Although acute renal failure usually connotes previously normal kidneys, diagnosis and management are the same for a child with a known renal abnormality whose function becomes suddenly worse.

ETIOLOGY

A review of 455 infants and children with both medical and surgical conditions disclosed that 63 per cent of all cases of acute renal insufficiency were the result of intrinsic renal disease, 26 per cent followed hypoperfusion, and 10 per cent developed from obstructive uropathy (Table 4–1). All possible causes must be considered in the differential diagnosis of the surgical patient. For example, the most common medical reason for acute renal failure is the hemolytic uremic syndrome, accounting for 23 per cent of cases (Table 4–1). It can present dramatically with acute abdominal signs suggesting colitis, intussusception, or appendicitis. In one series of 25 patients, six children were suspected of having surgical intra-abdominal disease, and three actually underwent laparotomy.[26] In one of these children the characteristic red blood cell fragmentation, low platelet count, and hemolytic anemia did not appear until the day after surgery.[26] Failure to recognize a primary medical problem that is overshadowed by the surgical condition can lead to management errors, the most common of which is excessive replacement of fluids and electrolytes.[12, 26]

Postoperative renal failure occurs more commonly following cardiovascular surgery than after any other operative procedure.[4, 7, 12, 14] In general pediatric reviews of acute renal failure, such surgery accounts for approximately 17 per cent of all cases in which hypoperfusion can be implicated (Table 4–1). Acute renal failure will develop in approximately 8 per cent of patients undergoing cardiac surgery.[7] Poor cardiac function, hypotension, poor tissue perfusion, and hypoglycemia are recognized as important contributing factors.[7, 14] Most patients will have been in congestive heart failure preoperatively, and renal failure will become evident within the first 8 hours following the surgical procedure.[7] Anuria in the absence of urinary tract obstruction is more common in this group than in any other postoperative patients. Persons who have had cardiac surgery share with those who have received burns and major trauma to soft tissue the special plight in which sequestration or loss of colloid contributes to hypoperfusion and subsequent renal injury.[17] Metabolic derangements such as hypoxia, acidosis, and conduction abnormalities also appear to be important contributing factors.[7]

The most common provocation of acute renal failure in the general surgical patient is, likewise, hypoperfusion, which is often related to transfusion reactions, operative

54

TABLE 4–1 MEDICAL AND SURGICAL CAUSES OF ACUTE RENAL FAILURE*

Etiology	Number of Patients	Number of Deaths	Death Rate (%)[†]
Hypoperfusion			
Dehydration	58	11	19
Low effective plasma volume	26	6	23
Vascular accidents	18	6	33
Congenital heart disease	16	14	88
Subtotal	118 (26%)[‡]	37 (30%)[§]	31
Intrinsic Renal Disease			
Hemolytic uremic syndrome	106	29	27
Glomerular disease	70	8	11
Tubular injury	46	15	34
Infection	33	11	33
Cortical necrosis	10	5	50
Other	21	7	33
Subtotal	288 (63%)[‡]	75 (62%)[§]	26
Obstructive Uropathy			
Hydronephrosis	23	1	4
Bladder outlet	16	4	25
Ureter-ureterovesical	3	1	33
Other	2	0	—
Subtotal	44 (10%)[‡]	6 (5%)[§]	14
Unknown	7 (1%)[‡]	4 (3%)[§]	57
Total	455 (100%)[‡]	122 (100%)[§]	27

*Data extracted from references 6, 8, 12, 14, 17, 19, and 29.

$\dagger\left(\dfrac{\text{Number of deaths}}{\text{Number of patients}}\right) \times 100.$

‡Per cent of total number (455).

§Per cent of total deaths (122).

shock, or septic shock.[6] As many as 83 per cent of intrinsic renal injuries such as tubular necrosis, vascular occlusion, and cortical necrosis represent the sequelae of hypoperfusion, severe dehydration, and electrolyte disturbances.[12] Hypernatremia, particularly in infants, contributes to as many as 10 per cent of the episodes of tubular injury.[12] Myocardial performance is known to be depressed by hypoxia and acidosis, which often accompany hypoperfusion, contributing still further to the decreased renal blood flow and to tubular injury.[7] Postoperative hypoperfusion in the child is also commonly associated with pre-existing nephropathy or obstructive uropathy, particularly if the child's renal concentrating ability or salt-retaining capacity is limited.[15] Patients with obstructive uropathy can experience acute renal failure in association with urinary tract infections and septicemia.[14]

Acute renal failure following burns and major trauma to soft tissue has become less common in recent years.[8] Similarly, nephrotoxic drugs[6, 10] have become a more common cause of direct tubular injury than accidental poisoning.[6, 19] Halothane and other anesthetic agents have been implicated in acute renal failure, with the usual manifestations being jaundice and altered urine output 1 to 2 weeks postoperatively.[5] Hemoglobinuria and myoglobinuria occasionally contribute to postoperative renal failure. The increased use of aggressive chemotherapy for patients with leukemia and lymphoma has led to a greater prevalence of renal failure secondary to hyperuricemia from rapid tumor lysis and accompanied by hyperkalemia and hypercalcemia.[14, 16]

In the newborn, renal failure may be the first sign of a congenital or structural abnormality.[2, 3, 15, 22, 24] Such infants often have other major congenital malformations. Anuria in the newborn is ominous, indicating either renal agenesis, aplasia, complete ob-

TABLE 4–2 MEDICATIONS USED IN MANAGEMENT OF CHILDREN WITH ACUTE RENAL FAILURE

Medication	Indication	Usual Dose*	Dose Interval/ Duration	Expected Result	Comment
Isotonic fluid (saline solution, albumin, blood, etc.)	Decreased intravascular volume	15–25 ml/kg IV	Over 1 h, repeat as needed	Maintain blood pressure, central venous pressure	
Mannitol	Diagnostic challenge Maintain urine output	0.5 gm/kg IV	1–2 doses only 1–2 hr	Increased urine output	Do not exceed 1 gm/kg if unexcreted Not for congestive heart failure
Furosemide	Diagnostic challenge Maintain urine output	1–2 mg/kg IV	1–2 doses only 1–2 hr	Increased urine output	Ototoxicity possible Not for decreased vascular volume
Kayexalate	Hyperkalemia	1 gm/kg in 70% sorbitol PO/PR	As needed	Remove 1 mEq K^+ per gm of resin	Gastrointestinal obstruction; 1 mEq Na^+ exchanged for 1 mEq K^+
Insulin/glucose	Hyperkalemia	0.25–1.0 unit/kg insulin, 1 ml/kg 50% glucose	One time	Decreased serum K^+	K^+ not removed
NaHCO$_3$	Hyperkalemia Acidosis	2–3 mEq/kg IV 1 mEq/kg IV/PO	One time As needed	Decreased serum K^+ Increased serum HCO_3^- (2 mEq/l)	K^+ not removed Correct to 15 mEq/l; Na^+ overload possible
Calcium gluconate	Hyperkalemia	0.5 ml/kg IV (10% solution)	One time	Prevent arrhythmia	K^+ not changed
	Hypocalcemia	30 mg/kg/day elemental Ca^{++}, IV or PO	Every 2–6 hr	Increased serum Ca^{++}	May cause asystole Transient increase in serum Ca^{++}
3% NaCl	Hyponatremia	12 ml/kg	Over 12–24 hr	Increased serum Na^+ (10 mEq/l)	May produce pulmonary edema

*IV = intravenously; PO = by mouth; PR = by rectum.

struction, or a vascular accident.[3, 15] Renal insufficiency is often associated with the respiratory distress syndrome and thus may be unrelated to the surgical procedure.[9]

INITIAL ASSESSMENT AND SUPPORT

The degree of derangement of renal function will vary considerably between patients. Problems requiring immediate attention include hyperkalemia, circulatory collapse, sepsis, metabolic acidosis, hypertension, severe hypervolemia, hypocalcemia, and osmolar dysequilibrium.[3, 13, 17] Successful therapy requires the integration of several interrelated functions[13]; dialysis is but one aspect of the care of these patients.[12] A summary of medications used in conventional management of these children is presented in Table 4–2.

The full extent of renal function cannot be evaluated until one is certain that plasma volume is adequate.[3, 13, 17] Changes in weight are the most accurate and easily obtained indicators of the patient's overall fluid status.[3, 13, 17] Another important, yet simple, measurement is that of the electrolyte composition of the urine.[8, 19] One can usually differentiate between hypoperfusion and intrinsic renal damage (Table 4–3), although a sharp demarcation is not always possible.[8, 19] Similarly, there is no guarantee that all patients with a low urinary sodium concentration, a high urinary osmolality, and a high ratio of urinary creatinine to plasma creatinine will automatically improve with fluid replacement. In one series, almost 25 per cent of children whose initial urinary sodium concentration was less than 20 mEq/l required dialysis at some time during the course of their disease.[8] Other

indicators of fluid status that must be assessed include central venous pressure, hematocrit, serum osmolality, and skin turgor.[8] Whatever the assessment, the goal in the child with short-term oliguria or uremia remains the dynamic maintenance of appropriate plasma volume and renal perfusion, thereby preventing the development of intrinsic renal damage.[3, 19]

If the patient's fluid replacement is clearly adequate, further attempts to increase plasma volume are inappropriate.[13] Hypovolemia, when present, should be corrected intravenously over 1 to 3 hours, allowing a definite rise in central venous pressure or weight, with 15 to 25 ml/kg of either isotonic fluids (e.g., normal saline solution, albumin, blood) or 5 per cent dextrose containing 75 mEq/l sodium, 50 mEq/l chloride, and 25 mEq/l bicarbonate. If urine output fails to increase, a trial of intravenous mannitol, 0.2 to 0.5 gm/kg, or a loop diuretic such as furosemide or ethacrynic acid, 1 mg/kg, can be initiated.[17] Again, the major goal is to preserve renal perfusion rather than just to ensure adequate flow of urine.

Lack of response to these diuretics is compelling evidence of intrinsic renal dysfunction. To attempt to increase urine output by overhydration or continued administration of diuretics is to invite disaster.[13] If urine output increases to greater than 10 ml/kg over 4 hours, diuretic agents may be continued for 2 to 3 days.[17] However, care must be taken to replace accurately urinary losses of both fluids and electrolytes. Repeated administration of mannitol without appropriate excretion can exacerbate the hyperosmolar state of uremia and precipitate pulmonary edema, cerebral edema, convulsions, and coma. Furosemide and ethacrynic acid have precipitated renal failure when administered to hypovolemic patients and have been associated with severe ototoxicity.[13] Finally, the use of any of these agents may lead to a diuretic response without improvement in renal function, thus giving the physician a false sense of security.

TABLE 4–3 TYPICAL URINARY BIOCHEMICAL COMPOSITION IN "HYPOPERFUSION" AND "INTRINSIC" ACUTE RENAL FAILURE

Urine Value	Hypo-perfusion	Intrinsic Renal Failure
Volume (ml/kg/hr)	< 0.5	0.5–1.5
Sodium concentration (mEq/l)	< 10	> 20
Creatinine U/P*	> 20	< 10
Osmolar U/P	1.3–3	< 1.2
Urea U/P	> 5	< 3
Specific gravity	> 1.015	≤ 1.010

*U/P = urine-to-plasma concentration ratio.

FLUID AND SODIUM MAINTENANCE

Fluid management designed to match output capabilities becomes paramount.

The total quantity of fluid administered should be balanced with urine output, insensible losses, gastrointestinal losses, losses through surgical drains, endogenous water of oxidation, and preformed water. Urine output can be measured over 6 to 8 hours and used, in conjunction with accurate weighing of the patient, to determine the requirement for the next 6 to 8 hours. Usual insensible losses from skin, stool, and lungs amount to 300 ml/M^2 body surface area/24 hr.[17] This figure is increased in the presence of fever, hyperventilation, and hypercatabolic states, and it is decreased in a humidified environment or when the patient is hypothermic. Insensible losses should be returned as electrolyte-free water. Endogenous water produced by the oxidation of carbohydrates and fat is usually equivalent to an intake of 100 ml/M^2/24 hr. Preformed water is the fluid present in otherwise "solid" food, representing 50 to 60 per cent of the weight of most natural foodstuffs.

Weight should be stable in the patient whose caloric intake is sufficient. However, a patient not receiving adequate alimentation should lose 0.5 to 1 per cent of body weight each day.[13, 17] In fact, stable weight despite starvation indicates progressive overhydration as lean body mass is replaced by endogenous water. The patient's actual daily fluid intake often must be adjusted for appropriate weight loss to occur.

Once adequate plasma volume is assured, fluid is often administered during the early phases as 10 per cent dextrose in water without added electrolytes. Solute as required can be added thereafter, depending upon changes in serum levels and measured urinary losses. All fluids given, including blood and blood products, must be counted as intake. None of the measurements commonly used to estimate fluid balance is a substitute for frequent, accurate weighing.[3, 17] In fact, accurate recording of fluid input and measured output combined with weighing of the patient at least twice daily allows more precise planning of fluid therapy than does any biochemical measurement.[19] With the bed scales currently available it is possible to weigh even the most critically ill postoperative patients.

Sodium balance is usually maintained with 1 mEq/kg/day or less.[13] When fluid balance is accurately maintained, sodium requirements can be derived from changes in serum levels and urinary losses. Hypernatremia, often a result of vigorous sodium replacement, occurs in approximately 10 per cent of patients.[8] Hyponatremia, on the other hand, occurs in about 13 per cent of patients and usually represents overhydration.[8]

Urinary sodium concentration is generally high in patients with acute renal failure and does not itself reflect sodium balance. Therefore, accurate measurement of the total urinary sodium loss is more important in the determination of daily requirements. Sodium depletion can be intensified by gastrointestinal losses through nasogastric suction, enterostomy, or diarrhea. A rapid fall in serum sodium concentration to less than 120 mEq/l can be apparent clinically as lethargy, stupor, or convulsions. Rapid intravenous correction can be obtained, when required, with 3 per cent sodium chloride; 12 ml/kg should raise the serum sodium concentration by 10 mEq/l.[13]

HYPERKALEMIA

Hyperkalemia almost invariably develops in patients with renal failure. During anuria, serum potassium concentrations increase 0.4 to 0.8 mEq/l/24 hr. This rise is intensified by hemolysis, acidosis, blood accumulation, tissue necrosis, infection, catabolism, or malnutrition. The major consequence of hyperkalemia is cardiac arrhythmia.

Administered fluids should be free of potassium until the patient's ability to avoid hyperkalemia is firmly established. Beyond that, potassium replaced through diet and parenteral fluids must not exceed urinary losses. Efforts should maintain serum potassium concentrations of less than 6 mEq/l. If restricted intake is insufficient to prevent rises in the serum potassium concentration, potassium can be removed with sodium polystyrene sulfonate (Kayexalate); 1 gm/kg of the exchange resin will decrease serum potassium levels 1 mEq/l over a period of 1 to 3 hours.[11] The resin is usually dissolved in 70 per cent sorbitol to prevent fecal impaction. It can be given either orally or rectally. To be effective, the enema must be retained for at least 30 minutes. Oral doses have a slower onset of action. It should be appreciated that the resin causes the retention of

1 mEq of sodium for each mEq of potassium removed; therefore, hypernatremia and vascular congestion can be produced, and the amount of sodium retained should enter into calculations of sodium balance.

When serum potassium concentrations cannot be maintained below 6 mEq/l, more efficient therapy is necessary, particularly if arrhythmia develops or if the serum concentration rises abruptly. Rapid forms of treatment include sodium bicarbonate (2 to 3 mEq/kg intravenously), glucose and insulin (0.25 unit of insulin and 0.5 gm of glucose/kg intravenously), and intravenous calcium gluconate (0.5 ml/kg of a 10 per cent calcium gluconate solution). These emergency measures either shift potassium temporarily from one body compartment to another or counteract its cardiotoxic effect; none effects a net removal of potassium. Therefore, all must be supplemented by either exchange resins or dialysis. In only rare circumstances is the patient so hypercatabolic that peritoneal dialysis is insufficient.[8] This can become a problem, however, in patients with florid rhabdomyolysis or burns and in some patients who have undergone cardiac surgery. In these circumstances hemodialysis is preferred. Although infants seem to tolerate hyperkalemia better than older children, vigilance is still mandatory.[12]

METABOLIC ACIDOSIS

Renal failure typically produces metabolic acidosis from continued protein catabolism. As with hyperkalemia, acidosis can be lessened by provision of adequate nonprotein calories, prompt treatment of infection, and elimination of devitalized tissues or accumulated blood. Acidosis can usually be managed by intravenous administration of 1 to 3 mEq/kg/day of sodium bicarbonate or sodium lactate or by oral administration of the same amounts of sodium bicarbonate or citric acid/sodium citrate.[13] Generally, the goal is to maintain serum bicarbonate levels of between 15 and 20 mEq/l. Attempts to correct the serum values totally or to correct them too rapidly can produce complications. Children are generally able to tolerate acidosis with serum bicarbonate levels as low as 10 mEq/l.

As with therapy for hyperkalemia, the correction of acidosis usually involves sodium-containing agents.[13] Unless this sodium is included in the calculations of total sodium balance, hypervolemia, hypernatremia, pulmonary congestion, or cardiac failure may result. It is not unusual for dialysis to be dictated by the patient's inability to tolerate the therapeutic sodium load rather than by specific problems with either potassium or hydrogen ion.

HYPERTENSION

Although intrinsic causes of hypertension exist occasionally in postoperative acute renal failure, the most frequent cause is fluid and sodium excess. Reduction of total fluid intake and administration of diuretics may be sufficient management. Severe fluid excess, coupled with anemia, can be treated with a partial exchange transfusion utilizing packed red blood cells. Antihypertensive agents are indicated if the hypertension fails

TABLE 4–4 ANTIHYPERTENSIVE MEDICATIONS

Drug	Route of Administration*	Dose	Interval	Usual Maximum Dose
Hydralazine	IV	0.2 mg/kg	4 hr	10–15 mg/dose
	PO	0.1–1 mg/kg	6 hr	300 mg/day
Diazoxide	IV (rapid)	3–5 mg/kg	4–24 hr	
Nitroprusside	IV	0.5–8 mg/kg/min	Continuous infusion	
Methyldopa	IV or PO	5–10 mg/kg	6 hr	2 gm/day
Propranolol	PO only	0.1–2 mg/kg	6 hr	300 mg/day

*IV = intravenously; PO = by mouth.

to respond to volume depletion or is the result of intrinsic renal disease. Drugs in common use, and their dosages, are outlined in Table 4–4. Diazoxide and nitroprusside are extremely reliable in the acute situation when a prompt response is required. However, care should be taken to avoid reducing blood pressure too rapidly, since that may exacerbate renal hypoperfusion. In addition, prolonged use of nitroprusside by patients with renal failure can lead to the accumulation of toxic metabolites of the drug, notably thiocyanate.

NUTRITION

It is of utmost importance that children with acute renal failure have sufficient caloric intake. Starvation can contribute appreciably to uremic symptoms, increased endogenous protein catabolism, endogenous water production, hyperkalemia, acidosis, and hyperphosphatemia and can complicate wound healing and recovery from infection. A minimum of 20 to 40 calories/kg is needed to minimize tissue breakdown. As much as 60 per cent of the usual daily caloric requirement may be necessary to reduce endogenous urea generation.[1] Nonetheless, provision of a satisfactory nutritional intake presents a difficult challenge in the presence of severe fluid, sodium, potassium, and phosphorus restrictions.

The nutrient intake of the nondialyzed child should include large quantities of carbohydrate and fat while avoiding protein sources. For children on regular dialysis, nutritional and fluid restrictions can be lessened, which on occasion may prompt an earlier initiation of dialysis therapy.

Oral feedings provide more calories with less fluid than does parenteral alimentation. The protein concentration should be adjusted according to the patient's dialysis status, and potassium, sodium, and phosphorus should be restricted as much as possible. For children who are unable to eat, intravenous alimentation must be provided. The solutions usually given must be modified for patients with renal failure to avoid fluid overload, hypercalcemia, and hyperphosphatemia. Intravenous administration of essential amino acid solutions to patients with renal failure has been advocated. Some studies suggest that these solutions promote protein synthesis, avert rapid rises in blood urea concentration, and may, in fact, speed recovery of renal function.[1, 7] However, these solutions have not been as well studied in children and have been associated with hyperammonemia and metabolic acidosis.[21] For children undergoing hemodialysis, the provision of a total amino acid solution should not lead to significant complications.[21]

CALCIUM AND PHOSPHORUS

Therapy of hyperphosphatemia is of prime importance because attempts to raise the serum calcium concentration when the serum phosphorus concentration is elevated may lead to metastatic calcifications. Intake of phosphorus is controlled by limiting protein intake and by preventing intestinal absorption with oral aluminum hydroxide, 50 to 100 mg/kg/day, taken with meals. Hypocalcemia is usually asymptomatic but may become clinically manifest as tetany or convulsions. Correction by intravenous infusion of 10 per cent calcium gluconate (0.5 ml/kg over 5 minutes) will improve serum calcium levels for only a few hours.[13] More prolonged correction generally requires oral calcium sufficient to supply 20 to 30 mg/kg/day of elemental calcium.

DRUG THERAPY

Many pharmaceuticals are excreted or metabolized by the kidney. Therefore, dosages should be adjusted in relation to renal function as indicated in Table 4–5.

ANEMIA

Although acute renal failure is often associated with mild anemia, the patient can generally tolerate a hematocrit as low as 18 per cent.[6] Transfusion may be associated with severe hypertensive crises, pulmonary edema, and seizures. Patients with severe anemia tolerate transfusion best when packed red blood cells are given as a partial exchange transfusion or during dialysis.

TABLE 4–5　DRUGS AND RENAL FAILURE

Drug	Elimination		Half-Life (hr)		Dose Change for Renal Failure	Loss with Dialysis
	Hepatic	Renal	Normal	Anephric		
Penicillin	Slight	75–90%	1	7–20	Interval q 12 hr	Slight
Ampicillin	Slight	50–90%	1	6	Dose 20 mg/kg/day	Moderate
Isoxazolyl penicillin	Moderate	40–70%	0.5	1	None	Slight
Carbenicillin	Moderate	50%	1	16	¼ dose q 12 hr	Moderate
Cephalothin	30%	70%	0.5	15	Interval q 12–24 hr	Considerable
Cephalexin	Slight	90%	1	20	Interval q 24–60 hr	Considerable
Cefamandole	—	90%	0.5	9	q 12 hr	Slight
Cefazolin	—	60–90%	2	40	Interval q 48 hr	Considerable
Cephradine	—	80%	1.3	15	25% dose	Considerable
Chloramphenicol	Major	—	3	3–7	None	Considerable
Aminoglycosides	—	100%	2–4	4–100	Follow levels	Considerable
Erythromycin	Major	<15%	1–2	4–6	None	Slight
Tetracycline	Slight	45%	6–12	35–75	Avoid	Slight
Aspirin	Variable	—	2–5		Avoid	Considerable
Acetaminophen	Major	—	2	2	None	Considerable
Opiates	Major	<15%	3	?	None	Unknown
Digitalis	Moderate	60%	36	120	25% dose; follow levels	Slight
Diazepam	Major	<20%	30	?	None	Slight
Phenobarbital	Major	<10%	50	120	Interval q 12 hr	Considerable
Phenytoin	Major	<15%	15	8	None	Slight
Hydralazine	Major	10–50%	2	8	Interval q 8–24 hr	Slight
Methyldopa	Moderate	>50%	2–8	3–16	Interval q 12–24 hr	Moderate

DIALYSIS THERAPY

Dialysis is indicated for patients with (1) severe hyperkalemia not correctable by exchange resin; (2) severe acidosis; (3) intractable fluid overload, especially if accompanied by pulmonary edema or hypertension; or (4) signs of encephalopathy. Although absolute levels of urea or creatinine are not specific indications for dialysis, it is prudent to keep the blood urea nitrogen below 150 mg/dl. A preference for either hemodialysis or peritoneal dialysis is not yet evident.[12-14] Hemodialysis is more efficient, which may be an advantage in critically ill patients. However, there is a lower risk of dysequilibrium or vascular instability with peritoneal dialysis, which is also easier to start and supervise.[14, 15] Clearly, if one method is technically impossible, the other becomes the only alternative. Often, the choice between peritoneal dialysis and hemodialysis depends on the size of the patient and the experience of the medical team.

Hemodialysis

Hemodialysis is an efficient technique that allows control of both clearance and ultrafiltration within narrow limits. The experienced physician can dialyze even small infants and newborns without difficulty.[18] Some form of vascular access allowing sufficient blood flow is necessary for hemodialysis treatment. For older children, temporary dialysis can be undertaken through a catheter placed percutaneously into the femoral or subclavian vein.[28] One radiopaque, polyethylene catheter* presently used generally permits blood flow at a rate of at least 200 ml/min. A single catheter can be used with either a unipuncture control system or a double-headed pump system for blood delivery. Generally, the "single needle" system is not satisfactory when the rate of blood flow is less than 75 ml/min because of blood recirculation. Two catheters should be placed for children who cannot tolerate a blood flow of more than 75 ml/min. Catheters inserted by careful septic technique can be retained in place between dialyses, with their patency maintained by either periodic clearing with a dilute heparin solution or continuous flows using an infusion pump. Patients with femoral catheters must remain immobilized, but those with subclavian catheters may ambulate, maintaining catheter patency with the small battery-operated infusion pump. Temporary catheters are routinely changed once weekly over a guide wire. More permanent vascular access may be obtained by the use of either standard Scribner or Thomas[27] femoral shunts; the latter entails a more prolonged surgical procedure, however.

Hemodialysis is undertaken with small dialyzers appropriate for the child's size.[18] Because of the small size of the blood compartment of many newer dialyzers, it is rarely necessary to prime the dialyzer with blood. Blood and dialysate flow rates are generally adjusted to permit a urea clearance of 2 to 3 ml/min/kg of body weight, while dialysis time is regulated to permit both adequate removal of metabolites and ultrafiltration. Short daily dialyses are frequently used early in the course of treatment to prevent dysequilibrium syndrome. As the patient becomes adapted to the procedure, longer and more vigorous treatments can be undertaken every 2 to 3 days.

If dialysis is insufficient, the patient will remain uremic and experience all the attendant consequences of that condition. Two common complications occur if dialysis is too vigorous or if the dialyzer is too large. First, seizures may result from dysequi-

---

*Surgimed Corp., Somerville, South Carolina.

TABLE 4–6 ESTIMATION OF UREA REMOVAL DURING HEMODIALYSIS

Desired Urea Removal (% of Total)	$\dfrac{KT*}{W}$
10	63
20	134
30	214
40	306
50	415
60	549
70	722
80	965
90	1381

*K = urea clearance of dialyzer (ml/min); T = duration of dialysis treatment (min); W = body weight (kg).

librium syndrome. Second, serious disturbances of acid-base balance may occur because of excessive absorption of acetate. Generally, it is safe to prescribe treatment so that less than 50 per cent of the patient's urea burden is removed during the first treatment. Subsequent treatments are increased until 75 to 80 per cent of urea is removed with each treatment. The percentage of urea removed from an individual patient can be estimated from the patient's body weight, the duration of treatment, and the dialyzer's urea clearance, as shown in Table 4–6.

The major complications of hemodialysis include the dysequilibrium syndrome, bleeding from heparinization, shock from too-vigorous ultrafiltration, and infection of the vascular access. Most of these can be obviated by careful attention to technical details.

Peritoneal Dialysis

Peritoneal dialysis is less efficient and less controllable than hemodialysis, but it can be undertaken with fewer preparations and with less highly trained personnel.[15] It is technically simpler to perform in infants and small children. Because it is less efficient, peritoneal dialysis usually does not produce the problems of rapid fluid and osmotic shifts that occur with hemodialysis. Although recent surgery or peritonitis does not contraindicate peritoneal dialysis,[6] children who have poor perfusion or who are in shock may not have adequate exchange at the peritoneal membrane.

The technique of peritoneal dialysis has been well described.[2, 7, 29] After the urinary bladder is emptied by a catheter, the peritoneal cannula is placed percutaneously with aseptic technique in the midline just below the umbilicus, and then is directed downward to the abdominal gutter (in younger children) or the pelvis (in older children). A direct surgical placement of the catheter is preferable when there is ileus, bowel distention, or a coagulation defect. Warmed dialysate, 20 ml/kg, is infused into the peritoneum, then drained by gravity flow after 5 to 10 minutes to ensure the adequacy of flow and the integrity of the system. If flow or drainage is poor, the catheter or patient or both are repositioned. The amount of fluid infused during each cycle is gradually increased to 40 to 50 ml/kg as tolerated by the patient. The fluid is instilled rapidly, allowed to remain in the peritoneal cavity for 15 to 20 minutes, and drained by the flow of gravity as rapidly and completely as possible. Each full cycle therefore requires 30 to 45 minutes.

Since the amount of solution used for children is frequently small, fluid for each cycle must be appropriately warmed to body temperature. Careful measurement of the amount of fluid instilled and extracted, coupled with frequent weighing of the patient, is mandatory for accurate maintenance of fluid balance.

The complications of peritoneal dialysis include peritonitis, hypothermia, perforation of the bowel or bladder, intraperitoneal hemorrhage, failure to adequately recover dialysate, hyperglycemia, and hypoproteinemia. Most problems can be avoided if careful attention is given to technical details.

RECOVERY

Gradual return of renal function usually occurs over several days to weeks. A diuretic phase often precedes evidence of functional improvement. Thus, despite increasing urine output, the patient may demonstrate continuing azotemia, hyperkalemia, and acidosis. Surveillance of the patient's state of hydration and his electrolyte status is equally important throughout this period, since large quantities of sodium, potassium, and water can be lost. Allowing the child free access to salt and water will frequently prevent dehydration, since thirst at this stage is an excellent indication of excessive loss. Daily re-evaluation of fluid replacement is important, as inappropriate restriction of fluid intake during diuresis can lead to significant dehydration, hypoperfusion, and perpetuation of renal dysfunction. As renal function improves, medication dosages are readjusted.

OUTCOME

Death rates from acute renal failure associated with surgical conditions are still alarmingly high. Postoperative mortality among children within the last decade has varied between 60 and 83 per cent,[14] compared with an overall mortality in acute renal failure of less than 30 per cent (Table 4–1). Death, however, is the consequence more of severe and complicated disease than of the mode of treatment or the severity of the renal failure.[8] This is emphasized by recent data showing that the mortality among patients requiring dialysis for acute primary medical diseases is less than 10 per cent,[14] whereas mortality among patients whose renal failure has followed cardiac surgery approaches 74 per cent.[3, 7, 14] There is no essential difference between survivors and nonsurvivors relative to age, sex, indications for dialysis, type or frequency of dialysis, peak levels of blood urea, serum creatinine levels, serum potassium concentrations, serum osmolarity, or time from the onset of symptoms to the first dialysis.[14] The cause of death in postoperative renal failure is often severe neurologic injury, prolonged hypotension, severe cardiac dysfunction, multiple intra-abdominal operations, or undiagnosed serious infection.[14] Most patients who die of acute renal failure resulting from medical conditions have underlying disorders such as respiratory failure or cardiac failure that are severe enough to be fatal themselves.[14, 17]

One encouraging fact is that mortality from acute renal failure of all causes, both medical and surgical, has fallen in recent years.[8] It is not clear, however, that survival of the kidneys has changed. Approximately 15 per cent of survivors of acute renal insufficiency have chronically impaired renal function. In one series, for example, 47 per cent of kidneys or patients failed to recover fully.[8] In another series involving newborns, 36 per cent died, but more than half the survivors continued to have impaired renal function.[2] Nevertheless, the general overall improvement in the outcome of this group of postoperative patients, largely due to the availability of adequate dialysis, mandates continued emphasis on careful and aggressive management.

References

1. Abitbol, C. L., and Holliday, M. A.: The effect of energy and nitrogen intake upon urea production in children with uremia and undernutrition. Clin. Nephrol. 10:9, 1978.
2. Anand, S. K., Northway, J. D., and Crussi, F. K.: Acute renal failure in newborn infants. J. Pediatr. 92:985, 1978.
3. Barratt, T. M.: Renal failure in the first year of life. Br. Med. Bull. 27:115, 1971.
4. Barratt, T. M.: Post-operative complications of children with congenital heart disease. Bull. Assoc. Eur. Pediatr. Cardiol. 9:54, 1973.
5. Blackmore, W. B., Erwin, K. W., Weigand, O. F., et al.: The influence of halothane on cardiovascular and renal function. Anesthesiology 21:489, 1960.
6. Broyer, M.: Acute renal failure. *In* Royer, P., et al. (eds.): Pediatric Nephrology. Philadelphia, W. B. Saunders Co., 1974, pp. 343–357.
7. Chesney, R. W., Kaplan, B. S., Freedom, R. M., et al.: Acute renal failure: An important complication of cardiac surgery. J. Pediatr. 87:381, 1975.
8. Counahan, R., Cameron, J. S., Ogg, C. S., et al.: Presentation, management, complications and outcome of acute renal failure in childhood: Five years' experience. Br. Med. J. 1:599, 1977.
9. Daniel, S. S., and James, L. S.: Abnormal renal function in the newborn infant. J. Pediatr. 88:856, 1976.
10. Falco, F. G., Smith, H. M., and Arcieri, G. M.: The nephrotoxicity of aminoglycosides and gentamicin. J. Infect. Dis. 119:406, 1969.
11. Fleisher, D. S.: Cation exchange resin therapy for hyperkalemia in infants and children. J. Pediatr. 58:436, 1961.
12. Griffin, N. K., McElnea, J., and Barratt, T. M.: Acute renal failure in early life. Arch. Dis. Child. 51:459, 1976.
13. Grupe, W. E.: Glomerulonephritis. *In* Gellis, S. S., and Kagan, B. M. (eds.): Current Pediatric Therapy — 9. Philadelphia, W. B. Saunders Co., 1980, pp. 375–380.
14. Hodson, E. M., Kjellstrand, C. M., and Mauer, S. M.: Acute renal failure in infants and children: Outcome of 53 patients requiring hemodialysis treatment. J. Pediatr. 93:756, 1978.
15. Jain, R.: Acute renal failure in the neonate. Pediatr. Clin. North Am. 24:605, 1977.
16. Kjellstrand, C. M., Campbell, D. C., vonHartitzsch, B., et al.: Hyperuricemic acute renal failure. Arch. Intern. Med. 133:349, 1974.
17. Lieberman, E.: Management of acute renal failure in infants and children. Nephron 11:193, 1973.
18. Mauer, J. M., and Lynch, R. E.: Hemodialysis techniques for infants and children. Pediatr. Clin. North Am. 23:843, 1976.
19. Meadow, S. R., Cameron, J. S., Ogg, C. S., and Saxton, H. M.: Children referred for acute dialysis. Arch. Dis. Child. 46:221, 1971.
20. Mofenson, H. C., and Greensher, J.: Peritoneal dialysis, an outline of the procedure. Clin. Pediatr. 11:534, 1972.
21. Motil, K., Harmon, W. E., and Grupe, W. E.: Complications of intravenous essential amino acid hyperalimentation in children with acute renal failure. J. Parenter. Enter. Nutr. 4:32, 1980.
22. Norman, M. E., and Asadi, F. K.: A prospective study of acute renal failure in the newborn infant. Pediatrics 63:475, 1979.
23. Ogg, D. S., and Cameron, J. S.: Renal failure and cardiac surgery. Bull. Guy's Hosp. 118:85, 1969.
24. Reimold, E. W., Dom, T. D., and Worthen, H. G.: Renal failure during the first year of life. Pediatrics 59(Suppl.):987, 1977.
25. Robinson, G. C., and Wong, L. C.: Acute tubular necrosis in infancy and childhood. Am. J. Dis. Child. 95:417, 1958.
26. Smith, C. D., Schuster, S. R., Grupe, W. E., and Vawter, G. F.: Hemolytic uremic syndrome: A diagnostic and therapeutic dilemma for the surgeon. J. Pediatr. Surg. 13:597, 1978.
27. Thomas, G. I.: A large-vessel applique arteriovenous shunt for hemodialysis. Trans. Am. Soc. Artif. Intern. Organs 15:288, 1969.
28. Uldall, P. R., Dyck, R. F., Woods, F., et al.: A subclavian catheter for temporary vascular access for hemodialysis or plasmaphoresis. Dial. Trans. 8:963, 1979.
29. Wiggelinkhuizen, J., and Pokroy, M. V.: Acute renal failure in infancy and childhood. S. Afr. Med. J. 48:2129, 1974.
30. Williams, G. S., Klenk, E. L., and Winters, R. W.: Acute renal failure in pediatrics. *In* Winters, R. W. (ed.): The Body Fluids in Pediatrics. Boston, Little, Brown & Co., 1973, pp. 523–557.

5 | MALNUTRITION AND WOUND HEALING

Arnold G. Coran, M.D.

The major deterrents to primary wound healing following surgery are malnutrition and infection.[1, 19, 25] Infection has been recognized for many years as a cause of surgical wound disruption and improper healing. It can be prevented by the use of proper aseptic technique and the appropriate perioperative administration of antibiotics. Malnutrition, however, has until recently been recognized as a cause of inadequate healing of surgical wounds only in its severest form. Until the past decade, moderate to mild nutritional deficiency was not considered a major factor in the proper healing of surgical wounds. The introduction of parenteral nutrition in the middle 1960's caused physicians to become increasingly aware of the importance of nutrition in the management of their patients. This, in turn, led to more aggressive treatment of nutritional deficiencies in the preoperative and postoperative periods.

NORMAL WOUND HEALING

The initial biologic response in a healing wound is inflammation.[21] The tissue destruction and hemorrhage caused by trauma produce an open wound through which bacteria and foreign substances from the external environment gain entrance. Inflammation is a vascular and cellular response that acts to dispose of the microorganisms, the foreign material, and the dying tissue in preparation for the subsequent repair process. The basic inflammatory response is nonspecific; it is the same whether the injury is caused by heat, cold, radiant energy, mechanical energy, or bacterial infection. Immediately after an injury occurs,

there is transient vasoconstriction of the local vasculature, followed by significant vasodilatation with increased blood flow. Vasodilatation is accompanied by increased permeability of small vessels, especially the venules. The vascular changes of inflammation are thought to be mediated by substances released at the wound site during injury, most notably histamine. Lymphatics are also involved in inflammation. Local lymphatic channels are occluded by fibrin plugs arising from escaping plasma, thus preventing drainage of fluid from an injured area and localizing the inflammatory reaction.

During inflammation, a highly cellular environment develops around the wound. Polymorphonuclear leukocytes and mononuclear leukocytes leave the vessels by diapedesis and then engage in active phagocytosis. The ingested bacteria are partially digested by enzymes contained within the leukocyte lysosomes. As the polymorphonuclear leukocytes die, their intracellular enzymes and debris are released into the wound area and become part of the wound exudate or pus. Monocytes are transformed into macrophages and ingest materials that have not been solubilized by the polymorphonuclear leukocytes. If an excessive amount of pus accumulates, wound healing can be impaired. Successful macrophage function usually heralds the end of the acute inflammation. In most clean wounds, the acute inflammatory response subsides within several days. Some wounds, however, become contaminated with bacteria or retained foreign material, have a persistent inflammatory response, and remain unhealed. They represent chronic inflammation in which mononuclear leukocytes predominate. These leukocytes eventually

65

transform into macrophages or form multinucleate giant cells.

Removal of foreign material by the white blood cells, toward the end of inflammation, is accompanied by other events in wound healing. At the surface of the wound, epithelial cells begin to cover the tissue defect. Epithelialization occurs within 24 hours in a well-sutured incision. In the depths of the wound, migratory fibroblasts enter the area and begin synthesizing scar tissue, primarily collagen and protein polysaccharides.[11, 15, 16, 20, 21] This period of scar tissue formation is known as *fibroplasia*. Significant amounts of collagen are synthesized by the fibroblasts at the wound site starting approximately 4 or 5 days after injury and continuing for about 2 to 4 weeks. During the period of fibroplasia, the wound becomes grossly and microscopically recognizable as granulation tissue.[14] The characteristic vascularity and redness of the granulation tissue are due to the formation of capillaries by endothelial budding. In addition, the ingrowth of granulation tissue is accompanied by lysis of the fibrin network. These migratory fibroblasts evolve from undifferentiated mesenchymal cells from nearby sites and move into the wound. The fibroblasts are the source of a variety of substances essential to wound repair. Initially, they manufacture glycoproteins and mucopolysaccharides, which are major components of the ground substance of connective tissue. Later, the fibroblasts manufacture collagen. As the amount of collagen at the wound site increases, the glycoprotein and mucopolysaccharide content decreases.

The biochemical events related to fibroplasia are the major function of the fibroblasts.[11, 21] The normal sequence of events controlling protein synthesis initiates the process of collagen formation. Briefly, this sequence of biochemical events is as follows: Messenger RNA is synthesized within the nucleus of the fibroblast from a template of DNA; messenger RNA molecules enter the cytoplasm and attach to ribosomes along the endoplasmic reticulum; ribosomes translate the nucleotide sequence of the messenger RNA into an amino acid sequence. In this manner, a polypeptide chain of several amino acids in a specific sequence is assembled. The completed polypeptide chain is detached from the ribosome and enters the cisternae of the endoplasmic reticulum for transport to the extracellular space. The collagen molecule is a complex helical structure whose mechanical properties are largely responsible for the strength and rigidity of the scar tissue. The units of collagen protein manufactured by fibroblasts are triple helical chains called tropocollagen. Outside the fibroblasts, the tropocollagen units unite with one another into chains of increasing length and diameter.[21]

It is during the period of fibroplasia that the tensile strength of the wound increases most rapidly. The tensile strength increases at a rate proportional to the rate of collagen synthesis. As a sufficient quantity of collagen is produced, the number of fibroblasts in the wound diminishes. The disappearance of fibroblasts marks the end of the fibroblastic phase and the beginning of the maturation phase of wound healing.

During the maturation phase, pronounced changes in the form, bulk, and strength of the scar occur. The strength of the wound continues to increase despite the disappearance of fibroblasts from the wound and the consequent reduction in the rate of collagen synthesis. Remodeling is a spontaneous process and may continue for several years.[4] The extent to which a scar remodels varies from patient to patient and depends on a person's age at the time of injury. When the rate of collagen breakdown exceeds the rate of production, the scar becomes soft and smooth. When the rate of collagen synthesis exceeds the rate of breakdown, a keloid or hypertrophic scar results.

Wound healing may be a beneficial or a detrimental process. Examples of detrimental wound healing with scarring are hepatic cirrhosis, duodenal ulcer with gastric outlet obstruction, myocardial infarction, valvular heart disease, and cerebral repair.

SPECIFIC NUTRITIONAL REQUIREMENTS OF THE HEALING WOUND

The first correlation between wound healing and malnutrition was made by Lind more than 200 years ago during his treatment of scorbutic sailors aboard the English ship H.M.S. *Salisbury*. Poor nutrition impedes all phases of wound healing by interfering with normal cellular function and protein synthesis. Moreover, specific nutritional requirements of the healing wound distinguish it from other body tissues. Carbohydrate metabolism, collagen and mucopolysaccharide synthesis, replication, and some lipid synthetic pathways are involved. Repair requires essential vitamins, minerals, proteins, lipids, and adequate calories.

Vitamins

Vitamin A is probably required for wound healing, although its specific role in the process is not known. It plays an essential part in cell differentiation and protein synthesis. Severe deficiency of vitamin A in animals substantially retards repair.[13]

The B vitamins have not been proved essential to wound repair. Severe deficiencies of these vitamins would adversely affect the reparative process. Niacin forms nicotinamide adenine dinucleotide (NAD) and is therefore important in energy metabolism, in which fibroblasts and white blood cells participate. Thiamine is a cofactor in decarboxylation, which is an important part of the fibroblast's metabolism.

Vitamin C, or ascorbic acid, is a hydrogen donor and an essential cofactor (together with iron, alpha-ketoglutarate, and molecular oxygen) in the hydroxylation of proline in collagen. If this step is not completed, collagen synthesis is blocked; therefore, collagen cannot leave the fibroblasts, and the wound cannot gain any substance or strength. In scurvy, wounds that apparently have healed may break down. Clinical scurvy is now a rare condition that occurs only after several months of vitamin C deficiency. However, latent deficiency of ascorbic acid may become manifest under conditions of stress, such as a major surgical procedure. Vitamin C deficiency can be detected by measuring the concentration of ascorbic acid in the buffy coat of centrifuged blood.

Vitamin D does not seem to be essential to normal healing of soft tissue but is critically important in skeletal repair. Deficiency can lead to osteomalacia and poor fracture healing.

Vitamin E appears to have a detrimental effect on normal wound healing. It is an anti-inflammatory agent similar to steroids. The presence of vitamin E may retard normal wound inflammation and, subsequently, normal wound healing. Therefore, it should not be given to the stressed or traumatized patient.

Protein and Calories

A deficiency of protein and nonprotein calories impairs normal wound healing. Recent experience with parenteral and enteral nutrition supports this concept. Enterocutaneous fistulae and disrupted wounds in the severely malnourished patient begin to heal promptly with the institution of major nutritional support. Studies in animals suggest that protein depletion resulting in loss of approximately 20 per cent of body weight interferes with the repair of wounds. Lesser degrees of protein deprivation combined with other factors detrimental to wound healing may result in a synergistic interference with the normal reparative process.

In general, some type of wound repair can be expected to occur in all but the most debilitated patients. However, rates of dehiscence and failure of primary wound healing appear to correlate with the level of serum albumin, which tends to fall as protein deficiency occurs. If weight loss exceeds 15 to 20 per cent of body weight, elective surgery should be postponed until protein and calorie deficiencies have been corrected through some type of nutritional support. Specific deficiencies of certain amino acids may affect wound repair more adversely than a general protein deficiency. The specific amino acids involved are lysine, proline, and methionine. Breakdown of collagen into hydroxyproline and hydroxylysine is not followed by reutilization of these amino acids for new collagen synthesis. They cannot be reconverted to proline and lysine; therefore, a source of these two amino acids other than breakdown of old collagen is required. Subclinical nutritional deficiency in a patient who is not stressed may suddenly become clinically significant when the stress of surgery, trauma, or sepsis is added.

Oxygen and Hemoglobin

Oxygen deficiency, even if marginal, can significantly retard collagen synthesis. Several factors are important in the oxygen supply to the healing wound. These are blood volume, cardiac output, arterial P_{O_2}, and the state of the local wound circulation. Iron deficiency anemia has been shown to retard wound repair only in immature animals.[18] Provided that normal protein level, blood volume, cardiac output, and P_{O_2} are maintained, the anemia itself does not appear to inhibit normal wound healing in the human subject or in the experimental animal model.

Trace Elements

Direct correlations between blood levels of the trace elements manganese, copper, and zinc and wound repair have been made in recent years. Of these trace elements, zinc has been studied most extensively. Zinc appears to be necessary for adequate wound repair, but the exact mechanism of action is unknown. Zinc is a necessary cofactor for many enzymes and appears to be actively involved in cell division and turnover. There are increased losses of zinc in the urine as a consequence of injury and inflammation. The consensus is that zinc deficiency inhibits and zinc administration enhances normal repair. Chronic skin ulceration is one of the signs of zinc deficiency. Patients with severe diarrhea, prolonged nasogastric drainage, burns, severe infection, or grossly inadequate nutrition are likely to become zinc deficient. A deficiency can be detected by measuring serum zinc; levels of less than 100 μg/dl have been related to poor repair.

Calcium is essential to fracture repair and to the prevention of pathologic fractures in severely ill, debilitated, bedridden patients. Despite adequate intravenous infusions of calcium, immobilization will result in excretion of most of the administered calcium into the urine without significant incorporation of exogenous calcium into new bone formation. The most effective means of providing calcium deposition into healing bone is mobilization.

NUTRITIONAL SUPPORT OF THE INFANT AND CHILD

Nutritional management of the infant and child differs from that of the adult because of growth considerations.[6] The nutritional requirements of children and teenagers do not differ significantly from those of adults. The infant, by contrast, has unique nutritional requirements.

Nutritional Requirements

Water and Calories. The water content of the infant body is higher than that of the adult (70 to 75 per cent of body weight versus 60 to 65 per cent). Requirements for water are related to caloric consumption, so the infant must consume much larger amounts of water per unit of body weight than the adult (Table 5–1). The caloric requirements of the newborn and young infant are also far greater than those of the older child and adult. In fact, the caloric requirements closely parallel the water requirements, which in turn decrease as age increases (Table 5–2).

Protein. Most of the increase in body stores of nitrogen occurs during the first year of life. The major protein requirements of infants are shown in Table 5–2. Twenty amino acids have been identified, nine of which are essential in the infant (Table 5–3). New tissue cannot be formed unless all the essential amino acids are present in the diet simultaneously; the absence of only one essential amino acid will result in a negative nitrogen and protein balance. Protein requirements vary with the age of the patient; they are highest in the neonate. Total plasma protein in the normal child ranges from 6 to 7.6 gm/dl, with somewhat lower values in newborns and premature infants.

Carbohydrate. The greatest part of the body's caloric need is supplied by carbohy-

TABLE 5–1   WATER REQUIREMENTS

3-kg Infant	70-kg Adult
220 gm/kg body weight	90 gm/kg body weight
220 gm/100 calories consumed	210 gm/100 calories consumed

TABLE 5-2 CALORIE AND PROTEIN
REQUIREMENTS

Age (yr)	Calories/kg Body Weight	Protein (gm/kg Body Weight)
0–1	90–120	2.0–3.5
1–7	75–90	2.0–2.5
7–12	60–75	2.0
12–18	30–60	1.5
>18	25–30	1.0

TABLE 5-3 ESSENTIAL AMINO ACIDS

Threonine
Leucine
Isoleucine
Valine
Lysine
Methionine
Phenylalanine
Tryptophan
Histidine*
Tyrosine
Cystine†

*Essential only in infancy.
*May be essential in the premature baby.

drate. Carbohydrates are stored chiefly as glycogen in the liver and muscle but account for no more than 10 per cent of body weight. Since the infant's liver and muscle mass is proportionately much smaller than that of the adult, his glycogen or carbohydrate reserve is significantly smaller.

Fat. Fats constitute the body's other major source of nonprotein calories and also supply the essential fatty acid, linoleic acid. A deficiency of this fatty acid will result in a typical skin rash with desquamation.

Minerals and Vitamins. The rapidly growing infant needs more minerals than does the adult. This is especially true for phosphorus and calcium because of the exceptional growth of the infant's skeleton. Vitamins are required in minute amounts for normal cellular metabolism. They must be supplied wholly or in part exogenously. Table 5–4 lists the daily requirements at various ages for two common minerals, calcium and iron, and for the more common vitamins.

Nutritional Assessment

To determine nutritional requirements, the surgeon must adequately assess the patient's nutritional state prior to injury.[6] This can be done quite simply by taking the history and performing physical examination and a few laboratory tests. In the neonate, infant, and preschooler, nutrition can be assessed by measuring weight, length, head circumference, chest circumference, triceps skinfold thickness, and serum albumin level. After the age of 6 years, chest and head circumference are not useful measurements of nutrition. Serum albumin is probably the most sensitive and useful measurement. Serum albumin levels between 2.8 and 3.5 gm/dl indicate moderate malnutrition.

Nutritional Management

The most effective way of supplying nutrients to the patient is in the form of regular food passed through the gastrointestinal tract. This can often be accomplished without resorting to sophisticated nutritional-support techniques. In many situations, however, especially in infants and

TABLE 5-4 MINERAL AND VITAMIN REQUIREMENTS

Age (yr)	Minerals		Vitamins						
	Ca (gm)	Fe (mg)	A (IU)	Thiamine (mg)	Riboflavin (mg)	Niacin (mg)	Ascorbic Acid (mg)	D (IU)	B (mg)
Infancy	0.7	6	1500	0.4	0.6	6	30	400	0.3
1–3	1.0	8	2000	0.6	0.9	8	40	400	0.2
4–6	1.0	10	2500	0.8	1.2	10	50	400	0.2
7–9	1.2	12	3500	1.0	1.5	12	60	400	0.2
10–12	1.2	14	4500	1.2	1.8	14	70	400	0.2
13–15	1.4	16	4500	1.4	2.0	16	80	400	0.2
16–19	1.4	18	5000	1.6	2.2	18	90	400	0.2

TABLE 5–5 COMPOSITION OF ELEMENTAL DIETS*

	Vivonex High Nitrogen and Vivonex Standard (Eaton)	Flexical (Mead Johnson)
Form	Powder	Powder
Carbohydrate	Glucose and glucose oligosaccharides	Sucrose, maltodextrin, citrate
Fat	Safflower oil	Soy oil, MCT oil
Protein	Crystalline amino acids	Supplemented protein hydrolysate
Essential amino acids	36.25%	49.3%
Nonessential amino acids	63.75%	50.7%

*Both products are available in various flavors. Neither product contains sufficient vitamins; these must be supplemented.

children with major gastrointestinal anomalies, this approach is ineffective. Provided that the gastrointestinal tract is intact and has adequate length and normal absorptive capacity, predigested or elemental diets can be given orally or by a nasogastric feeding tube, a gastrostomy tube, or a jejunostomy tube. In 1969, Stephens and Randall report-

TABLE 5–6 CONTENTS OF ELEMENTAL DIETS

	Units	Vivonex Standard (Eaton)	Vivonex High Nitrogen (Eaton)	Flexical (Mead Johnson)
Calories		1000	1000	1000
Caloric concentration	calories/ml	1.0	1.0	1.0
Osmolality	mOsm	500.0	844.0	724.0
Protein	gm	20.44 equivalent	41.69 equivalent	22.5
Nitrogen	gm	3.27	6.67	7.2
Amino acids	% by weight	7.9	16.8	9.92
Carbohydrate	% by weight	84.9	78.9	67.89
Fat	% by weight	0.54	0.33	14.98
Normal dilution		80 gm/300 ml	80 gm/300 ml	454 gm/2000 ml
Resulting % dilution		26.67%	26.67%	23.0%
Calcium	mEq	22.17	13.31	30.0
Iron	mEq	0.199	0.119	0.33
Copper	mEq	0.0339	0.020	0.03
Magnesium	mEq	16.0	9.58	17.0
Manganese	mEq	0.0567	0.034	0.09
Potassium	mEq	29.96	17.94	32.0
Sodium	mEq	37.40	33.52	15.0
Zinc	mEq	0.21	0.127	0.3
Chloride	mEq	50.86	52.47	29.0
Iodine	mEq	0.00063	0.00038	0.00075
Phosphate (as P)	mEq	43.03	25.83	15.0
Sulfate (as S)	mEq	0.398	0.239	0.42
Acetate	mEq	0.35	0.21	0.0
Sorbate	mEq	4.47	2.68	0.0
Vitamin A		2777.8 USP	1666.0 USP	2500.0 IU
Vitamin D		222.2 USP	133.3 USP	200.0 IU
Vitamin E	IU	16.67	10.0	23.0
Ascorbic acid	mg	38.87	23.33	150.0
Folic acid	μg	55.5	33.0	200.0
Niacin	mg	7.39	4.43	25.0
Riboflavin	mg	0.66	0.4	2.2
Thiamine	mg	0.58	0.35	1.9
Pyridoxine	mg	1.1	1.1	2.5
Vitamin B_{12}	μg	2.76	1.67	7.5
Pantothenic acid	mg	5.05	3.03	12.5

ed results of a study in which eight patients with severe malnutrition resulting from gastrointestinal tract disease or sepsis were fed a chemically defined diet consisting of essential and nonessential amino acids, simple sugars, minimal fat, minerals including trace elements, and vitamins.[26] Since that time, many reports on the use of elemental diets have been published. This technique of administering a chemically defined, bulk-free diet via the gastrointestinal tract is as effective as parenteral feeding if even a small portion of intestine is functional. These diets are usually administered by tube because the material is unpalatable. A constant infusion using a pump is the preferred mode of administration because the high osmolarity of these diets produces nausea, vomiting, cramps, and diarrhea if bolus feeding is used. Initial feedings are started with half-strength formula and are increased by increasing the volume over a 24-hour period. During the next 24-hour period, the concentration is increased to three-quarters strength. If this is well tolerated during the third 24-hour period, full-strength formula is given. Once the patient is receiving full-strength formula at full volume, intravenous fluids are no longer required, since all the fluid, electrolyte, and nutritional requirements can be met with the elemental diet alone. Patients receiving elemental diets should be monitored in the same way as those who are receiving parenteral nutrition. Unfortunately, infants and neonates tolerate chemically defined diets less well than do older children and adults. Such diets are infrequently employed in neonatal and infant surgery. Two commonly used elemental diets are described in Tables 5–5 and 5–6.

TOTAL PARENTERAL NUTRITION (TPN)

If the patient cannot be nourished through the gastrointestinal tract with the techniques outlined in the preceding section, intravenous nutrition should be initiated. There are three approaches to intravenous nutrition in infants and children: (1) central infusion of hypertonic glucose solutions; (2) peripheral infusion of moderately hypertonic solutions of glucose along with a fat emulsion; and (3) peripheral infusion of moderately hypertonic glucose in large volumes.[5] Each of these techniques is effective in producing nitrogen retention and weight gain. In a difficult patient, all three techniques may be required over a long period.

Parenteral nutrition is reserved for those infants and children whose lives are threatened because feeding by means of the gastrointestinal tract is impossible, inadequate, or hazardous. In some instances, such as in infants with chronic nonspecific diarrhea, allowing the gastrointestinal tract to rest for a prolonged period is curative. In others, the restoration and maintenance of adequate nutrition will permit subsequent corrective surgery. Although intravenous nutrition is used to replete the malnourished child, it may be started prophylactically in clinical situations in which prolonged starvation is expected. A prime example of this is the infant with gastroschisis.

The composition of the basic solution for central intravenous nutrition used at the Mott Children's Hospital is shown in Table 5–7.[9, 10, 12, 17] The solution contains 25 per

TABLE 5–7 SOLUTION FOR CENTRAL INTRAVENOUS NUTRITION

Each 1000 ml is prepared by mixing 500 ml of $D_{50}W$ and 500 ml of 7% Aminosyn* and adding appropriate amounts of electrolytes and vitamins. The general contents are as follows:

Crystalline amino acids	35.0 gm
Dextrose	250.0 gm
Potassium	12.0 mEq
Sodium	15.0 mEq
Calcium	27.0 mEq
Phosphorus	155.0 mg
Magnesium	7.6 mEq
Chloride	10.8 mEq
Folic acid	0.5 mg
Multivitamins†	5.0 ml
Vitamin K_1	0.2 mg
Vitamin B_{12}	6.6 μg
Trace elements‡	2.0 ml

*Abbott Laboratories, North Chicago, Illinois.

†M.V.I. (USV Pharmaceutical Corp., Tuckahoe, New York). Each 10 ml contains ascorbic acid (C), 500 mg; vitamin A, 10,000 IU; vitamin D, 1000 IU; thiamine, 50 mg; riboflavin, 10 mg; pyridoxine, 15 mg; niacin, 100 mg; dexpanthenol, 25 mg; vitamin E, 5 IU.

‡Trace element solution (manufactured at University of Michigan Pharmacy Department). Each ml contains zinc, 2 mg (0.060 mEq); copper, 0.4 mg (0.030 mEq); manganese, 0.2 mg (0.015 mEq); iodide, 0.056 mg (0.00044 mEq).

cent glucose and a crystalline amino acid preparation. Electrolytes, vitamins, and trace elements are added to the solution. The infusion of 100 to 110 ml/kg/day of this solution into a central vein provides a mixture of glucose, amino acids, and other nutrients sufficient to meet the normal infant's needs for tissue repair and growth. This volume is also safe in the older child whose basic caloric requirements are less. For the first day or two, the parenteral nutrition solution is diluted with equal volumes of 5 per cent dextrose and water to allow the patient to adapt to the osmotic load, thus preventing osmotic diuresis and hypertonic dehydration. As the patient's tolerance develops, as judged from diminishing glucosuria, full-strength solution is used. Iron requirements are met either by weekly intramuscular injections of iron-containing dextran or by blood transfusions. Essential fatty acids can be supplied by the daily application of sunflower seed oil to the skin[23] or by the infusion of small amounts of a commercial fat emulsion.

Hypertonic infusates must be delivered through a central venous catheter to prevent peripheral venous inflammation and thrombosis. In the older child the central venous catheter is inserted by percutaneous puncture of the subclavian vein. In the infant a silicon rubber catheter is passed through the internal or external jugular vein to the superior vena cava by means of a venous cutdown. This procedure is best carried out in an operating room or a cardiac catheterization laboratory where proper instruments and strict aseptic conditions are available. To minimize contamination of the blood stream, the venous catheter is tunneled from the entry point in the vein to an exit site in the skin 2 to 4 inches away. In the infant it is brought out on the scalp, whereas in the older child the exit site may be the neck, the chest wall, or the upper extremity (Fig. 5–1). Every 2 days, the dressing is removed, the skin is cleansed with an antiseptic, and povidone-iodine ointment (which is antibacterial and antifungal) and sterile dressings are reapplied. A 0.22-μm

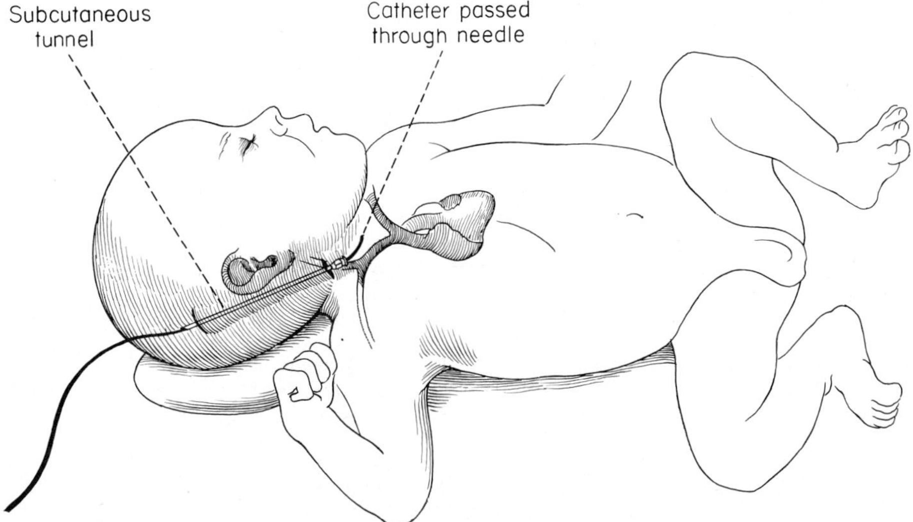

Figure 5–1 A transverse incision is made over the lower portion of the medial border of the sternocleidomastoid muscle, and the external or internal jugular vein is prepared for cannulation. The external jugular vein is preferred and can usually be cannulated even in the premature infant. If the external jugular vein has been used or is too small, the internal jugular vein is used. A long, hollow needle with an obturator in place is passed beneath the skin of the neck from the incision to the scalp. After the obturator is removed, the silicon rubber catheter is passed through the needle, and the needle is withdrawn. The external jugular vein is ligated distally. If the internal jugular vein has been selected, ligature of the vein can sometimes be avoided by passing the catheter into the vein through an incision made in the center of a pursestring suture. The catheter is advanced so that the tip lies at the junction of the superior vena cava and right atrium (approximately 5 cm in an infant). This position is confirmed by roentgenogram in the operating room. The catheter is secured to the subcutaneous tissue of the neck incision with a silk suture to prevent it from sliding out of the vein easily. An antibacterial and antifungal ointment is applied to the exit site incision, and the entire area is then covered with a sterile dressing. A coil of the catheter is included in the dressing to avoid accidental displacement.

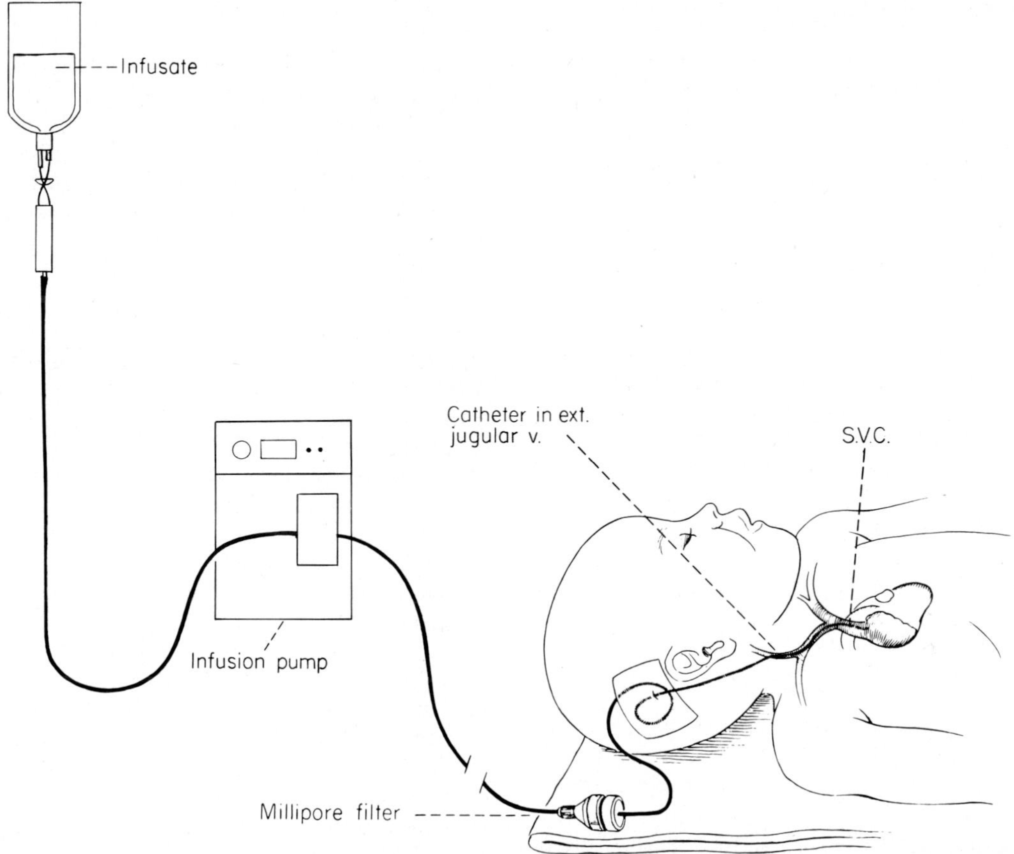

Figure 5–2 System for long-term central total parenteral nutrition. An infusion pump and a calibrated buret ensure uniform hourly flow rates. The Millipore filter in the circuit will remove any particulate matter, bacteria, and fungi. The catheter tip is positioned at the junction of the superior vena cava and right atrium, which is confirmed by roentgenogram.

Millipore filter* is placed in line to remove particulate matter and microorganisms. A calibrated buret is necessary to monitor the volume delivered. All intravenous tubings and the bottle of infusate are changed daily (Fig. 5–2).

Peripheral parenteral nutrition is administered through any convenient peripheral vein.[2, 3, 7, 8] No special equipment is required. Infusion pumps are used in infants and young children because they facilitate monitoring of the volume infused. The solution is composed of equal amounts of a 5 per cent crystalline amino acid solution† and 25 per cent glucose in water. This solution contains 2.5 per cent amino acids and 12.5 per cent glucose, which yields 0.60 calorie per ml. Electrolytes are added to the infusate to provide the recommended daily requirements plus additional needs based on the patient's clinical condition (Tables 5–8 and 5–9). The electrolyte and vitamin concentrations are essentially the same as those recommended for central infusions. When a fat emulsion is not used, the major portion of the essential fatty acids needed is supplied through the daily application of sunflower seed oil to the skin of the infant's chest. For infants, 160 to 200 ml/kg/24 hr of the fat-free solution is administered, providing 96 to 120 calories per day (Table 5–9). In older children the volume is reduced according to caloric needs. When Intralipid* is used, 40 ml (4 gm) of fat/kg/24 hr is administered to infants, and the nonlipid

---

*Millipore Corp., Bedford, Massachusetts.

†Aminosyn, Abbott Laboratories, North Chicago, Illinois.

*Cutter Laboratories, Berkeley, California.

TABLE 5–8 PERIPHERAL HYPERALIMENTATION
WITH FAT IN INFANTS

Constituent	Amount/kg/24 hr
Volume	160–200 ml
Intralipid	40 ml
Water	120–160 ml
Protein	3–4 gm
Glucose	15–20 gm
Fat	4 gm
Calories	116–140
Heparin	100 IU
Sodium	2–4 mEq
Potassium	2–3 mEq
Chloride	2–4 mEq
Magnesium	0.6 mEq
Calcium	1.0 mEq
Phosphate	3.5 mm
Multivitamins*	1.0 ml
Vitamin K_1	0.04 mg
Vitamin B_{12}	1.32 μg
Trace elements†	0.4 ml

*M.V.I., USV Pharmaceutical Corp., Tuckahoe, New
York.

†See Table 5–7.

solution is reduced by this amount (see
Table 5–8). This provides 116 to 140 calo-
ries/kg/day, which is more than adequate
for an infant to gain weight and grow. In
older children, Intralipid is given at the rate
of 2 gm/kg/24 hr, with the nonlipid solution
supplying the remainder of the caloric
needs. Intralipid meets all the essential fatty
acid requirements. The administration of
vitamins and iron is as described in the
central feeding program. Trace elements

TABLE 5–9 PERIPHERAL HYPERALIMENTATION
WITHOUT FAT IN INFANTS

Constituent	Amount/kg/24 hr
Water	160–200 ml
Protein	4–5 gm
Glucose	20–25 gm
Calories	96–120
Heparin	100 IU
Sodium	2–4 mEq
Potassium	2–3 mEq
Chloride	2–4 mEq
Magnesium	0.6 mEq
Calcium	1.0 mEq
Phosphate	3.5 mm
Multivitamins*	1.0 ml
Vitamin K_1	0.04 mg
Vitamin B_{12}	1.32 μg
Trace elements†	0.4 ml

*M.V.I., USV Pharmaceutical Corp., Tuckahoe, New
York.

†See Table 5–7.

are given routinely or as necessary. Figure
5–3 depicts the technique of peripheral intravenous nutrition with a fat emulsion. The
intravenous needle must be changed every 2
to 3 days because of infiltration, which is
usually bland and nonphlebitic. When no
fat is employed, needles are changed every
24 to 48 hours routinely, or more often if
signs of infiltration or phlebitis are observed.

Essential clinical measurements during
parenteral nutrition include daily body
weight, volume of urine, and volume of
other body fluid losses. Urine sugar and
acetone content are monitored with each
voiding. Important blood tests and recommended frequency in the routine patient
are listed in Table 5–10. Weight change
during the period of intravenous nutrition
will vary with the patient's overall clinical
status. Normal weight gain may be expected
in babies who are not severely malnourished
and in whom sepsis has not developed.
Weight gains observed with the three different techniques are comparable, averag-
ing 20 to 30 gm/day in the neonate.[22, 24]
Positive nitrogen balance has been observed
in most patients studied.

***Complications of Parenteral Nutri-
tion.*** The complications of parenteral nutrition can be classified as technical, infectious, and metabolic. Technical problems
are usually associated with the use of the
central venous catheter. The substitution of
nonreactive silicon catheters for polyvinyl
catheters has reduced the incidence of
sterile inflammation and thrombosis. Placing the tip of the catheter at the junction of
the superior vena cava and the right atrium,
rather than in the heart, has reduced the
incidence of arrhythmias. Insertion of the
central venous catheter under roentgenographic control ensures proper positioning.
The catheter does not usually become dislodged if it has been well secured during
placement. Thrombosis of the superior
vena cava is rare, but can cause serious
illness and even death. Pulmonary embolism is also rare but is occasionally seen in
infants when a central venous catheter is
present for a prolonged period. Phlebitis is
very rare in patients treated with Intralipid
peripherally, despite the fact that the entire
infusate is slightly hypertonic. Intralipid, in
some unknown fashion, appears to protect
the vein from phlebitis. When infiltration

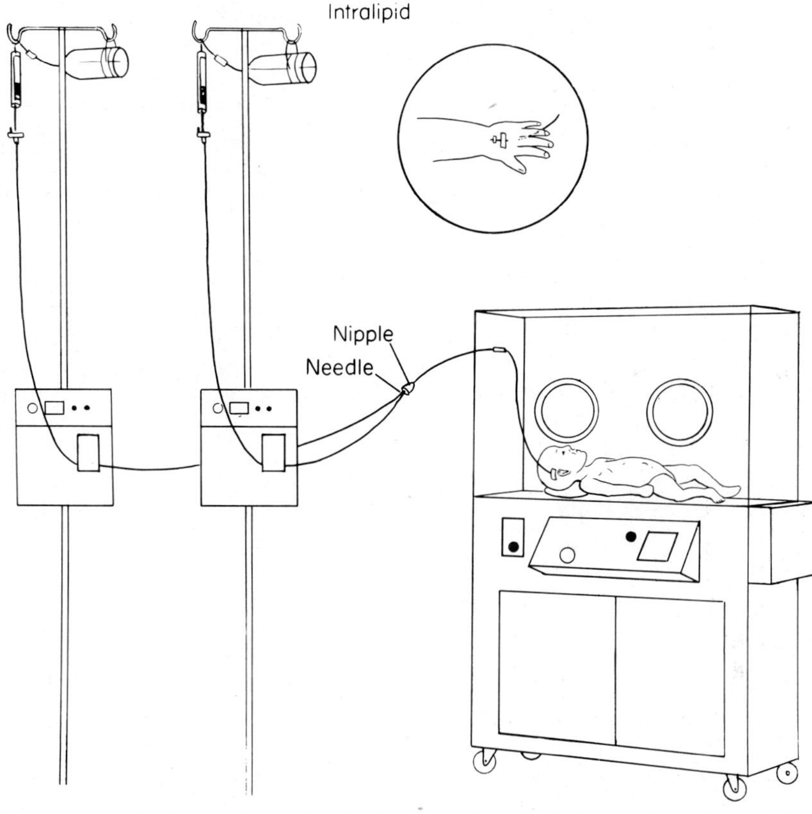

Figure 5–3 Peripheral intravenous feeding with Intralipid. The two solutions are infused simultaneously into a peripheral vein using a constant infusion pump. The scalp is generally used in the infant; the dorsum of the hand in the older child.

does occur, it is usually bland and the fluid is rapidly reabsorbed. Phlebitis is seen occasionally in patients fed peripherally without fat, but it disappears when the infusion site

TABLE 5–10 BLOOD VALUES MONITORED ROUTINELY DURING TOTAL PARENTERAL NUTRITION

	Frequency of Monitoring	
At Start of Therapy and Weekly	At Start of Therapy and Every 2 Weeks	As Indicated
Sodium, potassium, chloride	SGOT, LDH, alkaline phosphatase*	Copper
Urea	Bilirubin	Zinc
Glucose	Creatinine	Iron
Magnesium		Ammonia
Calcium, phosphorus		Osmolarity
Total protein		pH
Hemoglobin, hematocrit, white blood cell count, platelets		
Blood culture		
Candida precipitins		

*SGOT = serum glutamic oxaloacetic transaminase; LDH = lactic dehydrogenase.

is changed. Of 60 patients treated by peripheral hyperalimentation without fat, three had skin slough at the infusion site. Two of these healed spontaneously and one needed skin grafting.

Sepsis remains the major complication of central parenteral nutrition in patients of all ages, but especially in the infant. Indwelling venous cannulas that remain in place for a long time are a well-documented source of blood-stream infection. The catheter, a foreign body in the blood stream, may act as a focus for bacterial growth even when organisms enter from a distant septic site. Placement of catheters under aseptic conditions and meticulous daily care of the catheter site significantly reduce the incidence of this complication. In addition, minimal use of the catheter for blood drawing will reduce the risk of contamination. The *parenteral nutrition team* has led to a significant decrease in the incidence of sepsis, which is directly related to the duration of therapy. For each week of therapy beyond the first week, and in spite of the strictest precautions, the incidence of catheter sepsis ranges between 3 and 8 per cent. Fever, leukocytosis, or unexplained glucosuria is often the first indication of sepsis. Infection is confirmed by culturing microorganisms from blood obtained through the central venous catheter line and from another venous site. If no other site of sepsis is found, the catheter should be removed. No antibiotics are administered unless fever persists longer than 24 hours after removal of the catheter. During the early era of parenteral nutrition, bacteria were responsible for most episodes of sepsis. For several years after that, *Candida* appeared to be the major cause of invasive sepsis. During the last few years, *Candida* sepsis has been rare and we are witnessing the return of bacterial sepsis. Invasive sepsis related to hyperalimentation was not seen in any of our 102 patients treated with Intralipid nor in any infants and children who received peripheral intravenous feeding without fat.

Table 5–11 lists the more common metabolic complications of parenteral nutrition. Some metabolic complications are unavoidable, but most can be prevented by appropriate adjustments of the infusate based on careful clinical monitoring. Most of the complications are related to the administration of too little or too much of the particular nutrient. In the absence of sepsis, significant hyperglycemia is usually observed only in the low-birth-weight infant. Temporary dilution of the infusate usually solves the problem. If it does not, exogenous insulin is administered. Hypoglycemia is a theoretical complication of the abrupt cessation of TPN solution, yet this complication is seldom

TABLE 5–11 METABOLIC COMPLICATIONS OF PARENTERAL NUTRITION

Persistent hyperglycemia and glycosuria
Osmotic diuresis
Postinfusion hypoglycemia
Acidosis
Hyperammonemia
Amino acid toxicity
Hypomagnesemia
Hypocupremia
Essential fatty acid deficiency
Hypocalcemia, hypercalcemia, hypophosphatemia
Hepatic impairment (toxic)
Hypercholesterolemia
Hypertriglyceridemia

seen. Metabolic acidosis is also rare. Amino acids in presently available TPN solutions challenge the patient with a large acid load, but few become acidotic. Hyperammonemia has been reported in infants less than 6 months of age. Clinical signs of essential fatty acid deficiency occur after 2 to 3 months of fat-free parenteral nutrition. A typical generalized skin rash develops. Chemical signs of essential fatty acid deficiency may occur after only 3 weeks of fat-free therapy. The classic chemical abnormality is an increased level of serum eicosatrienoic acid. Essential fatty acid deficiency can be prevented by providing 2 to 4 per cent of daily caloric needs in the form of linoleic acid.

Most patients receiving Intralipid have normal serum triglyceride and cholesterol levels; however, a few to whom hyperalimentation is given for longer than 1 month have serum triglyceride values in the range of 300 to 350 mg/dl (normal, 150 to 250 mg/dl) and serum cholesterol levels of 150 to 250 mg/dl (normal, 100 to 150 mg/dl). These mild elevations return to normal when Intralipid is discontinued.

Abnormalities in liver function have frequently been observed during parenteral nutrition. Variable and intermittent elevations in levels of serum glutamic oxaloacetic transaminase, lactic dehydrogenase, and bilirubin have occurred throughout the course of treatment in many patients. The histologic appearance of the liver fails to reveal any consistent pathologic alteration. Cholestatic jaundice has been described and appears to be far more common in the young infant than in the older child or adult. This may be related to the fact that the biliary excretory system of the infant is immature and more susceptible to damage. Liver abnormalities seen in patients receiving Intralipid are not different from those seen in patients whose parenteral feeding program does not include fat. Cholestatic jaundice usually clears within 2 to 3 weeks after cessation of intravenous nutrition.

A peripheral eosinophilia of 5 to 10 per cent develops in about 80 per cent of patients receiving Intralipid. In a few, this may rise to 35 per cent. There are no clinical manifestations of this abnormality.

Osmotic diuresis secondary to significant glucosuria occasionally occurs when 25 per cent glucose infusate is used. The premature infant with underdeveloped renal tubules is most susceptible to this complication. This phenomenon is not seen in patients who receive peripheral hyperalimentation because of the lower tonicity of the infusate.

CONCLUSION

Although most of the nutritional requirements for proper wound healing are poorly defined and even more poorly understood, there are a few specific nutrients that appear to be essential for proper wound healing, such as vitamin A, vitamin C, protein, calories, oxygen, and a few trace elements. Since adequate wound healing involves most of the metabolic processes that occur in other tissues and organs in the body, the normal healing of a surgical or traumatic wound will proceed most effectively under the conditions of balanced nutrition. Proper nutritional support of the patient by whatever means necessary will ensure a better clinical result and better wound repair.

References

1. Ballinger, W. F., Collins, J. A., Drucker, W. R., et al.: Manual of Surgical Nutrition. Philadelphia, W. B. Saunders Co., 1975.
2. Benner, J. W., Coran, A. G., Weintraub, W. H., and Wesley, J. R.: The importance of different calorie sources in the intravenous nutrition of infants and children. Surgery 86:429, 1979.
3. Borresen, H. C., Coran, A. G., and Knutrud, O.: Metabolic results of parenteral feeding in neonatal surgery: A balanced parenteral feeding program based on a synthetic L-amino acid solution and a commercial fat emulsion. Ann. Surg. 172:291, 1970.
4. Bryan, W. T., Greenwell, J. E., and Weeks, P. M.: Alterations in collagen during dilatation of the cervix uteri. Surg. Gynecol. Obstet. 126:27, 1968.
5. Coran, A. G.: The long-term intravenous feeding of infants using peripheral veins. J. Pediatr. Surg. 8:801, 1973.
6. Coran, A. G.: Total intravenous feeding of infants and children without the use of a central venous catheter. Ann. Surg. 179:445, 1974.
7. Coran, A. G.: Nutritional support of the pediatric surgical patient. In Holder, T. M., and Ashcraft, K. W. (eds.): Surgery of Infants and Children. Philadelphia, W. B. Saunders Co., 1980.
8. Coran, A. G., and Filler, R. M.: Total parenteral nutrition. In Ravitch, M. M., Welch, K. J., Benson, C. D., et al. (eds.): Pediatric Surgery. Chicago, Year Book Medical Publishers, 1979.
9. Dudrick, S. J., Wilmore, D. W., Vars, H. M., and Rhoads, J. E.: Long-term parenteral nutrition with growth, development and positive nitrogen balance. Surgery 64:134, 1968.
10. Dudrick, S. J., Wilmore, D. W., Vars, H. M., and Rhoads, J. E.: Can intravenous feeding as a sole means of nutrition support growth in a child, and restore weight loss in adults? An affirmative answer. Ann. Surg. 169:974, 1969.
11. Dunphy, J. W., and Udupa, K. N.: Chemical and histochemical sequence in the normal healing of wounds. N. Engl. J. Med. 253:847, 1955.
12. Filler, R. M., Eraklis, A. J., Rubin, V. G., and Das, J. B.: Long-term parenteral nutrition in infants. N. Engl. J. Med. 281:589, 1969.
13. Frieman, M. F., Seifter, E., Connerton, C., and Levenson, S. M.: Vitamin A deficiency and surgical stress. Surg. Forum 21:81, 1970.
14. Gabbiani, G., Herschel, B. J., Ryan, G. B., et al.: Granulation tissue as a contractile organ. A study of structure and function. J. Exp. Med. 135:719, 1972.
15. Gould, B. S.: Biology of collagen. In Ramachandran, G. N. (ed.): Treatise on Collagen. Vol. 2, Part I. New York, Academic Press, 1968.
16. Grant, M. E., Phil, D., and Prockop, D. J.: The biosynthesis of collagen (parts I, II, III). N. Engl. J. Med. 286:194, 242, 291, 1972.
17. Heird, W. C., and Winters, R. W.: Total parenteral nutrition: The state of the art. J. Pediatr. 86:2, 1975.
18. Heughan, C., Grislis, G., and Hunt, T. K.: The effect of anemia on wound healing. Ann. Surg. 179:163, 1974.
19. Lee, H. A.: Parenteral Nutrition in Acute Metabolic Illness. New York, Academic Press, 1974.
20. Madden, J. W., and Peacock, E. E., Jr.: Studies on the biology of collagen during wound healing. III. Dynamic metabolism of scar collagen and remodeling of dermal wounds. Ann. Surg. 174:511, 1971.
21. Peacock, E. E., Jr., and VanWinkle, W., Jr.: Wound Repair, 2nd edition. Philadelphia, W. B. Saunders Co., 1976.
22. Polley, T. Z., Jr., Benner, J. W., Rhodin, A. G. J., et al.: Changes in total body water in infants receiving total intravenous nutrition. J. Surg. Res. 26:555, 1979.
23. Press, M., Hartop, P. J., and Prottey, C.: Correction of essential fatty acid deficiency in man by the cutaneous application of sunflower seed oil. Lancet 1:579, 1974.
24. Rhodin, A. G. J., Coran, A. G., Weintraub, W. H., and Wesley, J. R.: Total body water changes during high-volume peripheral hyperalimentation. Surg. Gynecol. Obstet. 148:196, 1979.
25. Shils, M. E.: Guidelines for total parenteral nutrition. J.A.M.A. 220:1721, 1972.
26. Stephens, R. B., and Randall, H. T.: Use of a concentrated balanced liquid elemental diet for nutritional management of catabolic states. Ann. Surg. 170:642, 1969.

SURGICAL INFECTIONS AND ANTIBIOTICS

6

H. Harlan Stone, M.D.

Infection has always been and probably will forever remain the most common complication of any surgical procedure. Postoperative sepsis is occasionally fatal; however, even an apparently trivial infection of the incision causes the patient additional discomfort and increases his medical bill. Accordingly, efforts to prevent, minimize, and treat postoperative sepsis are exceedingly important if high-quality surgical care is to be provided.[13]

AREAS OF INFECTION

After trauma and during the postoperative period, fever is the most common initial indication that sepsis may be developing. The cause of the fever should be sought immediately by assessing four specific high-risk areas of the body. A routine survey of this type will disclose the presence and source of suspected infection in more than 95 per cent of patients, thus well justifying the effort.

Lungs

Although the occurrence of atelectasis and its subsequent progression to pneumonia are not as frequent in children as in adults, congestive pneumonitis still is common. Lobar consolidation is often caused by occlusion of the left main-stem bronchus during operation or assisted ventilation or by an endotracheal tube that is too deeply seated. Oversedation may also be responsible for an ineffective cough or for aspiration of vomited gastric contents.

Secondary pneumonitis, generally the result of hematogenous seeding during bac-

teremic episodes complicating sepsis elsewhere in the body, is almost uniformly diffuse and develops relatively late. Suppurative phlebitis and poorly controlled peritonitis are the most common primary foci.

The diagnosis of pneumonia is suggested by abnormalities noted on physical examination (e.g., dullness, rales, tachypnea) and is then confirmed by a chest x-ray film. Microscopic examination of a stained sputum smear and sputum culture are valuable guides to antimicrobial therapy, provided that the sputum sample consists of relatively pure bronchial secretions. Examination of the saliva is worthless. Organisms grown on blood culture are the most accurate bacteriologic determinants of the antibiotic to be administered.

Urinary Tract

Urinary tract infection may represent an acute exacerbation of a chronic process, or it may be a first attack caused by colonization from bacteremia or an indwelling drainage tube. The presence of bacteria alone rarely produces acute pyelonephritis. Urine stasis due to mechanical obstruction (e.g., anatomic block, reflux) or severe dehydration must also be present. Fluid therapy is therefore an important preventive as well as therapeutic measure. There is no substitute for the unobstructed, brisk flow of urine (2 to 3 ml/kg body weight/hr) in the prevention of urinary tract infection.

The diagnosis is usually made by microscopic examination of a spun urine sample obtained from a child who has an unexplained fever. Pyuria and, more especially, bacilluria are characteristic findings. Diagnostic confirmation is based upon a urine colony count of greater than 10^3/ml of urine. An intravenous pyelogram is obtained to rule out a pathologic condition that demands more detailed study (e.g., cystography and cystoscopy) and eventual surgical correction.

Treatment involves hydration and administration of an appropriate antibiotic— usually ampicillin until culture or sensitivity tests dictate otherwise.

Venous System

Colonization of the intravenous catheter, its connecting tubes, or the infusion solution is a common cause of hospital-acquired bacteremia.[1] The incidence is approximately equal to the square of the number of days that the intravenous line has been in place (e.g., 4 per cent at 2 days, 9 per cent at 3 days). However, by practicing strict asepsis during insertion of the cannula and by adhering to a daily maintenance schedule that includes cleansing with iodophor, application of a topical antimicrobial, and replacement of all external infusion apparatus, the risk of associated bacteremia can be reduced to as low as 1 per cent for each day of continued use of a given intravenous catheter.

Fewer than half the intravenous sites responsible for bacteremia will manifest any sign of local inflammation. Thus, otherwise unexplained sepsis should be managed initially by removing all intravenous lines and culturing the tip of the indwelling catheter. A new site of venous access is then established with a fresh, sterile set-up in the contralateral extremity.

Any segment of vein that is obviously suppurative must be either drained or excised. Persistence of bacteremia (usually staphylococcal) despite such measures demands that an appropriate beta-lactamase– resistant penicillin or cephalosporin be administered parenterally.

Wound

Infection of the wound occurs in one or both of two specific areas: the cavity explored or violated, and the incision or wound through which that particular cavity was entered.

INCISIONAL INFECTIONS

The individual bacteria participating in an infection determine the time of clinical onset of sepsis following inoculation (Table 6–1), the physical characteristics of the infectious process, and the likelihood of an attendant bacteremia.

Aerobic gram-positive coccal infections, especially those due to streptococci, become manifest within 1 or 2 days after seeding, just as do those infections caused by the anaerobic clostridia alone (Table 6–1). Although differentiation between the two is relatively easy, there may be confusion if the wound itself is not examined carefully for temperature, tenderness, and aroma of any liquid discharge (Table 6–2). Gaseous crepitation is noted in fewer than half of those patients with an early, yet pure, clostridial sepsis, and a smear of the tissue exudate often fails to contain identifiable pathogens.

Infection due to *Staphylococcus aureus* generally does not become clinically apparent until the third or fourth day, as do those infections caused by a polymicrobial flora of aerobic gram-negative rods mixed with various anaerobes. Isolated gram-negative sepsis seldom produces physical changes in the wound until the sixth or seventh day.

As a general rule, administration of antibiotics delays onset of symptoms and signs of infection by 1 to 5 days.

TABLE 6–1 POSTOPERATIVE INFECTION OF THE WOUND

Days Postoperatively	Pathogen	Type of Infection
1–2	Hemolytic streptococci Clostridia	Cellulitis Gas gangrene
3–4	*Staphylococcus aureus*	Abscess with halo cellulitis
5–6	Gram-negative rods plus anaerobes	Synergistic gangrene and/or abscess
7–12	Gram-negative rod alone	Abscess

TABLE 6–2 STREPTOCOCCAL INFECTION VERSUS GAS GANGRENE

	Streptococcal Infection	Gas Gangrene
Systemic Signs		
Fever	39–40° C	39–40° C
Orientation	Disoriented	Disoriented
Leukocytosis	Marked	Marked
Jaundice	Mild	Moderate
Anemia	Hemolytic	Hemolytic
Wound		
Odor	Slight	Putrid
Color	Hyperemic	Darkened
Temperature	Warm	Cool
Pain	Tender	Constant
Crepitation	Often	Rare
Blebs	As second-degree burn	Hemorrhagic
Discharge		
Color	Pink	Brackish
Smear	Gram-positive cocci	Gram-positive rods

The specific types of wound infection, their causative pathogens and distinctive features, and the preferred modes of therapy are listed in Table 6–3.

Cellulitis. Extreme, classic inflammation is characterized by cellulitis. Aerobic gram-positive cocci, particularly the streptococci, are the usual cause. An excellent blood supply guarantees that parenterally administered antimicrobial agents will reach the site of infection in adequate bactericidal concentrations. A relatively massive dose of penicillin G, given intravenously and repeated every 4 to 6 hours, is the treatment of choice. Erythromycin is given to patients who have a history of penicillin allergy.[9]

Abscess. Although a halo of cellulitis surrounds the abscess almost uniformly, its central locules of necrotic debris reflect the adequacy of host defenses in confining the process to a given space. Despite the fact that parenterally administered antibiotics are valuable in the control of an associated bacteremia and in preventing further tissue destruction, only incision and drainage will effect a cure. Positioning the patient or using a sump drain is exceedingly important, as only gravitationally dependent drainage will permit complete evacuation of the abscess cavity.

A second-generation cephalosporin (i.e., cefamandole or cefoxitin) provides an adequate antibacterial spectrum for protection whenever culture data are not available for use as a guide before operation. The intravenous route of administration is generally preferred.

TABLE 6–3 SPECIFIC TYPES OF WOUND INFECTION

Type	Pathogens	Presentation	Basic Treatment
Cellulitis	Hemolytic streptococci (*Staphylococcus aureus*)	Intense, diffuse inflammation	Penicillin alone (erythromycin)
Abscess	*Staphylococcus aureus* Gram-negative rods with or without anaerobes	Halo cellulitis with central locules of liquefied necrotic material	Incision and dependent drainage Selective antibiotic for operation, i.e., cephalosporin
Phlegmon	*Staphylococcus aureus* Gram-negative rods plus anaerobes	Diffuse cellulitis with multiple tiny abscess pockets	Division of partitioning septa, if subcutaneous Resection of organ, if deep Routine concomitant parenteral antibiotic
Gangrene	Clostridia Gram-negative rods plus anaerobes	Tissue necrosis with putrid exudate	Excision of all necrotic tissue, with delayed wound closure Routine appropriate parenteral antibiotic until wound closure
Toxemia	Tetanus *Pseudomonas* Diphtheria	Central nervous system toxin effect Reticuloendothelial system toxin effect Cardiac toxin effect	Wound excision, with delayed closure Routine topical and parenteral antibiotic until wound closure

Phlegmon. Inability of bacterial enzymes to digest host fascial barriers may lead to the compartmentalization of an abscess into innumerable small, macroscopic locules. The carbuncle, transmural gastritis and enterocolitis, bacterial pancreatitis, and the felon are classic examples. In many areas of the body, excision of the phlegmonous tissue (e.g., gastrectomy, colectomy) may be the most practical approach. However, for the felon and the carbuncle, division of the fibrous septa to create a single abscess pocket is the preferred method.

Subcutaneous phlegmons are usually due to *Staphylococcus aureus* alone or in combination with a hemolytic streptococcus. Accordingly, a beta-lactamase–resistant penicillin or cephalosporin is the preferred agent for local control of infection, both before and after drainage. Phlegmons of the alimentary tract, on the other hand, are most often caused by a polymicrobial aerobic-anaerobic flora and thus should be managed by either a second-generation cephalosporin (cefamandole or cefoxitin) or the combination of an aminoglycoside (gentamicin or tobramycin) and a macrolide (clindamycin or erythromycin).

Gangrene. Necrotizing infections always necessitate performance of relatively radical débridement as soon as possible.[7] There can be no exception to this rule. It is critical that there be bactericidal concentrations of an appropriate antibiotic in the blood to combat attendant bacteremia as well as to protect healthy tissues, freshly exposed as a result of surgical excision of the gangrenous lesion, from becoming reinfected.

Aerobic monomicrobial gangrene in the healthy child is usually due to a highly virulent strain of either a hemolytic streptococcus or *Staphylococcus aureus.* Massive doses of penicillin G plus a beta-lactamase–resistant penicillin analogue should be administered intravenously until more specific antimicrobial sensitivity data are available. Erythromycin and the cephalosporins are acceptable alternatives, but they should be used only if the patient is known to be allergic to penicillin.[9]

Pseudomonas gangrene, often referred to as pyoderma gangrenosum, occurs primarily in children with deranged immune mechanisms, antibody deficits (e.g., dysgammaglobulinemias), poor phagocyte function (e.g., leukemia, agranulocytosis), or less specific anergy complicating a major thermal burn or starvation.[14] Impairment of host resistance may be congenital or may be acquired as a result of medications, nutritional deficiency, exposure to radiation, stress, or other factors. Antimicrobial therapy should be parenteral with an aminoglycoside (gentamicin, tobramycin, or amikacin, depending upon results of recent sensitivity testing) as well as topical. For the latter, the ability of the agent to diffuse through tissue limits the selection to an aqueous solution or cream preparation of an aminoglycoside or to one of the topical antimicrobials that has proved efficacious in the treatment of burn wound sepsis.

Necrotizing enterocolitis is another example of aerobic bacterial gangrene. The responsible pathogens are almost uniformly one or more of the gram-negative rods, with or without participation by streptococci, staphylococci, or both.[16] Antibiotics used for therapy should then include some combination of an aminoglycoside (gentamicin or tobramycin) and penicillin or one of its penicillinase-resistant analogues.

Various fungi may also produce an infectious gangrene as a complication of invasion through the colonized open wound.[2] Aspergillosis and sporotrichosis are prime examples. Topical as well as parenteral amphotericin B appears to be the agent of choice.

Toxemia. Absorption of bacterial toxins is an almost routine occurrence in every type of infection. Nevertheless, certain toxemias are so overwhelming that they account for the majority of physical signs and symptoms of sepsis, as well as being the immediate cause of death in fatal cases. The classic examples are diphtheria, tetanus, and *Pseudomonas* wound sepsis.

Diphtheria occurs in otherwise healthy individuals who possess no acquired active or passive immunity. Although the site of infection by *Corynebacterium diphtheriae* is usually the pharynx, sporadic instances arising from wound colonization have been reported. Cardiac derangements are most impressive. Treatment includes wound excision and parenteral administration of penicillin to patients whose diphtheria is not of pharyngeal origin.

Tetanus is generally diagnosed on the basis of increased muscle tone, extreme irritability, and an unexplained convulsive disorder, primarily a tetanic seizure. The responsible focus can be identified in only 80 per cent of patients, and even then the usual wound of origin is a relatively innocuous-appearing lesion. Although gram-positive rods cannot always be seen or grown from a smear of wound exudate, an otherwise unsupported clinical diagnosis is sufficient to initiate energetic treatment measures. Penicillin and human antitetanus globulin are administered intravenously, the child is sedated, and complete wound excision is carried out as soon as possible.

Prophylaxis is far superior to any known treatment and should be implemented for all patients with wounds sustained in an uncontrolled environment.[5] Active immunization with tetanus toxoid as an initial course or booster, administration of homologous antitetanus globulin, and antibiotic therapy with penicillin are based upon the patient's immunization history, the massiveness of wound contusion and contamination, and the patient's known allergies. All children who have significantly destructive or dirty wounds or who live in an uncertain home situation should be admitted for observation after thorough surgical cleansing and débridement have been accomplished. If any doubt exists, the wound should be left open so that a delayed primary closure can be performed 2 to 4 days later.

Pseudomonas toxemia occurs only when a large proportion of body surface has been colonized by *Pseudomonas aeruginosa*.[14] The excretion of verdoglobin, caused by a metabolic block in the reticuloendothelial catabolism of hemoglobin, gives the urine an olive-green color. Treatment requires both parenteral and topical administration of aminoglycosides (gentamicin, tobramycin, or amikacin) and wound excision.

Bacteremia/Septicemia. Pathogens reach the blood stream by inoculation from a septic focus directly into an adjacent vein or by a more indirect route involving a tissue compartment, cavitary conduit, or lymphatic channel. The source or intermediary structure usually shows signs of inflammation (e.g., phlebitis, lymphangitis). Nevertheless, bacteremia and septicemia both may arise from a focus without external evidence of microbial colonization (contaminated intravenous fluids). The infected site may be within the central cardiovascular system (e.g., endocarditis).

Treatment is twofold: (1) Control the bacteremia with appropriate parenteral antibiotics, and (2) eradicate the primary focus of infection by drainage or excision or both.

INFECTION OF THE CAVITIES

Serosa-lined cavities are relatively resistant to limited bacterial contamination. The initial inflammatory response occurs rapidly and progresses at an accelerated rate. Its resultant exudate is rich in antibody, complement, and other noncorpuscular resistance factors of humoral origin. Phagocytes are immediately present in relatively large numbers. Fibrinous adhesions soon form between apposing serosal surfaces and, in effect, partition the infectious process into one or more locules, thereby protecting uninvolved areas of the parent cavity. There is then either complete resolution of all inflammatory response as the infection is eradicated or more solid isolation of the septic process into a well-defined abscess pocket. Failure to control the infection by one of these mechanisms allows sepsis to become more generalized, leading eventually to the death of the patient.

Parenteral antibiotics, selected on the basis of their effect against anticipated or already identified pathogens, have become the key to successful control of cavitary infections.[17] Accordingly, clinical assessments of the apparent bacteremia (Table 6–4) and of the anticipated source of original contamination (Table 6–5) are exceedingly important guides to intelligent choice of antibiotic before a culture report is in hand.

Intra-abdominal abscesses tend to collect in one of three major areas. Those in the *pelvis* are readily appreciated on rectal examination. After confirmation by inspection of a needle aspirate, thereby avoiding injury to the bladder, the abscess is drained transrectally.

The *midabdominal* abscess is diagnosed by the presence of a tender mass at any site along the anatomic horseshoe created by one abdominal gutter extending across the false pelvis to the contralateral gutter. Even when the process has decompressed by dis-

TABLE 6–4 CLINICAL DIFFERENTIATION OF SEPTICEMIA

	Gram-Positive	Gram-Negative	Anaerobic	Fungal
Sensorium	Irrational	Rational	Irrational	Rational
Temperature	Spiking to 39–40° C	Sustained, 38–39° C	Spiking to 39–40° C	Sustained, 38–39° C
Blood pressure	Gradual fall	Sudden fall	Gradual fall	Gradual fall
Urine flow	Gradual fall	Sudden oliguria	Gradual fall	Gradual fall
Jaundice	Hemolytic	Rare	Hemolytic	Rare
White blood cell count	>16,000	10,000–16,000	>14,000	>14,000
Urine microscopic findings	—	—	—	Yeast
Antimicrobial	Penicillin/ cephalosporin	Aminoglycoside/ second-generation cephalosporin	Erythromycin/ clindamycin/ cefoxitin	Oral nystatin/ amphotericin B

charge through the abdominal incision, it may still be inadequately drained because of its indirect path to the body surface. An extraperitoneal approach for drainage is preferred, with use of patient positioning or a sump drain to ensure dependent drainage and gravitational flow of pus.

Subphrenic abscesses, on the other hand, are often difficult to identify, especially with respect to exact location. Percussion tenderness along the costal margin, shoulder pain, and a pleural effusion are relatively late signs. The diagnosis is commonly suspected because an otherwise unexplained fever persists. Overpenetrated plain films of the thoracoabdominal region usually reveal the extraluminal bubbles of gas produced by an infecting flora containing anaerobes. Barium contrast studies can be used for confirmation. Liver-lung and gallium scans are of limited benefit. Surgical drainage is always indicated and may require a transperitoneal or transcostal approach.

PROPHYLACTIC MEASURES

The interaction of three factors determines the likelihood that infection will develop in a wound. These factors are the quantity and virulence of the microbial inoculum, the amount of nutrient media in which bacteria can grow, and the patient's resistance to infection.

TABLE 6–5 ANTIBIOTIC SELECTION ACCORDING TO SOURCE OF PERITONEAL CONTAMINANT

Source	Anticipated Pathogens	Preferred Parenteral Antibiotics
Esophagus Stomach	Gram-positive cocci Gram-positive rods	Penicillin/penicillin analogue/cephalosporin
Biliary Unobstructed small bowel	Gram-negative rods	Cephalosporin/aminoglycoside
Terminal ileum Obstructed small bowel Colon and its appendages	Gram-negative rods Enterococci Anaerobes	Aminoglycoside plus either cefoxitin, erythromycin, clindamycin, or chloramphenicol Cefamandole plus erythromycin
Acute pelvic inflammation	Gram-negative cocci	Penicillin
Chronic or recurrent pelvic inflammation	As with colon	As with colon

Inoculum

Quantity and virulence of the microbial inoculum best define the infectiousness of a specific contaminant. The absolute bacterial population within the immediate vicinity of the surgical incision is reduced by preparing the skin (mechanical scrub followed by application of a topical antiseptic), draping, and maintaining a sterile field through use of masks, gowns, scrubbed hands, and gloves. Any breach in technique, no matter how slight, must be corrected instantly. Should operation on the bowel be planned, mechanical cleansing of the gut followed by oral administration of nonabsorbable antimicrobials (neomycin or kanamycin plus erythromycin base) will provide an internal preparation that approximates what has been achieved at the skin level.[4]

If contamination has already occurred, meticulous removal of all foreign matter is important. Irrigation consistently fails to carry away the residual bacteria trapped in the fibrin peel on serosal and wound surfaces.[11] Only a parenterally administered antibiotic or a penetrable (non-protein-bound) topical antimicrobial will eliminate this source of future sepsis. Alternatively, the entire layer of fibrin can be removed by local application or parenteral administration of heparin, yet the problem of capillary ooze would appear to pose a greater threat.[10]

Nutrient Media

The manual skill of and the operative techniques employed by the surgeon can be correlated with the amount of necrotic tissue or blood clot left in the surgical wound.[13] Inexact use of the cautery, mass ligation of tissues, and closing the wound with sutures that cause significant local irritation all increase the amount of nutrient pabulum in which bacteria can grow and thereby reduce to a minimum the quantity and virulence of contaminant necessary to induce wound sepsis.

Drains cannot offset such consequences of faulty technique.[8] Instead, they merely guarantee a pathway for invasion of the wound depth by antibiotic-resistant bacteria resident in the hospital environment.

Resistance

Active immunization is practical against only a few bacterial species, primarily ones that produce an exotoxin with specific actions and for which a safe toxoid is available. Immunity that is inherently present can be lost if anergy is permitted to develop as a complication of continuing sepsis or malnutrition.[12] Intravenous hyperalimentation may then become an absolute necessity.[6]

Prophylactic antibiotics offer another means by which protection can be afforded. However, bactericidal concentrations of antibiotic with an appropriate spectrum for the anticipated pathogens must be in the blood as well as in the tissues at risk by the time contamination occurs.[3] Delay in administering antibiotics so limits the effectiveness of antimicrobial prophylaxis that no benefit can be noted beyond the third hour after inoculation.[15] Accordingly, administration of prophylactic agents must be begun just prior to operation and continued with repeated dosing every second half-life of the drug until the wound has been closed.

References

1. Bentley, D. W., and Lepper, M. H.: Septicemia related to indwelling venous catheter. JAMA 206:1749, 1968.
2. Bruck, H. M., Nash, G., Foley, F. D., and Pruitt, B. A., Jr.: Opportunistic fungal infection of the burn wound with phycomycetes and Aspergillus: A clinical-pathologic review. Arch. Surg. 102:476, 1971.
3. Burke, J. F.: The effective period of preventive antibiotic action in experimental incisions and dermal lesions. Surgery 50:161, 1961.
4. Clarke, J. S., Condon, R. E., Bartlett, J. G., et al.: Preoperative oral antibiotics reduce septic complications of colon operations: Results of prospective, randomized, double-blind clinical study. Ann. Surg. 186:251, 1977.
5. Committee on Trauma: A guide to prophylaxis against tetanus in wound management. Bull. Am. Coll. Surg., July 1979, pp. 19–20.
6. Copeland, E. M., MacFadyen, B. V., and Dudrick, S. J.: Effect of intravenous hyperalimentation on established delayed hypersensitivity in the cancer patient. Ann. Surg. 184:60, 1976.
7. Gorbach, S. L., and Bartlett, J. G.: Anaerobic infection. N. Engl. J. Med. 290:1177, 1237, 1289, 1974.
8. Haller, J. A., Jr., Shaker, I. J., Donahoo, J. S., et al.: Peritoneal drainage versus non-drainage for generalized peritonitis from ruptured appendicitis in children; a prospective study. Ann. Surg. 177:595, 1973.

9. Handbook of Antimicrobial Therapy. New Rochelle, Medical Letter, 1978.
10. Hau, T., Payne, W. D., and Simmons, R. L.: Fibrinolytic activity of the peritoneum during experimental peritonitis. Surg. Gynecol. Obstet. 148:415, 1979.
11. Hobson, W. B., Britt, L. G., Sherman, R. T., and Ledes, C. P.: The use of topical antibiotics in the prevention of experimental wound infection. J. Surg. Res. 8:261, 1968.
12. MacLean, L. D.: Host resistance in surgical patients. J. Trauma 19:297, 1979.
13. Pollock, A. V.: Surgical wound sepsis. Lancet 1:1283, 1979.
14. Stone, H. H.: Review of pseudomonas sepsis in thermal burns: Verdoglobin determination and gentamicin therapy. Ann. Surg. 163:297, 1966.
15. Stone, H. H., Haney, B. B., Kolb, L. D., et al.: Prophylactic and preventive antibiotic therapy: Timing, duration, and economics. Ann. Surg. 189:691, 1979.
16. Stone, H. H., Kolb, L. D., and Geheber, C. E.: Bacteriologic considerations in perforative necrotizing enterocolitis. South. Med. J. 72:1540, 1979.
17. Wang, M. S., and Wilson, S. E.: Subphrenic abscess: The new epidemiology. Arch. Surg. 112:934, 1977.

BURNS

James A. O'Neill, Jr., M.D.

7

Complications of burn injury are related not only to pathophysiology but also to the therapy necessary for the patient's recovery. Problems may occur at any time during the course of treatment, but those that occur late may be particularly dangerous since they are likely to go unnoticed. Virtually every organ system is in jeopardy, just as every system is affected by the trauma.

Complications may be divided into those related to infection and those related to other factors.

BURN WOUND INFECTION

Infection has always been the main cause of death in burn patients. Fortunately, knowledge about the characteristics of infection and the wound in which it occurs, as well as about factors involving host defense, has increased. Although the initial effect of heat is to sterilize skin, within 1 hour the wound surface becomes colonized by a multiplicity of bacterial organisms. Over a period of days there may be gradual involvement of skin appendages. Studies by Teplitz and others indicate that after 4 or 5 days in adults and after 2 or 3 days in children, infection may involve tissues around hair follicles to the point of focal invasion of adjacent underlying tissue.[28] Simultaneously, the bacterial flora may change from one that is predominantly gram positive to one that is gram negative and in which *Pseudomonas aeruginosa* predominates. This may progress to involvement of lymphatics and to bacterial vasculitis. The massive number of organisms may cause death even without embolic visceral involvement.

Topical antibacterial therapy was introduced in 1964 and has reduced the incidence of burn wound sepsis.[22] However, sepsis still occurs in patients with larger injuries and in those whose host defense is compromised. Alexander and his group have pointed out potential deficiencies at virtually every level of the immune arc.[2] Abnormalities of T-cell function, diminished production of immunoglobulin G, consumptive opsoninopathy, and altered neutrophil function have all been demonstrated. It is only by manipulation of all these factors that infection of burn wounds can be kept under control.

The diagnosis of burn wound infection is frequently best made by careful daily observation of the patient. Since the advent of topical antibacterial therapy, the classic clinical signs of burn wound sepsis have become more obscure (Fig. 7–1). Rather than presenting with classic wound degeneration and ecthyma gangrenosum, patients with burn wound sepsis now present with indolent wounds that fail to heal. Hypo- or hyperthermia and glucose intolerance may also occur. Blood cultures may be helpful. In contrast to gram-positive burn wound infection with early intravascular involvement, *Pseudomonas* invades the blood stream late. Quantitative bacterial analysis of burn wound biopsy specimens has proved to be one of the best guides to impending burn wound sepsis.[27] Biopsy should be performed weekly or twice weekly in patients at risk, particularly those with burns covering more than 40 per cent of the body surface. Quantitative bacterial counts in the range of 10^4 to 10^5 organisms per gram of tissue indicate that a change in therapy is in order. Patients with counts in the range of 10^6 to 10^7 organisms per gram have well-established sepsis. The options for therapy under these circumstances include a change in topical therapy, vigorous administration of systemic antibiotics, the use of subeschar clysis with specific antibiotics, and passive

86

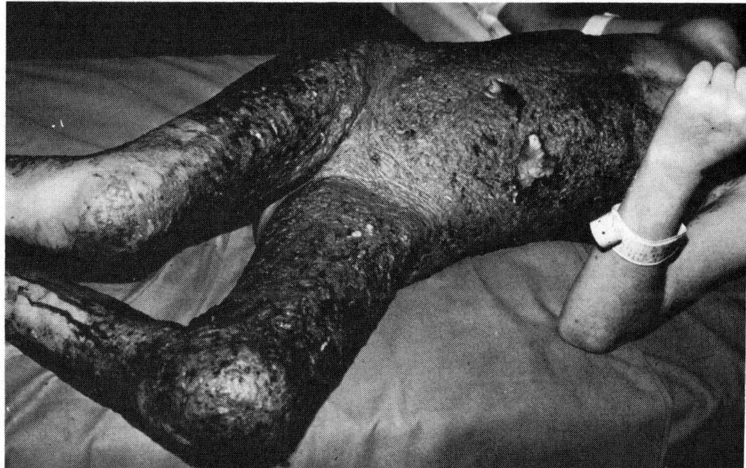

Figure 7–1 Child with burn wound sepsis. The classic clinical signs have been masked by topical antibacterial therapy. Quantitative bacterial analysis of burn wound biopsies is helpful in this regard.

immunization with *Pseudomonas* globulin.[7, 24] The last-named form of therapy has not yet been approved by the Food and Drug Administration but is known to be a valuable adjunct in the treatment of established *Pseudomonas* infection. It is advisable to perform weekly qualitative bacterial cultures for all patients in order to obtain information about the type of bacteria present and to determine antibiotic sensitivity should intensive therapy be needed later. This is becoming increasingly important, since the incidence of *Pseudomonas* infection has diminished somewhat and other opportunists such as *Klebsiella pneumoniae* and *Enterobacter cloacae* are appearing in numbers. Infections due to *Providencia stuartii* and *Serratia marcescens* are appearing in epidemic clusters. Although there may be some question about the efficacy of isolation techniques in the general care of burn patients, it is well accepted that isolation is a valuable adjunct when unusual opportunistic organisms appear.[8]

Systemic antibiotic therapy is sometimes helpful in the management of patients who have invasive infection, but unless there is sequential monitoring, the physician will not be aware of changing patterns of antibiotic sensitivity. Weekly reassessment is necessary in patients receiving systemic antibiotics to prevent the emergence of resistant organisms. Unless a patient is in imminent danger of dying of sepsis, antibiotics should be administered only after precise cultures have been obtained (Table 7–1). The patient's own gastrointestinal tract is usually the source of bacterial colonization; how-ever, bacteria may also gain access to the wound from the respiratory tract of the patient or ward personnel or from cross-contamination. Although isolation of each patient may not be practical, avoidance of cross-contamination is important.

The aim of topical therapy is to control the number of organisms within the burn wound and to prevent invasion with bacteremia. Bacteriologic surveillance is mandatory. Burn wound sepsis ordinarily occurs during the first 2 weeks following burn injury. Invasion is uncommon once a granulating bed has become established, even though the wound may appear suppurative.

Although topical antibacterial therapy can often suppress bacterial flora to noninvasive levels, the patient remains susceptible to repeated bouts of infection if the eschar is allowed to remain for a long time. Janžekovič has described a method of tangential excision of deep partial-thickness burns, but the technique is equally applicable to full-thickness burns.[14] Excision of eschar beginning about 7 days postburn and temporary coverage with biologic dressings prior to autografting are recommended in the management of patients with extensive burns

TABLE 7–1   PRINCIPLES OF ANTIBIOTIC USE IN BURN PATIENTS

Short-term prophylaxis for débridement
Sudden clinical deterioration
Appearance of signs of bacteremia
Positive blood culture
Quantitative bacterial count greater than 10^5/gm
Pneumonia or urinary tract infection

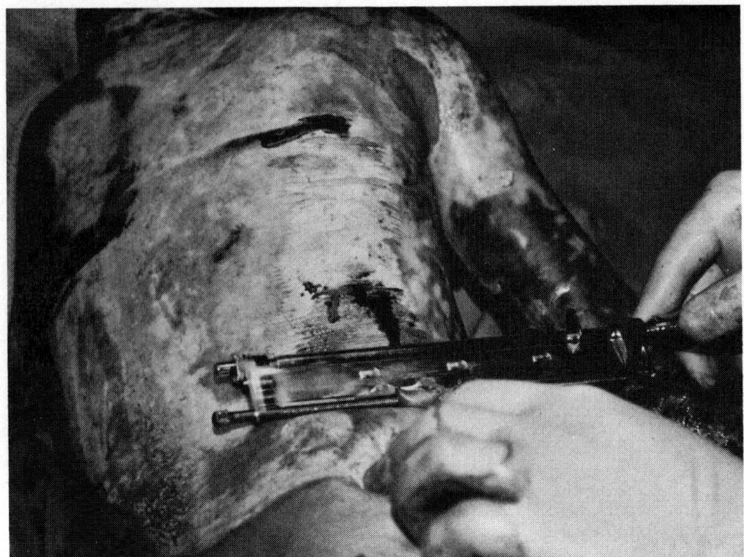

Figure 7–2 Tangential excision of deep partial-thickness burn 3 to 4 days postburn or of full-thickness burn approximately 7 days postburn is helpful in controlling infection and permitting expeditious wound coverage.

(Fig. 7–2). Initial efforts along these lines involved the use of enzyme débridement, but this has been shown to be associated with an increased incidence of sepsis.[13]

Topical antibacterial therapy itself may produce complications. Silver nitrate 0.5 per cent soaks, introduced by Moyer and associates, are used less often today because they necessitate use of dressings and cause undesirable staining of the environment.[22] In addition, since silver nitrate is applied in water, absorption of electrolyte-free water occurs, resulting in dilutional hyponatremia, hypochloremia, and hypokalemia. This may require determination of serum electrolyte levels every 4 to 6 hours initially and the administration of large amounts of salt and potassium. Use of mafenide acetate 10 per cent cream twice daily is associated with diuresis and inhibition of carbonic anhydrase, resulting in excretion of large amounts of bicarbonate and retention of chloride. As a consequence, hyperchloremic acidosis may occur and patients may present with hyperventilation. This can be minimized by applying mafenide only once daily after the first 2 or 3 days postburn. The administration of sodium bicarbonate or tromethamine may help correct the metabolic upset. Silver sulfadiazine 1 per cent cream applied twice daily produces the fewest complications. Although methemoglobinemia occurs in some patients with use of silver sulfadiazine cream, this is not ordinarily of clinical significance. Silver sul-

fadiazine must be used cautiously in patients with renal failure. Allergic sensitivity in the form of a maculopapular rash is noted in approximately 8 per cent of patients when mafenide or silver sulfadiazine is used. The rash may be controlled with modest doses of diphenhydramine hydrochloride. Superinfection or bacterial breakthrough may occur with any of the topical agents. Bacteriologic surveillance should indicate when a change in topical therapy is necessary.

Donor site infection is uncommon but disastrous because it represents a full-thickness skin loss. We prefer to cover donor sites with a single thickness of fine mesh gauze that is allowed to dry and gradually separate over a period of a week or so. When patients must lie on donor sites, the sites should be exposed at least every 6 hours. If donor sites appear infected, topical antibacterial therapy and local care are required.

METABOLIC COMPLICATIONS

Early metabolic complications are related primarily to fluid and electrolyte balance. During the first 24 hours postburn, 3 to 4 ml/kg/per cent burn of Ringer's lactate solution appears to meet most closely the fluid and sodium needs of the burned child.[6] If fluid administration is inadequate, particularly during the first 8 hours, nonoliguric or oliguric renal failure may ensue.[9] Careful monitoring of hourly urinary output and cardiac output and serial determinations of serum electrolyte levels and urea nitrogen concentration will ordinarily give the physician sufficient information to prevent this complication. After the first 24 hours, administration of half-normal saline solution in amounts appropriate to maintain urinary output in the range of 1 ml/kg/hr is ordinarily sufficient. The most common error in fluid and electrolyte therapy occurs after the second day postburn when evaporative water loss is the prime consideration in fluid therapy.[21] By this time, most patients are able to receive either oral or tube-administered feedings. Some confusion may occur then because urinary diuresis ordinarily begins at about this time. Hypernatremia and hyperosmolarity are the most common manifestations of inadequate replacement of free water lost by evaporation. This complication may be avoided by daily weighing of the patient and determination of serum electrolyte levels. Our method of correcting insensible water loss is to provide either oral fluid or intravenous 0.2 per cent normal saline in 5 per cent glucose solution in the range of 1 to 2 ml/kg/per cent burn/24 hr in addition to estimated normal daily maintenance requirements.

Virtually all burn patients have significant urinary potassium loss. If this potassium is inadequately replaced, cardiac arrhythmias may occur. From the standpoint of fluid balance, the majority of children who have sustained extensive burns will gain approximately 15 to 20 per cent of basal weight over 2 days and then lose it over the next 2 to 5 days. This approximate guideline is helpful in estimating the volume of fluid replacement.

Other mineral disturbances are ordinarily related to either long-term immobilization or extensive gastrointestinal secretory loss. Weekly determinations of serum calcium, phosphorus, and magnesium levels are required in such patients. In rare instances, patients who have been unable to take enteral feedings may become zinc deficient and have delayed wound healing.

The usual metabolic response of the burn patient is hypermetabolism.[29] Patients cared for in the ordinary hospital environment will have persistent fever (100 to 101°F), a reflection of increased metabolic rate. The hormonal mechanism consists of increased catecholamine and glucagon output with diminished insulin output. At the same time, there is increased oxygen consumption and glucose flow. This may lead to significant hyperglycemia and associated urinary loss of water with resultant dehydration. Determination of the serum glucose level is the key to managing this problem, which is accentuated in the child. The same factors cause negative nitrogen balance and rapid, extensive loss of lean body mass. Although diminished wound healing is one of the obvious consequences of diminished protein synthesis and negative nitrogen balance, another important consideration is the increased incidence of septic complications associated with malnutrition. Careful attention to provision of adequate amounts of calories and nitrogen has been shown to reverse negative nitrogen balance. Patients who are adequately nourished have a much lower incidence of lethal sepsis than do those who are malnourished.[18] Stress pseudodiabetes usually will not develop after the first week postburn. If it does occur later, the condition is most often associated with extensive surgical procedures or a septic complication. Continued monitoring of serum glucose levels may be helpful in anticipating the onset of sepsis, which might otherwise go unnoticed.

GASTROINTESTINAL COMPLICATIONS

Most children who have been seriously burned hyperventilate for the first several hours following injury. This may result in acute gastric dilatation, vomiting, and pulmonary aspiration. The early passage of a nasogastric tube is an important feature of care, particularly in patients who are to be transported. In addition to this, the circulatory changes associated with serious burn injury are such that cardiac output is distributed to areas of priority. The splanchnic circulation tends to suffer in this regard, with resulting intestinal ileus during the first 24 hours postburn.

Gastroduodenal endoscopy during the first 24 hours postburn has indicated that some degree of gastroduodenal ulceration occurs in most patients with serious burns.[19] In the past, serious bleeding occurred in 10 to 15 per cent of burn patients, particularly if sepsis was present. Since the advent of early milk feedings and the occasional use of intravenous cimetidine, the incidence of life-threatening bleeding has been dramatically reduced. Unfortunately, uncontrollable bleeding or even perforation will still occur in some patients. Duodenal ulcers account for the majority of these serious complications. Significant hemorrhage usually occurs during the first 10 days after injury in children with burns covering more than 40 per cent of the body surface, particularly when sepsis is present. Vagotomy, antrectomy, and excision of the ulcer, if possible, is the preferred surgical approach when conservative measures have failed.[26] The decision to operate should be based on the same criteria in burn patients as it is in other patients who have life-threatening hemorrhage of the upper gastrointestinal tract. Routine acid prophylaxis is clearly helpful. Frequent milk feedings satisfy this purpose while improving nutrition and fluid balance.

Elevation of hepatic enzymes has been noted in most patients, yet this is seldom clinically significant. Patients who have sustained major burn injury associated with early shock and hypoxemia may experience jaundice and cholestasis.[10] Some will demonstrate prolonged glucose intolerance and inability to metabolize drugs that are ordinarily well detoxified by the liver.

Overwhelming pancreatitis or acalculous cholecystitis may develop in patients who are seriously dehydrated as a result of inadequate replacement of evaporative water losses.[15] Sepsis may potentiate these problems. Diagnosis of these conditions is ordinarily delayed, particularly in those patients who have burns of the abdominal wall. The diagnosis is based on clinical suspicion plus abdominal tenderness in a patient who has gastric retention, ileus, sepsis, and perhaps disseminated intravascular coagulation. Determination of serum amylase and bilirubin levels is diagnostically helpful.

A late problem that may occur in burned children who have lost weight is obstruction of the duodenum by the superior mesenteric artery.[15] This syndrome is characterized by projectile, bile-stained vomiting following feedings. An upper gastrointestinal tract roentgenographic series reveals the characteristic picture of obstruction of the third portion of the duodenum. Obstruction is typically incomplete and may be associated with duodenal ulcer. Fortunately, the majority of these patients may be treated by positioning them in either the prone or the left lateral decubitus position and passing a feeding tube into the jejunum. Jejunal feedings and gastric decompression will ordinarily allow resolution of this problem as adequate weight is regained. Intravenous hyperalimentation is sometimes necessary. Occasional patients who do not respond to nutritional therapy within 10 to 14 days will require operative intervention and duodenojejunostomy.

Nasogastric feeding tubes are routinely required in children with extensive burns if adequate amounts of calories and protein are to be provided. The smallest tube possible should be used, and the head of the bed should be slightly elevated to minimize the effects of gastroesophageal reflux. Esophageal stricture may occur if this is not taken into account. Another complication related to indwelling nasogastric tubes is parotitis due to staphylococcal infection of the parotid gland. This is treated with appropriate antibiotics.

CARDIORESPIRATORY COMPLICATIONS

Cardiac complications are uncommon in the burned child as compared with adults. Bacterial endocarditis may develop in children with congenital cardiac disease if inadequate attention is paid to bacteriologic control and sepsis.[5] Intravenous catheters that have been left in place for long periods may cause infected vegetations on cardiac valves or around septal defects. *Staphylococcus aureus, Pseudomonas,* and *Candida albicans* are the most common organisms associated with this complication. The sudden appearance of a cardiac murmur or a change in character of a murmur already present is pathognomonic. Intensive long-term antibiotic therapy is necessary.

Cardiac arrhythmias due to hypokalemia should be suspected in any patient in whom sudden circulatory collapse and cardiac arrest occur. Patients with alkalosis and those taking digitalis are particularly at risk.

At present, respiratory complications are the most common cause of death in burn patients and occur immediately after burn injury or after the first week.[1] Upper airway obstruction is likely to occur in children as a result of edema of the head and neck or of the upper airway. Critical airway obstruction should be anticipated in such patients since placement of a naso- or orotracheal tube may be extremely difficult once edema has become established. Tracheostomy should be avoided at this stage since temporary endotracheal intubation ordinarily suffices. Patients who have been burned in an enclosed space may have inhaled noxious combustion products that result in tracheobronchial mucosal sloughing and obstruction. There may be significant hypoxemia. One of the best guides to therapy at this stage is the frequent determination of blood pH, P_{CO_2}, and P_{O_2}. Occasional patients may require tracheostomy, preferably with Silastic or molded plastic tubes. Endotracheal and tracheostomy tubes may cause ulcerative tracheobronchitis with bacterial invasion. Patients with upper airway obstruction and those with inhalation injury either die or are much improved by the end of the first week postburn. Treatment involves vigorous attention to tracheobronchial toilet, bronchoscopy, and assisted ventilation.

After the first week postburn, pulmonary complications are due to infection. Radiographs show atelectasis that may be explained by immobilization, plugging of endotracheal tubes, aspiration of vomitus, or even iatrogenic introduction of infection (Fig. 7–3). The ideal treatment of these late respiratory complications is to prevent them. During the second week postburn, spotty bronchopneumonia is usually due to burn wound sepsis with invasion. Careful bacteriologic monitoring of tracheobronchial secretions and appropriate antibiotic therapy form the basis for treatment along with intensive ventilatory support and tracheobronchial toilet. Steroids are to be avoided in these patients because they potentiate infection. Inhalation injury complicated by infection usually presents as a widely confluent bronchopneumonia. The causative organisms are ordinarily those found in the burn wound, with *Staphylococcus aureus* and *Pseudomonas* being most common. At this stage, tracheostomy may be lifesaving, but the risks and benefits of this procedure must be considered carefully. Pneumothorax may be avoided if tracheostomy is performed over an indwelling

endotracheal tube. Late-appearing, spotty pulmonary infiltrates are characteristic of hematogenous pneumonia. Multiple blood cultures should be performed and a careful search made for an extrapulmonary site of infection such as focal burn wound sepsis, soft tissue infections, or septic phlebitis.

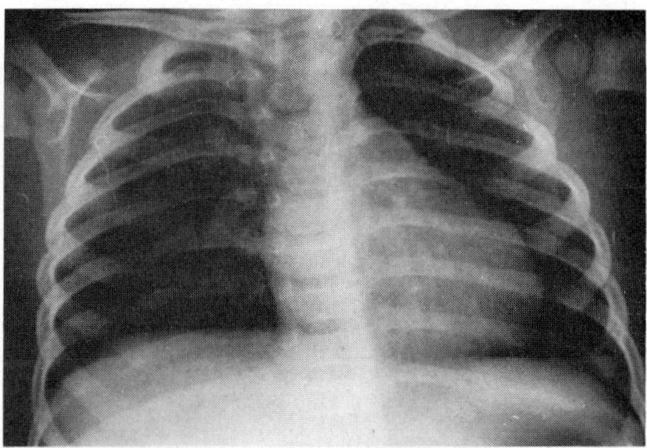
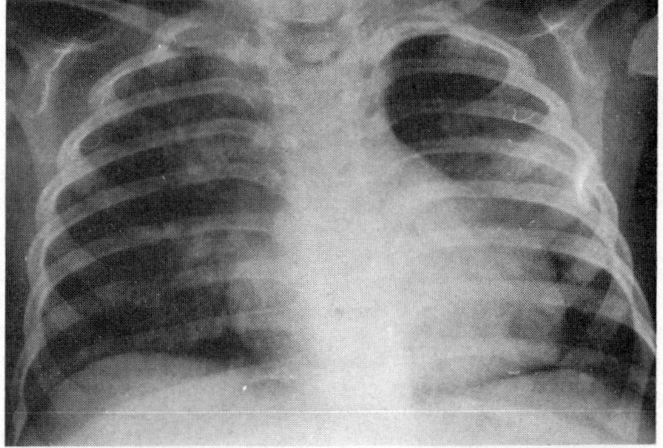
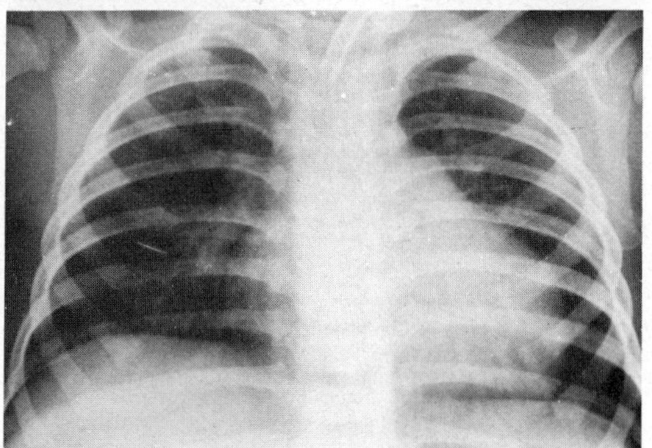

Figure 7–3 Chest radiographs showing normal lung fields at the time of hospital admission (*upper panel*). There are patchy, bilateral infiltrates and atelectasis typical of bronchopneumonia of the airborne type 10 days postburn (*middle panel*). Clearing occurred within 3 days with vigorous tracheobronchial toilet and antibiotic therapy (*lower panel*).

VASCULAR COMPLICATIONS

The most common problem related to the vascular tree is compression of arterial supply to the distal portions of the extremities by circumferential third-degree eschar. Although cyanosis of the distal digits, diminished capillary refill, the appearance of paresthesias, and coolness are helpful clinical signs indicating arterial compromise, the most helpful guide at present is the use of the Doppler ultrasonic flowmeter.[23] Blood flow should be evaluated hourly for the first 48 hours in patients who have circumferential burns of the extremities. Elevation and frequent active exercise are helpful. When there is any suspicion of inadequate arterial flow, escharotomy is indicated. The procedure involves incision through the eschar on the lateral and medial aspects of the extremities throughout the area of full-thickness burn. No anesthesia is required. Before escharotomy, the wound should be cleansed with povidone-iodine. Topical antibacterial agents should be applied over the escharotomy site after the procedure. Blood loss is rarely significant. Fasciotomy may be associated with invasive infection and should be avoided except in patients who have extremely deep burns or electrical injuries. Occasional patients will have deep injuries of the lower extremities that result in edema of the anterior compartment of the lower leg.[4] Fasciotomy may be necessary to prevent muscular necrosis in this restricted space.

One of the most common causes of sepsis after the first week postburn is suppurative thrombophlebitis.[25] This lethal complication results from colonization of a venous catheter and ordinarily does not become manifest until several days after removal of the catheter. Patients who have this condition present with unexplained fever or hematogenous pneumonia. Local signs of phlebitis may be present in only one of four patients with this complication. Suppurative thrombophlebitis may be avoided by sterile placement of intravenous catheters in unburned sites, careful daily care, and removal of such catheters as soon as possible after enteral feedings have been established. All intravenous catheters should be cultured when removed so that infection may be anticipated. If infection is present, gram-positive and gram-negative organisms are ordinarily found. When suppuration occurs, *Staphylococcus aureus* is the most common organism involved. In patients suspected of having suppurative thrombophlebitis, previously cannulated veins and cutdown sites must be explored and the involved vein totally excised (Fig. 7–4). Lesser forms of therapy are not effective. When pus is not encountered, systemic antibiotic therapy is sufficient. When long incisions have been required for

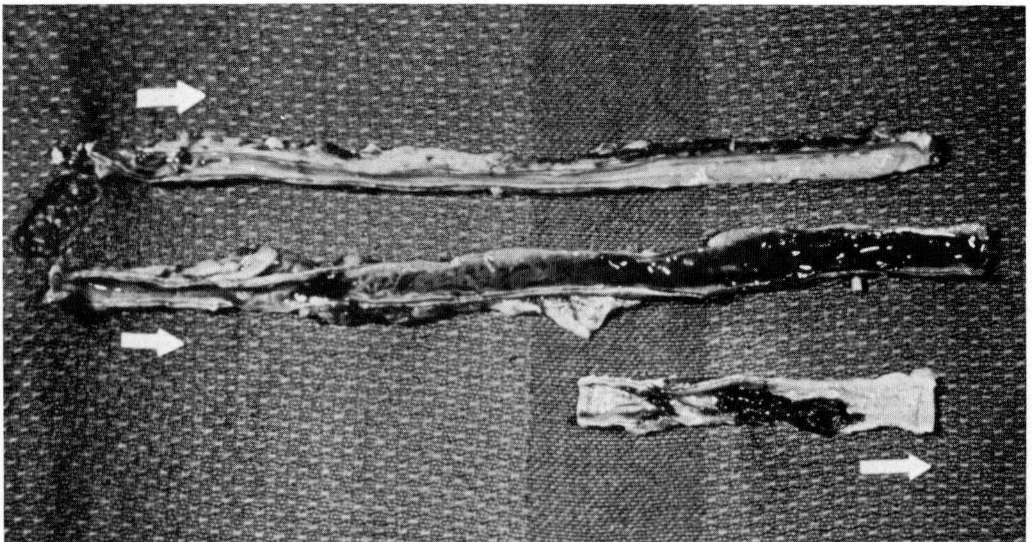

Figure 7–4 A pathologic specimen of the greater saphenous vein with the typical findings of pus and infected clot. Vein excision is the most effective treatment for suppurative thrombophlebitis.

excision of veins, they may be closed secondarily 5 to 7 days later. Infection of central veins that cannot be excised may result in septic pulmonary embolism or bacterial endocarditis. Under these circumstances, systemic heparinization in addition to intensive long-term intravenous antibiotic therapy may be helpful.

GENITOURINARY COMPLICATIONS

Reference has already been made to renal failure as a consequence of inadequate resuscitation during the shock phase immediately following burn. An additional early problem in patients with deep thermal burns is hemoglobinuria with distal tubular necrosis. Renal complications may be avoided by administration of appropriate doses of mannitol, provision of adequate intravenous fluids, and judicious use of diuretics such as furosemide. Renal flow will be reestablished within 4 to 6 hours if appropriate therapy is given.

Urinary catheters are used to monitor early intravenous therapy in children with extensive burn injury and should be removed as soon as possible. Although Foley-type catheters may be used in girls, such balloon catheters may be dangerous in small boys because associated trauma may result in stricture of the membranous urethra. Plain catheters or plastic feeding tubes are preferred. If urinary catheters are not removed soon enough, cystitis or pyelonephritis may occur. When prolonged catheter drainage is required, periurethral abscess may result, presenting in the perineum. Early mobilization helps to prevent calculi, which may cause pain and hematuria.

CONTRACTURES AND MUSCULOSKELETAL COMPLICATIONS

Hypertrophic scarring and contracture formation are common problems that may occur in spite of early active movement, early skin coverage, and splinting. The neck, axillae, and elbows are commonly involved (Figs. 7–5 and 7–6). Larson and coworkers have demonstrated that hypertrophic scarring is the result of contraction of an abnormal number of myofibroblasts that cause newly deposited collagen in the healing burn wound to fuse in an unfavorable manner.[17] They have shown that the ratio of contracting myofibroblasts to normal fibroblasts in the burn wound reaches a peak at about 3 months following healing and that this ratio declines over the following 6 to 9 months. For this reason, they suggested that compression dressings might be helpful. Ingenious compression garments and similar devices are currently available and have remarkably diminished the need for revisionary plastic surgical procedures. Compression garments should be used for 9 to 12 months following healing (Fig. 7–7).

In patients whose joints are immobilized

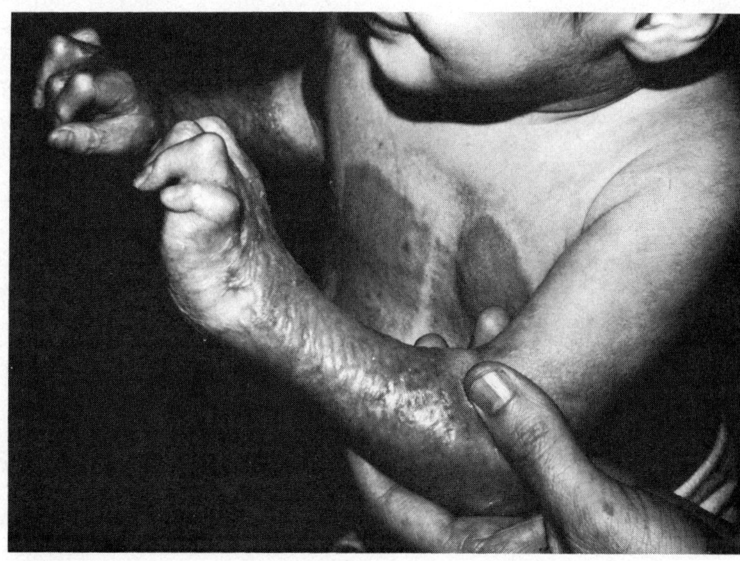

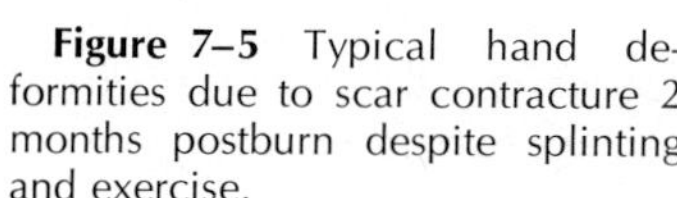
Figure 7–5 Typical hand deformities due to scar contracture 2 months postburn despite splinting and exercise.

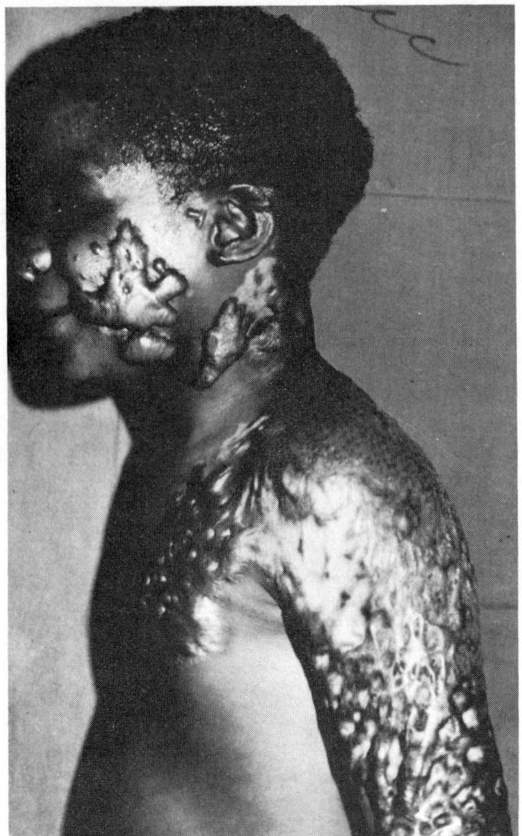

Figure 7–6 Severe hypertrophic scarring has developed in areas of healed deep partial-thickness burn, but there is very little scarring on the back, which was mesh grafted. Some deep partial-thickness burns are best treated by grafting because spontaneous healing may take too long.

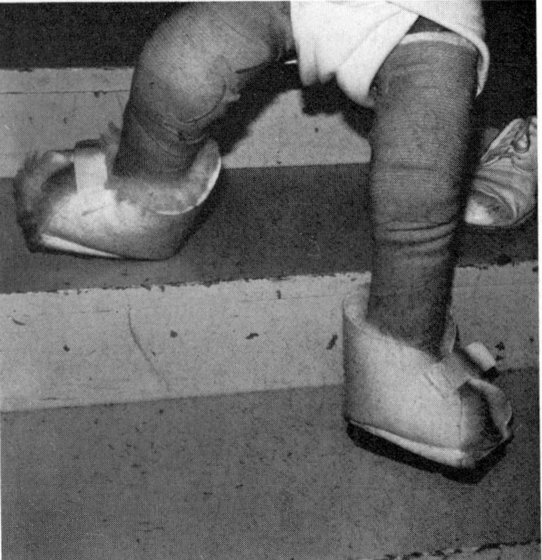

Figure 7–7 Compression dressings shown here followed by use of Jobst compression garments have provided substantial improvement in wound maturation, scar prevention, and avoidance of later contracture release.

for long periods, pericapsular calcification and heterotopic tendinous ossification may occur (Fig. 7–8).[12] Excision of calcified tissue and intensive mobilization therapy are required. Complications related to the joints themselves include ankylosis and dislocation, particularly of the hips. Septic arthritis may occur in persons in whom many femoral venipunctures have been performed. These children are seriously ill, requiring drainage of the hip and traction. Deep burns of the hands or feet may result in ankylosis of the distal joints, loss of articular cartilage or the epiphysis, soft tissue and muscle contracture with subluxation of phalangeal joints, and syndactyly.[16] Most of these problems may be avoided if the hands are given priority in early wound care and autograft coverage, followed by intensive physical therapy including dynamic splinting, active movement, and compression. Later growth disturbances such as scoliosis and inequality of the extremities may be avoided by long-term observation and correction of the cause of the deformity, usually a contracture.

Decubitus ulcers may develop in patients who have sustained extensive weight loss and who must remain immobilized in one position for long periods. The most common location of the ulcers is over the sacrum. Decubitus ulceration should be anticipated in patients who cannot be turned or moved about on a regular basis. Daily observation, which may be done most effectively at the time of hydrotherapy, is the key to prevention.

NEUROLOGIC COMPLICATIONS

Seizures may occur in children who have been bathed in hexachlorophene soap. This substance should be used minimally or not at all at the time of initial débridement and subsequent hydrotherapy treatment. Seizures may also occur later in the postburn period for no apparent reason. There is often a sudden upward or downward shift in the serum sodium level in these patients. Rarely, hypocalcemia or hypomagnesemia

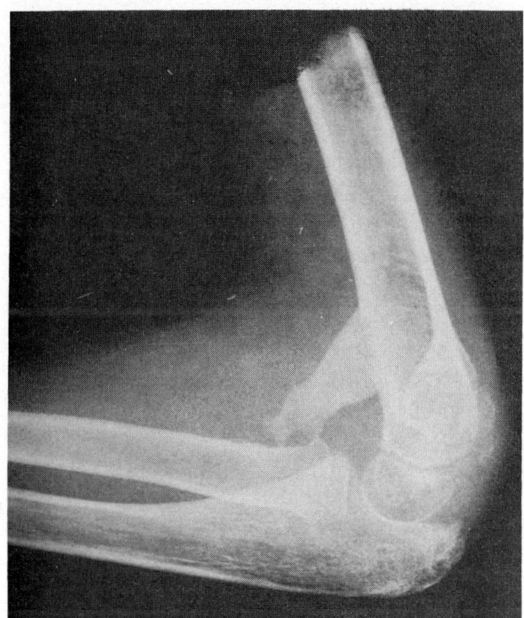

Figure 7–8 This radiograph demonstrates heterotopic peritendinous calcification after 6 weeks of elbow joint immobilization for burns.

may be responsible for neurologic complications in patients who have extensive gastrointestinal losses associated with sepsis. Peripheral neuropathies may occur in patients in whom inadequate mobilization has caused pressure over peripheral nerves. They may also occur as a result of improperly applied splinting devices or a constricting eschar, or as part of the anterior compartment syndrome.

COMPLICATIONS RELATED TO EYES AND EARS

Thermal damage to the cornea is, fortunately, unusual. If corneal ulceration is superficial, repeated application of antibiotic ophthalmic ointment and frequent cleansing are ordinarily sufficient for recovery within 7 days. In severe cases, it is necessary to suture the eyelids closed to allow for healing. More commonly, there will be a full-thickness burn of the lid in association with facial burns. This may result in ectropion since the skin of the eyelids is thin. Ectropion is of little consequence with respect to later appearance, but if it results in drying of the conjunctiva and cornea, a

corneal ulcer may develop. Secondary infection is frequent under these circumstances. It is best to anticipate this complication by performing tarsorrhaphy. Depending upon the stage at which this is required, tarsorrhaphy may be associated with the application of partial-thickness skin grafts to the upper and lower lids following incisional release of the contracted skin.[20] It is important to overcorrect the defect if permanent correction of the ectropion is to be accomplished.

If the thin skin covering the ears is damaged by burn, chondritis may occur. Although the incidence of this complication has decreased since the advent of topical antibacterial therapy, it still is seen occasionally. Suppurative chondritis frequently appears after the third week postburn with clinical signs of pain, tenderness, swelling, and fever. Once suppuration has occurred, the only effective form of therapy is to bivalve the skin of the ear and to excise all involved cartilage, leaving the wound open.[11] The ear should be dressed daily, splinting the bivalved edges with a dressing until granulation occurs, at which time healing can be completed. Unfortunately, major reconstructive procedures are required to replace the lost cartilage.

EMOTIONAL COMPLICATIONS

Follow-up studies of seriously burned patients indicate that the incidence of long-term psychiatric complications is low.[3] Characteristically, children who are under severe chronic stress, particularly when pain is involved, regress to more primitive stages of development. Disorientation occasionally occurs. Frequently, young children demonstrate hostility toward their parents and those who are caring for them. However, a compassionate nurse or other person who is spending a great deal of time with the child is usually able to break through and alleviate this type of behavior. It takes great understanding on the part of the parents in their response to this hostility. Reassurance by the physician may be helpful since hostility invariably disappears as the child recovers. A manifestation of psychosis in seriously burned children is self-destructive behavior in the form of bruxism with loss of teeth, biting of the tongue, and dislodgement of healed skin grafts. Gentle management and a sincere display of understanding and support by the entire burn team in conjunction with the family are vital. Use of effective, gentle restraint devices and judicious administration of drugs such as diazepam are helpful. Diazepam may minimize the need for narcotics, which may potentiate disorientation. Fears about deformity and mutilation may lead to serious depression. The hospital environment must be appropriate for children, and the regular introduction of toys and games may make the child's world more acceptable. Fortunately, our long-term experience has been that the overwhelming majority of children have recovered with little or no emotional disability.

References

1. Achauer, B. M., Allyn, P. A., Furnas, D. W., et al.: Pulmonary complications of burns: The major threat to the burn patient. Ann. Surg. 177:311, 1973.
2. Alexander, J. W., Ogle, C. K., Stinnett, J. D., and Macmillan, B. G.: A sequential, prospective analysis of immunologic abnormalities and infection following severe thermal injury. Ann. Surg. 188:809, 1978.
3. Andreasen, N. J., Noyes, R. J., Hartford, C. E., et al.: Management of emotional reactions in seriously burned adults. N. Engl. J. Med. 286:65, 1972.
4. Asch, M. J., Flemma, R. J., and Pruitt, B. A., Jr.: Ischemic necrosis of tibialis anterior muscle in burn patients: Report of three cases. Surgery 66:846, 1969.
5. Baskin, T. W., Rosenthal, A., and Pruitt, B. A.: Acute bacterial endocarditis: A silent source of sepsis in the burn patient. Ann. Surg. 184:618, 1976.
6. Baxter, C. R.: Fluid volume and electrolyte changes of the early postburn period. Clin. Plast. Surg. 1:693, 1974.
7. Baxter, C. R., Curreri, P. W., and Marvin, J. A.: The control of burn wound sepsis by the use of quantitative bacteriologic studies and subeschar clysis with antibiotics. Surg. Clin. North Am. 53:1509, 1973.
8. Burke, J. F., Quinby, W. C., Bondoc, C. C., et al.: The contribution of a bacterially isolated environment to the prevention of infection in seriously burned patients. Ann. Surg. 186:377, 1977.
9. Cameron, J. S., and Miller-Jones, C. M. H.: Renal function and renal failure in badly burned children. Br. J. Surg. 54:132, 1967.
10. Czaja, A. J., Rizzo, T. A., Smith, W. R., Jr., et al.: Acute liver disease after cutaneous thermal injury. J. Trauma 15:887, 1975.
11. Dowling, J. A.: Chondritis in the burned ear. Plast. Reconstr. Surg. 42:115, 1968.
12. Evans, E. B.: Musculoskeletal Changes Secondary to Burns. Philadelphia, W. B. Saunders Co., 1969, p. 347.
13. Hummel, R. P., Kautz, P. D., MacMillan, B. G., et al.: The continuing problem of sepsis following enzymatic debridement of burns. J. Trauma 14:572, 1974.
14. Janžekovič, Z.: A new concept in the early excision and immediate grafting of burns. J. Trauma 10:1103, 1970.
15. Kirksey, T. D., Moncrief, J. A., Pruitt, B. A., Jr., et al.: Gastrointestinal complications of burns. Am. J. Surg. 116:627, 1968.
16. Krizek, T. J., Robson, M. C., and Flagg, S. V.: Management of burn syndactyly. J. Trauma 14:587, 1974.
17. Larson, D. L., Abston, S., Evans, E. B., et al.: Techniques of decreasing scar formation and contractures in the burned patient. J. Trauma 11:807, 1971.
18. Lennard, E. S., Alexander, J. W., Craycraft, T. K., et al.: Association in burn patients of improved antibacterial defense with nutritional support by the oral route. Burns 1:98, 1975.
19. McAlhany, J. C., Czaja, A. J., Villarreal, Y., et al.: The gastric mucosal barrier in thermally injured patients: Correlation with gastroduodenal endoscopy. Surg. Forum 25:414, 1974.
20. Moncrief, J. A.: Burns of specific areas. J. Trauma 5:278, 1965.
21. Moncrief, J. A., and Mason, A. D.: Evaporative water loss in the burned patient. J. Trauma 4:180, 1964.
22. Moyer, C. A., Brentano, L., Gravens, D. L., et al.: Treatment of large human burns with 0.5% silver nitrate solution. Arch. Surg. 90:812, 1965.
23. Moylan, J. A., Jr., Inge, W. W., Jr., and Pruitt, B. A., Jr.: Circulatory changes following circumferential extremity burns evaluated by ultrasonic flowmeter: An analysis of 60 thermally injured limbs. J. Trauma 11:763, 1971.
24. O'Neill, J. A., Jr., Nance, F. C., and Fisher, M. W.: Heptavalent pseudomonas vaccination in seriously burned children. J. Pediatr. Surg. 6:547, 1971.
25. O'Neill, J. A., Jr., Pruitt, B. A., Jr., Foley, F. D., et al.: Suppurative thrombophlebitis — a lethal complication of intravenous therapy. J. Trauma 8:256, 1968.
26. O'Neill, J. A., Jr., Pruitt, B. A., Jr., and Moncrief, J. A.: Surgical treatment of Curling's ulcer. Surg. Gynecol. Obstet. 126:40, 1968.
27. Pruitt, B. A., Jr., and Foley, F. D.: The use of biopsies in burn patient care. Surgery 73:887, 1973.
28. Teplitz, C.: Pathogenesis of Pseudomonas vasculitis and septic lesions. Arch. Pathol. 80:297, 1965.
29. Wilmore, D. W.: Metabolic changes in burns. *In* Artz, C. H. P., Moncrief, J. A., and Pruitt, B. A., Jr. (eds.): Burns: A Team Approach. Philadelphia, W. B. Saunders Co., 1979, pp. 120–131.

HEAD AND NECK | 2

8

CENTRAL NERVOUS SYSTEM

Ken R. Winston, M.D.

Early and accurate diagnosis of complications depends upon personal knowledge, the experience of others, and alertness to possibilities and probabilities. The most important things to know about neurosurgical complications are how to avoid them and how best to manage them when they do occur. The central nervous system is relatively unforgiving of technical errors and insult. The increased technical difficulty of operating upon the relatively small neural structures in children is partially counterbalanced by the remarkable ability of the young to recover from injury.

Complications that occur exclusively or most commonly in children will be considered; however, not all of them can be included. Some complications deserve discussion because of the frequency with which they occur, others because something special has been learned through painful experience. Complications that occur in patients of all ages are discussed in more comprehensive works such as *Postoperative Complications in Neurosurgical Practice* by Horwitz and Rizzoli.[42] Many complications of pediatric neurosurgery are described in Matson's textbook.[52]

All surgical procedures, indeed all therapeutic endeavors, involve some risk of complication. Examined retrospectively, most complications occurring in pediatric neurosurgery could have been avoided. Surgical complications and unsatisfactory results are *not* synonymous. There is no substitute for experience and knowledge of the disorder being treated.

COMPLICATIONS OF SHUNTS FOR DIVERSION OF CEREBROSPINAL FLUID

The most common operation in pediatric neurosurgery is the insertion (or revision) of a tube to divert cerebrospinal fluid (CSF) from the ventricles to some distal site. Discussion of complications of CSF shunts in children without considering the reason for the shunt is disturbingly artificial. Shunts are inserted in patients with tumor, trauma, infection, hemorrhage, and congenital anomaly. The majority of complications of pediatric neurosurgery are, in one way or another, related to these operations.

Failure to detect a child's need for a shunt is a well-recognized error. Less well known are the problems resulting from insertion of shunts in children who never needed the device. Some children with achondroplasia have received shunts that they did not need. Most achondroplastic children have a head circumference that is greater than the 97th percentile and ventricles that are larger than normal, but few have elevated intracranial pressure or symptoms and signs thereof. Once a shunt has been inserted and left in place for months or years, the patient typically becomes "shunt dependent" and is permanently exposed to the risks associated with shunts.

Symptoms of Shunt Failure

Shunt failure most often produces symptoms of elevated intracranial pressure but may present in other ways. Occasionally shunt failure occurs without symptoms. Children who are unable to make their symptoms known (those less than 2 years of age, the retarded, and those whose ability to communicate is impaired) must be watched closely for evidence of shunt failure.

Shunt failure in a patient who is wholly dependent on the shunt produces sudden symptoms and signs of elevated intracranial pressure, with rapid neurologic deterioration. If the patient is not treated, cardiorespiratory arrest may occur within 1 or 2 hours. There is no more urgent situation in

99

neurosurgery. Delay in diagnosis and treatment can result in permanent neurologic dysfunction or death. Resuscitation from cardiorespiratory arrest due to elevated intracranial pressure can be difficult or impossible until the intracranial hypertension is reduced.

Patients who are not totally dependent on their shunts have less acute symptoms. Fortunately, most patients are in this category. The intracranial pressure rises but neither as high nor as rapidly as in a patient who is totally shunt-dependent. Elevated intracranial pressure in patients in the first group does not significantly alter CSF production.

Infants with shunt failure often become irritable and cannot be calmed. The anterior fontanelle appears full and veins may become more prominent over the scalp and forehead. "Spitting up" or vomiting may occur. Fever may accompany shunt failure; if it does, infection must be suspected. Lethargy and anorexia are common. Parents often report a change in the eyes such as "the eyes have become crossed," "one eye is lazy," or "the eyes look glassy."

Children who are able to describe their symptoms complain of headache that is typically, but not necessarily, midfrontal in location. It may be intermittent or constant and may occur only in the early morning or in the evening. It is often described as pounding in character and, in contrast to low pressure headache, may be accentuated when the patient lies down. Unlike migraine it is rarely unilateral and may be associated with photophobia.

Nausea, vomiting, and anorexia are common symptoms of shunt failure in older children. Many experience a diminished state of alertness or consciousness. Blurred vision and diplopia are common. Stiff neck, cervical spinal pain, and low back pain are uncommon. Seizures may indicate shunt failure, particularly in patients with a history of such attacks. Swelling or discomfort along the subcutaneous course of the shunt, usually at the upper end or near the valve, may occur.

Signs of Shunt Failure

Examination of an open fontanelle or craniectomy site provides a reliable means of estimating intracranial pressure. With the patient supine, the head is tilted upward until the fontanelle becomes flat. The *vertical* difference between the anterior fontanelle and the central venous pressure, which is approximately zero at the midpoint of the clavicle, is then measured. Normal intracranial pressure in an infant is 0 to 40 ml of CSF — far below normal for an adult.[95] A bulging fontanelle that is palpably taut is a sign of very high intracranial pressure.

There are several less direct indicators of intracranial pressure. The most useful of these is an examination of the optic fundi. Papilledema is a useful sign when present, but it is not commonly seen in very young children with shunt failure. A funduscopic examination is difficult or impossible in an uncooperative infant for whom sedation is contraindicated and mydriatics are not advisable. The absence of papilledema is not a very useful sign in these patients.

Abducens palsy (unilateral or bilateral) is a nonspecific indication of elevated intracranial pressure. Defects of the visual field and loss of acuity are less common. Oculomotor palsy, facial palsy (occasionally bilateral), and impaired hearing have been observed. Paralysis of the vocal cords has been reported in myelodysplastic children with shunt failure.

Measurement of maximum circumference of the head can be useful in identifying patients with chronically elevated intracranial pressure. An increase that exceeds the value predicted from a standard growth chart suggests failure of the shunt. Hyperelevation of the lids ("setting sun eyes") is often present with inability to gaze upward[78]; in its most severe form there is forced downward deviation of the eyes with hyperelevation of the lids. Spasticity and hyperreflexia, particularly in the lower extremity, may be caused by ventricular dilatation, which compresses and stretches the supratentorial portion of the corticospinal tracts.

Decorticate and decerebrate posturing, when due to elevated intracranial pressure, is probably caused by downward transtentorial herniation that may stretch or tear perforating vessels. Bradycardia, systolic hypertension, elevated pulse pressure, and disturbances in respiration are not common in infants. The physician should never await these signs before taking action, because they are really signs of impending death of the brain stem.

Fluctuance along the shunt that can be obliterated or displaced by manual pressure indicates that cerebrospinal fluid has leaked into the subcutaneous tissue and suggests infection or a disconnected shunt.

Crusts that develop over the shunt, particularly along one of the incisions, should be cleared away and the area inspected because this may be a sign of erosion of some part of the shunt through the skin. This is particularly likely to occur at the site of abrasion by a cast, in the very thin skin of premature infants, and in patients who lie on the shunt for long periods (e.g., severely retarded children, those with very large heads, and neglected children).

Direct measurement of intracranial pressure is accomplished by inserting a needle into a CSF-containing space that communicates with the ventricular system. If there is uncertainty about communication between the ventricles and the lumbar theca, lumbar puncture may expose the patient to an unnecessary risk of brain herniation. It is usually safer, quicker, and easier to measure the intracranial pressure through a needle inserted into the reservoir proximal to the valve. If the ventricular tube is obstructed and the child's intracranial pressure is critically elevated, a spinal needle can be inserted into the ventricular system by passing it through or adjacent to the reservoir.

Assessing a Child with a Shunt

A child with a shunt should be examined regularly. In a relatively uncomplicated case with a shunt inserted a few days after birth, I would evaluate the patient at age 1 month, 3 months, every 6 months until age 5 years, yearly for about 5 years, and every 2 years thereafter. This should be adjusted according to the child's diagnosis, condition, and age; the physician's perception of the parent's reliability in detecting problems and the physician's familiarity and experience with such patients. The purposes of regularly scheduled appointments with a neurosurgeon are (1) to anticipate difficulties with the shunt and thereby avoid them and (2) to identify shunt failure that has not been recognized by the patient or family. It

is the practice in this institution to schedule an elective revision (lengthening) of the appropriate parts of the shunt a few months before an anticipated failure.

Each examination of a child with a shunt must be done with an underlying suspicion that the shunt may be malfunctioning. Shunt failures may be total, partial, or intermittent and do not necessarily cause symptoms. If the anterior fontanelle is open, the intracranial pressure can be estimated on the basis of clinical criteria. Head circumference should be measured and compared with past measurements (if available) using a standard graph. The function of extraocular muscles should be checked and a funduscopic examination attempted. The child should not be sedated nor should pupils be routinely dilated. Any decrease in level of consciousness that is not well explained is highly significant. It is unwise to attribute such a finding to fatigue or lack of sleep. Many of the symptoms of shunt failure, particularly in infants, are also symptoms of the common disorders of childhood.

A persistent, unexplained problem such as fever of undetermined origin, anemia, failure to thrive, change in personality, or deterioration of school performance may be related to shunt failure or to a chronically infected shunt.[25]

Symptoms that could be due to shunt failure should never be ignored. Antibiotics and other medications should not be prescribed without definite indications. Patients who have symptoms but few if any signs of shunt failure are best managed by an overnight stay in the hospital for observation. The attribution of symptoms to psychological problems (e.g., school phobia) is ill-advised.

NEURODIAGNOSTIC TESTS

Radiographs of the shunt (usually lateral and anteroposterior views of the skull and of the abdomen or chest) are often helpful in evaluating a child with shunt failure and are occasionally diagnostic.[2]

Most of the shunts currently in use are radiopaque, but occasionally a patient with a radiolucent shunt is encountered. If it becomes important to visualize the shunt in these patients, a water-soluble radiopaque material can be injected carefully into the system.[16, 32, 51, 74]

Computed tomography of the head will show ventricular size and shape, information that may be useful — particularly if there is an earlier scan for comparison. Computed tomography can be very useful in identifying size, shape, and location of CSF-containing cavities and the position of the ventricular catheter. It does not provide direct information about pressure, but a change in ventricular size gives reliable indirect information.

It is occasionally useful to evaluate function using a radiopharmaceutical material.[28]

PUMPING THE VALVE

The evaluation of a shunt by manually pumping the valve is frequently a source of misunderstanding and misinterpretation. A single manual compression of the pumping mechanism can force (suck) tissue (choroid plexus or ependyma) into the openings of the ventricular catheter and cause an immediate total obstruction of the shunt in a child who came to the examiner with an adequately functioning shunt. In children with small ventricles the valve should not be pumped as part of the routine examination. In other children the valve should be cautiously compressed once to about the halfway point and released.

Little useful information is gained by repeatedly compressing the valve (or flushing device) and seeing or feeling its refill.[62] If the valve *cannot* be compressed manually, the shunt is not functioning. The possibility of this finding is the only justification for pumping the valve in an asymptomatic child. The observation that the valve is "easy to compress" has little value. "Slow refill," depending upon the definition of "slow," occurs in nearly half of all patients with adequately functioning shunts. Very slow refilling (one-half hour or more) does not necessarily mean that the shunt is malfunctioning but may reflect a very low intracranial pressure. Conversely, we have seen patients with proven shunt failure whose valves were easily compressed and then quickly refilled; the pumping action moved fluid "to and fro" within a totally occluded system.

Infection Involving a Shunt

Infection involving a CSF shunt was the most common complication occurring in neurosurgical patients of all ages until the middle 1970's. Approximately 10 to 20 per cent of patients with shunts had at least one infection involving the nervous system, and approximately 10 per cent of all CSF shunt operations were followed by infection.[27, 30, 33, 47, 69, 77, 79, 82] At present, a new infection develops in approximately 2 per cent of patients undergoing shunt surgery.[94, 96] Reduction of the infection rate resulted in great part from a better understanding of the problem. The most common offending organism is *Staphylococcus epidermidis,* which is abundantly present on normal skin and is rarely pathogenic in other settings. The bacteriophage type of *Staphylococcus epidermidis* responsible for the infection is usually on the patient's skin. Most shunt infections become apparent within a few days or weeks after an operation on the shunt.[30] There is no effective host resistance within the lumen of the shunt. Most shunt infections result from contamination at the time of operation by organisms from the patient's skin.[7-9, 88] The list of organisms that have been involved in shunt infections is extensive. Hematogenous spread from other sites of infection is well known.

In all patients in whom shunt infection is suspected, ventricular fluid must be examined microscopically and bacteriologically. Usually the best place to obtain fluid is from the reservoir proximal to the valve or from the valve itself using a small-gauge needle inserted through skin that has been shaved and cleaned well. Bacteria identified on Gram stain or by culture of this fluid give conclusive evidence of infection. The presence of more than five to 10 white cells suggests infection. It is our custom to inject 1 to 2 mg of gentamicin sulfate (Garamycin) in a volume of 2 to 4 ml at the completion of each shunt tap.

TECHNIQUE FOR INSERTION OF A SHUNT

Insertion of a CSF shunt is, in principle, a simple procedure, but perhaps the simplicity accounts for many of the complications. A small break in sterile technique can and often does lead to infection; error in the assembly and placement of the shunt will probably lead to mechanical failure. In most patients at the Children's Hospital Medical Center in Boston, CSF is diverted from the lateral ventricles to the peritoneal cavity. Shunts diverting CSF into the peritoneal cavity require fewer revisions and have fewer complications than do shunts that enter the venous system.

The prophylactic use of antibiotics is one of the most important measures in preventing shunt infections. The following regimen is used at the Children's Hospital Medical Center[94, 96]:

1. Oxacillin 25 mg/kg intravenously every 4 hours for 1 or 2 days. The first dose is given during induction of anesthesia. In newborns the dose is 50 mg/kg and is repeated every 12 hours for the same duration.

2. Gentamicin sulfate (Garamycin) 3 to 5 mg (1 or 2 mg/ml) is injected into the ventricular catheter through the reservoir just before the skin is closed (a single dose).

3. All wounds are irrigated with polymyxin B 0.2 mg/ml and neomycin 0.4 mg/ml in 0.9 per cent saline solution immediately before closure (but after the peritoneum is closed).

All buried sutures used in closing the skin should be absorbable. Poorly approximated skin edges and unnecessarily tight sutures delay healing, increase the risk of infection, and produce excessive scar tissue.

TREATMENT OF CHILD WITH INFECTED SHUNT

The best method of treating a child with an infected shunt is a subject of disagreement. Some authors have recommended that antibiotics be administered and that the shunt not be changed; others have advocated antibiotics and a single operation to replace the shunt.[55, 61, 66] We use the following approach. The entire shunt is removed, and a new ventricular catheter is inserted and connected to a subcutaneous reservoir. The skin is closed. A needle is inserted percutaneously into the reservoir and connected by a tube to a bottle for continuous ventricular drainage (CVD).[75] All connections in the CVD are covered with povidone-iodine

(Betadine) ointment and wrapped with a dressing sponge (taped in place) to ensure a sterile connection and to discourage disconnection for examination. The bottle should be changed daily, and CSF is cultured and examined microscopically (cell count) every 1 to 2 days. It has been our practice to give oxacillin intravenously from the time the infection is discovered; gentamicin sulfate (Garamycin) is injected intraventricularly each day. This regimen of antibiotics may have to be changed after the organism is identified and its sensitives determined. Typically the CVD remains in place for about 1 week, but it has been used for 4 weeks or longer. The site of needle puncture should be changed every 4 to 6 days: A new shunt is inserted after the infection has been eliminated.

If infection persists despite adequate concentrations of appropriate antibiotics in ventricular fluid,[91, 97] infection probably exists in a site protected from the antibiotic. Two possibilities must be considered: (1) The ventricular catheter has become colonized, or (2) there is a CSF-containing compartment that does not communicate with the one being drained. Fluid may collect in subdural spaces, or the patient may have one or more isolated ventricles or a subarachnoid cyst.

Isolated Compartments. If one or more CSF-containing spaces (ventricles or cysts) are not in communication with the ventricle being drained by the shunt, the patient may have symptoms and signs suggesting shunt failure. The presence of a shunt may predispose to stenosis or occlusion of the aqueduct of Silvius.[26] Occasionally this results in an isolated fourth ventricle that requires a shunt.[37] Intracranial herniations (transfalx or transtentorial) may develop. If the ventricles do not communicate, two or more ventricular catheters, each with its own reservoir, must be inserted. It is important that all be brought together proximal to a single valve. This eliminates the risk of intracranial herniations due to differences in performance of valves.

Complications Involving the Ventricular Catheter

Careful attention to the length of a catheter and to the direction of its advancement into the brain usually avoids penetration of thalamus, brain stem, or internal capsule. Such complications occur most often in children with small ventricles in whom multiple attempts are made through a parietal burr hole to achieve proper placement. Not only does a malpositioned catheter fail to function but the lesion produced by its insertion may also cause severe neurologic deficits such as hemiparesis.

If white matter overlies the proximal holes of the ventricular catheter, tissue will enter the lumen of the catheter and occlude it. This complication could result from the insertion of a catheter that is too short or too long, from normal growth of the brain, or from re-expansion of a compressed brain. Initially the catheter may not appear too long; however, the catheter tip can become embedded as the ventricles decrease in size owing to re-expansion of the brain or as the entire shunt migrates downward (Fig. 8–1). A catheter in which the holes are too far back from the tip runs the risk that at least some of the holes will be surrounded by white matter. It is best to choose a catheter with holes that are confined to the distal 1 to 1.5 cm.

The most common cause of shunt failure is obstruction of the ventricular catheter by choroid plexus that has grown into the lumen. This can happen only when the perforated portion of the ventricular catheter is in contact with the choroid plexus. The frontal and occipital horns do not contain choroid plexus; therefore, either site is satisfactory. The temporal horn is probably the worst intraventricular location, but the body of the lateral ventricles should also be avoided. In some children with very small ventricles it may be necessary to accept a less desirable site because no other site is available. In so doing the surgeon should recognize the increased risk of shunt failure from obstruction of the ventricular catheter.

Tissue that enters the ventricular catheter either during the insertion of a new catheter or at some later time[12] can obstruct the outflow from the reservoir. Such tissue can be removed only by an operation.

Occasionally a nonfunctional ventricular catheter cannot be removed easily during surgery. If the catheter cannot be removed by several seconds of firm traction, it is best to leave it in place and insert a new catheter. Growth of the choroid plexus into and around catheters with phalanges produces the firm attachment. Removal of such a catheter often produces a small intraventricular hemorrhage. The hemorrhage usually

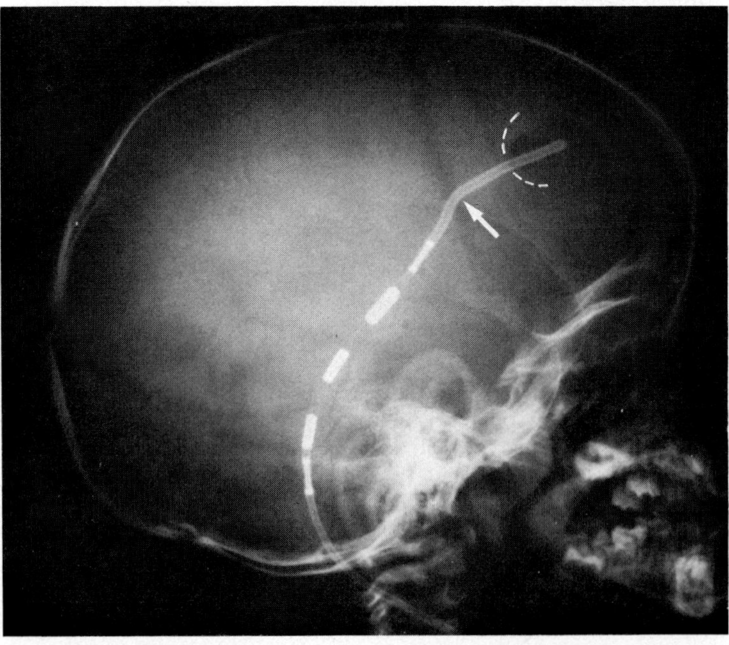

Figure 8–1 The ventricular catheter is in a very poor position. The entire shunt has been retracted downward. Note that the angle in the catheter (*arrow*) should be at the edge of the burr hole. This system contains a Hakim (pediatric-size) valve and reservoir.

stops quickly but is always a source of concern because blood in the ventricular fluid can impair the functioning of the valve.

SHUNT FAILURE DUE TO SLIT VENTRICLES

This serious complication is occurring with increasing frequency. Its pathophysiology is not well understood. Typically the patient presents with shunt failure, and evaluation reveals obstruction of the ventricular catheter. Computed tomography, if done, demonstrates abnormally small ventricles. Sometimes no ventricles are apparent. Slit ventricles are probably one result of chronic exposure to abnormally low intracranial pressure; the brain and calvarium grow in such a way that the ventricles become progressively smaller.[19, 45] The ependymal surface of the ventricle comes into contact (or nearly so) with the holes in the ventricular catheter. Minor changes in pressure (e.g., as produced by manual pumping of the valve) may occlude the holes in the catheter; once occluded, intracranial pressure rises very rapidly in such a small cavity.

At operation, minor changes in length or position of the catheter may appear to solve the problem but often do not. The insertion of a higher-pressure valve may relieve the problem. Several authors have reported success with subtemporal craniectomies.[20, 41]

DISCONNECTED VENTRICULAR CATHETER

Occasionally a ventricular catheter becomes disconnected from the remainder of the shunt. If the external tip of the catheter is near the dura, it may be possible to retrieve it with a hemostat or a curved needle. If the catheter is free within the ventricular cavity, it is best to leave it since it rarely causes difficulty. Catheters have been removed with the aid of a ventricular scope, but this requires a new and larger opening through the brain and, in the absence of infection, is usually not justified. This complication can be avoided by making a secure connection between the ventricular catheter and the next portion of the shunt.

Other Discontinuities in the System

Discontinuities in the shunt, whether caused by disconnection or by break, are

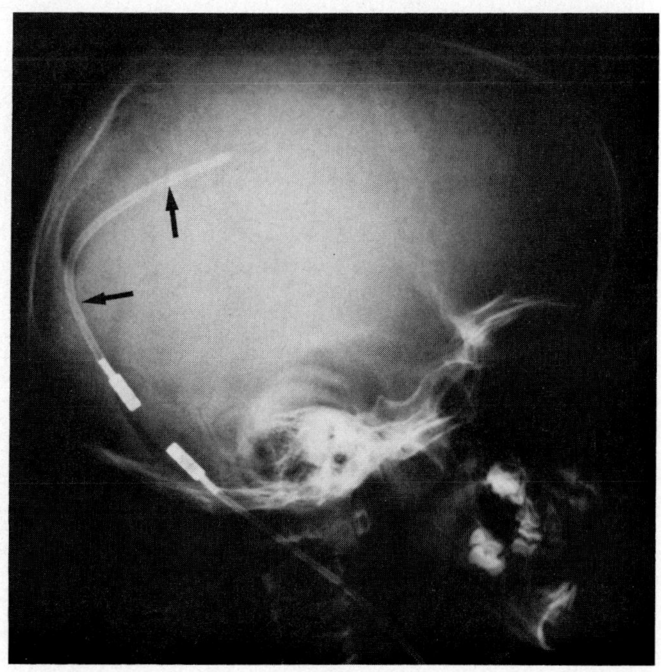

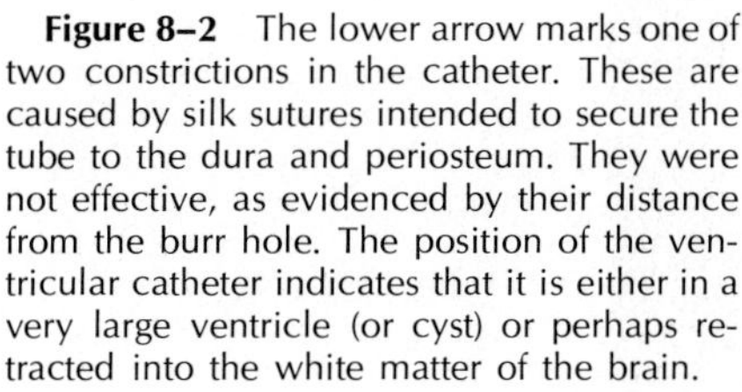

Figure 8–2 The lower arrow marks one of two constrictions in the catheter. These are caused by silk sutures intended to secure the tube to the dura and periosteum. They were not effective, as evidenced by their distance from the burr hole. The position of the ventricular catheter indicates that it is either in a very large ventricle (or cyst) or perhaps retracted into the white matter of the brain.

common causes of shunt failure. If the ligature is too tight, it will constrict (Fig. 8–2) or cut circumferentially through the Silastic. Most connectors are made of metal, but some are of radiolucent plastic.

Another cause of disconnection is the separation of the Silastic cap from the funnel-shaped portion of the reservoir (not all are manufactured this way). Downward traction on the shunt caused by surgical manipulations, trauma, or normal growth can pull the Silastic cap off the reservoir. Palpation of a disconnected reservoir sometimes discloses an abnormal amount of mobility. On several occasions the cap has been disconnected from the metallic portion by a needle inserted for the purpose of obtaining fluid from the reservoir. Once disconnected, the only treatment is an operation to reconnect the two parts.

A disconnected tube often migrates along the track of the shunt. Catheters have been found free in the peritoneal, pleural,[13] and ventricular cavities, in the scrotum,[69, 70] and in the superior vena cava, heart, and pulmonary artery (see later).

A discontinuity in the shunt system due to a break is unusual, but when this happens it tends to be near a valve or connector. Physi-

cal disruption of the valve (Fig. 8–3) is also rare.

The pumping mechanism for some brands of shunts is discoid in shape and is positioned directly over the burr hole. These systems may not contain a separate reservoir. The outflow arm of either system may rotate 90 degrees or more in the early postoperative period (i.e., before it is securely locked in place by fibrous tissue); this kinks and usually occludes the outflow arm of the reservoir. This complication can sometimes be detected by palpation of the system but should be obvious on a radiograph. It can be prevented by attaching the system to the pericranium with one or more sutures.

Complications Related to the Valve

There are many types of valves in use today. Most of these lie beneath the scalp and distal to the site of exit of the ventricular tube. Partial or complete obstruction within the valve may result from blood or solid tissue within the valve but is often due to mechanical failure of the valve itself (Fig. 8–4). It is easy to check the operating

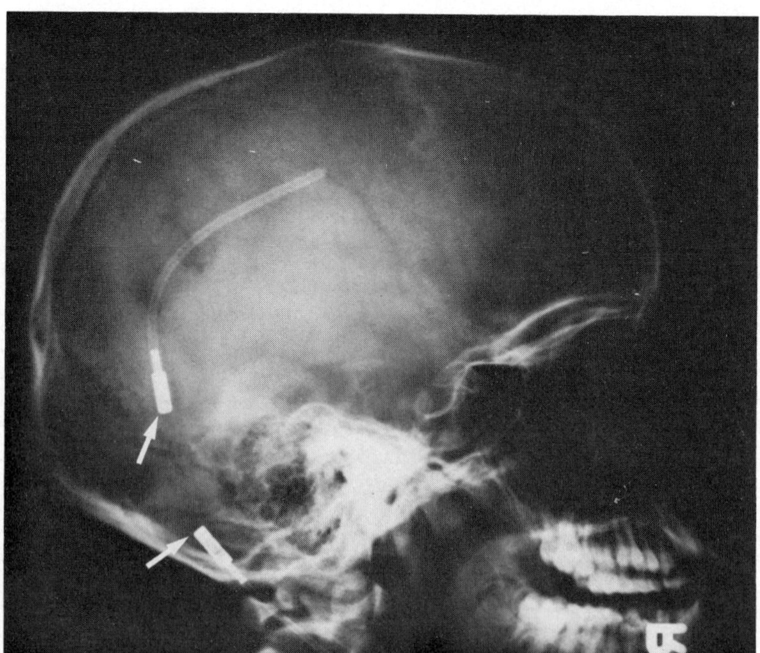

Figure 8–3 This valve has separated, which is apparent from the abnormal distance between the parts of the valve and from their orientation. Position of the ventricular catheter strongly suggests that the lateral ventricle is very large.

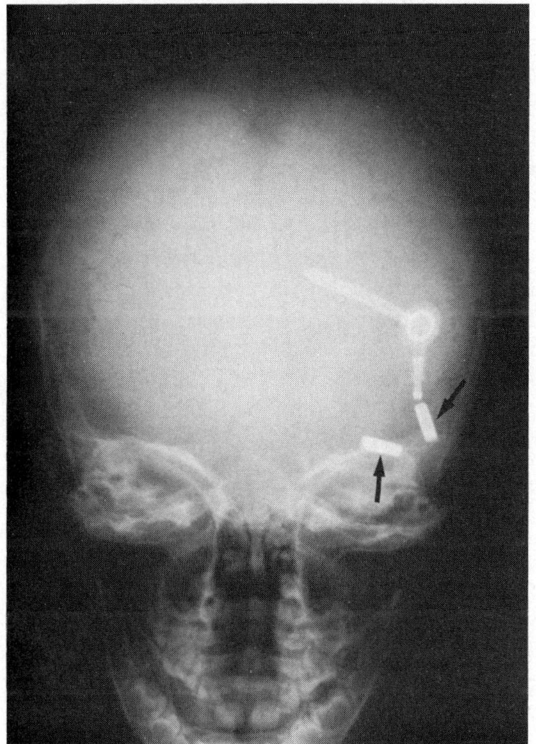

Figure 8–4 The Hakim (pediatric-size) valve is kinked. Note the malalignment of the two metallic portions. The system contains a Rickham reservoir. The tube distal to the valvue is radiolucent.

characteristics of the valve at the operating table. This should be done for every valve just prior to insertion, according to the manufacturer's instructions.

Most valves in common use today actually consist of two valves in series. Either can malfunction, a fact that must be kept in mind when interpreting the results of taps of the reservoir and valve during the evaluation of a child with suspected shunt failure.

Valves currently in use are differential pressure valves. This means that CSF flows through the valve whenever the pressure above the valve exceeds the pressure below by an amount determined by the characteristics of the valve itself.

Some patients, particularly those who have received cranial radiation, may not tolerate an intracranial pressure above 100 mm of CSF. A valve with excessive resistance (for a given patient) will cause symptoms and signs of elevated intracranial pressure. A valve with too little resistance increases the risk of subdural hematoma, low pressure headaches, and the problems of slit ventricles.

Complications Related to the Distal Tubing

Obstruction within the distal tubing is rare. A break in the distal tubing can be easily identified on a radiograph because most tubing now available is radiopaque. Surprisingly, this complication can be missed on physical examination because fibrous tissue around the tubing may feel exactly like the tube itself. Radiolucent segments of old tubing or a connector can be misinterpreted as a break in tubing. Tiny indentations on each side of the tip of a radiopaque tube may be the only clue to the site of a ligature. Metallic parts may be disconnected.

In infants and children who were born prematurely it is easy to mistake the properitoneal space for the peritoneal cavity. One should insist on seeing the free edge of the liver.

FORESHORTENED PERITONEAL TUBE

Foreshortened tubing in a growing child is common and should be considered a complication only if it goes unrecognized until malfunction occurs. It can be produced suddenly by an operation to correct scoliosis. We are now inserting an entirely new tube, making the connection at the lower end of the valve (parieto-occipital area).

The peritoneal end of the tubing should be inserted in a caudal direction so that the tubing will lie free in the peritoneal cavity. If the catheter lies over the left lobe of the liver, the patient may complain of pain in the lateral chest or in the left shoulder.

Intraperitoneal Complications

Intraperitoneal complications of shunts are uncommon. Shunts with slit valves in the distal end are prone to obstruction by the omentum, whereas obstruction of straight, open-ended catheters is very rare.

Occasionally a patient with a shunt presents with an intra-abdominal mass, with or without shunt failure. A large cyst filled with CSF can often be demonstrated in these patients.[22, 25, 64] The cause of this complication is unknown, but this may be a response to chronic peritoneal inflammation and a walling-off of a portion of the peritoneal cavity. Treatment consists of draining the CSF from this cavity and reinserting the peritoneal tubing into another part of the peritoneal cavity.

Some children are not able to absorb CSF as fast as it enters the peritoneal cavity. "Ascites" and clinical evidence of shunt failure then develop.[3, 14, 71, 92]

In patients who have had many abdominal operations (e.g., many shunt revisions and perhaps several operations involving the urinary tract) there may be no free peritoneal cavity. In such patients there is a high risk of causing accidental injury to intraperitoneal structures while searching for the peritoneal cavity.

Many other complications have been reported: volvulus of the gut[73]; perforation of the bowel,[72, 98] bladder,[34] gallbladder,[67] and vagina[58, 65]; and extrusion through the umbilicus[1, 69] and abdominal incision.[15] The catheter has become knotted within the peritoneal cavity.[34]

Inguinal hernias occur in about 16 per cent of children with ventriculoperitoneal shunts.[33, 34] It is not unusual for the surgeon repairing the hernia to encounter the peritoneal tubing within the scrotum.[69] The tube should be returned to the peritoneal cavity and the repair continued as planned. Patients with shunts who are undergoing herniorrhaphy should receive prophylactic intravenous antibiotics for 48 hours. Inflammatory pseudotumor of the mesentery has also been reported.[46]

Iatrogenic Failure of Peritoneal Shunts

Intra-abdominal pressure rises and the shunt malfunctions in the child whose bowels are severely impacted with feces. This complication occurs most often in children with myelodysplasia. Following evacuation of the large intestine, intracranial pressure falls rapidly.

A spica cast may cause elevated intra-abdominal pressure; the problem is resolved by making an abdominal window in the cast.[31]

Metastases Through Shunt

Malignant tumors of the brain, particularly medulloblastomas, may metastasize to the peritoneum through a ventriculoperitoneal shunt.[40] A filter can be placed in the shunt of patients with tumors that are likely to metastasize. If the filter is located within the field of radiation, the incidence of occlusion by tumor cells can be reduced.

Complications of Ventriculovenous Shunts

Cerebrospinal fluid is seldom shunted directly into the venous system today[82, 83]; however, many patients still have these types of shunts. Most vascular shunts enter a vein in the neck, and the lower end of the tubing lies within the superior vena cava. If the catheter enters the heart, the tip will move with each cardiac contraction and can produce cardiac arrhythmias. If the tubing goes through the tricuspid valve, it may, in the presence of bacteremia, cause valvulitis or endocarditis.[11, 76] Endocarditis has also been encountered with very long catheters that pass through the right atrium and into the inferior vena cava. Myocardial perforation,[17, 86] cor pulmonale,[84] and thrombosis of the inferior vena cava and hepatic vein have been reported.[63]

The catheter tip migrates in a cephalad direction with normal growth. As the tip passes above the level of the fourth rib, it becomes increasingly likely that the shunt will be occluded by tissue growing over the tip of the catheter. Elective revision before shunt failure occurs is recommended.

If a catheter becomes disconnected within the venous system, it usually lodges in the heart but may pass through the heart and lodge in the pulmonary artery, causing pulmonary valvular dysfunction.[43] Usually such a free tube can be removed by a catheter containing a snare inserted through the femoral vein and guided under fluoroscopic control.[53, 85] Venous catheters that become kinked after insertion can sometimes be straightened by percutaneous catherization techniques.[56, 59, 60]

The distal catheter is occasionally very difficult to remove at the time of revision. Sometimes the only reasonable and safe decision is to abandon the catheter and divert the CSF elsewhere. A method has been described for removing such catheters by prolonged traction.[57]

Patients who, for whatever reason, cannot have a ventriculoperitoneal shunt or a ventriculovenous shunt can have a shunt inserted directly into the cardiac atrium.[23] Complications and problems associated with these shunts have been reviewed by Anderson.[4]

Shunt nephritis is a severe complication of ventriculovascular shunts that has recently been reviewed by Wald and McLaurin.[90]

Complications of Ventriculopleural Shunts

Some patients with ventriculopleural shunts absorb CSF more slowly than the fluid enters the pleural space.[89] The result is a massive pleural "effusion" that can be drained easily, but treatment must include removal of the shunt from the pleural space.

Complications of Lumboureteral and Lumboperitoneal Shunts

Insertion of a lumboureteral shunt originally required a nephrectomy and is no longer performed. Patients with this type of shunt may still be seen and occasionally have complications.[18] More recently, a technique that does not require nephrectomy has been described.[80] The patency of the shunt can be confirmed by finding glucose in the urine. A urinary tract infection can lead to meningitis. A urinary catheter should not be inserted in such patients unless it is absolutely necessary. Syringomyelia has been reported in a few patients with lumboureteral shunts.[24]

Very small spinal subarachnoid spaces develop in many patients with lumbar shunts and can make revision difficult. Several patients have developed kyphoscoliosis[50] and hyperlordosis,[81] which usually improves or becomes stable after the shunt is removed.

Low Pressure Headache

After the insertion of a shunt, some children, particularly those with large ventricles, complain of headache when the head is elevated for 5 to 10 minutes. This problem is usually self-limiting but may persist for days or even weeks. The headache is characteristically most intense when the patient is in the upright position and is relieved or diminished when he lies down for a few minutes. In rare instances it becomes necessary to replace the valve with one of higher resistance. Severe headache after the insertion of a shunt also raises the possibilities of shunt failure, infection, and subdural hematoma. Epstein et al. have addressed the problem of headache in adolescents with shunts and small ventricles.[21]

Intracranial Hematoma

Subdural hematoma as a complication of a shunt usually occurs in a child with very large ventricles.[39, 44, 69] It is often recognized within a few days or weeks after a shunt is inserted but may appear months or years later. Regardless of the cause, the bleeding is into a subdural space with very low, perhaps even subatmospheric, pressure when the patient is upright.[54] The hematoma enlarges as ventricular fluid is displaced. An infant can exsanguinate as a result of bleeding into the subdural space.

The treatment of subdural hematomas in children with shunts can be very difficult and may require multiple procedures. It is often necessary to raise intraventricular pressure to re-expand the brain and obliterate the subdural space. This can be done by removing or occluding the shunt or by inserting an anti-siphon or an "on-off" device.[68] Recurrence is common.

Epidural hematoma has also been reported as a complication of ventricular decompression.[93]

Leaking Cerebrospinal Fluid

A leak of cerebrospinal fluid through the skin occurs most often in the very early postoperative period and necessarily leads to contamination. A few skin sutures will control the leak, but the incidence of infection is high. It is our practice to remove the shunt immediately, place the patient on CVD for a few days, and reinsert a new shunt after we are confident that the patient has no infection.

A subcutaneous leak of CSF indicates that the shunt is not functioning properly and that the CSF has found an alternate path that offers less resistance. In such patients the shunt should be revised. The most common site of leakage is through the dura adjacent to the catheter. In children with an absent or a very thin mantle of brain, it is particularly important that only a very tiny opening be made in the dura so that the catheter will fit snugly.

Rarely, a sheath may form around the end of the peritoneal catheter. Cerebrospinal fluid may then flow through the catheter, into the sheath, and back out of the peritoneal cavity around the shunt.

MYELODYSPLASIA

Myelodysplasia in most patients is unmistakable at birth; however, it may be confused with sacrococcygeal teratoma in patients who have large lesions in the sacral region.

Decisions about the early treatment of newborns with myelodysplasia must be made with the understanding that most children who have this disorder, even those with severe neurologic deficits, live for many years. An unrealistically pessimistic approach is not in the patient's best interest.[10] Prolonged delays in repair of a leaking myelomeningocele and management of hydrocephalus increase the risks of additional neurologic damage.

Complications that may occur in the closure of myelomeningoceles include infection in the operative site, meningitis, breakdown of the closure, and persistent leaking of CSF. It is usually necessary to reduce the intracranial pressure temporarily to prevent CSF from leaking through the site of closure. A complete CSF shunt should not be inserted until the repair site is well healed because of the risk of infection. If large skin flaps are elevated or if skin is undermined excessively, necrosis of the skin may follow. With the techniques now available to close very large defects, lateral relaxing incisions and rotation skin flaps are rarely, if ever, necessary.[97]

Hydrocephalus usually becomes apparent within the first few days or weeks of life but may be delayed for months or years. Two such patients were seen at age 26 years. Some have unusual symptoms and signs such as severe back pain or paralysis of the vocal cords.[29, 48]

In patients with myelodysplasia, progressive weakness, spasticity, or scoliosis may develop many years later.[6, 87] These abnormalities are usually due to elevated intracranial pressure, hydromyelia,[6, 36] or a tethered spinal cord. In most (probably all) children with myelodysplasia, the spinal cord is firmly attached at the site of closure, but this will not necessarily cause trouble.

Removal of Spinal Cord in Children with Myelodysplasia

These patients have severe scoliosis, and surgeons may choose to remove the neurologically nonfunctional spinal cord and use the lower part of the spinal canal as a site for fusion. The spinal cord in children with myelodysplasia can function as a conduit. In some children this is the only channel available for the egress of CSF. It is difficult to detect a malfunctioning shunt in such children because the failure of the shunt may produce no symptoms or signs. If the dura and spinal cord are ligated at a level that is neurologically nonfunctional, and the patient's only fuctional "shunt" has been occluded, intracranial pressure rises rapidly, leading to cardiac arrest and death.[99] It is imperative that the patency of the shunt be demonstrated unequivocally in all patients undergoing this operation. The spinal cord should not be ligated; instead, the dura should be opened, the nonfunctional spinal cord transected, and the dura closed to form a pouch several millimeters distal to the cord transection. This allows CSF to flow from the hydromyelic cavity into the spinal subarachnoid space until the patient recovers from anesthesia and perhaps for much longer.

CRANIOSYNOSTOSIS

Most operations for synostosis are done with the patient in the lateral or supine position, but occasionally a patient undergoing surgery for bilateral lambdoidal stenosis, particularly patients with Crouzon's disease, may be operated on in the prone position. Pressure on the face, particularly on the forehead, can cause necrosis of the skin. The risk of this complication is enhanced by moisture and by the increased weight of wet drapes. The face must be kept dry, and the anesthesiologist should carefully raise the child's head every 10 to 15 minutes and record this on the anesthetic record.

It is essential that the full length of the closed portion of the cranial suture be removed. To ensure that this is done, bone can be removed for several millimeters beyond the apparent end of the suture. This is particularly true for the sagittal suture anteriorly and posteriorly.

The loss of blood from bone may be greater than appreciated. Therefore, replacement may be inadequate. Patients should be monitored closely during the postoperative period because of the possibility of continuing loss of blood. Deaths have occurred because of failure to provide volume replacement.

Craniosynostosis has been reported as a complication of operation for hydrocephalus.[5, 49]

LIPOMENINGOCELE

It is very difficult to secure a watertight closure between malformed dura and adipose tissue after the subtotal removal of a lipomeningocele. The surgeon should anticipate this difficulty and make every effort to avoid a CSF leak. In some patients the dura can be opened, leaving a cuff that can be more easily approximated during closure.

Nerve roots or spinal cord may be damaged in the course of removal of adipose tissue from the spinal cord.

References

1. Adeloye, A.: Spontaneous extrusion of the abdominal tube through the umbilicus complicating peritoneal shunt for hydrocephalus. Case report. J. Neurosurg. 38:758, 1973.
2. Alker, G. J., Glasauer, F. C., and Leslie, E. V.: The radiology of cerebrospinal fluid shunts and their complications. Br. J. Radiol. 46:496, 1973.
3. Ames, R. H.: Ventriculo-peritoneal shunts in the management of hydrocephalus. J. Neurosurg. 27:525, 1967.
4. Anderson, F. M.: Ventriculocardiac shunts: Iden-
   tification and control of practical problems in 143 cases. J. Pediatr. 82:222, 1973.
5. Anderson H.: Craniosynostosis as a complication after operation for hydrocephalus. Acta Paediatr. Scand. 55:192, 1966.
6. Batnitzky, S., Hall, P. V., Lindseth, R. E., Wellman, H. N.: Meningomyelocele and syringohydromyelia. Radiology 120:351, 1976.
7. Bayston, R.: Antibiotic prophylaxis in shunt surgery. Dev. Med. Child Neurol. 35(Suppl.):99, 1975.
8. Bayston, R., and Lari, J.: A study of the sources of infection in colonized shunts. Dev. Med. Child Neurol. 32(Suppl.):16, 1974.
9. Bayston, R., and Penny, S. R.: Excessive production of mucosal substance in staphylococcus SIIA: A possible factor in colonization of Holter shunts. Dev. Med. Child Neurol. Suppl 27:25, 1972.
10. Black, P. M.: Selective treatment of infants with myelomeningocele. Neurosurgery 5:334, 1979.
11. Bruce, A. M., Lorber, J., Shedden, W. I. H., and Zachary, P. B.: Persistent bacteremia following ventriculo-caval shunt operations for hydrocephalus in infants. Dev. Med. Child Neurol. 5:461, 1963.
12. Collins, P., Hockley, A. D., and Woolam, D. H. M.: Surface ultrastructure of tissues occluding ventricular catheters. J. Neurosurg. 48:609, 1978.
13. Cooper, J. R.: Migration of ventriculoperitoneal shunt into the chest. Case report. J. Neurosurg. 48:146, 1978.
14. Dean, D. F., and Keller, I. B.: Cerebrospinal fluid ascites: A complication of ventriculoperitoneal shunt. J. Neurol. Neurosurg. Psychiatry 35:474, 1972.
15. DeSousa, A. L., and Worth, R. M.: Extrusion of peritoneal catheter through abdominal incision: Report of a rare complication of ventriculoperitoneal shunt. Neurosurgery 5:504, 1979.
16. Dewey, R. C., Kosnik, E. J., and Sayers, M. P.: A simple test of shunt function: The shuntgram. Technical note. J. Neurosurg. 44:121, 1976.
17. Dzenitis, A. J., Mealey, J., Jr., and Waddell, J. R.: Myocardial perforation by ventriculoatrial shunt tubing. JAMA 194:1251, 1965.
18. Eisenberg, H. M., Davidson, R. I., and Shillito, J., Jr.: Lumboperitoneal shunts. Review of 34 cases. J. Neurosurg. 35:427, 1971.
19. Engel, M., Carmel P. W., and Chutorian, A. M.: Increased intraventricular pressure without ventriculomegaly in children with shunts: "Normal volume" hydrocephalus. Neurosurgery 5:549, 1979.
20. Epstein, F. J., Fleischer, A. S., Hochwold, G. M., and Ranshoff, J.: Subtemporal craniectomy for recurrent shunt obstruction secondary to small ventricles. J. Neurosurg. 41:29, 1974.
21. Epstein, F., Martin, A. E., and Wald, A.: Chronic headache in the shunt-dependent adolescent with nearly normal ventricular volume: Diagnosis and treatment. Neurosurgery 3:351, 1978.
22. Fischer, E. G., and Shillito, J., Jr.: Large abdominal cysts: A complication of peritoneal

shunts. Report of three cases. J. Neurosurg. 31:441, 1969.

23. Fischer, E. G., Shillito, J., Jr., and Schuster, S.: Ventriculo-direct atrial shunts. J. Neurosurg. 36:438, 1972.

24. Fischer, E. G., Welch, K., and Shillito, J., Jr.: Syringomyelia following lumboureteral shunting for communicating hydrocephalus. J. Neurosurg. 47:96, 1977.

25. Fokes, E. C., Jr.: Occult infections of ventriculo-atrial shunts. J. Neurosurg. 33:517, 1970.

26. Foltz, E. L., and Shurtleff, D. B.: Conversion of communicating hydrocephalus to stenosis or occlusion of the aqueduct during ventricular shunt. J. Neurosurg. 24:520, 1966.

27. Forrest, D. M., and Cooper, D. G. W.: Complications of ventriculo-atrial shunts. A review of 455 cases. J. Neurosurg. 29:506, 1968.

28. Frick, M., Roesler, H., and Kinser, J.: Functional evaluation of ventriculoatrial and ventriculoperitoneal shunts with $^{99}Tc^{m}$-pertechnetate. Neuroradiology 7:145, 1974.

29. Gendell, H. M., McCallum, J. E., and Reigel, D. H.: Cricopharyngeal achalasia associated with Arnold-Chiari malformation in childhood. Childs Brain 4:65, 1978.

30. George, R., Leibrock, L., and Epstein, M.: Long-term analysis of cerebrospinal fluid infections. A 25 year experience. J. Neurosurg. 51:804, 1979.

31. Gerber, A. M.: Iatrogenic failure of a ventriculoperitoneal shunt. Case report. J. Neurosurg. 46:830, 1977.

32. Globl, H. J., and Kaufmann, H. J.: Shunts and complications. *In* Kaufmann, H. J. (ed.): Progress in Pediatric Radiology. Part II. Skull, Spine and Contents. Vol. ô. Basel, S. Karger, 1978, pp. 231–271.

33. Grosfeld, J. L., and Cooney, R. R.: Inguinal hernia after ventriculo-peritoneal shunt for hydrocephalus. J. Pediatr. Surg. 9:311, 1974.

34. Grosfeld, J. L., Cooney, D. R., Smith, J., and Campbell, R. L.: Intra-abdominal complications following ventriculoperitoneal shunt procedures. Pediatrics 54:791, 1974.

35. Gutierrez, F. A., and Raimondi, A. J.: Peritoneal cysts. A complication of ventriculoperitoneal shunts. Surgery 79:188, 1976.

36. Hall, P. V., Campbell, R. L., and Kalsbeck, J. E.: Meningomyelocele and progressive hydromyelia. J. Neurosurg 43:457, 1975.

37. Hawkins, J. C., Holtman, H. J., and Humphreys, R. P.: Isolated fourth ventricle as a complication of ventricular shunting. J. Neurosurg. 49:910, 1978.

38. Hemmer, R.: Surgical treatment of hydrocephalus, complication, mortality, developmental prospects. Z. Kinderchir. 22:443, 1977.

39. Hemmer, R., and Potthoff, P. C.: Subdurales Hamatom als begleitercheinung des ventrikuloaurikularen shunts. Neurochirurgia 12:102, 1965.

40. Hoffmann, H. J., Hendrick, E. B., and Humphreys, R. P.: Metastasis via ventriculoperitoneal shunt in patients with medulloblastoma. J. Neurosurg. 44:562, 1976.

41. Holness, R. O., Hoffman, H. G., and Hendrick,

E. B.: Subtemporal decompression for the slit-ventricle syndrome after shunting in hydrocephalic children. Childs Brain 5:137, 1979.

42. Horwitz, N. H., and Rizzoli, H. C.: Postoperative Complications in Neurosurgical Practice: Recognition, Prevention and Management. Baltimore, Williams & Wilkins Co., 1967.

43. Hougen, T. J., Emmanoulides, G. C., and Moss, A. J.: Pulmonary valvular dysfunction in children with ventriculovenous shunts for hydrocephalus: A previously unreported complication. Pediatrics 55:836, 1975.

44. Illingworth, R. D.: Subdural haematoma after the treatment of chronic hydrocephalus by ventriculo-caval shunts. J. Neurol. Neurosurg. Psychiatry 33:95, 1970.

45. Kaufman, B., Weiss, M. H., Young, H. F., and Nulsen, F. E.: Effects of prolonged cerebrospinal fluid shunting on the skull and brain. J. Neurosurg. 38:288, 1973.

46. Keen, P. E., and Weitzner, S.: Inflammatory pseudotumor of mesentery: A complication of ventriculoperitoneal shunt. Case report. J. Neurosurg. 38:371, 1973.

47. Keucher, T. R., and Mealey, J.: Long-term results after ventriculoatrial and ventriculoperitoneal shunting for infantile hydrocephalus. J. Neurosurg. 50:179, 1979.

48. Kirsch, W. M., Duncan, B. R., Black, F. O., and Stears, J. C.: Laryngeal palsy in association with myelomeningocele, hydrocephalus, and the Arnold-Chiari malformation. J. Neurosurg. 29:207, 1968.

49. Kloss, J. L.: Craniosynostosis secondary to ventriculoatrial shunt. Am. J. Dis. Child. 116:315, 1968.

50. Kushner, J., Alexander, G., Davis, C. H., and Kelly, D. L.: Kyphoscoliosis following lumbar subarachnoid shunts. J. Neurosurg. 34:783, 1971.

51. Lee, F. A., and Gwinn, J. L.: Complication of ventriculoperitoneal shunts. Ann. Radiol. 18:471, 1975.

52. Matson, D. D.: Neurosurgery of Infancy and Childhood. Springfield, Ill., Charles C Thomas, Publisher, 1969.

53. McCulloch, G. A. J., and Cartledge, J. M.: Retrieval of detached shunt catheter from the heart. Case report. J. Neurosurg. 42:98, 1975.

54. McCullough, D. C., and Fox, J. L.: Negative intracranial pressure hydrocephalus in adults with shunts and its relationship to the production of subdural hematoma. J. Neurosurg. 40:372, 1974.

55. McLaurin, R. L.: Treatment of infected ventricular shunts. Childs Brain 1:306, 1975.

56. McSweeney, W. J.: Intravascular repositioning of a ventriculoatrial shunt. Technical note. J. Neurosurg. 36:512, 1972.

57. Morantz, R., Kim, G., and Epstein, F.: The trapped distal shunt catheter: Removal by graded skin traction. Case report and technical note. J. Neurosurg. 38:521, 1973.

58. Mozingo, J. R., and Cauthen, J. C.: Vaginal perforation by a Raimondi peritoneal catheter in an adult. Surg. Neurol. 2:195, 1974.

59. Natelson, S. E.: Percutaneous restoration of a kinked shunt. Case report. J. Neurosurg. 50:391, 1979.

60. Natelson, S. E., and Molnar, W.: Malfunction of ventriculoatrial shunts caused by the circulatory dynamics of coughing. J. Neurosurg. 36:283, 1972.

61. O'Brien, M., Parent, A., and Davis, B.: Management of ventricular shunt infection. Childs Brain 5:304, 1979.

62. Osaka, K., Yamasaki, S., Hirayama, A., et al.: Correlation of the response of the flushing device to compression with the clinical picture in the evaluation of the functional status of the shunting system. Childs Brain 3:25, 1977.

63. O'Shea, P.: Inferior vena cava and hepatic vein thrombosis as a rare complication of ventriculoatrial shunt. Case report. J. Neurosurg. 48:143, 1978.

64. Parry, S. W., Schuhmacher, J. K., and Llewellyn, R. C.: Abdominal pseudocysts and ascites formation after ventriculoperitoneal shunt procedures. Report of four cases. J. Neurosurg. 43:476, 1975.

65. Patel, C. D., and Matlaub, H.: Vaginal perforation as a complication of ventriculoperitoneal shunt. Case report. J. Neurosurg. 38:761, 1973.

66. Perrin, J. C., and McLaurin, R. S.: Infected ventriculoatrial shunts. A method of treatment. J. Neurosurg. 27:21, 1967.

67. Portnoy, H. D., and Croissant, P. D.: Two unusual complications of a ventriculoperitoneal shunt. Case report. J. Neurosurg. 39:775, 1973.

68. Portnoy, H. D., Schulte, R. R., Fox, J. L., et al.: Anti-siphon and reversible occlusion valves for shunting in hydrocephalus and preventing post-shunt subdural hematomas. J. Neurosurg. 38:729, 1973.

69. Raimondi, A. J., Robinson, J. W., and Kuwamura, K.: Complication of ventriculoperitoneal shunting and a critical comparison of the three-piece and one-piece systems. Childs Brain 3:321, 1977.

70. Ramani, P. S.: Extrusion of abdominal catheter of ventriculoperitoneal shunt into the scrotum. Case report. J. Neurosurg. 40:772, 1974.

71. Rosenthal, J. D., Golden, G. T., Shaw, C. A., and Hanes, J. A.: Intractable ascites: A complication of ventriculoperitoneal shunting with a Silastic catheter. Am. J. Surg. 127:613, 1974.

72. Rubin, R. C., Ghatak, N. R., and Visudhipan, P.: Asymptomatic perforated viscus and gram-negative ventriculitis as a complication of valve-regulated ventriculoperitoneal shunts. Report of two cases. J. Neurosurg. 37:616, 1972.

73. Sakoda, T. H., Maxwell, J. A., and Brackett, C. E., Jr.: Intestinal volvulus secondary to a ventriculoperitoneal shunt. Case report. J. Neurosurg. 35:95, 1971.

74. Savoiardo, M., Solero, C. L., Passerini, A., and Migliavacca, F.: Determination of cerebrospinal fluid shunt function with water-soluble contrast medium. J. Neurosurg. 49:398, 1978.

75. Scarff, T. B., Nelson, P. B., and Reigel, D. H.: External drainage for ventricular infection following cerebrospinal fluid shunts. Childs Brain 4:129, 1978.

76. Schimke, R. T., Black, P. H., Mark, V. H., and Swartz, M. N.: Indolent *Staphylococcus albus* or *aureus* bacteremia after ventriculoatriostomy. Role of foreign body in the initiation and perpetuation. N. Engl. J. Med. 264:264, 1961.

77. Schoenbaum, S. C., Gardner, P., and Shillito, J.: Infections of cerebrospinal fluid shunts: Epidemiology, clinical manifestations, and therapy. J. Infect. Dis. 131:543, 1975.

78. Shallat, R. F., Pawl, R., and Jerva, M. J.: Significance of upward gaze palsy (Parinaud's syndrome) in hydrocephalus due to shunt malfunction. J. Neurosurg. 38:717, 1973.

79. Shurtleff, D. S., Christie, D., and Foltz, E. L.: Ventriculoauriculostomy — associated infection. A 12 year study. J. Neurosurg. 35:686, 1971.

80. Smith, J. A., Lee, R. E., and Middleton, R. G.: Ventriculoureteral shunt for hydrocephalus without nephrectomy. J. Urol. 123:224, 1980.

81. Steel, H. H., and Adams, D. J.: Hyperlordosis caused by the lumboperitoneal shunt procedure for hydrocephalus. J. Bone Joint Surg. 54A:1537, 1972.

82. Steinbok, P., and Thompson, G. B.: Complications of ventriculo-vascular shunts: Computer analysis of etiologic factors. Surg. Neurol. 5:31, 1976.

83. Strenger, L.: Complications of ventriculovenous shunts. J. Neurosurg. 20:219, 1963.

84. Syamansundar, R., Molthan, M. E., and Lipow, H. W.: Cor pulmonale as a complication of ventriculoatrial shunts. Case report. J. Neurosurg. 33:221, 1970.

85. Tatsumi, T., and Howland, W. J.: Retrieval of a ventriculoatrial shunt catheter from the heart by a venous catheterization technique. Technical note. J. Neurosurg. 32:593, 1970.

86. Tsingoglou, S., and Eckstein, H. B.: Pericardial tamponade by Holter ventriculoatrial shunts. J. Neurosurg. 35:695, 1971.

87. Turnbull, F. A.: Syringomyelic complications of spina bifida. Brain 56:304, 1933.

88. Venes, J. L.: Control of shunt infection. Report of 150 conservative cases. J. Neurosurg. 45:311, 1976.

89. Venes, J. L., and Shaw, R. K.: Ventriculopleural shunting in the management of hydrocephalus. Childs Brain 5:45, 1979.

90. Wald, S. L., and McLaurin, R. L.: Shunt associated glomerulonephritis. Neurosurgery 3:146, 1978.

91. Wald, S. L., and McLaurin, R. L.: Cerebrospinal fluid antibiotic levels during treatment of shunt infections. J. Neurosurg. 52:41, 1980.

92. Weidmann, M. J.: Ascites from a ventriculoperitoneal shunt. Case report. J. Neurosurg. 43:233, 1975.

93. Weiss, R. M.: Massive epidural hematoma compli-

cating ventricular decompression. J. Neurosurg. 21:235, 1964.

94. Welch, K.: The prevention of shunt infection. Kinderchirurgie 22:465, 1977.

95. Welch, K.: Cerebrospinal fluid pressure (letter to the editor). Surg. Neurol. 10:253, 1978.

96. Welch, K.: Residual shunt infection in a program aimed at its prevention. Kinderchirurgie 28:374, 1979.

97. Wilson, H. D., Bean, J. R., James, H. E., and Pendley, M. M.: Cerebrospinal fluid antibiotic concentrations in ventricular shunt infections. Childs Brain 4:74, 1978.

98. Wilson, C. B., and Bertan, V.: Perforation of the bowel complicating peritoneal shunt for hydrocephalus. Report of two cases. Am. Surg. 32:601, 1966.

99. Winston, K., Hall, J., Johnson, D., and Micheli, L.: Acute elevation of intracranial pressure following transection of non-functional spinal cord. Clin. Orthop. 28:41, 1977.

100. Winston, K. R., Schuster, S. R., and Mickle, P.: Management of large skin defects in newborn children with myelodysplasia. J. Pediatr. Surg. 13:303, 1978.

101. Zidan, A. H., and Girvin, J. P.: Effect on the Cushing response of different rates of expansion of a supratentorial mass. J. Neurosurg. 49:61, 1978.

9

EYES AND LIDS

J. S. Crawford, M.D.

Ophthalmic surgery has advanced greatly in recent years as a result of both clinical experience and research. New instruments, new sutures with better needles, new techniques, and new drugs are changing our concepts of eye surgery and leading us to revise our ideas about the proper management of complications.

This chapter discusses the surgical procedures in current use. Because it is assumed that the reader is aware of the actual techniques, only a summary of the principles is presented. Problems related to ophthalmic surgery are also discussed, since the real test of the surgeon's skill occurs not when things go smoothly but when they go wrong. Knowing how to handle complications helps prevent them and enables one to obtain a satisfactory result. It is hoped that the information presented here will help the reader avoid complications or manage them better when they arise.

INJURIES OF THE LID

Two of the most important structures to be considered in lid injuries are the levator muscle and the lacrimal drainage system.

With upper lid lacerations, the levator muscle may be cut (Fig. 9–1). Occasionally the skin and superficial structures are reapproximated and a cut levator is not discovered until later. Before surgical repair is undertaken, the physician should have the patient look up and down to ensure that the levator muscle is functioning well. If levator action is absent or limited, the muscle should be explored during repair and resutured if necessary.

Laceration of the lid necessitates careful approximation of the lid border followed by suturing of the skin and deep structures. A figure-of-eight suture should be used to reduce the possibility of notching the lid border (Fig. 9–2).

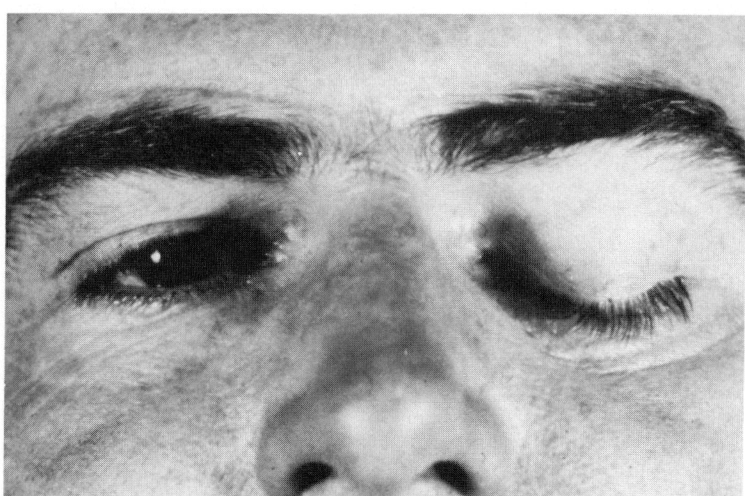

Figure 9–1 This patient's left upper lid was caught on a hook as he ran through a barn. The hook caught the upper bony margin of the orbit and avulsed the levator muscle. The lid laceration was sutured. Later the patient was found to have a nonfunctioning levator muscle.

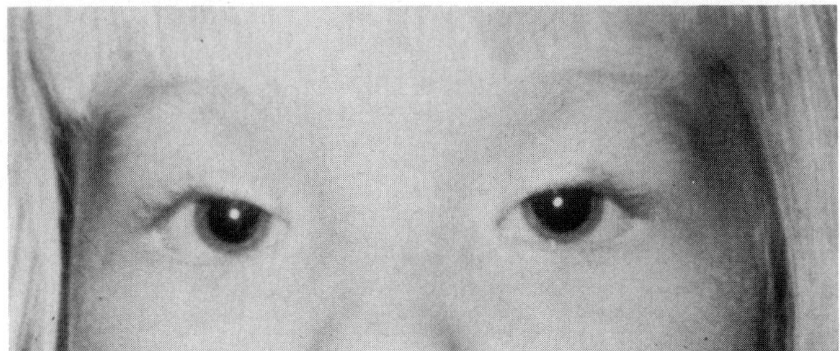

Figure 9–2 Notching of right upper lid after repair of lid laceration. A figure-of-eight suture reduces the possibility of notching.

Recently I saw a child whose lid laceration had been sutured using 5–0 plain gut. The wound was carefully approximated, but the knots were tied on the posterior surface of the lid. A severe corneal abrasion resulted, and the sutures had to be removed. A subcuticular suture is useful. Fine gut sutures may be used, provided that the knots are tied deep in the wound so as not to rub the cornea.

Laceration of the lid borders may result in division of the canaliculi. If this is suspected, a Bowman probe should be passed along the canaliculus, and saline solution may be irrigated through the lacrimal system.

Occasionally the medial end of the cut canaliculus may be difficult to find; however, it may be located by injecting milk into the other uncut punctum and canaliculus of the same eye. Milk is useful because it can be seen coming out of the cut end of the canaliculus and does not stain cut tissue as does methylene blue.

Stainless steel rods, polyethylene tubing, and pieces of catgut have been used to maintain the patency of the canaliculus. The best results are obtained with silicone tubing (Fig. 9–3). Intubation is carried out using silicone tubing attached to a stainless steel wire probe with a knob on the end.[3] The knob is engaged by a special hook used to draw the wire out from under the inferior turbinate of the nose. Silicone tubing (inside diameter 0.063 cm, outside diameter 0.119 cm)* is attached to a light stainless steel wire, 0.05 mm in diameter, that is flexible enough to be deflected easily through a 90-degree angle from the nasolacrimal duct out through the nostril. The wire has an en-

larged, rounded end that prevents damage to the tissues and can be picked up by a special hook. If the lower canaliculus is cut, a wire probe attached to the silicone tubing is passed through the punctum and out through the cut end of the canaliculus. The medial end of the cut canaliculus is located by means of a microscope or by injecting milk through the upper canaliculus and seeing where it comes out. The wire is then passed down through the nasolacrimal duct and brought out through the nostril. The

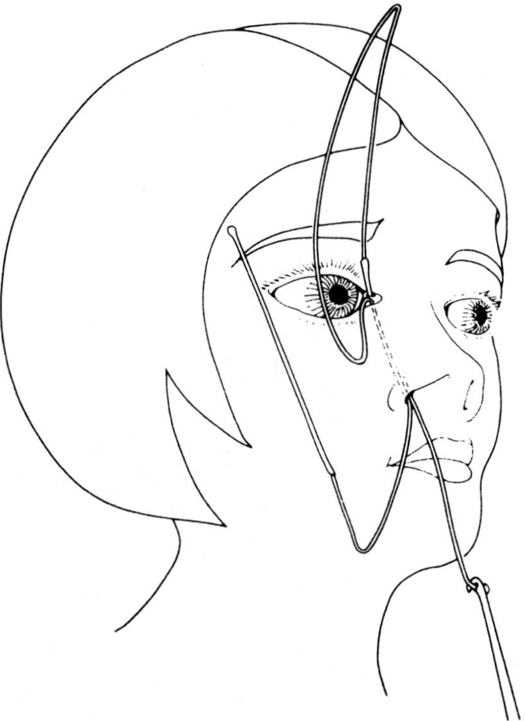

Figure 9–3 Silicone tubing is inserted through upper and lower canaliculi and brought out through nostril by hook.

---

*Dow Corning Corporation Medical Products Division, Midland, Michigan.

other end is passed into the upper canaliculus and brought down and out through the nostril. The ends are cut and tied together with a nonabsorbable suture such as 5–0 Prolene. The tubing is well tolerated by the patient.

INJURIES OF THE GLOBE

Various eye injuries, for example, laceration of the conjunctiva, may appear trivial. They usually heal quickly and cause very few symptoms. Most superficial injuries do not necessitate surgery. Deeper injuries may lead to complications, for example, rupture of the sclera. Consequently, all wounds of the conjunctiva must be carefully appraised. Deeper injuries should be closed with fine Dexon or Vicryl sutures.

Contusion injuries to the eyeball may result from direct impact on the globe, with the greatest effect occurring where the blow was received. A transmitted force may send a wave of pressure through the vitreous contents of the eye and produce a contrecoup injury to the posterior portion of the globe, resulting in retinal edema, rupture of the choroid, or even rupture in the posterior portion of the sclera.

Perforating Wound of the Eye

Perforating wounds may be small punctures, such as those caused by darts, or extensive lacerations. Penetrating injuries of the cornea are frequently complicated by a prolapse of the intraocular contents.

In dealing with perforating wounds, one must remember that the affected eye is extremely painful. If an attempt is made to pull the lids open, the patient will squeeze his lids closed involuntarily. This may result in herniation of orbital contents through the wound. If there is an obvious perforating wound, the eye should be covered with a clean pad and taped shut; the patient should be admitted to a hospital and placed under general anesthesia so that the wounds may be examined more carefully. Suturing may not be necessary for clean perforating wounds of the cornea, such as those produced by a knife, if there is no herniation of ocular contents. However, larger, irregular

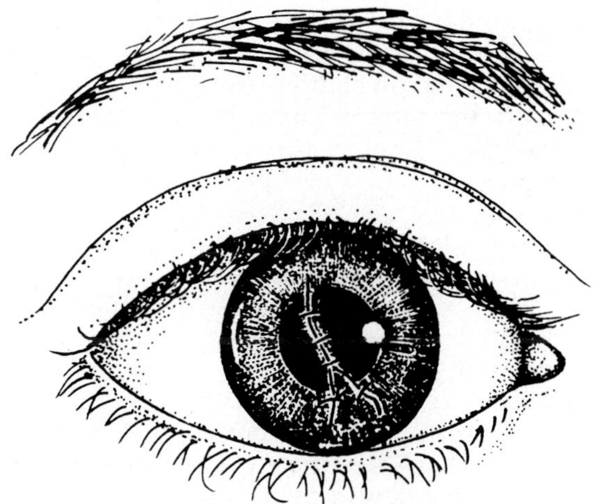

Figure 9–4 Irregular corneal wound requiring direct suturing with fine sutures.

corneal wounds necessitate direct suturing of the corneal tissues with fine silk (8–0, 9–0, or 10–0) (Fig. 9–4).

If the wound is not carefully approximated, herniation of the iris may occur between the sutures. In this case, it may be necessary to reposition the iris or excise the prolapsed iris. Depending on the site of the corneal laceration, it may be necessary to constrict or dilate the pupil.

Frequently the lens capsule has been torn, resulting in a traumatic cataract. The lens becomes swollen as the aqueous leaks into it, and glaucoma may result. This complication can be avoided by aspirating the lens at the time of injury, using either a 21-gauge needle or a suction cutter. When the lens is allowed to absorb by itself, a thick membrane that requires discission often develops.

An attempt should be made to restore vision and binocular function; otherwise, a secondary strabismus may result. The patient must be fitted with a contact lens as soon as all the lens material is absorbed.

Vitreous hemorrhages are frequently associated with both nonpenetrating and penetrating eye injuries. Bleeding occurs from the ciliary region and collects in the retrolental space. Hemorrhage may occur in the substance of the vitreous, occasionally giving an almost black fundus reflex. Vitreous hemorrhages either are gradually absorbed or become organized. They take weeks or months to disappear.

Treatment of vitreous hemorrhages consists of waiting to see whether the hemorrhage clears. Recently, procedures for replacing the vitreous have been carried out after the cloudy vitreous has been removed.[7]

Rupture of the Sclera

Rupture of the sclera may be due either to contusion or to a foreign object passing through the globe. With contusion ruptures, it is important to ensure that there is only one break in the external coat of the eye. After a rupture is found and sutured, resolution of the injury is sometimes complicated by a posterior rupture that has not been closed. If the eye is hypotensive, it may be necessary to anesthetize the child before incising the conjunctiva and examining the sclera. Often the rupture is too far back to be sutured and enucleation of the eye may be necessary.

Retinal Tears

Retinal tears may occur in young, healthy patients, but they are more frequent in patients with myopia or other retinal degenerative conditions associated with old age.

Localized dialysis of the ora serrata is common, usually in the inferotemporal quadrant of the globe. Retinal detachment may be associated with rupture of the globe or may be due to choroidal hemorrhage. To avoid the problems associated with this complication of contusion, it is necessary to locate any retinal holes, drain the subretinal fluid, seal the retinal holes, and approximate the retina to the choroid.

Hyphema

Most hyphemas (free blood in the anterior chamber) (Fig. 9–5) are caused by blunt ocular trauma. They may also result from penetrating ocular injury and less commonly from surgery (for cataracts or glaucoma). Hyphemas may occur in certain systemic diseases, such as leukemia, hemophilia, or scurvy, or after bleeding from an intraocular neoplasm, for example, juvenile xanthogranuloma. The prognosis is excellent; most hyphemas are clear of gross blood within 5 days. Secondary hemorrhages into the anterior chamber are more serious because secondary glaucoma fre-

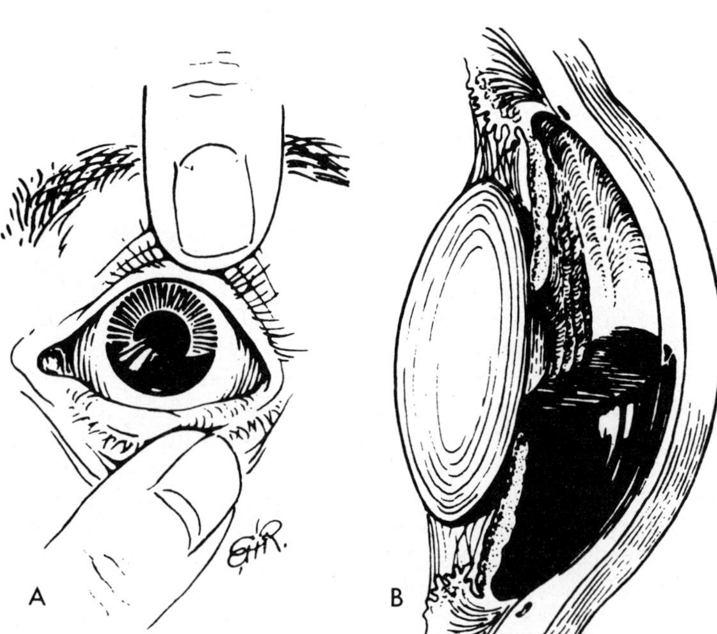

Figure 9–5 Hyphema showing layered blood in the anterior chamber.

quently ensues, followed by blood staining of the cornea. Secondary glaucoma occurs in about 25 per cent of patients with secondary hemorrhages but in less than 1 per cent of those with primary hemorrhages. About 77 per cent of secondary hemorrhages occur on the third or fourth day after injury. Almost none occur later than the fifth day.

The complications of hyphema may be serious, in some cases leading to the loss of an eye. Patients with hyphemas, even if they are very young, must be put to bed and sedated. Binocular bandages may be used, but in very small patients they may be disturbing and may have to be removed.

Mydriatics and miotics have proved ineffective with hyphemas. However, when a hyphema reaches the stage of absorption, a secondary uveitis results from the breakdown of the blood products. At this stage a mydriatic drug and a steroid should be administered. Ocular hypotensive agents such as mannitol are of doubtful value but may be necessary before irrigation of the anterior chamber when glaucoma is present.

Hyphemas may be divided into three categories according to the amount of blood in the anterior chamber: Grade I, microscopic amounts to one third of chamber filled (Fig. 9–6); Grade II, one third to one half of chamber filled; and Grade III, more than half of chamber filled.

Conservative management is advised with hyphema of Grades I and II to see whether the hemorrhage will be absorbed. With Grade III hyphema, rebleeding, raised intraocular pressure, and complications are more frequent. Management should be conservative for 48 hours, but if the anterior chamber is filled with blood and the intraocular pressure is elevated, the clot should be washed out. The best time to remove the clot is 4 days after injury.

Many patients with hemorrhage in the anterior chamber are given aspirin or aspirin-containing compounds. The inhibitory effect of acetylsalicylic acid on platelet function is well documented; one normal therapeutic dose of aspirin will prolong the bleeding time and interfere with platelet aggregation for 5 days or more.[8] The incidence of rebleeding in patients with Grade I hyphema has been shown to be significantly higher among those who had taken aspirin than among those who had not.[6] Aspirin-containing compounds should not be used in patients with pain from intraocular hemorrhage; however, acetaminophen (Tempra) or codeine may be given because neither has the deleterious effect of aspirin.

If complete hyphema with blood filling the entire anterior chamber remains for many days, the cornea may become stained with blood as a result of hemosiderin being forced into and deposited in the corneal stroma. Small amounts of hemosiderin will disappear, but in many cases the blood staining is permanent.

Sympathetic Ophthalmia

Sympathetic ophthalmia (Fig. 9–7) is a low-grade uveitis occurring in one eye after a penetrating injury to the other eye. It is thought to be a sensitivity reaction of the uveal pigment. In its early stages, it is characterized by insidious uveitis involving the anterior or posterior segment of the eye and by a disproportionate and early decrease in visual acuity in an eye that does not seem particularly red or painful. Early signs are the presence of cells and flare in the anterior chamber of the second eye, along with photophobia. Keratic precipitates, swelling in the iris, papillitis, or scattered yellowish spots in the fundus may occur early; all eventually lead to panuveitis. The process in the exciting eye may begin at any time from

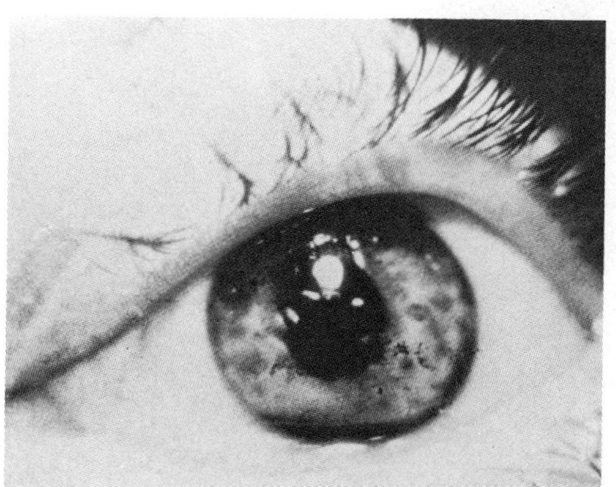

Figure 9–6   Grade I hyphema.

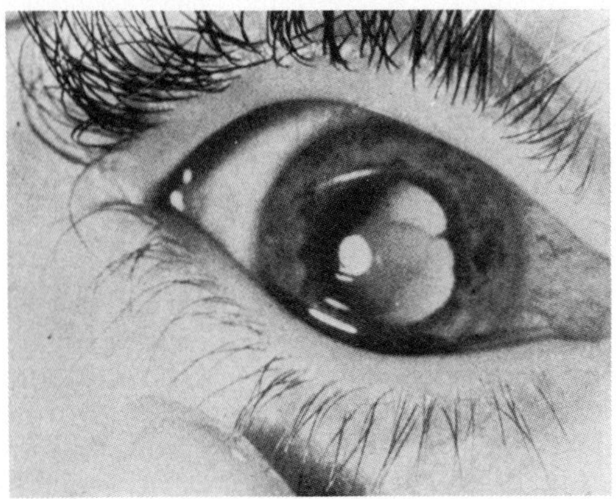

Figure 9–7 Sympathetic ophthalmia resulting from a stick penetrating the eye.

9 days to many years after the accident. The sympathizing eye becomes involved shortly thereafter.

Sympathetic ophthalmitis may begin to develop 10 days after a penetrating injury. In 80 per cent of patients it develops within 3 months. If the injured eye is enucleated within 10 days after injury, the development of sympathetic ophthalmia is extremely unlikely.

Sympathetic ophthalmia is less hazardous today than it was in the past. It may be resolved or controlled by administration of systemic corticosteroids, immunosuppressive agents, or both. However, remissions and exacerbations may follow.

The wound of a penetrating injury is sutured, and the eye is observed for 10 days. At that time, depending on the patient's visual function, a decision is made about whether to enucleate the eye. The risk of sympathetic ophthalmia must be explained to the parents at this time, and the surgeon and parents must decide whether enucleation or continued treatment of the eye is indicated.

Blow-Out Fractures of the Floor of the Orbit

This discussion is restricted to blow-out fractures of the floor of the orbit and will not deal with other fractures involving bones of the middle third of the face and associated with fractures extending into the floor of the orbit. Fractures of the malar-zygomatic complex or crushing injuries of the intraorbital rim may cause a comminution of the orbital floor, but they are not true blow-out fractures because they do not interfere with the motility of the globe to any great extent.

A pure blow-out fracture involves sudden pressure over the orbit that increases intraorbital pressure, leading to a blow-out of the thin portion of the floor. The blow-out is a safety feature that allows the periorbital structures to herniate into the opening and helps prevent rupture of the globe. It occurs when an object such as a fist, ball, or similar missile strikes the eye; usually it saves the globe.

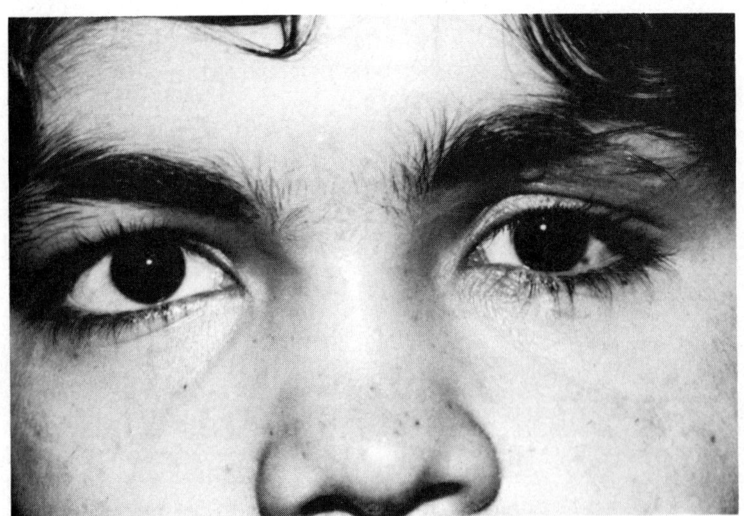

Figure 9–8 Left enophthalmos following fracture of orbital floor.

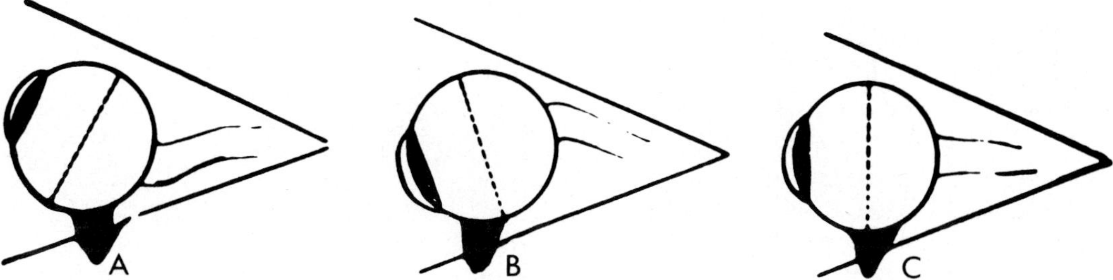

Figure 9–9 Blow-out fracture of orbital floor. *A,* Inferior rectus caught posterior to equator. *B,* Inferior rectus caught anterior to equator. *C,* Inferior rectus caught at equator.

PHYSICAL FINDINGS

Examination may show inability to elevate the globe, depression of the globe, vertical diplopia, hypesthesia over the distribution of the infraorbital nerve, and edema and hemorrhage that may cause proptosis. When the edema and hemorrhage subside, enophthalmos may be noted (Fig. 9–8).

The punched-out piece of bone usually allows orbital fat, Tenon's capsule, the inferior rectus muscle, and/or the inferior oblique muscle to herniate downward. Linear fracture may trap some muscle tissue. If the inferior rectus muscle is trapped posterior to the equator of the globe, the eye will be held in an elevated position (Fig. 9–9*A*); if it is caught anteriorly, the eye will be fixed in a depressed position (Fig. 9–9*B*); and if it is caught at the equator, the eye will be held in the straight-ahead position (Fig. 9–9*C*).

Tomograms of the orbital floor (Fig. 9–10) are usually required to visualize the fracture. They may show a "hanging drop" density in the roof of the antrum. This must be differentiated from a hematoma under the periosteum in the roof of the antrum, which may give the same picture.

A traction test is done under local anesthesia, using a thumb forceps and securing a bite of conjunctiva and episcleral tissue below the cornea. This shows a definite restriction of passive movement.

A Hess Screen or Lees Screen test (Fig. 9–11), as done in the orthoptic department, is very helpful in determining the actual ocular movements and provides a good record for comparison after surgery.

Surgery may not be as urgent as was previously thought. Many of the symptoms are due to damage to the extraocular muscles caused by hemorrhage and may gradu-

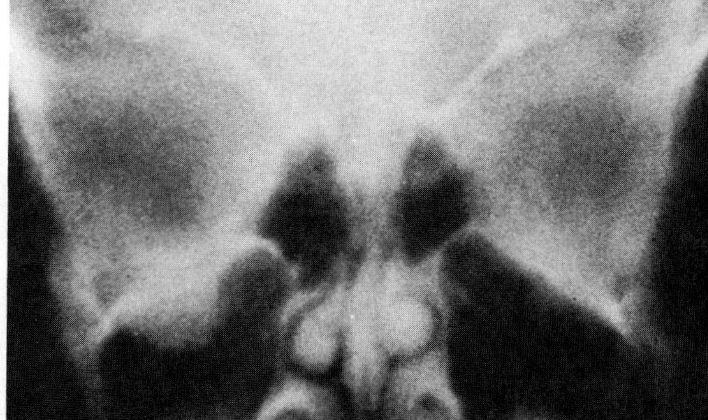

Figure 9–10 Tomogram of orbital floor showing typical "hanging drop" density in roof of antrum.

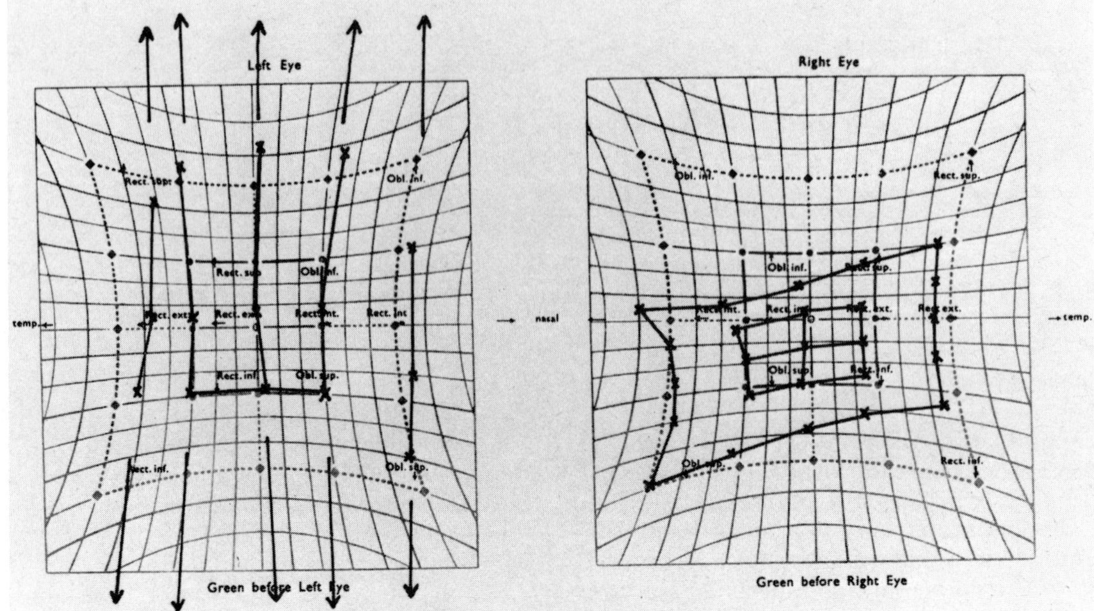

Figure 9–11   Lees Screen test showing restricted up-and-down movement of right eye.

ally disappear. When indicated, however, the surgical procedure consists of making a skin incision at the junction of the lower lid and the cheek. The incision is carried down through the periosteum below the rim of the orbit. The periosteum is then raised from the floor of the orbit, and, with the aid of suitable retractors, the hole in the orbital floor can usually be located. A small polytetrafluoroethylene (Teflon) or silicone rubber plate 1 mm thick is placed over the defect on the orbital floor and wired to the rim of the orbit with stainless steel; the ends of the wire are tucked under the plate. It is important to use the right size of plate for the injury, since one that is too long may press on the optic nerve, causing blindness. A small degree of ptosis of the upper lid may occur after repair of an orbital-floor fracture; this may be treated successfully using a modified Fasanella-Servat operation.[2]

PTOSIS

Meticulous care must be taken in assessing the patient so that the correct ptosis operation is performed. If the ptosis is correctly classified, the surgeon can avoid under- or overcorrection. The goals of surgery must be decided before the operation is begun. Ideally, ptosis surgery should achieve the following:

1. Symmetry of both lids in terms of (a) position and contour of lid margins, (b) position and length of lid fold, and (c) width of palpebral aperture
2. Complete uncovering of both pupils
3. Maintenance of normal, synchronous blinking
4. Eyelids that remain closed during sleep
5. Absence of any complications such as (a) notching of the lid margins, (b) distortion or absence of lashes, and (c) exposure keratitis

Perfect results can be expected only in patients with mild ptosis and good function of the levator muscle. When levator function is limited, the lid cannot be placed in its proper position and will not have normal excursion; the patient's appearance can be considerably improved, but the lid will not move up and down normally and the patient may sleep with the lid incompletely closed. The limitations of surgery should be explained to the patient and his parents before the operation so that they know what to expect. Complications of ptosis surgery

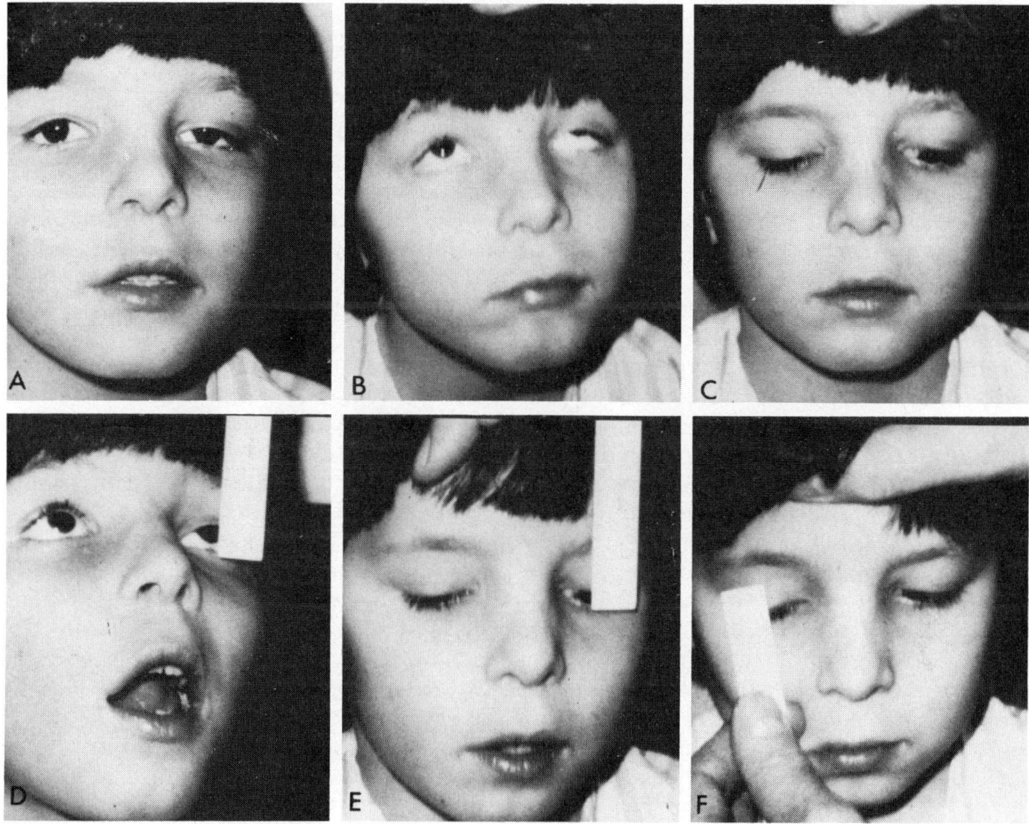

Figure 9–12   Measuring ptosis. *A,* Eyes straight. *B,* Looking up. *C,* Looking down. *D,* A ruler is held in front of the lid as the patient looks up. The ruler is held tightly against the forehead to prevent the frontalis muscle from acting. *E,* The patient looks down. The lid excursion is then determined. *F,* The position of the lid fold on the normal lid is measured.

are rare, but surgeons who perform the procedure frequently will occasionally encounter problems.[1]

Various postoperative problems may be avoided if the following questions are considered before surgery is undertaken:

1. Does diplopia occur if the ptotic lid is raised?

2. Is the affected eye amblyopic?

3. Is corneal sensation normal?

4. Is there good Bell's phenomenon?

After checking the presence or absence of these important characteristics, we must then assess the ptosis to decide what type of operation is appropriate. The following questions should be answered:

1. Is the ptosis unilateral or bilateral?

2. How much lower than normal is each lid margin? (Fig. 9–12)

3. How good is the levator function?

4. Is the superior rectus function normal?

5. Are there any associated syndromes such as blepharophimosis syndrome, the Marcus Gunn syndrome, or the congenital fibrosis syndrome?

TABLE 9–1   OPERATION OF CHOICE FOR DEGREES OF PTOSIS

Operation	Amount of Ptosis	Excursion of Lid
Modified Fasanella-Servat[2]	1–3 mm (slight)	10–15 mm
Levator resection through skin[1]	3–5 mm (moderate)	8–10 mm
Fascial suspension to frontalis[4]	5–7 mm (large)	<6 mm

After the ptosis has been assessed and measured, the surgical procedure is determined, as shown in Table 9–1.

Complications of Ptosis Surgery

Undercorrection.   Undercorrection is the most frequent complication of ptosis surgery. It can be avoided by using the correct procedure. Occasionally a parent does not want his child's lid suspended to the frontalis muscle and elects to have a levator resection done when there is limited levator function. In such cases, the parent must be made to understand that undercorrection is very likely and that the operation may have to be repeated or another procedure used.

Overcorrection.   Overcorrection is not common and usually occurs with acquired ptosis. For many years, a Berke levator tenotomy was the operation of choice to reduce overcorrection. This simple procedure consists of everting the lid on a Desmarres retractor. An incision is made through the tarsus about 1 mm from its upper edge. The incision is deepened until the tarsal tissues separate by about twice the amount of the desired correction. A silk suture is then placed in the edge of the upper lid and taped to the cheek to keep the lid on the downward stretch. The upper edge of the wound may be held in its new position by placing a 6–0 plain catgut suture through the edge of the wound and tying it on the skin of the lid. A second suture is passed through the other wound edge and also tied on the skin of the lid.

I have found that the most satisfactory method of getting consistent results is to use a scleral graft[5] (Fig. 9–13). The upper lid is everted on a Desmarres retractor. A horizontal incision is made at the upper border of the tarsus from one side of the lid to the other through all the structures except the skin. A piece of fresh or bank sclera is placed in the wound between the cut margins. Fresh sclera is usually used for the graft, which can be one from which a corneal graft has been taken. The graft should be 2 mm wider and 2 mm longer than the amount of lowering the lid requires. During suturing, the graft is temporarily held in place with 4–0 silk sutures at each end and in the center above and below. Suturing is done with 6–0 plain gut and a ⅜ reverse cutting needle, starting at one end of the graft and taking a bite into the edge of the tarsus but not through it, and then taking a bite into the edge of the graft but not through it. The suture is woven in this way between the graft and the host until the other end of the graft is reached. The needle is then passed through the skin of

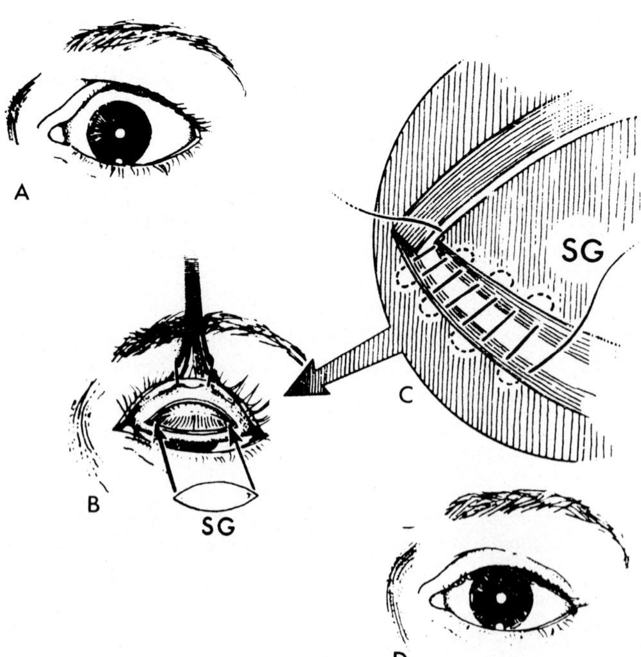

Figure 9–13   Repair of retracted lids. *A,* Upper lid retracted. *B,* Horizontal incision made across top of tarsus through all lid structures except skin. *C,* Scleral graft **(SG)** is placed in wound and sutured with 6–0 plain gut suture, the knot being tied on skin surface. The upper lid is lowered to a more normal position.

the lid. The second needle of the double-armed suture is then passed in a similar way around the graft. When the opposite end is reached, the suture is also passed through the skin and the two ends are tied. The suture is placed in this way so that when it is pulled tight, the gut does not rub against the cornea. The temporary 4–0 silk sutures are then removed. A pad is applied to the eye with adhesive strapping; this is removed the next day.

Uneven or Irregular Lids. Uneven or irregular lids are seldom seen when both lids are operated on at the same time, since symmetry is easier to produce under those circumstances. If the lids do not match, massage of the higher lid may correct the asymmetry. If that proves unsuccessful, surgical correction is necessary.

The higher lid may be lowered by a Berke levator tenotomy as previously described. However, a more satisfactory result can be obtained by elevating the lower lid. An irregular border may be caused by uneven insertion of the sutures into the tarsus during levator resection. Care must be taken to place sutures evenly across the lid and not overlap them.

Lagophthalmos and Exposure Keratitis. Some degree of lid lag follows many levator resections, especially when levator function is poor, because the muscle is composed of more fibrous tissue and less muscle and will not relax sufficiently to allow proper lid depression. This problem should be explained to the parents before surgery so that they will expect some lagophthalmos.

Lagophthalmos is inevitable after brow suspension surgery. There is some improvement within a year, but a unilateral repair remains noticeable; when repair is bilateral, there is no cosmetic defect. Thus, patients with unilateral ptosis who require a brow suspension should have a bilateral procedure.

Lagophthalmos often results in exposure keratitis. This should be treated by frequent instillation of 1 per cent methylcellulose drops during the day and taping of the lower lid upward at night. The corneal epithelium gradually becomes resistant to the exposure.

Entropion. Entropion is a rare complication; I have seen it only when the fascia was placed too deeply in the lid after fascial repair. It can be avoided by placing the

fascia lata more anteriorly in the substance of the orbicularis muscle.

Lid Pulled Away from Globe. After fascial repair of ptosis, the lid may pull away from the globe when extreme elevation of the lid is attempted. This does not seem to be a serious problem; patients soon learn to elevate the frontalis muscle less.

Loss of Lashes. Lashes are seldom lost if the anatomic position of the eyelash follicles is kept in mind during surgery. Dissection should stop at least 2 mm short of the follicle level. Loss of lashes is sometimes associated with excessive swelling of the lid after surgery, apparently as a result of damage to the lash follicles. In time, partial regrowth of lashes may occur. If it does not, lash grafts may be taken from the brow. Unfortunately, this procedure is not satisfactory.

Absorption of Stored Fascia. This complication was reported in a recent study of more than 100 patients who had received stored fascia for ptosis repair.[4] Within 3 months after surgery, the tissue was absorbed and ptosis recurred in 10 per cent of patients. In such cases, the patient's own fascia should be taken and the operation repeated.

Poor Lid Fold. The usual eyelid fold is about 5 mm above the eyelid margin and represents the level of attachment of the levator aponeurosis fibers to the skin. A good lid fold is cosmetically important. The incision on the surface of the ptotic lid should match the position of the lid fold on the normal side. It is almost impossible to change an eyelid fold that is not positioned properly.

If the lid fold is poor, an incision may have to be made in the desired position, and it is possible that some skin above the incision will have to be removed. Pang sutures consist of sutures placed through the full thickness of the lid and tied over the incision to produce an adhesion to the deeper tissues and a type of lid fold.

Wound Infection. Wound infection is extremely rare, but when it does occur, the patient should be hospitalized and treated with high doses of antibiotics.

When stored fascia is used, serous fluid often collects around the brow wounds and may give the appearance of a sterile abscess. These wounds are usually not infected and should be left alone, as the reaction will subside and a good result will be obtained. When stored fascia is used, I always close the brow wounds with 6–0 Dexon or Prolene, which holds the wound together until the reaction has subsided; when autogenous fascia is used, I close the brow wounds with 6–0 plain catgut.

Other Infections. Infection is one of the more serious complications following ophthalmic surgery. Today, antimicrobial agents (including penicillin, gentamicin, neomycin, tetracycline, chloramphenicol, bacitracin, erythromycin, polymyxin, isoniazid, rifampin, nystatin, and sulfonamides) reduce the problem, and new antibiotics are constantly being introduced. The multiplicity of antibiotics makes selection necessary. Antibiotics are chosen for their effectiveness, toxicity, ease of administration, and cost. The first essential of successful antibiotic therapy is accurate diagnosis of the infectious etiology of the disorder; the red eye of acute glaucoma will not respond to an antibiotic. It is extremely important to identify the causative organism by appropriate cultural and biochemical techniques and to determine its antibiotic sensitivity.

One of the most important physiologic features in the penetration of drugs is the blood–aqueous barrier. This barrier resists the entry of water-soluble ions into the eye. Penicillin, for example, penetrates the eye extremely poorly. The blood–aqueous barrier exists at the walls of the iris and retinal blood vessels, at the epithelial surfaces of the cornea and ciliary body, and at the retinal pigment epithelium. Hence, the cavity of the eye containing the aqueous, vitreous, and lens is a sheltered area within which invading microorganisms may be protected from systemic or topical antibiotic therapy. This barrier is particularly significant in prophylactic antibiotic treatment of an eye after a penetrating wound. The blood–aqueous barrier is permeable to lipid-soluble drugs such as chloramphenicol. For this reason, chloramphenicol is extremely effective against intraocular infections.

The extraocular tissues are outside the blood–aqueous barrier. Hence, the general principles of antibiotic therapy applicable to treatment of infections of any other part of the body are equally relevant to the treatment of an orbital infection.

Sensitivity testing of bacterial strains isolated from patients with ocular disorders indicates the superiority of drugs whose use is limited to topical application. Such drugs include bacitracin, gramicidin, nitrofurazone, neomycin, and sulfacetamide and, for gram-negative organisms, polymyxin, gentamicin, and chloramphenicol. These drugs are best for prophylactic therapy, for example, after corneal abrasion.

Most superficial infections cause an accumulation of discharge. This should be carefully wiped away, and firmly adherent crusts should be softened with compresses and removed. Ointments should be used at night because of their longer action. During the day, drops may be used because they do not have the same blurring effect caused by ointments. The eye should be left open and cleaned with sterile water or saline solution. Hands should be washed before and after touching infected eyes to prevent spread to other patients.

With more serious infections, such as orbital cellulitis or endophthalmitis, prompt, vigorous treatment is required. Sensitivity studies should be carried out and therapy started immediately. A Gram stain may facilitate initial selection of an antibiotic. Dosage should be as high as that used in treating serious systemic diseases. A penicillinase-resistant penicillin (such as methicillin) is the agent of choice against resistant *Staphylococcus aureus* unless the patient is allergic to penicillin. Ampicillin, a synthetic penicillin with a broad spectrum of antibacterial activity, is absorbed orally. Useful levels of ampicillin do not enter the normal vitreous.

There is a problem of toxicity associated with chloramphenicol, and severe anaphylactic reactions sometimes occur with penicillin. Since 5 per cent of the population is allergic to penicillin, the physician should make sure that the patient has not had previous adverse reactions to this drug.

Polymyxin B is bactericidal against most gram-negative microorganisms, such as Pseudomonas. It is one of the most effective antibiotics available for treating gram-negative infections on the ocular surface.

Corneal abrasions are sometimes complicated by a herpes simplex infection. In the past it was impossible to treat viral infections, but today idoxuridine, which inhibits the growth of herpes simplex virus, may be used. A 0.5 per cent ointment is applied five times a day for several weeks.

With intraocular infections it is usually necessary to dilate the pupil. This can be accomplished most effectively with 1 per cent atropine in the form of either drops or an ointment. Atropine may be combined with a steroid if there are no contraindications. Steroids are used in the treatment of viral infections only during the late healing stage.

References

1. Beard, C.: Ptosis, 2nd ed. St. Louis, C. V. Mosby Co., 1976, p. 156.
2. Crawford, J. S.: Repair of blepharoptosis with a modification of the Fasanella-Servat operation. Can. J. Ophthalmol. 8:19, 1973.
3. Crawford, J. S.: Intubation of obstructions in the lacrimal system. Can. J. Ophthalmol. 12:289, 1977.
4. Crawford, J. S.: Repair of ptosis using frontalis muscle and fascia lata: A 20-year review. Ophthalmic Surg. 8(4):31, 1977.
5. Crawford, J. S., and Easterbrook, M.: The use of bank sclera to correct lid retraction. Can. J. Ophthalmol. 11:304, 1976.
6. Crawford, J. S., Lewandowski, R. L., and Chan, W.: The effect of aspirin on rebleeding in traumatic hyphema. Am. J. Ophthalmol. 80:543, 1975.
7. Klein, R. M., and Katzin, H. M.: Microsurgery of the Vitreous. Baltimore, Williams & Wilkins Co., 1978, p. 55.
8. Stuart, R. K.: Platelet function studies in human beings receiving 300 mg of aspirin per day. J. Lab. Clin. Med. 75:463, 1970.

SOFT TISSUES

John B. Mulliken, M.D.
Joseph E. Murray, M.D.

10

Soft tissue complications are painfully apparent to both patient and physician. Skin necrosis, wound sepsis, and hematoma all call forth the same question: "Is this the result of something I did wrong, an error in my technique, judgment, or management?" Only after this soul searching is answered can a soft tissue complication be rightfully ascribed to accidental injury or to the patient's disease.

Soft tissue problems share common pathophysiologic pathways: tension or hematoma, leading to inadequate perfusion and tissue necrosis, or sepsis with resultant delayed healing, and finally scarring, fistulae, contractures, or exposure of vital structures such as underlying bone, tendon, joints, or a vascular anastomosis.

This chapter identifies avoidable soft tissue problems and discusses the management of established soft tissue complications.

PREVENTION

Systemic Factors

Systemic factors associated with soft tissue complications act to impair the host's resistance to infection, diminish the wound healing process, or interfere with the circulation in the soft tissues. Systemic problems should be corrected, whenever possible, before elective incision and dissection of soft tissues. Nutritional deficiencies, particularly those causing hypoalbuminemia and vitamin deficiency states, increase the incidence of soft tissue complications and impaired healing. Factors that decrease general circulation and lower tissue oxygen tension, such as diminished cardiac output, diabetes,

venostasis, and lymphatic obstruction, also cause lowered nutritive blood flow to the skin.

Local Factors

Most soft tissue complications are the result of local factors. Tissue perfusion may be jeopardized by injury secondary to trauma or an operative dissection. In either case, the result is a lowered resistance of tissues to growth of endogenous or exogenous microorganisms. The balance between bacterial contamination and local resistance and blood supply can be tipped favorably to minimize the chances of sepsis, soft tissue loss, or both.

Management of Contaminated Wounds

There are two principles for the prevention of sepsis in a contaminated wound: (1) maintenance of host defenses and (2) reduction of the level of the bacterial inoculum. Host defenses are supported by attention to systemic factors such as respiratory function, gas exchange, acid-base equilibrium, and fluid-electrolyte balance. Systemic prophylactic antibiotics are not useful after bacterial contamination has occurred (see Chapter 6). Aseptic principles and proper management of an already contaminated wound are paramount. Wounds that are heavily contaminated with bacteria, are badly contused, or are seen more than 6 hours after injury usually contain dangerously elevated levels of bacteria. It is now accepted that it is the *number* of bacteria within the tissue rather than the *type* of bacteria present that determines whether or not a wound will subsequently become infected.[11] The critical or significant number of bacteria is 10^5 per gram of tissue. Below this level, wounds generally heal in predictable fashion, whereas at greater levels, wounds often become infected, delayed primary closure will be unsuccessful, and skin grafts will not vascularize. Rapid slide techniques are now available for quantitation of wound bacteria within 1 hour after the specimen is taken.[12] Wounds seen 6 hours after an accident have been shown to harbor elevated levels of tissue bacteria — a confirmation of the empirical "golden period" after which primary healing is unpredictable.

Wound débridement, irrigation, and antibacterial therapy are directed toward reducing the bacteria to less than the critical 10^5 organisms per gram of tissue. Devitalized tissue must be thoroughly and accurately excised. In addition to the bacterial inoculum, the colloidal fraction of dirt is also a prime potentiator of wound sepsis.[24] Vigorous irrigation will remove these particles along with bacteria. When dirt is embedded in a wound, removal with a brush or forceps is necessary to prevent tattooing (Fig. 10–1*A, B*).

Fleming warned that antiseptics do more harm to wound tissue than to bacteria in the wound.[9] Irrigation with detergents has been shown to have adverse effects on the wound's microcirculation.[7] The best irrigant is buffered balanced solution, e.g., Ringer's lactate or Tis-U-Sol,* rather than unphysiologic saline solution. In addition, pulsating jet lavage helps to dislodge contaminants from a wound.[3, 23] In the presence of heavy bacterial contamination, irrigation with a topical antibacterial agent, e.g., povidone-iodine, may well be useful. Povidone-iodine may cause low-grade inflammation[1]; however, it does not affect subsequent wound healing.[20]

If there is any question about the potential for primary healing, a contaminated wound should be covered with an occlusive

----

*Travenol Labs., Inc., Deerfield, Illinois.

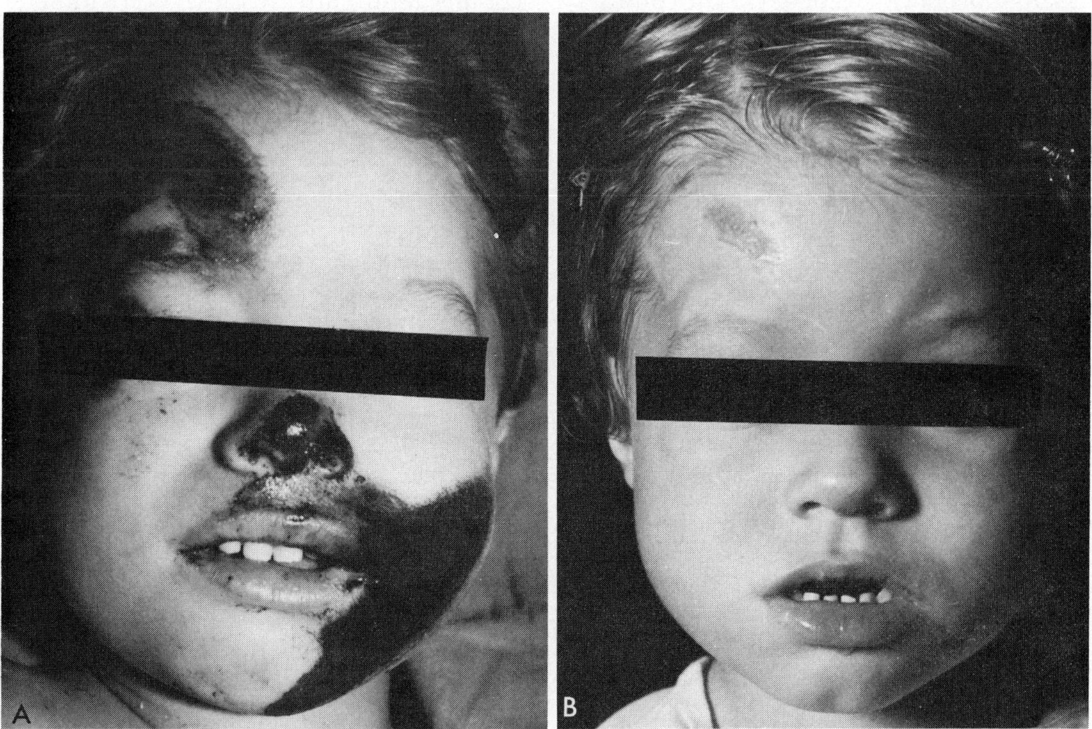

Figure 10–1   *A,* Deep abrasion wounds of the face with embedded dirt. *B,* The wounds were cleansed with a brush and were healed within 1 week.

dressing and not examined for possible delayed primary closure until 4 days later. A contaminated wound that has been irrigated, débrided, and judged favorable for primary healing should be closed with care. The minimum number of absorbable sutures, e.g., polyglycolic acid sutures, should be used in such wounds. Knots should also be kept to a minimum to avoid creating interstices for bacterial growth and to limit the amount of foreign material in the wound. The common practice of closing off "dead space" with subcutaneous sutures has been demonstrated to potentiate sepsis in the experimentally contaminated wound.[6] Sutures should be placed near the free edge of the wound to minimize strangulation of enclosed tissue. Micropore tape will minimize the number of sutures needed and may tip the balance in favor of primary healing.

Thermograms have documented the well-accepted clinical fact that blood supply is most abundant in the head and neck region and diminishes toward the extremities. For this reason, heavily contaminated bite wounds on the face, even human bite wounds, usually heal primarily if the wound has been properly cleaned. On the contrary, moderately contaminated wounds of the lower extremities, despite the best efforts of the surgeon, often heal slowly and frequently become infected.

Management of Avulsion Wounds

Wounds with actual loss of tissue, called avulsion wounds, have a traumatized bed and ragged edges. Thin, compromised tissue margins should be trimmed conservatively. On rare occasions a full-thickness avulsion wound can be closed with minimal undermining and without undue tension. One should always remember that a split-thickness graft is an expedient form of primary closure of an avulsion wound.

Closure Technique

Primary wound closure may be done by side-to-side approximation or by application of a split-thickness skin graft or pedicled flap. Undermining is a time-honored maneuver recommended whenever there is tension on a skin closure. It should not be practiced in the presence of a contaminated wound. Undermining is always done with a "double edged blade" and should be in the subcutaneous, not the intradermal, plane. This may allow for some relaxation of the closure; however, it also creates more potential dead space and may further compromise the vascularity of the elevated skin edges. It is usually preferable to take tension off the approximated skin margins by proper placement of deep sutures. Excessive tension on a skin closure will cause necrosis. A tangential tensile force of 25 gm applied to a skin flap increases interstitial tissue pressure enough to interfere with dermal blood flow.[25] If an incised or avulsion wound cannot be closed by appropriate suturing techniques, a skin graft or flap may be necessary. The split-thickness skin graft should be considered the "workhorse" of wound closure. It is always the simplest and best way to substitute for skin loss. Later, after healing, the grafted area can often be excised and the wound closed by direct approximation.

Although not usually thought of as a complication, suture tract scars are unnecessary and avoidable. Percutaneous sutures leave tract scars when they are placed under excessive tension and when they are not removed before 1 week. Caliber is unimportant, provided that the sutures are removed early.[4]

Planning Elective Incisions

To minimize wound tension, scar hypertrophy, and contracture, the skin incision should be planned to lie within the *relaxed skin tension lines*. Incisions should never cross a flexion crease. Relaxed skin tension lines are obvious about the face of an older patient and usually lie at right angles to the underlying pull of the muscles. If there is any question about the axis of the relaxed skin tension lines, a simple puncture wound or circular incision can be made; the resulting wound will elongate into an ellipsoid shape to indicate the tensile forces within the skin and the axis of skin closure. Movement of nearby joint structures and underlying muscles will affect this axis and must be considered in planning an incision.

An incision should also be devised with consideration of the circulation of its wound edges; this is particularly important in the design of flaps. Recent appreciation of the anatomy of the blood supply of skin has led to conception of more predictable flaps. The cutaneous blood supply throughout the body follows two basic anatomic patterns. The important difference is the level at which the longitudinally oriented artery lies (Fig. 10–2).[5, 17] In the most common pattern, the skin's circulation is provided by branches of musculocutaneous arteries with perpendicular perforating vessels to the skin and perfusion through the dermal and subdermal plexuses. This is the predominant blood supply of the skin, and flaps based on this type of circulation are known as *random pattern flaps*. The second pattern of skin circulation occurs in special areas of the body where segmental arteries perforate past the muscle layers and lie in a longitudinal orientation deep in the subcutaneous tissue, directly supplying the dermal and subdermal plexuses. These are called direct cutaneous arteries. Examples include the superficial temporal artery, anterior perforating branches of the internal mammary arteries, the superficial circumflex iliac artery, the dorsal artery of the penis, and the dorsalis pedis artery. Flaps based on these systems are known as *axial pattern flaps*. Flaps ought to be planned in terms of these vascular patterns rather than on the basis of empirical length-to-width ratios. Conventional skin flaps are of the random type and survive according to the number and type of vessels located within the base of the flap, or

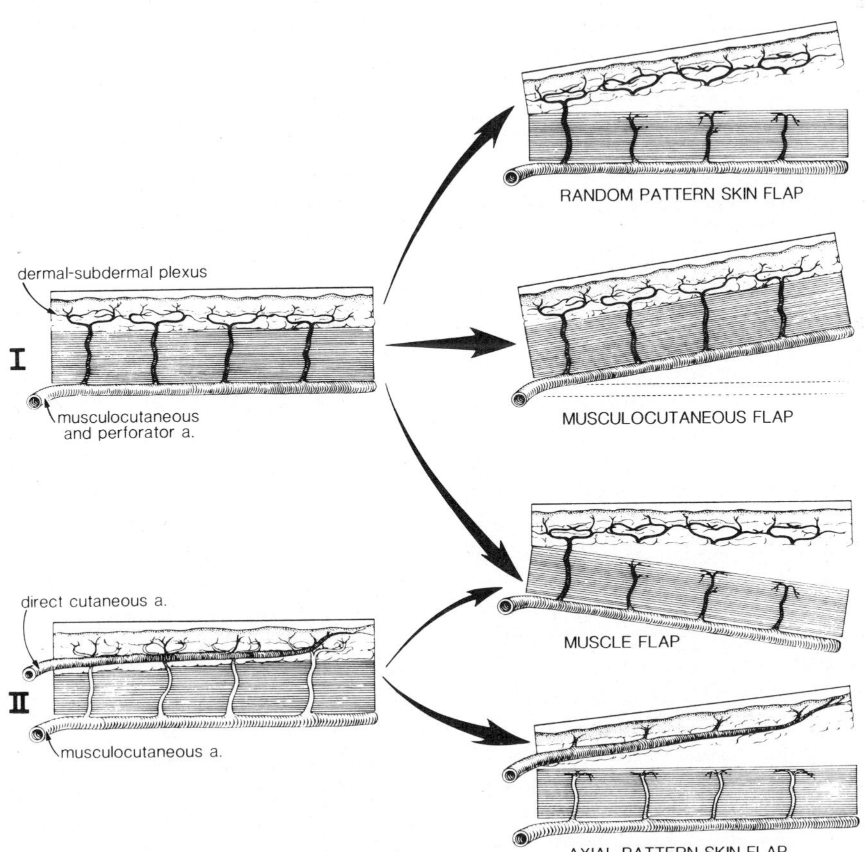

Figure 10–2 Blood supply to the surface of the body is provided by musculocutaneous arteries and perforating branches (I) or by direct cutaneous arteries (II). With knowledge of vascular anatomy, various types of flaps can be designed.

pedicle. Perfusion occurs through the dermal and subdermal plexuses; therefore, these flaps can be thinned of underlying fat as long as enough is left to shelter the subdermal plexus. The more specialized axial or arterial flaps can be raised irrespective of length-to-width ratio.[18] It is the central or lateral direct cutaneous artery that must be preserved. Arterial flaps also have a distal area with a random cutaneous plexus that can be included in the flap beyond the anatomic termination of the direct cutaneous artery.

Intravenous fluorescein has been used to delineate cutaneous vascular territories in animal and cadaver dissections.[16, 22] It is also extremely useful clinically in assessment of soft tissue viability following crush or avulsion injuries or after elevation of a random or axial flap. An intravenous bolus of 10 per cent fluorescein sodium (15 mg/kg) is given. After a 15- to 20-minute waiting period, an ultraviolet light source (Wood's light) is used to assess the fluorescence. Although there is considerable experience with this technique in adults, the Food and Drug Administration has not yet approved intravenous fluorescein for use in neonates.

Dressings

Well-conceived dressings will minimize the risk of soft tissue complications. Each dressing must be planned with several purposes in mind: protection of the wound, absorption of drainage, immobilization, compression, and observation for tissue viability.

Closed Wounds. Freshly closed wounds with minimal oozing of serosanguineous fluid can often be dressed with an axial or multiple transverse Steri-Strips.* However, if a sutured wound is oozing it should not be sealed with tape or an impermeable plastic sheet that would cause maceration and collection of fluid in which bacteria could grow. Instead, a nonadherent layer of petrolatum-impregnated gauze, covered with a layer of absorbent gauze, will keep the wound dry and protected. Whichever dressing technique is used, some effort must be made to protect the wound from the prying fingers of the child.

---

*3M Company, St. Paul, Minnesota.

Abrasion Wounds. Abrasion wounds should be dressed with a petrolatum-impregnated layer covered by absorbent gauze and a protective dressing. This technique is designed to prevent desiccation of the exposed dermal layer and subsequent formation of eschar. Epithelial cells migrating from adnexal structures would have to burrow beneath the eschar to resurface the denuded dermis. This is a slow process with more attendant dermal scarring than occurs with rapid epithelialization over moist dermis. Epithelialization is the basis for healing of a split-thickness skin graft donor site. If the protective dressing curls at the edge or becomes prematurely dislodged, the healing time is prolonged and hypertrophic scars tend to form in this area.

Immobilization Techniques. Children, of course, have a way of wriggling out of even the most cleverly constructed dressing. In the upper extremity, a cast should be extended above the flexed elbow to prevent a tiny hand from slipping out of the cylinder. When a graft is used to cover a wound, immobilization is critical, not so much for vascularization of the graft as for compression to minimize hematoma formation. The time-honored bolster or stent dressing is particularly useful for a freshly grafted wound. Nevertheless, if a graft is to be placed over a wound located in an area of movement, e.g., the chest wall, particularly over the scapula, an open grafting technique is preferred (Fig. 10–3). The traditional bolster dressing in these areas creates a shear force that is certain to dislodge the graft. The graft need not be sutured or taped; these techniques only add to the shear forces on a graft. For some areas of motion, immobilization with a polyurethane foam sponge, sutured about the perimeter of the graft, is useful. Whenever a skin graft fails, the loss is all too often ascribed to infection. Motion and hematoma are far and away the most common reasons for loss of a skin graft; both are the responsibility of the surgeon. If the bed is bleeding excessively, the wound should be covered with an occlusive compression dressing. The grafts can be simply applied 48 to 72 hours later. Meshed skin grafts are useful if the granulating bed has an irregular contour or is somewhat untidy.

Circumferential dressings, particularly elastic-type dressings around an extremity,

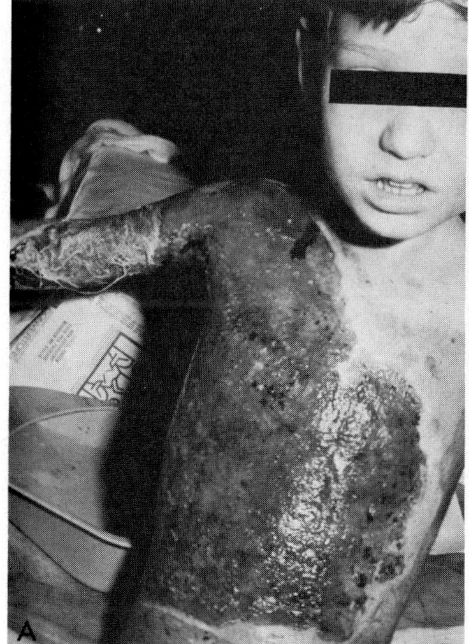

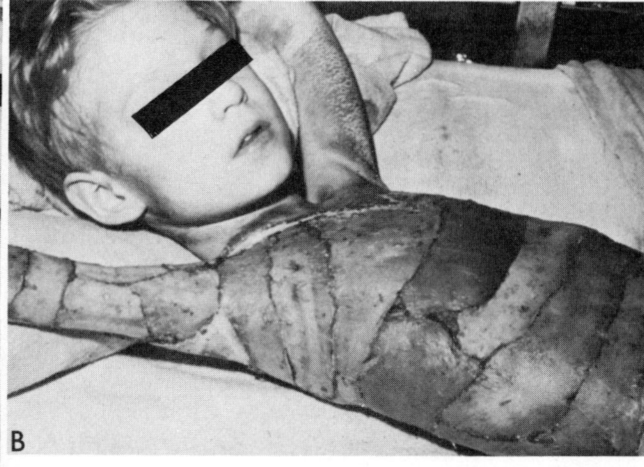

Figure 10–3 Granulation tissue following separation of a full-thickness burn eschar *(A)* and after coverage with split-thickness skin grafts *(B)*. The grafts were placed in an open (onlay) fashion with their axis along muscle groups and relaxed skin tension lines.

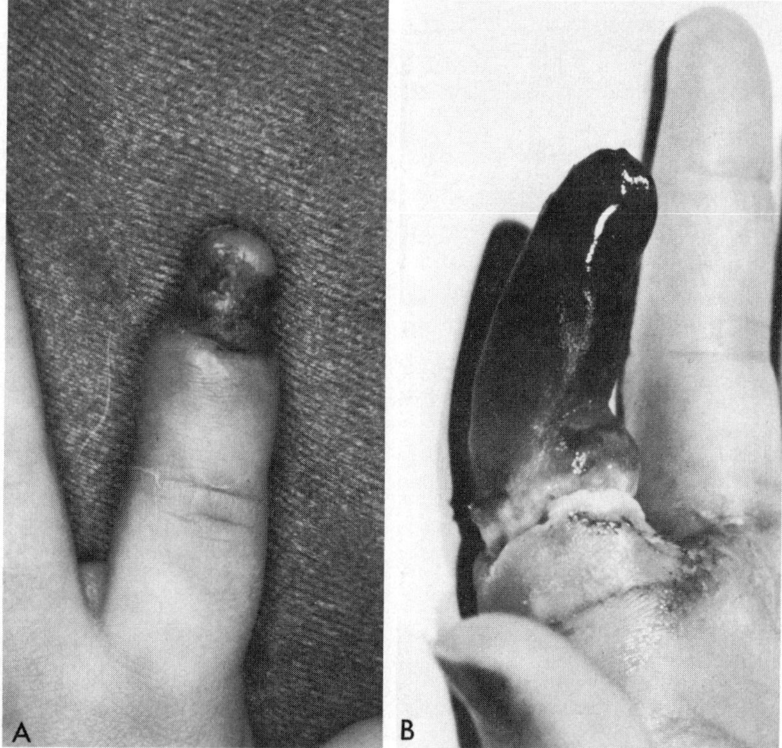

Figure 10–4 *A,* A circumferential bandage caused this full-thickness skin loss of the distal phalanx. (Courtesy of Joseph Upton, III, M.D.) *B,* Necrosis of the index finger secondary to an improperly managed rubber-band tourniquet. (Courtesy of John J. Byrne, M.D.)

should always be used with care. They tend to cinch up and twist, resulting in a tourniquet effect that may occlude circulation (Fig. 10–4). Circumferential dressings also create pressure, which is especially accentuated over points of bony prominence. This may result in ischemic necrosis of the subcutaneous fat and skin overlying these points. The radial and ulnar borders of the forearm are particularly vulnerable to pressure effects from tension caused by an Ace bandage. If one is willing to risk the inherent dangers of an elastic dressing, the addition of a wide splint will minimize the pressure exerted in the more convex radial and ulnar surfaces.

MANAGEMENT

Hematoma

It is a well-known fact that necrosis of the skin edge often occurs in the presence of underlying hematoma (Fig. 10–5). In the past this phenomenon was ascribed to a pressure effect on the dermal plexus. Recent studies of an experimental model have demonstrated that the mechanism of hematoma-related necrosis is neither pressure nor sepsis but a direct toxic effect of a component of blood on the circulation of the overlying skin. Hematomas must be evacuated promptly to diminish the extent of tissue necrosis. In the experimental model, evacuation must be accomplished within 4 hours to prevent necrosis. If 12 hours elapse, flap death is inevitable.[19]

There is increasing evidence that compromised circulation to muscle and skin can be improved pharmacologically. Isoxsuprine, a beta-agonist, has been used experimentally to improve survival of flaps. When it is administered early enough, there is evidence of improved survival of an ailing flap.[8] It is presumed that isoxsuprine acts by relaxing vascular smooth muscle within skeletal muscle and probably the subdermal

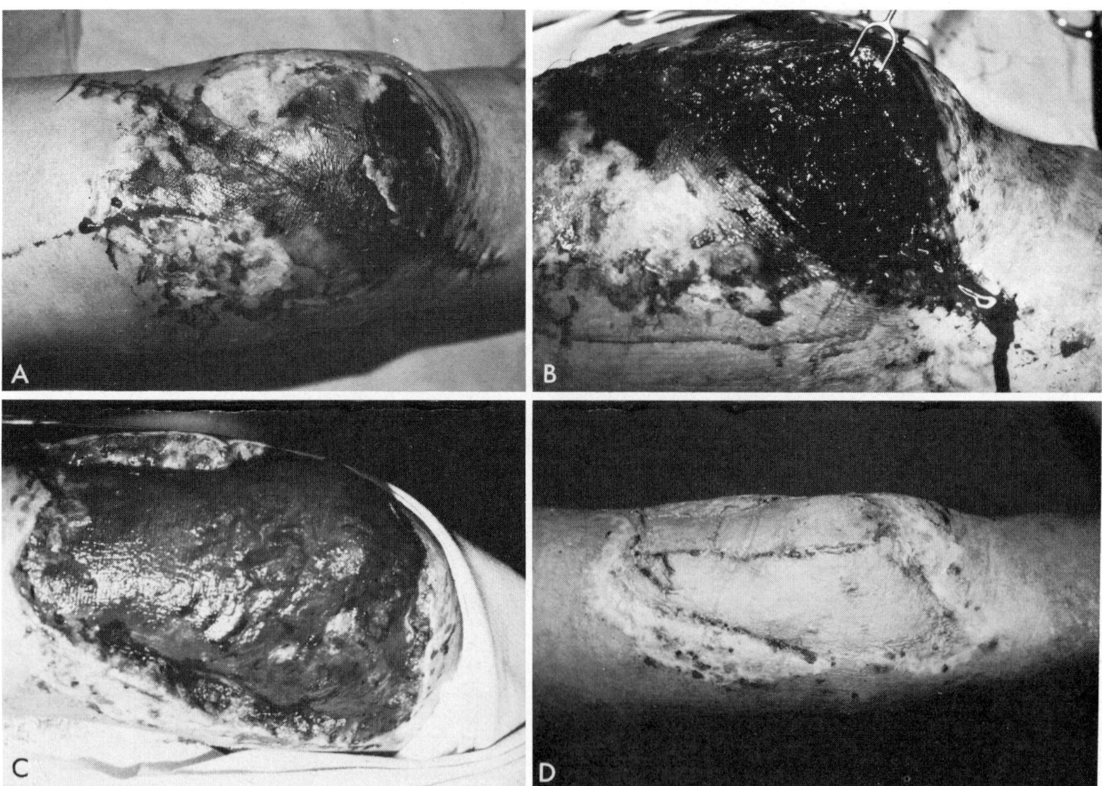

Figure 10–5 *A and B,* Postoperative hematoma of the knee after contour excision of a vascular malformation. *C and D,* After débridement of necrotic skin flaps, a skin graft was used to cover the granulating bed.

plexus as well. Recently, isoxsuprine has been used to salvage experimental flaps overlying hematoma.[10] Radiographic examination has demonstrated restoration of the microcirculation with this pharmacologic regimen.

Wound Disruption

Management of a disrupted wound depends on an accurate diagnosis of the basis for its occurrence. If disruption was caused by tension, e.g., postoperative abdominal wound dehiscence secondary to ileus or pulmonary complications, the wound may be resutured. A clean wound that gapes as the result of hematoma can be closed after evacuation of the hematoma and trimming of the ischemic wound edges. Wounds that disrupt secondary to wound sepsis should be left open and dressed frequently with fine mesh gauze and absorbent dressings. Once the granulating wound edges appear healthy, which can be documented by quantitative bacteriologic study, secondary closure may be undertaken. If the wound is large and the patient's condition necessitates rapid closure, an onlay split-thickness skin graft is best. If time is not important, closure by wound contraction can be relied upon, particularly in areas where the soft tissues are lax (healing by third intention).

Infiltration Wounds

Serious soft tissue loss can result from extravasation of peripheral intravenous fluids, blood transfusions, chemotherapeutic agents, or other medications. Infiltrations occur frequently in children, usually in the distal extremities where tenuous intravenous lines are placed. Fortunately, necrosis and slough of skin are uncommon considering the frequency with which intravenous extravasation is seen on a busy pediatric service.[2] Serious infiltration wounds are associated with the use of mechanical infusion pumps and with the administration of hypertonic or antitumor agents.[26] Tiny children cannot complain of a painful intravenous site. The best treatment is prevention, which requires hourly monitoring of intravenous lines. Securing an intravenous apparatus with clear tape (Dermaclear*) allows easy visibility and increased stretchability of the tape if an infiltration occurs.

Partial- or full-thickness extravasation wounds begin insidiously. The examining physician is often lulled into a false sense of security when only small intraepidermal blisters appear during the first 48 hours after extravasation. To date, there is no indication that intradermal steroids or specific antidotal solutions should be used to treat infiltration wounds. Instead, to minimize edema, the extremity should be elevated and, in the case of a hand, immobilized in the "position of advantage" with the wrist dorsiflexed 30 degrees, the metacarpophalangeal joints flexed 70 degrees, and the thumb abducted from the palm.

---

*Johnson &Johnson Co., New Brunswick, New Jersey.

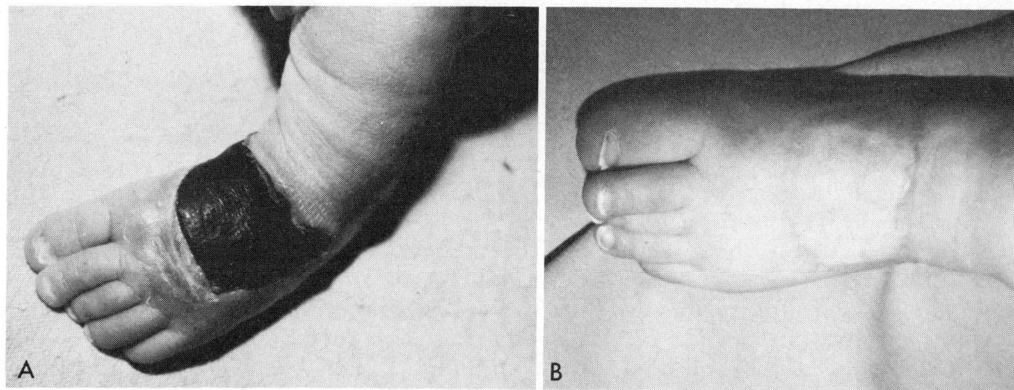

Figure 10–6   *A,* Infiltration of an intravenous fluid containing concentrated potassium chloride solution caused this full-thickness skin loss of the foot. *B,* One year after excision and closure with a split-thickness skin graft.

If the skin demonstrates only erythema or a few blisters, a simple dressing with petrolatum gauze and a layer of absorbent gauze is all that is necessary. Application of warm, moist compresses too often leads to maceration of the skin and necrosis. If the wound appears to be deep partial thickness or full thickness, povidone-iodine or silver sulfadiazine ointment can be used to minimize the chances of secondary sepsis. These wounds are often slow to epithelialize. When full-thickness loss is obvious, it is best to proceed with removal of the eschar and coverage with a split-thickness skin graft (Fig. 10–6). If prolonged intravenous therapy is necessary, the serious consequences of infiltration of chemotherapeutic agents can be minimized by vascular access shunts. A saphenous vein-to-superficial femoral artery loop fistula has been used in young children at this institution. Thomas shunts have also been needed in patients, such as those undergoing bone marrow transplantation, who require large volumes of medications, blood, or blood products.

Burn Wounds

Accidental thermal damage to the skin, whatever the cause, always presents with similar evidence. Secondary or partial-thickness burns, if superficial, result in blistering. Blisters should not be opened, because it has been shown that epithelialization occurs rapidly if the vesicle remains intact. If the blister fluid subsequently becomes infected, as evidenced by the presence of pus and surrounding cellulitis, it is mandatory that the bleb be opened and necrotic skin excised. Deep partial-thickness and full-thickness burns should be treated with a topical antibacterial agent, e.g., silver sulfadiazine, to minimize the chances of sepsis and further tissue loss. If a deep partial- or full-thickness eschar is obvious, early excision and closure with a split-thickness graft should be considered.

Burns can also occur in the operating room. The surgeon must be alert to this possibility (Fig. 10–7). Ground plates should be well secured and lubricated. Skin preparation solution should not be allowed to pool near the ground plate or in intertriginous areas. Whenever the electric cautery is

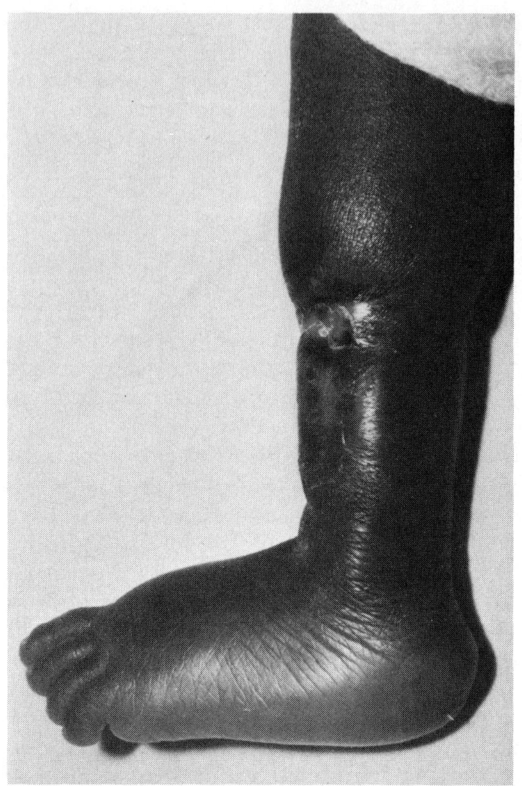

Figure 10–7 Circumferential scarring of a child's leg resulted from an electrical burn at the site of an electrocardiographic lead.

in use, the skin edge should be within view to prevent a burn. Tiny full-thickness burns of the skin edge should be excised before wound closure.

Hypertrophic Scars and Keloids

There is understandable confusion regarding the proper terminology for abnormal scar formation. In general, *hypertrophic scars* remain within the area of original skin injury and improve with time (Fig. 10–8). On the other hand, true *keloid scars* invade normal tissues beyond the injured area and usually do not improve with time (Fig. 10–9).[21] This is a practical definition useful in the management of scar problems. Hypertrophic scars, such as those seen after a burn injury, will respond to pressure; remodeling of collagen bundles results in softening and flattening. It has been shown that elastic pressure must be maintained for 12 months to be of lasting benefit. Hypertrophic scars

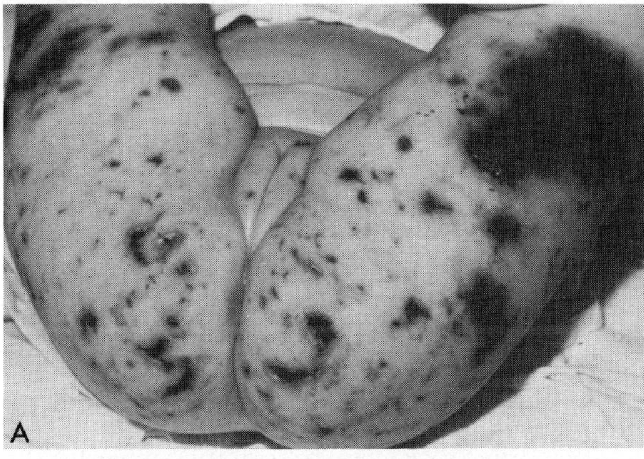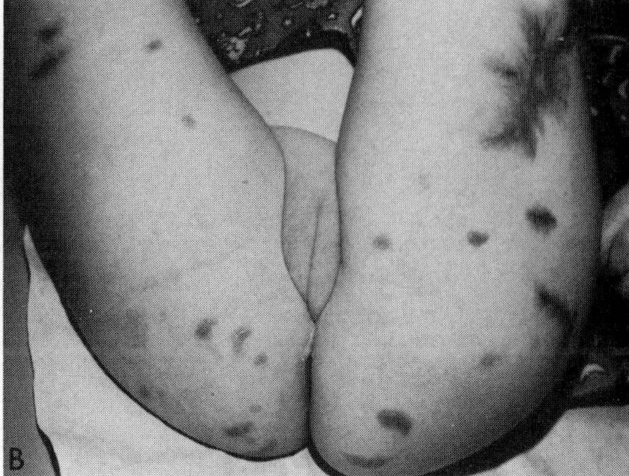

Figure 10–8 Purpuric, ecchymotic skin lesions of meningococcal septicemia. *B,* After healing, there is residual hypertrophic scarring of the most severely damaged areas.

also respond to intralesional steroid injections. Pruritus can be controlled in most instances with a series of intralesional steroid injections. Hypertrophic scars will also soften and mature more rapidly after

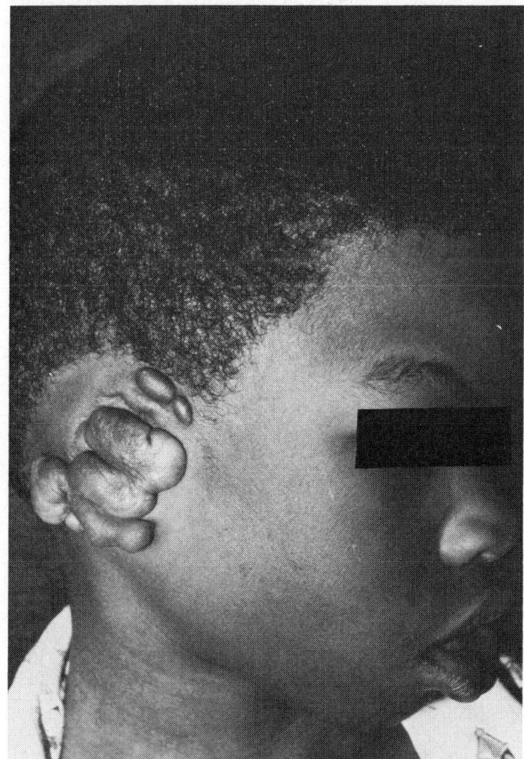

Figure 10–9 A true keloid scar following construction of an external ear. The keloid has invaded normal skin, with dissolution of the underlying autogenous cartilage graft.

such treatment. There are complications of intralesional steroid injections that must be weighed against the benefits. Local anesthetic should be injected initially. The usual dose of intralesional triamcinolone (10 to 25 mg/cc) for children should be no more than 40 to 50 mg per visit. The patient should be seen again in 6 weeks for consideration of further injections. A fine-gauge needle seems to permit better distribution and delivery of steroid than do air-pressure mechanical injections. Hypopigmentation, atrophy of the scar, telangiectasia, and clumping of the steroid beneath the scar are all signs of steroid effect. They usually improve with time.

True keloids do not respond to pressure. There will be some initial softening of a keloid with repeated intralesional steroid injections, but collagen remodeling and relief of pruritus are less predictable than with hypertrophic scars. Ear-lobe keloids can be managed by injection of steroid 1 to 2 weeks before excision and by injection of steroid into the wound edges at the time of closure. Keloids of the deltoid and sternal area are particularly vicious. They should not be excised, although intralesional steroids can be worthwhile.

Difficult Wound Problems

Each large, indolent wound challenges the surgeon in the application of established principles of wound care based on an understanding of wound biology. Any open wound, whatever its history, contains remnants of dead tissue, or eschar, that must be removed. A sharp blade is the best way to excise such necrotic tissue. The edges of the wound should be cleansed daily with soap and water to remove crusts that harbor bacteria. Dressings, consisting of a single layer of fine mesh gauze and an overlying absorbent layer, should be changed three or four times a day for mechanical removal of detritus from the wound. If a wound is heavily contaminated with bacteria, the local use of antiseptics such as hypochlorite solution (Dakin's solution) or povidone-iodine is useful. If a wound is, indeed, infected (i.e., if there are more than 10^5 organisms per gram of tissue), antiseptics will not be sufficient to handle the infection. Local antibacterial therapy is indicated instead. Once granulation tissue appears in the wound, one should not sit back and hope that it will

fill the wound cavity and replace the missing soft tissue. Granulation tissue, even healthy granulation tissue, is a clinical manifestation of inflammation. It is abnormal tissue, containing bacteria and acting as a metabolic drain on the patient. Application of split-thickness skin grafts is the quickest method of closing such a wound. Clinical judgment is usually sufficient for determining when to apply a graft. If a wound is ready for grafting, a close look at the edge of the wound will disclose an advancing blue-gray edge of epithelium. Otherwise, a quantitative culture can be taken; if the wound bed contains more than 10^5 organisms per gram of tissue, the graft will not adhere and become vascularized. Another method is to place a small allograft to make certain that the granulating bed is ready to accept an autograft. If the granulations remain untidy and closure is imperative, a meshed graft may be used. Application of split-thickness

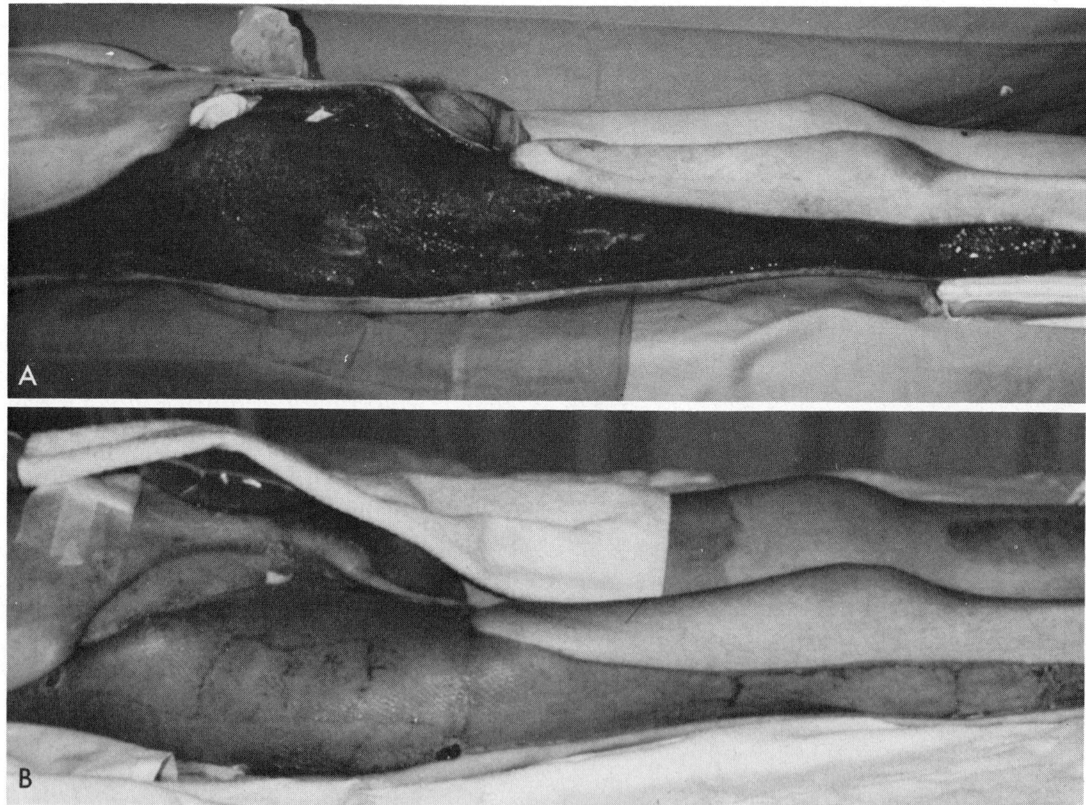

Figure 10–10 *A,* A 16-year-old boy contracted streptococcal fasciitis secondary to belatedly diagnosed traumatic bowel perforation. Colostomy and wide drainage resulted in an open wound from flank to lateral malleolus. *B,* This wound was closed with meshed split-thickness skin grafts, including the exposed bowel. (Courtesy of Richard A. Carter, M.D.)

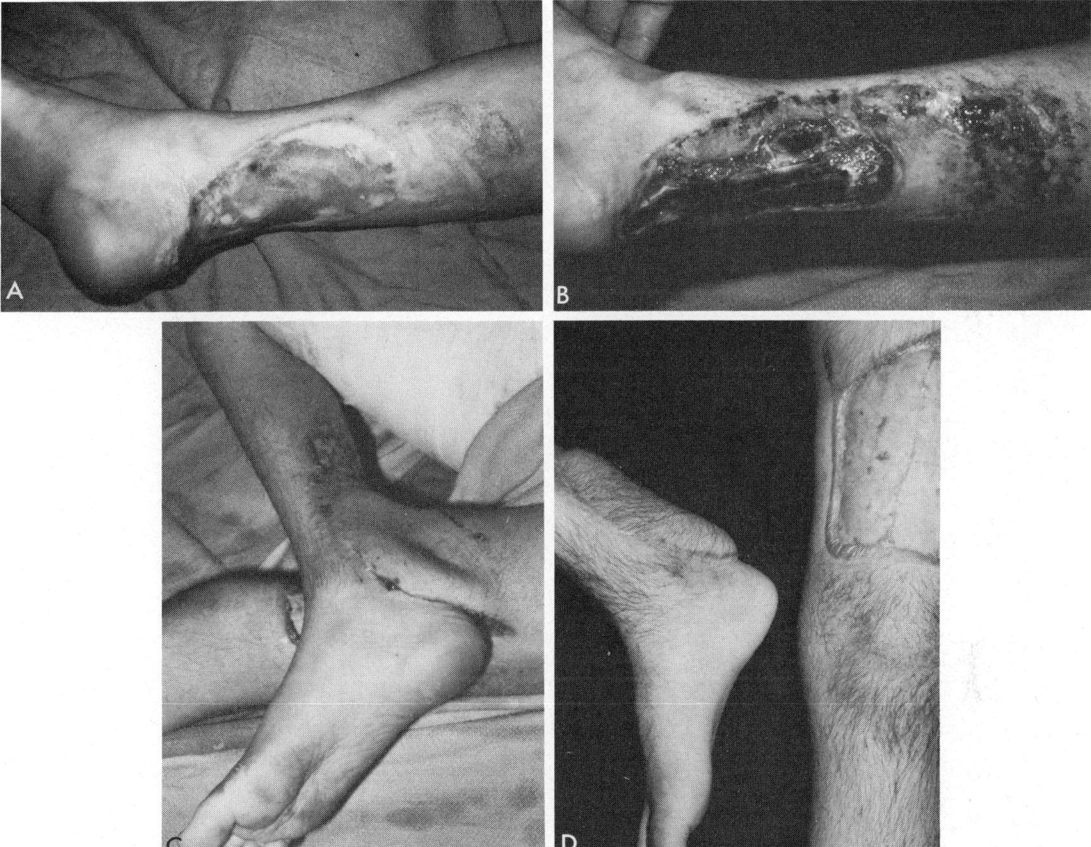

Figure 10–11 *A*, A, 9-year-old boy burned his leg against a hot muffler when his tractor turned over. *B*, Early tangential excision of the burn eschar and closure with a skin graft was unsuccessful. *C* and *D*, A cross-thigh flap was needed to cover the exposed Achilles tendon and provide long-term protection. A microvascular transfer of a groin flap would be an alternative method of coverage.

skin grafts should always be the first maneuver in closure of a difficult wound. This should be done as soon as possible to bring the wound and the patient under metabolic control (Fig. 10–10).

There are other wounds for which split-thickness grafts cannot be used. When tendons, joints, bone, or central nervous system tissue is exposed, flap coverage may be indicated (Fig. 10–11). Older skin flap techniques, often requiring multiple stages, are now used infrequently. On the basis of their

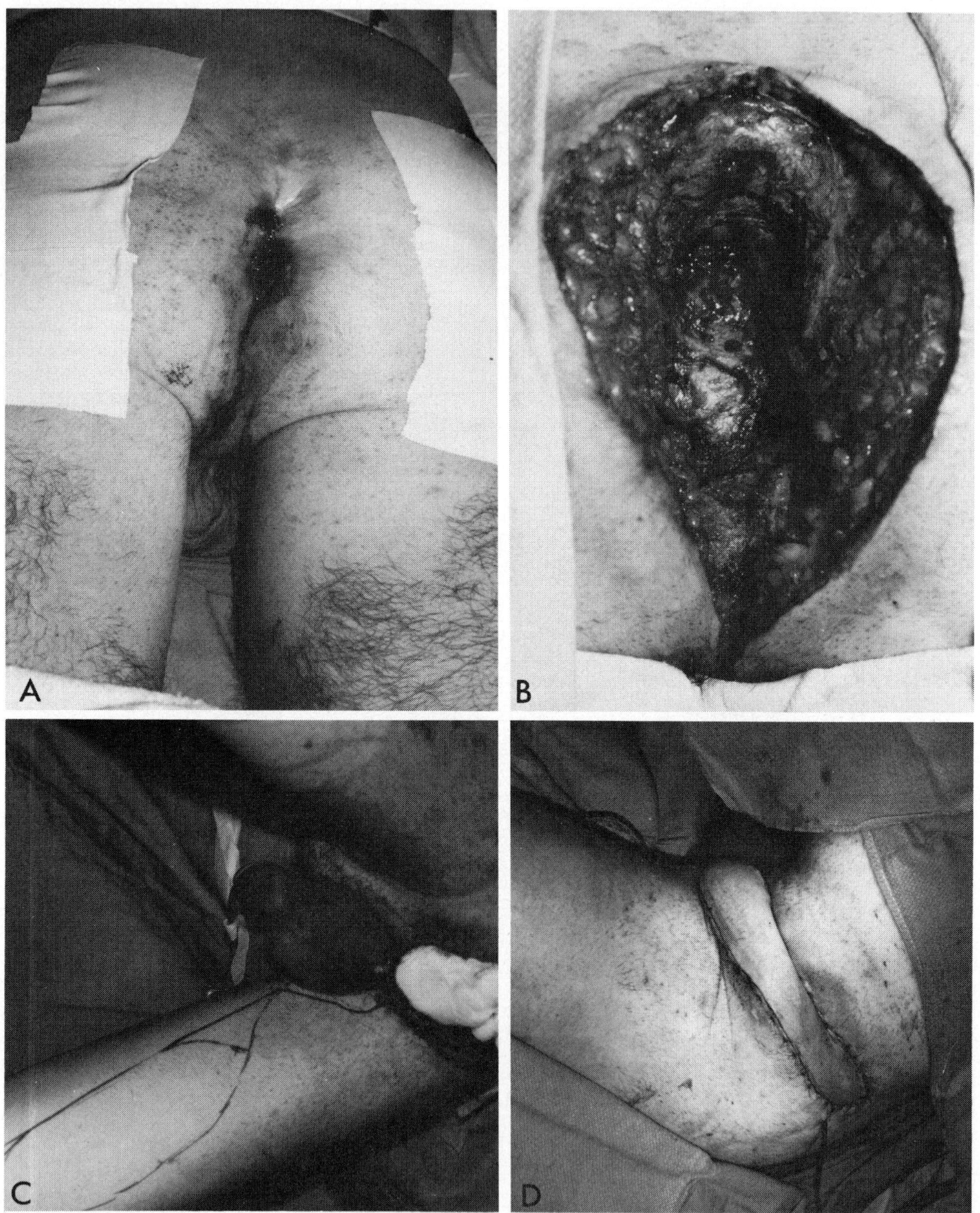

Figure 10–12　A 5-year-old boy underwent coloproctectomy and coloproctostomy (Swenson procedure) for Hirschsprung's disease. A pelvic hematoma and sepsis developed. *A,* Over the ensuing 10 years, the perineal wound failed to heal despite combined anterior-posterior resection, end colostomy, and numerous attempts at excision of the perineal sinus tract. *B,* After excision of the scarred perineum and multiple sinuses, the cavity extended from the bladder to the sacral hollow. *C* and *D,* The cavity was filled with a medially based gluteus maximus muscle flap (based on superior gluteal artery) and gracilis musculocutaneous flap (based on a branch of the profunda femoris artery). The wound has remained healed during a 3-year follow-up period.

new appreciation of the anatomy of blood supply to the skin, as noted earlier in this chapter, reconstructive surgeons may choose to utilize the musculocutaneous flap concept. The skin overlying a muscle is supplied by perforating vessels; a cutaneous paddle may be carried "piggyback" on the underlying muscle. This composite mass of tissue is supported by the vascular pedicle that nourishes the muscle (Fig. 10–12). Some muscles have a single or dominant blood supply; others have variable segmental arteries. Clinically useful musculocutaneous territories have been defined throughout the body.[13-15] The muscle is disconnected from its insertion and, if necessary, from its origin so that it can be transposed to cover a nearby wound. Now many challenging wounds can be predictably covered with these revolutionary "new" muscle and compound skin-muscle flaps (Fig. 10–12).

References

1. Brånemark, P. I., and Ekholm, R.: Tissue injury caused by wound disinfectants. J. Bone Joint Surg. 49A:48, 1967.
2. Brown, A. S., Hoelzer, D. J., and Piercy, S. A.: Skin necrosis from extravasation of intravenous fluids in children. Plast. Reconstr. Surg. 64:145, 1979.
3. Brown, L. L., Shelton, H. T., Bornside, G. H., and Cohn, I., Jr.: Evaluation of wound irrigation by pulsatile jet and conventional methods. Ann. Surg. 187:170, 1978.
4. Crikelair, G.: Skin suture marks. Am. J. Surg. 96:631, 1958.
5. Daniel, R. K., and Williams, H. B.: The free transfer of skin flaps by microvascular anastomoses. An experimental study and a reappraisal. Plast. Reconstr. Surg. 52:16, 1973.
6. deHoll, D., Rodeheaver, G. T., Edgerton, M. T., and Edlich, R. F.: Potentiation of infection by suture closure of dead space. Am. J. Surg. 127:716, 1974.
7. Edlich, R. F., Schmolka, I. R., Prusak, M. P., and Edgerton, M. T.: The molecular basis for toxicity of surfactants in surgical wounds. I. EO: PO block polymers. J. Surg. Res. 14:277, 1973.
8. Finseth, F., and Adelberg, M. G.: Experimental work with isoxsuprine for the prevention of skin flap necrosis and for treatment of the failing flap. Plast. Reconstr. Surg. 63:304, 1979.
9. Fleming, A.: The action of chemical and physiological antiseptics in a septic wound. Br. J. Surg. 7:99, 1919.
10. Hillelson, R. L., Glowacki, J., Healey, N. A., and Mulliken, J. B.: A microangiographic study of hematoma-associated flap necrosis and salvage with isoxsuprine. Plast. Reconstr. Surg. 66:528, 1980.
11. Krizek, T. J., and Robson, M. C.: Evolution of quantitative bacteriology in wound management. Am. J. Surg. 130:579, 1975.
12. Magee, C., Haury, B., Rodeheaver, G., et al.: A rapid technique for quantitating wound bacterial count. Am. J. Surg. 133:760, 1977.
13. Mathes, S. J., and Nahai, F.: Clinical Atlas of Muscle and Musculocutaneous Flaps. St. Louis, C. V. Mosby Co., 1979.
14. McCraw, J. B., and Dibbell, D. G.: Experimental definition of independent myocutaneous vascular territories. Plast. Reconstr. Surg. 60:212, 1977.
15. McCraw, J. B., Dibbell, D. G., and Carraway, J. H.: Clinical definition of independent myocutaneous vascular territories. Plast. Reconstr. Surg. 60:341, 1977.
16. McCraw, J. B., Myers, B., and Shanklin, K. D.: The value of fluorescein in predicting the viability of arterialized flaps. Plast. Reconstr. Surg. 60:710, 1977.
17. McGregor, I. A., and Morgan, G.: Axial and random pattern flaps. Br. J. Plast. Surg. 26:202, 1973.
18. Milton, S. H.: Pedicled skin flaps: The fallacy of the length/width ratio. Br. J. Surg. 57:502, 1970.
19. Mulliken, J. B., and Healey, N. A.: Pathogenesis of skin flap necrosis from an underlying hematoma. Plast. Reconstr. Surg. 63:540, 1979.
20. Mulliken, J. B., Healey, N. A., and Glowacki, J.: Povidone-iodine and tensile strength of wounds in rats. J. Trauma 20:323, 1980.
21. Peacock, E. E., Jr., and Van Winkle, W., Jr.: Wound Repair, 2nd edition. Philadelphia, W. B. Saunders Co., 1976, p. 231.
22. Reinisch, J. F.: Pathophysiology of skin flap circulation. Plast. Reconstr. Surg. 54:585, 1974.
23. Rodeheaver, G. T., Pettry, D., Thacker, J. G., et al.: Wound cleansing by high pressure irrigation. Surg. Gynecol. Obstet. 141:357, 1975.
24. Rodeheaver, G. T., Pettry, D., Turnbull, V., et al.: Identification of the wound infection potentiating factors in soil. Am. J. Surg. 128:8, 1974.
25. Sundell, B.: Studies on the circulation of pedicle skin flaps. Ann. Chir. Gynaecol. Fenniae (Suppl. 53), 133:1, 1963.
26. Upton, J., Mulliken, J. B., and Murray, J. E.: Intravenous extravasation injuries. Am. J. Surg. 137:497, 1979.

SALIVARY GLANDS, LARYNX, AND OROPHARYNX

Gerald B. Healy, M.D.
Trevor J. I. McGill, M.D.

The common otolaryngologic complications likely to be encountered by the pediatric surgeon follow salivary gland surgery, tonsillectomy and adenoidectomy, and procedures involving the larynx and adjacent structures. The surgeon operating on the head and neck must be aware of these problems and of the various means of prevention and correction.

SALIVARY GLAND SURGERY

Parotid Gland

Most trauma, infection, and neoplasia affecting the salivary glands involves the parotid gland. Surgery of the parotid gland requires knowledge of the position of the facial nerve, which may vary, especially in children.

ANATOMY

The facial nerve exits from the skull at the stylomastoid foramen. In children the site of exit is more superficial than it is in adults; thus, incisions behind the angle of the mandible and below the ear lobe must not pass beneath the subcutaneous tissue layer without thought being given to the facial nerve. After turning forward from the stylomastoid foramen, the nerve enters the deep surface of the parotid gland and becomes more superficial as it passes across the masseter muscle. Within the parotid, the nerve usually divides into two branches, an upper temporofacial branch and a lower cervicofacial branch. These branches divide further and then anastomose to form a plexus (Fig. 11–1).

Submandibular Gland

The most common complications of surgery of the submandibular gland are injuries to the hypoglossal nerve, the lingual nerve, and the marginal branch of the facial nerve.

ANATOMY

The medial surface of the gland rests on the hypoglossal and lingual nerves. The

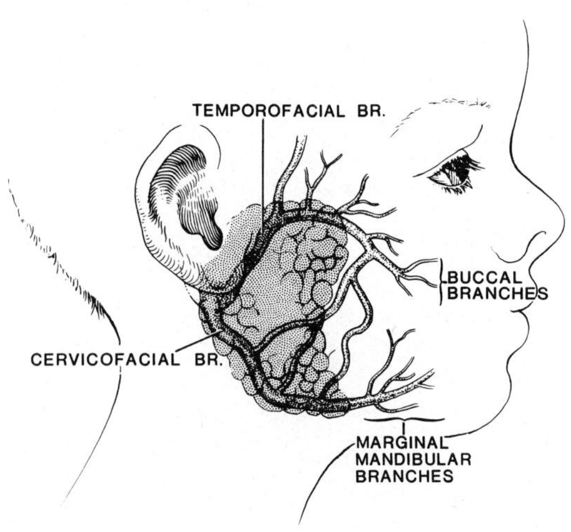

Figure 11–1 Common anatomic location and major divisions of the facial nerve.

hypoglossal passes beneath the posterior belly of the digastric muscle to the hyoglossus muscle. The lingual nerve is usually found at the uppermost surface of the gland just under the mandible. The mandibular branch of the facial nerve passes between the platysma and the facial vessels and usually runs through the capsule of the gland.

Complications

In parotid surgery, direct trauma to the facial nerve during dissection of the gland occasionally occurs. This may result in a temporary, partial, or complete paresis that usually resolves spontaneously. Such injury can frequently be avoided by careful dissection and the use of a nerve stimulator. In small infants, the use of magnification often helps to avoid such injuries.

Transection of the facial nerve is more likely to occur during procedures such as incision and drainage than it is when the nerve is carefully exposed, as in partial or total resection of the parotid gland.

Injuries to the nerves that are intimately related to the submandibular gland are much less frequent. The most commonly affected nerve is the marginal branch of the facial, which may be injured during incision and drainage of abscesses in this region. Trauma to the hypoglossal and lingual nerves is extremely rare during resection of the submandibular gland.

Transection of the parotid duct is an uncommon complication. Left untreated, it may lead to a salivary fistula, most often at the site of the original incision.

Flushing and sweating of the face, known as *gustatory sweating,* may occur after parotidectomy. It is thought to be the result of aberrant regeneration of nerve fibers to the sweat glands in the area of the parotid excision. Some believe that regenerating parasympathetic secretory fibers are misdirected and replace some of the divided sympathetic secretory nerves that previously innervated the sweat glands in the skin.[6]

TREATMENT

Injuries to the facial, lingual, or hypoglossal nerve that involve trauma but not transection are usually best treated by watchful waiting. If the nerve is intact, full resolution of paresis often occurs spontaneously within 2 to 3 months. It is best to reassure the patient or the family that recovery is probable.

When the nerve has been transected, immediate reanastomosis is indicated. If a large segment of the nerve has been removed so that end-to-end anastomosis is not feasible, nerve grafting is advisable.

Reanastomosis of the nerve involves placing fine monofilament (10–0) sutures in the epineurium. The nerve endings should be approximated without distortion so that there will be minimal aberrant regrowth and dyskinesia. The use of the operating microscope or magnifying loupes is advised. Soft Silastic tubing may be placed over the anastomosis to discourage ingrowth of scar.

If nerve grafting is necessary, the greater auricular nerve is conveniently available approximately 2 cm below the lobule of the ear overlying the sternocleidomastoid muscle. Use of the sensory elements of the cervical plexus has also been advocated in repairing injuries to the facial nerve or its divisions.[1]

Delayed repair of anatomic injuries is to be discouraged because the rapid ingrowth of scar tissue makes identification difficult.

Transection of the parotid duct requires reanastomosis and stenting with a fine polyethylene catheter, which may be brought out through the orifice of Stensen's duct and sutured in place inside the oral cavity. This catheter should be left in place for approximately 3 weeks and then removed. Occasional dilatation by a transoral approach may be necessary if slight stenosis occurs at the site of reanastomosis.

Gustatory sweating is a troublesome problem for which many treatments have been advised. At present, the most promising appears to be tympanic neurectomy. This involves interruption of the tympanic branch of the glossopharyngeal (Jacobson's) nerve, which contains the secretomotor preganglionic parasympathetic salivary fibers. This nerve may be interrupted by elevating the tympanic membrane and resecting the nerve as it courses through the middle ear space. This causes atrophy of the supplied glandular structures and, frequently, cessation of symptoms.[3]

DIAGNOSIS

When the nerve has merely been traumatized rather than transected, its status may be monitored by periodic assessment of nerve conduction by electrical testing or electromyography.[4]

LARYNX

Most laryngeal complications of pediatric surgery occur as a result of endotracheal intubation. The widespread use of the endotracheal tube for the delivery of anesthesia as well as for respiratory support has led to the recognition of laryngeal injuries secondary to use of this device.

Complications

The most common complication of endotracheal intubation is edema of the glottic and subglottic regions (Fig. 11–2). This commonly occurs as a result of excessive manipulation of the endotracheal tube. The placement of an endotracheal tube that is too large for the subglottic space may also be responsible. This problem is evident when

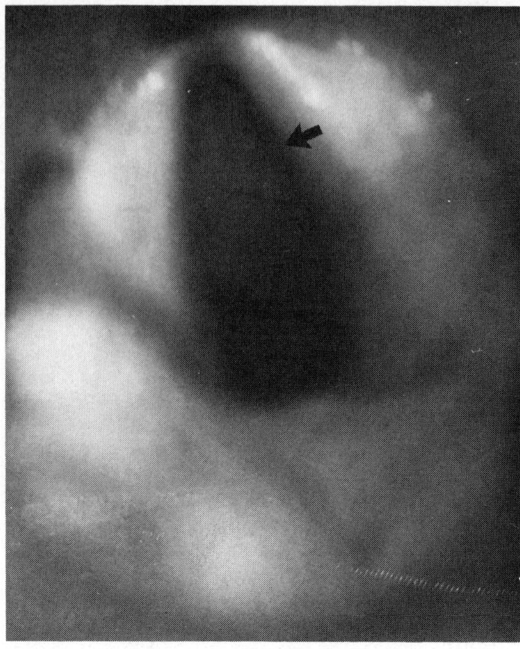

Figure 11–3 Chronic acquired subglottic stenosis with mature scar. *Arrow* points to organized scar below right vocal cord.

the tube is removed and the patient immediately experiences biphasic stridor and retractions.

Occasionally, more severe forms of chronic laryngeal injury result from the use of intubation. Marked scarring and constriction of the subglottis takes place, causing chronic acquired subglottic stenosis (Fig. 11–3). Glottic injury may also be present with webbing of the anterior or posterior commissure.

Laryngeal injuries may not be evident immediately upon removal of the endotracheal tube and may not become manifest for some weeks after extubation. With gradual maturation of scar tissue, there is a decrease in size of the lumen of the subglottic space. This is in contrast to the immediate closure seen with edema.

Occasionally, large amounts of granulation tissue may form around an endotracheal tube, especially in the posterior portion of the glottis. Upon extubation, this will cause immediate obstruction and the development of severe stridor, as with edema. The key to differentiating obturative obstruction due to granulation tissue from subglottic edema may be the quality of the

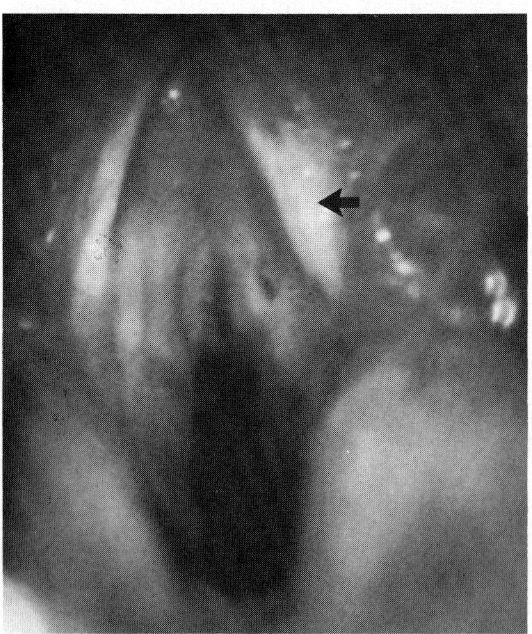

Figure 11–2 Edema of the subglottic space secondary to intubation (vocal cord at *arrow*).

stridor, which is usually inspiratory rather than biphasic.

Rarely, traumatic intubation may cause dislocation of the arytenoid cartilages or formation of hematoma in the supraglottic or glottic regions. This usually results in airway obstruction, which requires immediate treatment. Hoarseness or a change in voice may be the only sign of a dislocated arytenoid cartilage.

The recurrent laryngeal nerve may be injured during a variety of pediatric surgical procedures. These injuries may occur immediately adjacent to the larynx, as in surgery of the thyroid gland, repair of tracheoesophageal fistula, and tracheotomy. Injury may also occur at some distance from the larynx, as may be the case in cardiothoracic procedures. If the injury is unilateral, it is usually evidenced by a change in voice or hoarseness. Occasionally, very small children with this type of injury will display features of airway obstruction and stridor. In the occasional patient with bilateral injury, an adductor paralysis may cause severe airway obstruction necessitating tracheotomy. These patients may demonstrate a normal voice and cry. The surgeon should not be lulled into a false sense of security if this is the case. A patient may have severe obstruction from bilateral vocal cord paralysis and still have a normal voice and cry.

DIAGNOSIS

Various radiographic techniques, including xerography and fluoroscopy, may be useful in delineating the location and type of laryngeal injury. Fluoroscopy may help identify nerve injuries, while xerography may demonstrate the degree and location of laryngeal stenosis. Soft tissue radiography of the neck in both the lateral and the anteroposterior direction is useful in identifying subglottic edema immediately after intubation. This technique helps to differentiate subglottic edema from obstruction due to granuloma formation on the vocal cords.

If the child is old enough, indirect laryngoscopy will frequently be useful in identifying the problem and its cause. If the child is too young to undergo this, use of the flexible fiberoptic nasolaryngoscope is advised. This instrument can be employed even in the neonate for identifying lesions at or above the level of the true vocal cords (Fig. 11–4).

Direct laryngoscopy should be utilized whenever a diagnostic question cannot be answered by other means. This should be coupled with a complete evaluation of the airway, including bronchoscopy. Occasionally, simultaneous respiratory tract lesions are identified.

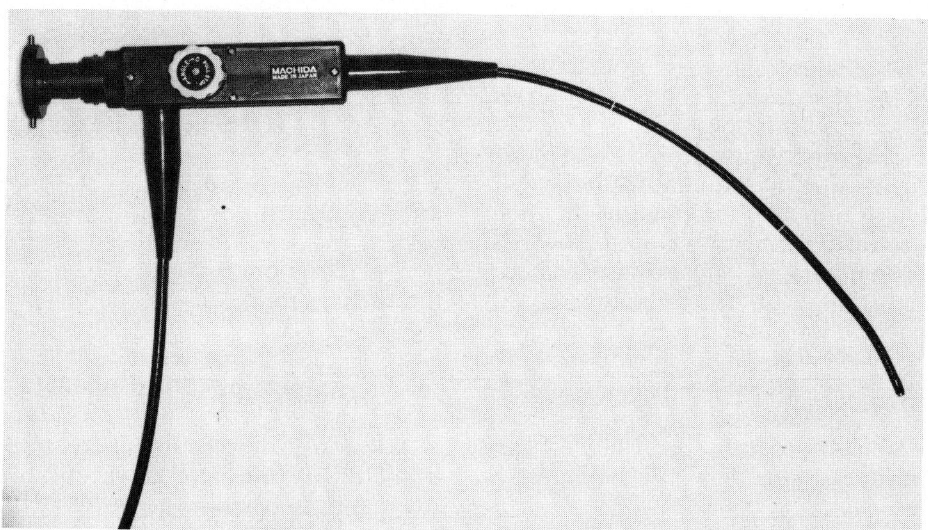

Figure 11–4 Flexible fiberoptic nasolaryngoscope useful for examination of the larynx.

TREATMENT

Corticosteroid therapy has proved useful in the treatment of acute laryngeal injuries. Racemic epinephrine may give temporary relief of mucosal swelling, but care must be taken to avoid a "rebound" phenomenon with the use of this medication. Humidification is always efficacious in improving ciliary function that has been diminished by swelling and inflammatory reaction.

Subglottic edema secondary to endotracheal intubation may by treated by a single intravenous bolus of dexamethasone (1 mg/kg; maximum dose, 30 mg). This may be accompanied by the use of racemic epinephrine until the blood level of dexamethasone has reached therapeutic levels.

Patients demonstrating glottic or subglottic granulomas secondary to intubation should undergo laryngoscopy with immediate removal of this tissue. This should be supplemented by administration of antibiotics for 7 days and diminishing doses of corticosteroids for 10 days. These lesions frequently have an inflammatory component. This regimen has been most useful in preventing recurrence by lessening formation of scar tissue.

When formation of hematoma or dislocation of the arytenoid cartilage is suspected, immediate direct laryngoscopy is required. If hematoma is found, it should be aspirated and the patient should begin receiving dexamethasone. Such patients must be observed carefully for airway obstruction. Occasionally, reintubation or tracheotomy may be required.

Paralysis of the vocal cords is a challenging problem. In cases of unilateral paralysis, watchful waiting is the best course of action if the airway is not compromised. The paralysis may be due to edema secondary to intubation or other systemic causes that may improve. In patients with bilateral paralysis, airway obstruction may necessitate immediate intervention with tracheotomy. If improvement is not evident over the long term, unilateral arytenoidectomy by either a transoral or an external approach may be indicated. Reinnervation techniques have been developed recently, but their efficacy in pediatric patients has not been established.[7]

The most difficult and perplexing problem for the airway surgeon is the correction of acquired subglottic stenosis. Many such injuries are secondary to prolonged intubation, and many methods of correction have been advocated.

Laryngeal dilatation does not seem to give satisfactory long-lasting results. Open operations with the use of stents and mucosal or skin grafts have been advocated by many.[2] Results have been most gratifying in some series, and this method of repair is probably the most reliable at present.

Recently, the introduction of the carbon dioxide laser for use in the pediatric airway has made it possible to employ a transoral approach in the correction of many of these troublesome lesions. The organized scar tissue in the subglottic space is resected with the laser. Frequently a soft Silastic stent is then placed for approximately 6 weeks. The patient is given antibiotics and corticosteroids while the stent is in place to reduce the amount of granulation tissue that may form in the area.[5]

Other methods such as cryosurgical removal of tissue and electrocautery are somewhat unpredictable. Injury to uninvolved tissue can occur because the depth of tissue destruction cannot be accurately controlled, as it can be with the laser.

It is obvious that many of these injuries are avoidable. Care must be taken by the surgeon and anesthesiologist whenever the airway of a small child is manipulated for any reason. Long-term intubation, especially of the neonate, has become popular. However, a tube may become the patient's worst enemy without proper care.

TONSILLECTOMY

Postoperative bleeding is the most common complication of tonsillectomy. It may occur in the immediate postoperative period (reactionary) or may be delayed until the fifth or tenth day (secondary).

Anatomy (Blood Supply)

The tonsil derives its blood supply from branches of the external carotid artery. Its main supply is from the tonsillar branch of the facial artery. It is also supplied by the

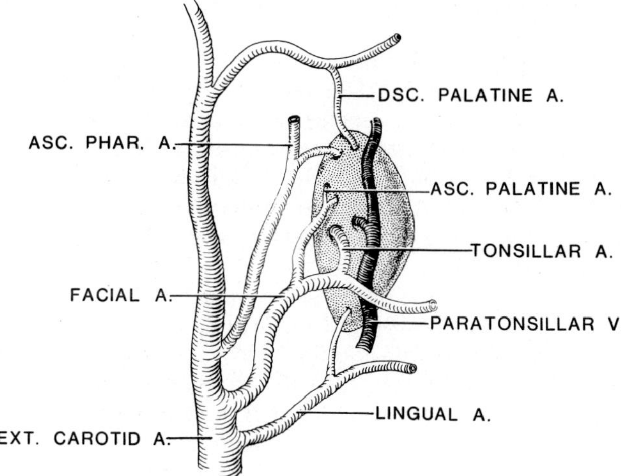

Figure 11–5 Major vascular supply of the tonsil.

ascending pharyngeal artery, the descending palatine artery, and the ascending palatine artery (Fig. 11–5). The paratonsillar vein emerges from the lateral surface of the tonsil and runs down its lateral surface outside the capsule. It then pierces the superior constrictor muscle and ends in the pharyngeal plexus. It may be a troublesome site of bleeding during or following tonsillectomy.

Reactionary Bleeding

Reactionary posttonsillectomy bleeding is usually due to a number of factors acting alone or in concert:

1. Failure to coagulate or ligate all bleeding vessels.

2. Inadequate operation leaving tonsillar remnants that prevent constriction of blood vessels.

3. Overzealous operative technique extending dissection to remove a section of the lingual tonsils at the base of the tongue. This area is difficult to visualize; therefore, it is difficult to secure hemostasis.

4. Excessive coughing and gagging during recovery from the anesthetic may cause a rise in blood pressure that dislodges an insecure thrombus.

CONTRIBUTING FACTORS

Active or recent respiratory tract infection increases the risk of bleeding from acutely inflamed tissues. Fibrosis of the tonsillar capsule after a peritonsillar abscess is also a common cause of failure of blood vessels to contract.

DIAGNOSIS

Frank blood coming through the nose or mouth indicates continued hemorrhage following tonsillectomy. Occasionally, the bleeding is more subtle and is manifest only by frequent swallowing movements in the pediatric patient. At times, the first indication of continued bleeding is the sudden vomiting of a large quantity of stale blood.

Continued hemorrhage may constitute a grave danger if it is unrecognized, because a large quantity of blood may be lost in a relatively short time. Skilled nursing surveillance, with quarter-hourly monitoring of pulse, blood pressure, and other signs of hypovolemia, is necessary.

Proper instruments must be available to inspect the oropharynx. These include a headlight, tongue depressor, and Yankauer sucker so that both hands of the physician are free to allow proper inspection of both tonsillar fossae.

TREATMENT

The oropharynx is inspected, and blood clot is removed from the tonsillar fossae with a Yankauer sucker. This alone may allow the tissue in the tonsillar fossae to retract and the bleeding to stop spontaneously.

Oozing from capillaries or veins may be stopped by applying pressure with a piece of cotton soaked in 0.5 per cent lidocaine (Xylocaine) and 1:200,000 epinephrine. The moistened cotton is held with Magill forceps in the tonsillar fossa, and counterpressure is applied with the hand on the side of the neck.

An alternative method is the use of Avitene,* a topically applied hemostatic agent. This microfibrillar collagen derivative is applied to the bleeding tonsillar fossa with a dry forceps. The tonsillar fossa is relatively insensitive for a few hours after tonsillectomy, and these measures may be repeated in a cooperative patient without causing undue pain.

If these simple measures fail to arrest the bleeding, it is necessary to return to the operating room and effect hemostasis under general anesthesia.

The indications for general anesthesia in patients with posttonsillectomy bleeding are as follows.

1. Uncooperative patient who continues to bleed

2. Continuous hemorrhage despite simple pressure methods described above

3. Arterial bleeding

The possibility of a coagulation defect must be considered, and a bleeding profile should be obtained. The patient's blood should always be typed and cross-matched as a precautionary measure. Intravenous fluid replacement with 5 per cent albumin in isotonic saline solution is started and continued until cross-matched blood is available. In patients with severe exsanguination, the use of O negative blood may be unavoidable.

With the patient under general anesthesia, the bleeding point is identified and ligated or coagulated with a bipolar cautery. Occasionally, it may be necessary to oversew the superior or the inferior pole of the tonsillar fossa if a definite bleeding point cannot be identified. In the rare event that bleeding cannot be controlled despite suturing, the fossa is packed with gauze and the two pillars are sutured together over the gauze.

---

*Avicon, Inc., Fort Worth, Texas.

Occasionally, all local attempts to control the bleeding fail, and the external carotid artery on the involved side must be ligated.

Secondary Hemorrhage

Secondary hemorrhage usually occurs 5 to 10 days postoperatively. It is caused by separation of a coagulum that has formed over the denuded tonsillar fossa. This is usually associated with local infection and should be anticipated whenever there is persistent postoperative pyrexia and increasing odynophagia.

DIAGNOSIS

Postoperative pyrexia usually persists, and the initial bleeding frequently presents as a slight tinging of the saliva. Later there may be continuous oozing of blood from either tonsillar fossa. Such bleeding is seldom severe and usually stops spontaneously.

TREATMENT

All patients with secondary posttonsillectomy hemorrhage should be admitted to the hospital for observation for 24 hours. Systemic antibiotics are administered. Simple pressure techniques, as outlined in the discussion of treatment of reactionary hemorrhage, usually effect complete hemostasis. Very occasionally, it may be necessary to return the patient to the operating room to control the bleeding. Edema of the tonsillar pillars and granulations in the base of the tonsillar fossa make ligation of a bleeding point extremely difficult. This is a situation in which suturing of both tonsillar pillars may be required.

ADENOIDECTOMY

Bleeding after adenoidectomy is more common than posttonsillectomy hemorrhage. It usually occurs during the first 24 hours after surgery. Secondary hemorrhage from the adenoid bed is extremely rare.

Postoperative hemorrhage is commonly

due to an incomplete removal of adenoid tags. These may be left on the posterior wall or roof of the nasopharynx. The adenoid bed should be inspected after removal of the lymphoid tissue, and a dry field should be obtained before the patient is allowed to leave the operating room.

Treatment

If bleeding occurs in the postoperative period, an attempt should be made to control it by administering 0.25 per cent phenylephrine hydrochloride drops through both nostrils. If the child is very restless, sedation is often required to control bleeding.

If bleeding persists, a postnasal pack must be inserted. This can sometimes be done in a cooperative child without anesthesia. Generally, however, it is necessary to return to the operating room and reanesthetize the patient.

The patient's blood is typed and cross matched. Intravenous therapy with 5 per cent albumin in isotonic saline solution is instituted. After induction of general anesthesia, the nasopharynx and oropharynx are cleared of blood and the nasopharynx is inspected. The cause of bleeding usually is a remnant of adenoid tissue that prevents proper contraction of blood vessels. Secondary curettage and packing often succeeds in arresting bleeding. If removal of the pack is repeatedly followed by bleeding, a postnasal pack may be left in place for 12 to 24 hours. The postnasal pack has three tapes attached to it. Two tapes in the anterior portion of the pack are led through the nostril and tied in front of the nose to hold it in position. The third tape is brought up through the mouth and attached to the cheek with paper tape, which facilitates removal.

UNUSUAL COMPLICATIONS

Posttonsillectomy submucosal bleeding may extend down the hypopharynx to involve the supraglottic larynx, necessitating airway intervention.

Laryngospasm may occur postoperatively. It is managed by holding the mandible forward and inserting an oral airway to keep the base of the tongue clear of the posterior pharyngeal wall. An oxygen mask is applied and manual inflation is attempted. Direct inspection of the larynx and aspiration of mucus or blood may be required.

Very rarely, surgical emphysema of the soft tissues of the neck is seen. This condition is due to air dissecting through the tonsillar fossa into the deep structures of the neck.

Pulmonary complications such as atelectasis, pneumonia, or lung abscesses may follow aspiration of mucus, blood, or teeth.

Occasionally, generalized pharyngeal and systemic infection follows tonsillectomy.

Exposure of aberrant blood vessels behind the posterior tonsillar pillar has been reported. This is usually an aberrant internal carotid or ascending pharyngeal artery.

Velopharyngeal incompetence causing hypernasality can result from adenoidectomy in the presence of an unrecognized submucosal cleft of the soft palate. Excessive scarring in the nasopharynx may damage the pharyngeal end of the eustachian tube. This can give rise to persistent dysfunction of the eustachian tube and chronic serous otitis media. Excessive scarring throughout the nasopharynx can cause nasopharyngeal stenosis and hyponasality requiring surgical intervention.

Atlantoaxial subluxation due to inappropriate manipulation during adenoidectomy has been reported.

Prevention of complications following tonsillectomy and adenoidectomy requires clear consideration of the cause of such complications. Preoperative hematocrit and coagulation studies should be performed to exclude an unrecognized bleeding tendency. Surgery should not be performed if the patient has had an upper respiratory tract infection within the previous 2 weeks. Attention to detail during the operation and skilled nursing monitoring in the first 24 postoperative hours will substantially reduce the incidence of most complications.

NASAL COMPLICATIONS

Postoperative nasal complications are rare and usually follow surgical measures to arrest epistaxis. The most common form of epistaxis in children is spontaneous bleeding from dilated blood vessels on the anterior nasal septum, usually associated with a mild upper respiratory tract infection. Epistaxis of this nature usually stops after pressure is applied at the lower end of the nose. In children, there is little or no need for electric cautery or cryosurgery of the nasal mucosa. Overzealous use of these methods can result in perforation of the anterior nasal septum with troublesome crusting and bleeding from the edges of the perforation.

Adventurous attempts at removal of foreign bodies within the middle meatus or superior meatus of a child's nose can lead to troublesome bleeding.

Prolonged nasotracheal intubation can cause mucosal changes within the nasal cavity. There are slight mucosal swellings initially, followed by ulceration and formation of granulation tissue with resulting synechiae. Sometimes these synechiae will have to be divided and a Silastic stent placed in the affected nasal cavity.

References

1. Conley, J. J.: Salivary Glands and Facial Nerve. New York, Grune & Stratton, 1975.
2. Cotton, R.: Management of subglottic stenosis in infancy and childhood. Ann. Otol. Rhinol. Laryngol. 86:789, 1977.
3. Friedman, W. H., and Pomarico, J. M.: The intratympanic correction of Frey syndrome. Arch. Surg. 108:366, 1974.
4. Gordon, A. S., and Friedberg, J.: Current status of testing for seventh nerve lesions. Otolaryngol. Clin. North Am. 11:301, 1978.
5. Healy, G. B., McGill, T., and Strong, M. S.: Surgical advances in treatment of lesions of the pediatric airway: Role of the carbon dioxide laser. Pediatrics 61:380, 1978.
6. Hemenway, W. G.: Gustatory sweating and flushing. Laryngoscope 70:84, 1960.
7. Tucker, H.: Reinnervation of the unilaterally paralyzed larynx. Ann. Otol. Rhinol. Laryngol. 87:649, 1978.

THE NECK

Samuel L. Cresson, M.D., F.A.C.S.
Harry Applebaum, M.D.

Complications of pediatric surgical procedures in the neck are uncommon if the surgeon is familiar with the types of lesions found in children, their natural history, and, in many cases, their embryology. A thorough knowledge and understanding of the anatomy of the neck and the pathologic conditions likely to be encountered is necessary. The surgeon should always remember that patients who have had previous neck surgery and those undergoing second-look cancer operations are at greatest risk of complications.

As in all head and neck procedures, obtaining and maintaining an adequate airway is of the greatest importance. Endotracheal anesthesia is almost always necessary because of the difficulty of intubating small children should it become necessary during a procedure, and because of the small size and easy compressibility of the child's trachea.

The preoperative use of ultrasound, scans, and angiograms often results in a safer operation, because better planning may make possible a less extensive procedure. Examination of frozen sections of tissue may alter the surgical procedure.

Meticulous care must be taken with the operation. Blood loss is relatively greater in a small child, and rough handling of tissue will lead to greater postoperative tissue induration and possible airway obstruction.

THYROID GLAND

Management of thyroid disease in children must be based on the knowledge that both benign and malignant diseases of the gland are associated with a nearly normal life expectancy if managed properly. Long-term consequences of any therapy must be considered.

Newborn Goiter

Large goiters can be seen in the neonates of mothers taking antithyroid medication and in children with inborn errors of metabolism.[5, 6] In the former, normal thyroid function and shrinkage of the gland will occur within several weeks without treatment. In the latter, thyroid replacement therapy will result in rapid shrinkage of the mass. Airway problems can generally be managed for that length of time with an endotracheal tube and without surgery.

Hyperthyroidism

Hyperthyroidism in children is usually best managed surgically. Although many adults can be treated successfully with either propylthiouracil or methimazole, children, especially teenagers, cannot be counted upon to take medication regularly.[12] In addition, long-term effects over a number of years are not well known. Although iodine 131 (^{131}I) is often utilized in adults, long-term studies have found that children treated with this substance have at least a 70 per cent incidence of hypothyroidism, again requiring medication to maintain a euthyroid state.[29] In addition, fears have been voiced concerning the potential long-term carcinogenic effects of the treatment, since it is well known that the thyroid gland is susceptible to carcinoma formation following external irradiation.[22] The treatment of choice in children has generally been bilateral subtotal thyroidectomy. In large series, complications of this procedure have included postoperative hypothyroidism in 5 to 10 per cent of patients, vocal cord paralysis in 5 per cent, and the need for tracheostomy in 5 per cent. Recently, however, there has been a renewed interest in the use of ^{131}I, because it has been shown that there may be as much as a 60 per cent incidence of postoperative hypothyroidism with subtotal thyroidectomy, roughly comparable to that produced by radioactive ablation.[29] Altman has proposed total thyroidectomy for patients with this illness.[1] Most authors do not agree, as there is a low incidence of recurrent hyperthyroidism (4 per cent) associated with a lesser procedure. Recurrent hyperthyroidism should be treated with ^{131}I because of the hazards of reoperation in this area.

Preoperative therapy in the hyperthyroid patient should consist of treatment with one of the antithyroid drugs until at least a semblance of euthyroidism is reached.[29] Most surgeons also use a 10-day course of Lugol's solution before surgery to reduce the vascularity of the gland. Recently, an increasing role for propranolol has been advocated.[9]

Carcinoma

Management of carcinoma of the thyroid gland in children should be planned with the knowledge that this disease, except in its more anaplastic forms, does not significantly alter life expectancy if treated in a reasonable manner.[7, 35] This is probably due to the fact that children's thyroid tumors seem to be more thyroid-stimulating hormone (TSH) dependent and that, with the addition of postoperative administration of thyroid hormone, the tumor and metastases are adequately suppressed. This indicates that radical surgical procedures should generally be avoided. We favor lobectomy and isthmusectomy as the procedure of choice. Node dissection is carried out only if clinically involved nodes are present. Although an effort is made to identify and preserve the recurrent laryngeal nerves, no attempt is made to dissect all tumor free, with possible nerve sacrifice. More radical procedures are carried out for poorly differentiated lesions.

Complications of the Thyroidectomy Procedure

RECURRENT-NERVE PARALYSIS

Both recurrent nerves must be visualized during dissection of the thyroid lobes. At least 50 per cent of patients will have multiple branches of at least one nerve. In general, damage to only one nerve will cause hoarseness. Damage to both nerves will cause airway obstruction because both vocal cords will remain in the adducted position. Tracheostomy is necessary for these patients. The cords should be examined and any hoarseness noted both pre- and postoperatively.

HEMORRHAGE

At the close of the procedure, following careful hemostasis, small Penrose drains are brought out through the midportion of the incision. Occasionally the drain tracts become occluded, resulting in formation of hematoma, which may obstruct the airway. Treatment consists of immediate opening of the incision and evacuation of the hematoma. Tracheostomy is rarely necessary (Fig. 12–1).

SUPERIOR LARYNGEAL NERVE PARALYSIS

Damage to the superior laryngeal nerves can occur with mass ligation of the superior thyroid vessels, as the nerves are found in close association with them. Careful dissection of the vessels is necessary to separate them from the nerves.

HYPOCALCEMIA

Hypocalcemia, if it occurs, will generally become manifest 48 to 72 hours postoperatively. Symptoms are discussed in the section of this chapter that concerns surgery of the parathyroid glands. The problem is caused by inadvertent removal of the glands or damage to their vascular supply during thyroidectomy dissection. Damage to the glands and to the recurrent laryngeal nerves

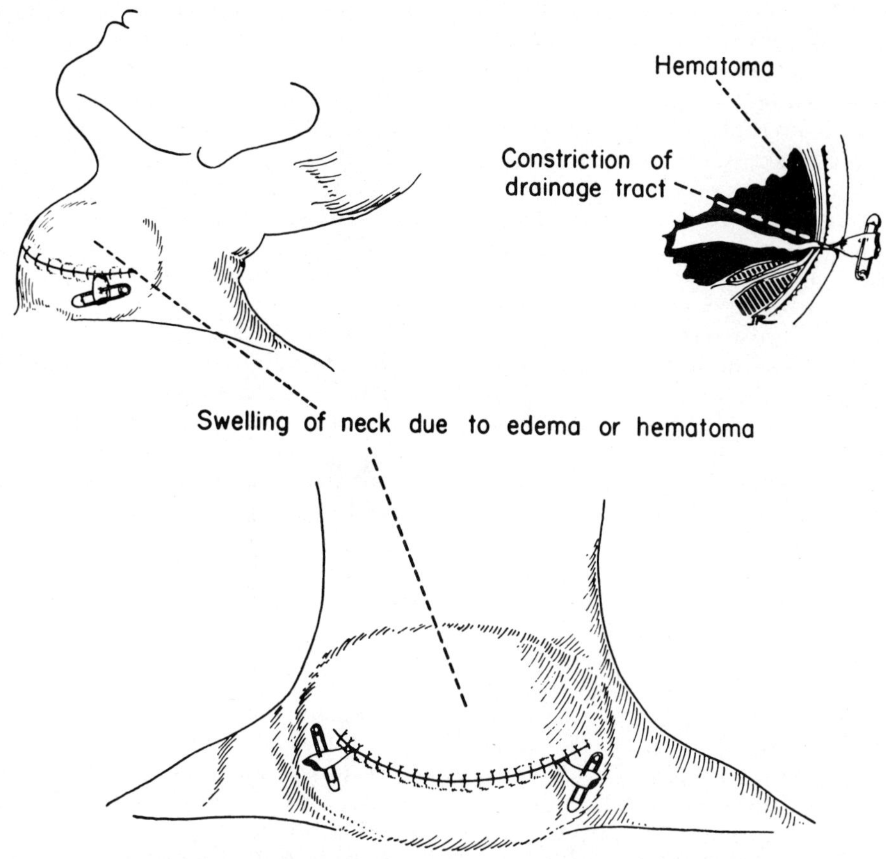

Figure 12–1 Hemorrhage into a thyroid wound. The swelling may be slight compared with the volume of blood that is present. The failure of drainage may be due to snug wound closure or clot formation. Postoperative evacuation of the hematoma may be necessary. The paramount consideration is asphyxia due to tracheal compression. A tracheostomy may be necessary following evacuation of the hematoma. (From Artz, C. P., and Hardy, J. D., eds.: Management of Surgical Complications, 3rd edition. Philadelphia, W. B. Saunders Co., 1975, p. 295.)

is more likely to occur during total thyroidectomy or during a secondary procedure. Vascular compromise or inadvertent removal of the glands is best avoided by leaving intact the posterior capsule of the thyroid gland on at least one side and ligating the inferior pole vessels close to the capsule of the gland.[10] Most postoperative hypocalcemia (serum calcium level less than 7 mg/dl or ionized calcium level less than 2.5 mg/dl) due to damage to parathyroid glands is temporary. Immediate treatment consists of injection of 2 ml/kg of 10 per cent calcium gluconate solution and cardiac monitoring to watch for bradycardia, followed by redetermination of serum calcium levels to assess the treatment.[20] When medication may be taken orally, vitamin D is added in a dose of 50,000 to 150,000 units per day. Oral calcium lactate or calcium carbonate is substituted for the intravenous form.

THE PARATHYROID GLANDS

Parathyroid surgery is associated with complications such as recurrent hyperparathyroidism resulting from inadequate surgery, hypoparathyroidism, and local wound problems including hematoma and infection. Another hazard is failure to recognize associated diseases of other endocrine glands (multiple endocrine adenomatosis).

During surgery for hyperparathyroidism, thorough neck exploration with positive identification of all four glands is an absolute necessity, as re-exploration is of course more hazardous and less rewarding in terms of finding residual parathyroid tissue. Tissue planes are no longer easy to find, and the recurrent laryngeal nerves are at considerable risk. As in thyroid surgery, we think it is preferable to always identify the recurrent laryngeal nerves. Glands should be identified by frozen section. The lower glands are less constant in location and may lie within the superior mediastinum. Superior retraction of the thymus through the cervical incision will often aid in identifying these glands if they should lie within the thymus. The lower glands are supplied by the inferior thyroid artery, and tracing of this vessel will often aid in locating the gland. In addition, a careful search of the tracheoesophageal groove and careful palpation of the thyroid lobe may be helpful. Occasionally resection of the thyroid lobe on the side of a missing gland will be rewarding. Attention has recently been drawn to the possibility of reducing the incidence of postoperative hypoparathyroidism by careful preservation of the blood supply of the glands left behind.[19] Preoperative intravenous injection of toluidine blue dye has been proposed to selectively stain parathyroid tissue.[13] Toluidine blue has caused cardiovascular problems in adults, but its use in children may be more promising. We have not used it.

If all four glands are not found and hypercalcemia remains a problem postoperatively, repeat neck exploration is the procedure of choice before mediastinal split for exploration of the mediastinum. Although a large number of mediastinal tumors have been found in adults, they are rarely found in children.[21] Selective parathyroid hormone radioimmunoassay with specimens obtained by selective venous catheterization has been particularly helpful in patients in whom hyperparathyroidism exists postoperatively, although this procedure is somewhat difficult in the smaller child.[32]

It is hoped that the tissue removed at surgery will be a solitary adenoma (or adenomas if a chance is obtained to explore all four glands). If only hyperplastic glands are found, the procedure of choice has been the removal of three and one-half glands. Recently introduced in this situation has been total parathyroidectomy with implantation of a portion of one of the glands into the forearm musculature after mincing of the tissue.[34] This tissue may be removed completely or in part should symptoms recur. If only one gland is removed, with a true adenoma, the remaining glands need not be marked with a nonabsorbable material. If an adenoma is not found, however, the glands should be marked in case further removal should prove necessary.

Postoperatively, serum calcium falls to its lowest level at 48 to 72 hours. Return to normal can be expected 2 to 3 days later. The sooner after surgery the drop in serum calcium level occurs and the longer it persists, the greater is the likelihood that all parathyroid glands have been damaged. Mental symptoms are common; patients are anxious, depressed, or occasionally confused. Clinically, the earliest manifestations are numbness and tingling in the circumoral region, fingers, and toes. Tetany may develop and is characterized by carpopedal spasm, tonic clonic convulsions, and laryngeal stridor. On physical examination, Chvostek's and Trousseau's signs may be present. Treatment is outlined in the section on thyroid surgery.

Parathyroidectomy incisions should be drained with Penrose drains for several days postoperatively as in thyroid surgery. This should avoid the possibility of airway compression should a wound hematoma occur. If this is not adequate, the wound will have to be opened and clot evacuated to restore the airway.

Special mention should be made of the multiple endocrine adenomatosis (MEA) syndromes, as they involve the parathyroid and thyroid glands to varying degrees. They tend to present in the second decade of life.

MEA-I includes concurrent disease of the pituitary gland and the parathyroids (usually hyperplasia) and islet cell tumors of the pancreas of the non-beta cell variety.[34] These are the most troublesome part of the syndrome other than the parathyroid disease, as gastrin is usually the hormone produced and ulcer diathesis is common. Measurement of serum gastrin level will help in screening for this part of the syndrome. Beta cell tumors of the pancreas may be present, although they are less common.

Proper visual field screening and computed tomographic scanning for pituitary abnormalities should be carried out.

MEA-II includes medullary carcinoma of the thyroid, parathyroid hyperplasia, and pheochromocytomas.[24] In children with parathyroid disease, thyrocalcitonin levels and urinary catecholamines should be measured as part of a planned long-term postoperative follow-up.

THYROGLOSSAL DUCT CYST

Complications of surgery of thyroglossal duct cysts include recurrence, possible removal of all functioning thyroid tissue, and wound infection and hematoma.

Recurrence is related to incomplete removal of the cyst and its tract. The midportion of the hyoid bone must be removed with the specimen, as the tract commonly passes through it.[25, 26] The specimen should include a comfortable margin of surrounding muscular tissue, particularly in the region between the hyoid bone and the foramen cecum, to ensure that no nests of cells are left behind. The index finger of the anesthesiologist, inserted into the patient's mouth and pressing the base of the tongue and foramen cecum forward, is a great aid in carrying dissection completely to the end of the tract. Drainage of the operative incision is necessary. We advise that it continue for 24 to 36 hours postoperatively.

The patient who has an infected cyst should be treated with antibiotics and warm soaks. Antibiotics should be effective against mouth organisms, as these are often involved because of the close communication between the cyst and the mouth by way of the foramen cecum. The cyst and tract should not be excised before the infection has been completely cleared for 6 weeks. An incidence of recurrence as high as 20 per cent has been reported in patients with these complicated cysts, as opposed to a 5 per cent recurrence rate in patients whose cysts were excised before becoming infected, probably because tissue planes and tract margins become less distinct and are operated on too soon after infection.[11, 23]

The thyroglossal duct cyst occasionally contains all of the patient's functioning thyroid tissue. In such a case, excision will result in postoperative hypothyroidism. Preoperative thyroid scanning has thus been recommended (Fig. 12–2). However, in most children, palpation of the thyroid gland is not difficult and will obviate the need for the radionuclide procedure. In any case, removal of all functioning thyroid tissue with a thyroglossal duct cyst is uncommon, but thyroid hormone replacement therapy has proved satisfactory should the need arise. Only two thyroglossal duct cysts containing thyroid tissue have been encountered at St. Christopher's Hospital for Children during the past 30 years. A scan is therefore mandatory only when thyroid tissue is found by frozen section before removal or in the specimen after removal. Furthermore, 35 cases of thyroid carcinoma arising from nonoperated thyroglossal duct cysts have been reported, six of them in children.[23] Twenty-nine were papillary adenocarcinomas arising from thyroid tissue, and six were squamous cell carcinomas.

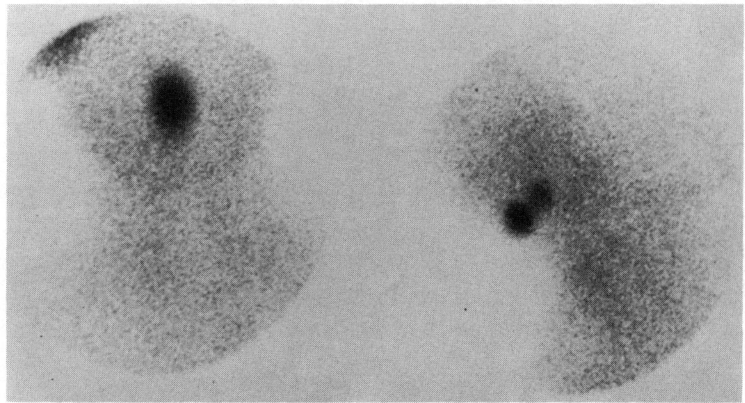

Figure 12–2 Thyroid scan. One-month-old infant with hypothyroidism determined by neonatal screening studies. A small amount of functioning thyroid tissue is contained in a thyroglossal cyst. Anterior-posterior and lateral views after thyroid scan using I^{123}.

All thyroglossal duct cysts should be removed when diagnosed and infection-free.

BRANCHIAL CLEFT REMNANTS

Surgery of branchial cleft remnants may result in complications such as recurrence due to incomplete removal, wound infection and recurrent abscess, damage to surrounding structures, and salivary fistulae.

Cysts encountered are usually those of the first or second branchial cleft or pouch, with those of the second being far more common.[4, 30] Operation should always take place when the patient is in a noninfected state. This is best accomplished either as soon as diagnosis is made or after a course of antibiotics, drainage, and warm soaks sufficient to clear the infection completely. Twenty-five per cent of cysts will become infected.[16] If a tract is present, preoperative study with radiologic contrast material will help to outline the full length of the tract and aid in planning complete excision. Injection of methylene blue at the time of surgery has been advocated by some, but we prefer not

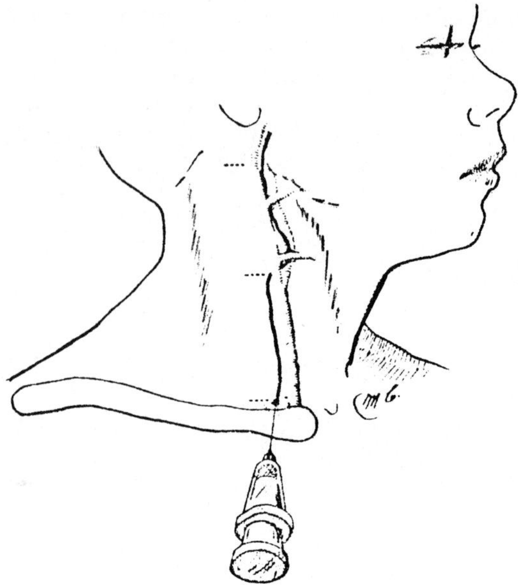

Figure 12–3 Injection of branchial sinus tract. Long tract may necessitate stepladder incisions, represented by dotted transverse lines. (From Artz, C. P., and Hardy, J. D., eds.: Management of Surgical Complications, 1st edition. Philadelphia, W. B. Saunders Co., 1961, p. 835.)

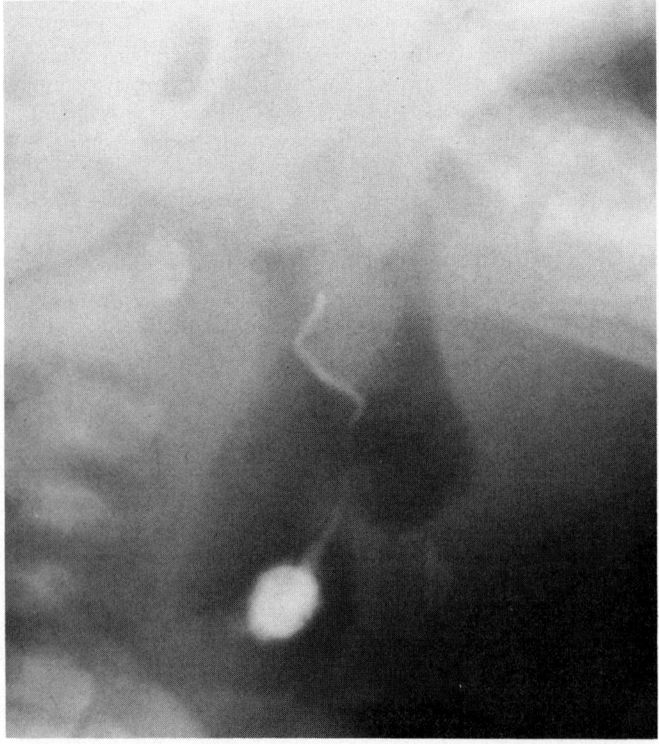

Figure 12–4 Branchial cyst and sinus tract, lateral view. Sinogram performed for an 11-month-old male infant who had a pinpoint-sized hole in the right side of the neck. The contrast material is noted to fill a small subcutaneous cyst and then to progress cephalad and medially toward the tonsillar fossa.

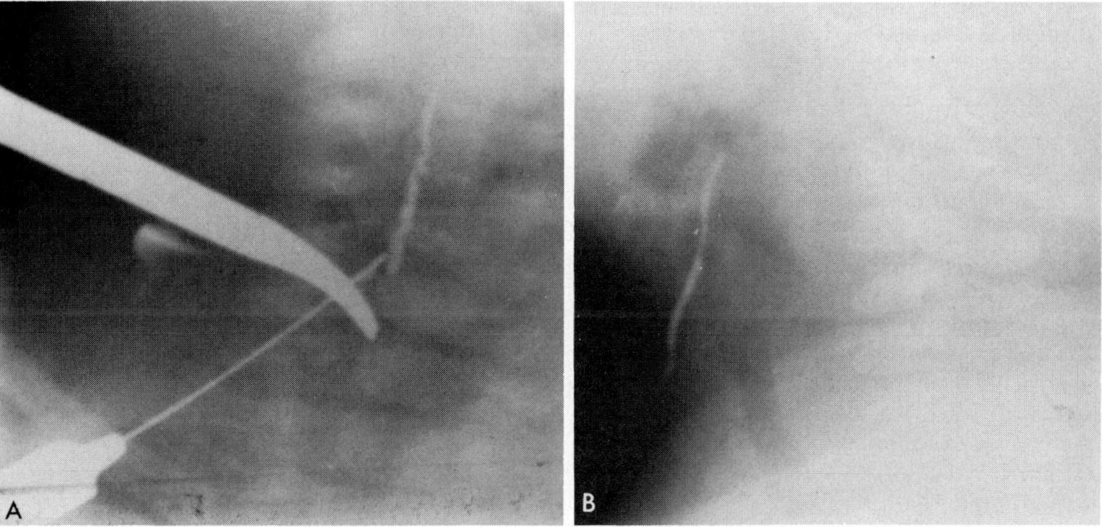

Figure 12–5   Branchial sinus tract. Frontal and lateral views of a 5-month-old male infant who had a pinpoint-sized opening in the neck. *A,* The blunt-ended cannula has been inserted into a small opening in the right side of the neck. *B,* There is a well-defined linear tract that extends from the opening in the neck cephalad toward the tonsillar fossa.

to use it, because staining of surrounding structures often makes dissection more confusing.

Cysts and sinuses of the second branchial cleft present along the anterior border of the sternocleidomastoid muscle and pass superiorly between the branches of the carotid bifurcation. The finger of the anesthesiologist, inserted in the patient's mouth and pressing against the tonsillar fossa, may aid in dissection of the proximal end of the tract. With this long type of tract, a somewhat higher, stepladder incision parallel to the main incision may greatly facilitate dissection (Figs. 12–3 to 12–5). Because of the many vital structures passing in the region of the carotid bifurcation, the initial procedure must be complete, as re-exploration in this area is likely to be exceedingly hazardous.

Remnants of the first branchial cleft appear in the region of the ear or in the submandibular area. Because of their location, the main trunk and branches of the facial nerve and the parotid gland are at risk during surgery (Fig. 12–6).

The more common preauricular cyst is of a less sophisticated embryologic derivation, and long tracts are not present. Simple excision when the patient is in a noninfected state should result in cure.[16] An asymptomatic dimple need not be excised except for cosmetic reasons.

A compelling argument for early excision of all branchial cleft remnants is the large number of carcinomas reported arising in adults from branchial cleft remnants.[15, 17]

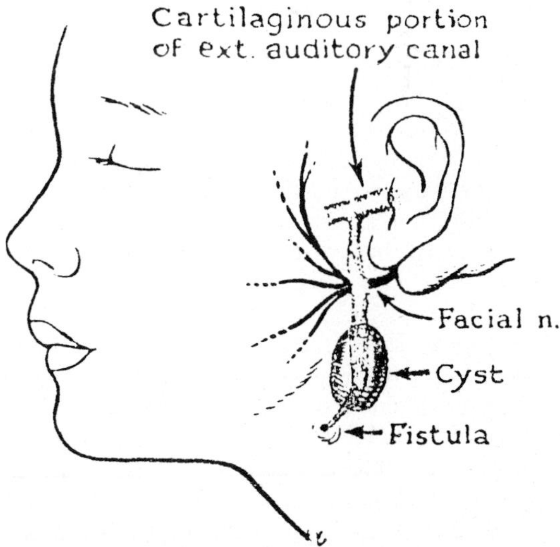

Figure 12–6   Cyst and fistula derived from first branchial cleft. The importance of the relation of the process to the facial nerve and external auditory meatus is shown. (From Bill, A. H., Jr.: Cysts and sinuses of the neck of thyroglossal and branchial origin. Surg. Clin. North Am. 36:1599, 1956.)

Following these procedures, the wound should be drained with a Penrose drain for 1 or 2 days postoperatively to avoid wound infection.

CYSTIC HYGROMA

Cystic hygroma is a lesion that arouses great anxiety in new parents. This often leads to attempts at extensive surgery when the patient is in early infancy, often with the idea of preventing further growth of the lesion and extension into surrounding structures. In fact, these lesions can usually not be excised in a single operation, and surgery may only serve to block still-functioning lymphatic channels. In the neonate, the only indication for early intervention is airway obstruction.

The timing of the surgery is of primary importance in the treatment of this lesion. The surgery is almost purely cosmetic in the great majority of patients. The larger the child, the safer the surgery in terms of preventing damage to vital nerve and muscular structures of the head and neck region. Infection is no longer the problem it once was because of frequent treatment of upper respiratory tract infections with antibiotics.

Three basic types of cystic hygromas may be identified when considering timing of surgery:

1. The pendulous, saccular lesion, often hanging low on the neck, has few attachments to deeper structures. This lesion may be safely removed relatively early in life. In fact, because of its floppy nature, it is susceptible to trauma with a resulting rapid increase in size due to hematoma formation.

2. The diffusely infiltrating type often presents initially in the floor of the mouth or at the base of the tongue, and usually shows a progressive increase in size during the first years of life. It usually is much more complicated in nature than one would judge from outward appearance, and involvement of deeper neck structures is the rule. Surgery in newborns should be reserved for relief of airway problems causing stridorous respiration.

Better cosmetic appearance can be achieved in the pre-school-age child, in whom an attempt to restore normal facial contours can be rewarding. By this age, further growth is not likely and the tumor has become smaller relative to the size of the child. A less extensive operation will often achieve acceptable results. Attempts at complete removal of the tumor are to be avoided, as a depression deformity will often result. Recently, with the advent of ultrasound and the computed tomographic scanner, better evaluation of the true size of the tumor and the structures invaded may be obtained preoperatively.

3. The hemangiolymphangioma, as its name implies, exhibits many of the characteristics of the hemangioma, the most important of which is its shrinkage with time. Although these tumors may be initially large and disfiguring, there is often marked regression of the vascular component of the tumor, frequently producing an acceptable cosmetic result without surgery. Bony, often mandibular, overgrowth may result from contact with the increased vascular supply and may dictate early surgery.

Surgical management of cystic hygromas is based on adherence to the concept that the goal of the procedure is restoration of facial contour and not complete removal of the tumor. Neck structures must be searched for and not merely recognized, as they are almost always attenuated and displaced from their normal course. Maintaining the cysts intact during dissection aids in identification of normal structures. All lymphatic channels encountered should be carefully ligated or cauterized. Because of the danger of entering the oral cavity during dissection of lesions in the floor of the mouth or base of the tongue, we routinely give patients with lesions in this area prophylactic doses of penicillin before surgery is begun. Should the mouth be entered, simple closure with absorbable sutures is carried out.

Drainage with small Penrose drains or closed suction systems is routinely employed, as it is impossible to ligate all lymphatic channels, and large areas of dead space are usually left in which fluid may accumulate. The drains are removed after several days when drainage has become minimal. Aspiration may have to be continued for several weeks after discharge as fluid reaccumulates. Meticulous care must be taken to avoid infection.

Tracheostomy was often employed routinely in the past when lesions of the anterior neck were removed. With the use of modern soft endotracheal tubes, it is almost always possible to maintain an airway with the tube for several days until the anticipated induration has receded.

The cure rate with complete excision has been reported at 81 per cent. Partial excision results in a cure in only 12 per cent of patients. However, it was found that 62 per cent of those with gross tumor remaining needed no further surgery for acceptable cosmetic results. Seventy-six per cent of significant recurrences occurred within 1 year.[27]

LYMPH NODES

Successful management of cervical lymph node disease is based on knowledge of the probable cause. Physical examination, the patient's age and background, and duration of symptoms are all important. Only a small percentage of children referred for surgical evaluation will require intervention. Malignant disease, frequently cited as an urgent reason for biopsy, is relatively uncommon as a cause of adenopathy, particularly in the younger child. Inflammatory disease, unless purulence develops, can usually be managed without surgery. Consequently, unless obvious fluctuance is encountered, a reasonable period of observation is the best course. During this time, a chest roentgenogram may be obtained and skin testing for tuberculosis performed if appropriate. A heterophil determination is useful if generalized adenopathy and splenomegaly are present, to rule out infectious mononucleosis.

All nodes in which fluctuance is present should be drained. Whereas the abscess due to the common gram-positive cocci will clear rapidly after appropriate drainage, the abscess due to acid-fast bacilli tends to form a chronic draining sinus. Needle aspiration of acid-fast lymphadenopathy is preferred. On physical examination, the acid-fast abscess will be fluctuant but will demonstrate only minimal tenderness and signs of inflammation. A tine tuberculin test will usually provide a definitive answer. Antituberculous chemotherapy is the treatment of choice, with surgery reserved for nonresponders. Further differentiation into typical and atypical acid-fast infections is also

useful, as the atypical mycobacterial lesions will not clear in the patient receiving antituberculous therapy, and earlier surgical excision is necessary. Recently it has become possible to differentiate between the two types of acid-fast infections by means of purified protein derivative (PPD).[2] The PPD-S skin test is positive in tuberculosis alone, while the PPD-B skin test is positive in both.[3] In all nonresponders to therapy in the tuberculous group, the atypical group, and those who have been inadvertently drained and in whom a sinus tract has formed, complete excision of the abscess, node, and sinus tract is the surgical treatment of choice.[36]

The bacterial abscess should be drained only when definite pointing exists. Earlier drainage is often inadequate and results in repeat abscess formation. Drainage should be carried out through the midpoint of the fluctuant area, with placement of packing or a drain to prevent closure and reaccumulation. The packing may be partially removed on the second day, and a little more may be removed each day thereafter until all is removed. Antibiotics that are effective against penicillin-resistant organisms are indicated when there is a significant area of surrounding inflammation. In the child with repeated abscesses, blood glucose concentration should be determined and immunologic testing performed.

Surgery for excision of nodal tissue to rule out malignant disease requires knowledge of the regional anatomy in relation to nerves, muscles, and glandular structures. The spinal accessory and hypoglossal nerves are particularly at risk during cervical node excision. The use of primarily blunt dissection will aid in the preservation of surrounding structures. When several groups of nodes seem to be involved with the same process, biopsy of the most easily accessible node is preferable. Advance planning must take place so that a sufficient number of representative samples are obtained for histologic, bacteriologic, and acid-fast studies, as well as for cell-marker and electron-microscopic studies when indicated.

Drainage of lymph node biopsy sites is generally not necessary unless pus has been encountered, and it is contraindicated when tumor is found because of the possibility of seeding the tract. In deep, inaccessible areas or those where hemostasis is possibly inadequate, a small Penrose drain may be left in place and removed on the first or second postoperative day. Incisions should be based on Langer's lines to produce an inconspicuous postoperative scar.

TORTICOLLIS

Many newborns have been referred to us because of a mass in the sternocleidomastoid muscle, often accompanied by contralateral gaze. There is often a history of breech or other difficult delivery. The diagnosis is usually made within several months after birth.[14] In more severe cases, plagiocephaly may be present. The mass may be expected to slowly disappear within 6 to 7 weeks in more than 80 per cent of patients if a careful plan of nonoperative management is followed.[8] We advise the mother to place the baby in the crib alternately head to foot, foot to head, and right to left and to approach the baby from the same side of the bed, talking as she approaches. The baby will turn his head toward her, thus slowly overcoming his torticollis (no active stretching or massage should be done).

Some older children and infants with torticollis need surgical correction because of neglect. Surgical treatment should be reserved for those patients who have facial hemihypoplasia or plagiocephaly. It consists of division of the involved muscle along with any accompanying fibrous constrictions. Division of the midportion of the sternocleidomastoid muscle through a transverse cervical incision is preferred. To ensure complete freedom of movement, the head must be turned before closure of the incision to make sure that there is no residual fibrosis involving the carotid sheath or omohyoid muscle. The spinal accessory nerve is at risk during this procedure, as it runs slightly superior to the region of the muscle division. The neck is held in an extended position for 7 to 10 days following surgery, when stetching exercises are begun to avoid recurrent fibrosis and contracture.

References

1. Altman, R. P.: Total thyroidectomy for the treatment of Graves' disease in children. J. Pediatr. Surg. 8:295, 1973.
2. Altman, R. P., and Margileth, A. M.: Cervical lymphadenopathy from atypical mycobacteria: Diagnosis and surgical treatment. J. Pediatr. Surg. 10:419, 1975.
3. Belin, R. P., Richardson, J. D., Richardson, D. C., et al.: Diagnosis and management of scrofula in children. J. Pediatr. Surg. 9:103, 1974.
4. Bill, A. H., Jr., and Vadheim, J. L.: Cysts, sinuses and fistulas of the neck arising from the first and second branchial clefts. Am. Surg. 142:904, 1955.
5. Blizzard, R. M.: Inherited defects of thyroid hormone synthesis and metabolism. Metabolism 9:232, 1960.
6. Bongiovanni, A. M., Eberlein, W. R., Thomas, P. Z., and Anderson, W. B.: Sporadic goiter of the newborn. J. Clin. Endocrinol. 16:146, 1956.
7. Buckwater, J. A., Thomas, C. G., Jr., and Freeman, J. B.: Is childhood thyroid cancer a lethal disease? Ann. Surg. 181:632, 1975.
8. Coventry, M. B., and Harris, L. E.: Congenital muscular torticollis. J. Bone Joint Surg. 41A:815, 1959.
9. Galoburda, M., Rosman, N. P., and Haddow, J. E.: Thyroid storm in an 11-year-old boy managed by propranolol. Pediatrics 53:6, 1974.
10. Gould, E. A., Hirsch, E., and Brecher, I.: Complications arising in the course of thyroidectomy. Arch. Surg. 90:81, 1965.
11. Gross, R. E.: The Surgery of Infancy and Childhood. Philadelphia, W. B. Saunders Co., 1953.
12. Hung, W., Williams, L., and Blizzard, R.: Medical therapy of thyrotoxicosis in children. Pediatrics 30:17, 1962.
13. Hurvitz, R. J., Perzik, S. L., and Morganstern, L.: In vivo staining of the parathyroid glands. Arch. Surg. 97:722, 1968.
14. Jones, P. G.: Torticollis in infancy and childhood. Springfield, Ill., Charles C Thomas, Publisher, 1967.
15. Katubig, D., and Damjanov, I.: Branchial cleft carcinoma. Arch. Otolaryngol. 89:750, 1969.
16. Lyall, D., and Stahl, W. M., Jr.: Lateral cervical cysts, sinuses, and fistulas of congenital origin, Internat. Abstr. Surg. Surg. Gynecol. Obstet. 102:417, 1956.
17. Martin, H., Morfit, H. M., and Erlich, H.: The case for branchiogenic cancer. Ann. Surg. 132:867, 1950.
18. Mason, G. R.: Care of patients with hypocalcemia after parathyroidectomy. Am. Surg. 42:23, 1976.
19. Reyes, J. M., Wright, J. R., and Rosenfield, R. L.: Prevention of hypocalcemia in children due to parathyroid infarction after thyroidectomy. Surg. Gynecol. Obstet. 148:76, 1979.
20. Root, A. W., and Harrison, H. E.: Disorders of calcium metabolism. J. Pediatr. 88:177, 1976.
21. Schwartz, D. L., Gann, D. S., and Haller, J. A.: Endocrine surgery in children. Surg. Clin. North Am. 54:363, 1974.
22. Sheline, G. E., Lindsay, S., and Bell, H. G.: Occurrence of thyroid nodules in children following I^{131} therapy for hyperthyroidism. J. Clin. Endocrinol. 19:127, 1959.

23. Shephard, G. H., and Rosenthal, L.: Carcinoma of thyroglossal duct remmants. Am. J. Surg. 116:125, 1968.

24. Sipple, J. H.: The association of pheochromocytoma with carcinoma of the thyroid gland. Am. J. Med. 31:163, 1961.

25. Sistrunk, W. E.: The surgical treatment of cysts of the thyroglossal tract. Ann. Surg. 71:12, 1920.

26. Snyder, W. H., Jr., and Pollock, W. F.: Thyroglossal cysts and midline clefts. *In* Mustard, W. T., et al. (eds.): Pediatric Surgery, 2nd edition. Chicago, Year Book Medical Publishers, 1969, chap. 22.

27. Stromberg, B. V., Weeks, P. M., and Wray, R. C., Jr.: Treatment of cystic hygroma. South. Med. J. 69:1333, 1976.

28. Tank, E. S., Bacon, G. E., and Lowrey, G. H.: Surgical management of thyrotoxicosis in children. J. Pediatr. Surg. 4:1, 1969.

29. Thompson, N. W., Dunn, E. L., Freitas, J. E., et al.: Surgical treatment of thyrotoxicosis in children and adolescents. J. Pediatr. Surg. 12:1009, 1977.

30. Toomey, J. M.: Cysts and tumors of the pharynx. *In* Paparella, M. M., and Shumrick, D. A. (eds.): Otolaryngology, 2nd edition. Vol. 3. Philadelphia, W. B. Saunders Co., 1980, pp. 2323–2342.

31. Ward, G. E., Hendrick, J. W., and Chambers, R. G.: Thyroglossal tract abnormalities. Surg. Gynecol. Obstet. 89:729, 1949.

32. Wells, S. A., Jr., Doppman, J. L., Bilezikian, J. P., et al.: Repeated neck exploration in primary hyperparathyroidism. Localization of abnormal glands by selective thyroid arteriography, selective venous sampling, and radioimmunoassay. Surgery 74:678, 1973.

33. Wells, S. A., Gunnells, J. C., Shelburne, J. D., et al.: Transplantation of the parathyroid glands in man: Clinical indications and results. Surgery 78:34, 1975.

34. Wermer, P.: Endocrine adenomatosis: Peptic ulcer in a large kindred. Am. J. Med. 35:205, 1963.

35. Winship, T., and Roxvall, R. V.: Thyroid carcinoma in childhood: Final report on a twenty year study. Clin. Proc. Children's Hosp. 26:11, 1970.

36. Wolinsky, E.: Nontuberculous mycobacterial infections of man. Med. Clin. North Am. 58:639, 1974.

THORAX | 3

13 # ENDOSCOPY

Samuel H. Kim, M.D.

The specialty of endoscopy is new in comparison with other specialties in medicine. Its late development was due to the problems of optics and lighting.[3] Initially, pediatric endoscopy was carried out with adult equipment, but this has changed since the introduction of the Hopkins lens system and fiberoptic lighting.[4] This advance has allowed endoscopic telescopes, sheaths, and accessory equipment to be miniaturized, enabling the endoscopist to diagnose and treat conditions accurately, safely, and without the previous hazards caused by utilization of adult instruments in infants and children.[14] With the Hopkins lens system, the endoscopist's view is magnified at the distal end of the telescope, permitting a much more precise view. With miniaturized catheters, grasping and biopsy forceps, and suction apparatus, procedures can be done with minimal risk. Adequate channels for administration of anesthetic agents and advances in pediatric anesthesia have contributed greatly to the safety of pediatric endoscopic procedures. However, even with all these advantages, endoscopic misadventure and iatrogenic injuries still occur.

LARYNGOSCOPY

Direct laryngoscopy is indicated for airway obstruction, hoarseness, stridor, and trauma.[5] In the newborn, general anesthesia is often not necessary, but in older infants and children, general anesthesia is required.

Complications

Use of an inappropriate laryngoscope blade can cause soft tissue injury including *swelling, laceration,* and *airway obstruction.* All facilities in which pediatric patients are cared for should have laryngoscope blades of appropriate size to accommodate all sizes of patients. Properly functioning suctioning apparatus, endotracheal tubes, Amboy bag and mask, and oxygen should be immediately available before a laryngoscopy is begun.

During inspection of the larynx without anesthesia in the newborn, *hypoxia* and *bradycardia* can occur quickly and easily. By preoxygenating the patient with mask oxygen, having another person monitor the patient's pulse and color, and allowing oxygen to flow into the corner of the patient's mouth during the procedure, these complications can be prevented. *Hypoxia* can also be produced by pharyngeal suctioning during the procedure. This can be prevented by keeping the period of suction short and limiting the duration of laryngoscopy. If more than visual examination is necessary in the newborn, general anesthesia should be utilized. Then, with a protected airway and operating room control, procedures requiring aspirating, unroofing, coagulating, or dilating can be done safely.

In the patient with upper airway obstruction, diagnostic laryngoscopy should be carried out without exception under general anesthesia. Attempts to visualize the larynx in the awake, hypoxic, partially obstructed patient may lead to complete airway obstruction, bleeding with aspiration, or respiratory and cardiac arrest. Whether due to a foreign body, infection (croup, epiglottitis, or laryngotracheobronchitis), or trauma, these complications can be avoided by inducing general anesthesia and carrying out direct laryngoscopy. Obviously, in a moribund patient, direct laryngoscopy with endotracheal intubation is lifesaving and can be accomplished with minimal trauma. In our own institution, every patient requiring intubation for croup undergoes general anesthesia and nasotracheal intubation with bronchoscopy stand-by. When there is cooperation among the neonatologists, anesthesiologists, and pediatric endoscopists, complications arising from airway obstruction can be minimized.

Recently, flexible fiberoptic laryngoscopes have become available for evaluation of the pediatric upper airway.[11] Introduction of the instruments can be accomplished in the awake or sedated patient through the nose and mouth. Complications are usually secondary to trauma and can be avoided by direct visualization and the use of general anesthesia when there is any question.

BRONCHOSCOPY

Until the advent of miniaturized bronchoscopy equipment, perhaps no other procedure had as high a morbidity as bronchoscopy in infants. With better lighting and optics, larger channels for administration of anesthesia, and appropriate-size forceps, biopsy equipment, and suction apparatus, bronchosopy in the pediatric patient is a very safe procedure today.

The indications for bronchoscopy include airway obstruction, atelectasis, foreign bodies, pulmonary toilet, biopsy, selective bronchography, and identification of fistulae.

Complications

Table 13–1 lists the complications of bronchoscopy. *Trauma* to the gingival ridge or to the teeth is caused by undue pressure

TABLE 13–1 COMPLICATIONS OF BRONCHOSCOPY

Dental trauma
Subglottic edema
Laryngeal laceration
Hypoxia
Respiratory acidosis
Atelectasis
Hypothermia
Infection
Bleeding
Pneumothorax
Bronchial tear
Pneumonia

from the bronchoscope. Loose teeth should be looked for and removed at the start of every procedure. Using a lower jaw bite block or resting the bronchoscope on the endoscopist's fingers, not on the patient's teeth, will avoid this problem.

Subglottic edema in the normal airway may be related to an underlying infection or to use of too large a bronchoscopic sheath. Using recommended endotracheal tube size, a bronchoscopic sheath of appropriate size can be selected and will usually avoid the complication. If there is significant subglottic edema following bronchoscopy, the use of oxygen, mist tent, and racemic epinephrine may relieve the airway obstruction. Occasionally, however, endotracheal intubation may be necessary, especially in patients with a very small airway.

Laryngeal laceration or *hematoma* is usually a result of introducing too large a bronchoscope or passing the instrument blindly. Bleeding from such injury usually stops spontaneously, but occasionally direct pressure through the bronchoscope may be required.

Hypoxia and *respiratory acidosis* are secondary to underventilation.[9] When the larger bronchoscopes are used, this problem is less likely to occur because of the larger channels for anesthesia gases. When the smaller bronchoscopes (2.5 and 3.0 mm) are used, the side channel for ventilation may not be adequate for gas exchange and simultaneous bronchoscopic evaluation. Under these circumstances, intermittent removal of the telescope and antifog sheath will allow appropriate ventilation through the bronchoscope and avoidance of these complications.

Atelectasis is due to retained secretions or too vigorous suctioning. The former can be avoided by removing all secretions during the endoscopic procedure and ventilating the patient well before removal of the bronchoscope. Too vigorous suctioning should be avoided at all times and is less likely if suctioning is done under direct visualization. When atelectasis is secondary to a foreign body, removal of the foreign body will relieve the condition. When the foreign body has been present for a long time and there is loss of lung parenchyma through infection, the atelectasis may not resolve.

Hypothermia may be more commonly associated with pediatric cystoscopy, but in the very small infant it is a real hazard.[8] Fortunately, operating rooms in which this problem is dealt with today have appropriate heating lamps and heating pads. When there is not an appropriate heating source, the infant should be wrapped to prevent hypothermia.

The introduction of *infection* is usually due to contaminated equipment and can be avoided by proper sterilization of equipment.[1] In the patient with infection, bronchoscopy may cause upper airway obstruction, necessitating a period of nasotracheal intubation.

Bleeding is an unusual complication of bronchoscopy. When there is an ongoing infection in the tracheobronchial tree, the mucosa may be friable and likely to bleed easily. Suctioning or the tip of the suction catheter may cause this bleeding. Careful suctioning with soft-tipped catheters or suctioning under direct vision will avoid this problem. Most bleeding is self-limiting and requires no specific direct action. In the case of a hemangioma of the trachea or larynx, the use of endoscopic electrocoagulation will eliminate the lesion and stop the bleeding as well. Granuloma formation from a long-standing foreign body may require not only electrocoagulation but also endoscopic resection of the granulation tissue to prevent a stenosis.

The presence of *pneumothorax, pneumomediastinum,* or *subcutaneous emphysema* after bronchoscopy may indicate a tracheal or bronchial laceration. This can be prevented by using an appropriate-size bronchoscope under direct visualization at all times. If a bronchial tear does occur, the patient should undergo a second bronchoscopy to visualize the injury. If no obvious injury is noted and the free air resolves, no further surgical treatment is necessary. If the tear is visualized and is of large size, direct repair should be carried out immediately by thoracotomy. Small leaks usually seal spontaneously but may require ipsilateral tube thoracostomy (Fig. 13–1).

Lipoid pneumonia has been associated with the use of oily contrast materials for bronchography. We have avoided this problem by draining off the supernatant oil and using a warm solution of the remaining contrast material in very small amounts, i.e., just enough to visualize the particular area of the lungs required. Using this technique, as little as 1 to 2 ml of contrast material is all that is required. At the end of the study, before the patient is wakened, saline irrigation and suctioning will decrease the

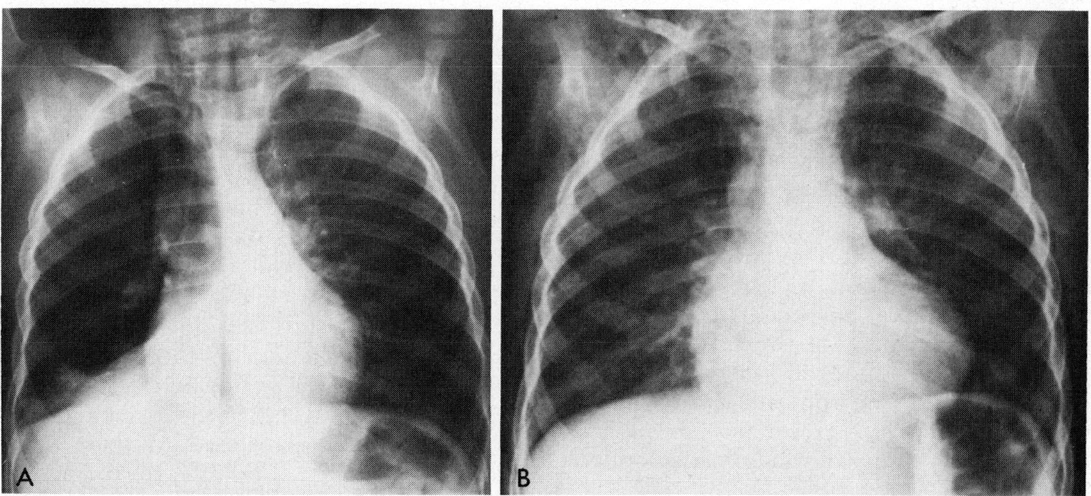

Figure 13–1   *A,* Perforation of right bronchus intermedius of a 20-month-old boy in unsuccessful attempt to remove vegetable foreign body (peanut). Note pneumomediastinum and cervical subcutaneous emphysema. There is right pneumothorax overinflation of the right upper lobe and collapse of the middle and lower lobes. Bronchoscopy using a #3½ Storz (Hopkins lens system) was repeated, and the foreign body was removed. The perforation sealed spontaneously. Right tube thoracostomy was required for 48 hours. *B,* Anteroposterior chest roentgenogram taken 72 hours later and showing normal inflation of both lungs, absent pneumothorax and pneumomediastinum, and subsiding subcutaneous emphysema.

amount of dye left in the tracheobronchial tree.

ESOPHAGOSCOPY AND GASTROSCOPY

Esophagoscopy and gastroscopy can be done with rigid or flexible instruments. In the infant and small child, general anesthesia should be utilized; in the cooperative older child, using the flexible instrument, the study can be accomplished under full sedation.[7] Indications for esophagoscopy include dysphagia, gastroesophageal reflux and esophagitis, strictures, hematemesis, lye ingestion, recurrent pneumonitis, and foreign bodies.[6] Gastroscopy is utilized most commonly for upper gastrointestinal tract bleeding and duodenoscopy for visualization of the bile and pancreatic ducts (endoscopic retrograde cholangiopancreatography.)[2, 10, 12, 13]

Complications

Table 13–2 lists the complications of esophagoscopy and gastroscopy. *Esophageal perforation* can be prevented by passing the instrument under direct vision. Most commonly, perforations occur during the dilatation of a stricture. This can be prevented by following a string or a small dilator through the stricture. In pediatric patients who require repeat dilatations, such as after repair of esophageal atresia, retrograde dilatation through a gastrostomy using Tucker dilators is much safer. If the gastrostomy has closed, filiforms and followers are used. Dilating a stricture too widely can also lead to perforation. This is best prevented by clinical judgment and by noting the first appearance of blood on the dilator. Obviously, it is better to repeat the dilatation and gradually increase the largest size of dilator used each time. Should a perforation occur, it may not be apparent at the time of the endoscopy. The presence of fever, leukocytosis, increasing dysphagia, hydropneu-

TABLE 13–2 COMPLICATIONS OF ESOPHAGOSCOPY AND GASTROSCOPY

Perforation
Tracheal obstruction
Bleeding

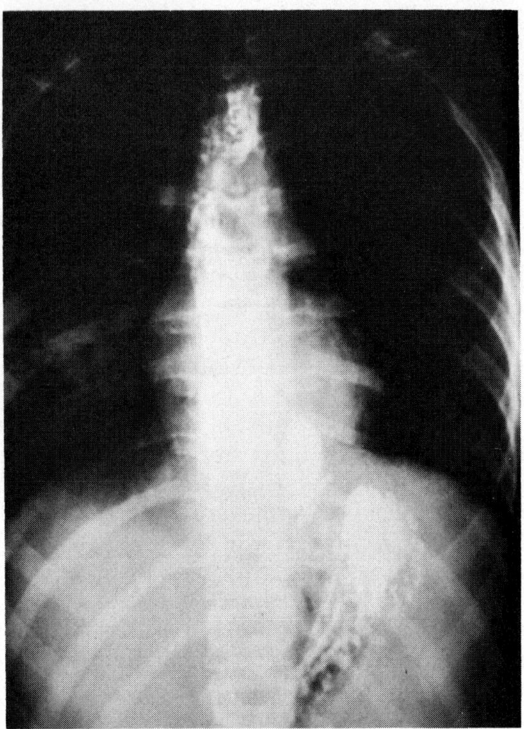

Figure 13–2 Esophageal perforation following stricture dilatation. Barium swallow shows extravasated contrast material. The perforation was recognized early and repair accomplished through a left thoracotomy with primary closure and drainage.

mothorax, or signs of sepsis following esophagoscopy should alert the clinician. Occasionally, a water-soluble contrast study is necessary to confirm the diagnosis (Fig. 13–2). Once the diagnosis has been made, a drainage procedure with repair of the laceration should be carried out. This is usually done through a left thoracotomy, and if the perforation is discovered early enough, a primary repair is accomplished. When diagnosis is delayed, the tissues may be too edematous for a primary repair. A pleural or pericardial flap should be used and drainage carried out. When the hypopharynx has been perforated, usually as a result of blind passage of the esophagoscope or dilator, immediate exploration with repair and drainage should be performed.

In infants and small children, rigid esophagoscopy can cause *tracheal compression* and *hypoxia* despite endotracheal intubation. The trachea is usually compressed when the esophagoscope is in the distal esophagus. This is due to the relative elasticity of the tracheal cartilages. This complication can be avoided if there is close cooperation between anesthesiologists and endoscopists.

Bleeding following esophagoscopy may be due to mucosal laceration, perforation, or areas of esophagitis. Other causes may be sites of biopsy or dilatation of esophageal varices. Bleeding from lacerations, esophagitis, and biopsy and dilatation sites will usually stop without direct action. Bleeding from varices may require the administration of vasopressin (Pitressin) or the use of balloon tamponade. Perforations should be repaired.

Perforation of the stomach requires immediate laparotomy and closure. This may be caused by the gastroscope or occasionally by overdistension of the stomach for visualization. Passing the instrument under direct vision should avoid instrumental perforation, and careful intermittent inflation will avoid overdistension. Bleeding from lacerations, gastritis, or biopsy sites is usually self-limited and does not require operative intervention.

Finally, inexperience is the leading cause of complications and must be minimized by appropriate supervision of trainees using pediatric endoscopic instruments.

References

1. Aelony, Y., and Finegold, S. M.: Serious infectious complications after a flexible fiberoptic bronchoscopy. West. J. Med. 131:327, 1979.
2. Ament, M. E., Gans, S. L., and Christie, D. L.: Experience with esophagogastroduodenoscopy in diagnosis of 79 pediatric patients with hematemesis, melena or chronic abdominal pain. Gastroenterology 68:858, 1975.
3. Benedict, E. B.: Endoscopy. Baltimore, Williams & Wilkins Co., 1951.
4. Gans, S. L., and Berci, G.: Advances in endoscopy of infants and children. J. Pediatr. Surg. 6:199, 1971.
5. Holinger, P. H.: Endoscopy. *In* Mustard, W. T., et al. (eds.): Pediatric Surgery. Chicago, Year Book Medical Publishers, 1969, p. 429.
6. Johnson, D. G.: Endoscopy. *In* Ravitch, M. M., Welch, K. J., Benson, C. D., et al. (eds.): Pediatric Surgery, 3rd edition. Chicago, Year Book Medical Publishers, 1979, p. 513.
7. Lux, G., et al.: Gastrointestinal fiberoptic endoscopy in pediatric patients and juveniles. Endoscopy 10:158, 1978.
8. Nelson, R. P., and Kinder, W.: Hypothermia during infant cystoscopy. J. Urol. 121:333, 1979.
9. Rah, K. H., Salzberg, A., Boyan, C. P., et al.: Respiratory acidosis with the small Storz-Hopkins bronchoscopes: Occurrence and management. Ann. Thorac. Surg. 27:197, 1979.
10. Riemann, J. F., and Koch, H.: Endoscopy of the biliary tract and pancreas in children. Endoscopy 10:167, 1978.
11. Silberman, H. D.: The use of the flexible fiberoptic nasopharyngolaryngoscope in the pediatric upper airway. Otolaryngol. Clin. North Am. 11:365, 1978.
12. Urakami, Y., Seki, H., and Kishi, S.: Endoscopic retrograde cholangiopancreatography (ERCP) performed in children. Endoscopy 9:86, 1977.
13. van der Spuy, S.: ERCP in children. Endoscopy 10:173, 1978.
14. Willital, G. H.: Significance of pediatric endoscopy. Endoscopy 10:153, 1978.

THE THORACIC PARIETES

Kenneth J. Welch, M.D.

14

ANTERIOR THORACIC DEFORMITIES

Discussion of the complications of repair of anterior thoracic deformities will be limited to pectus excavatum and pectus carinatum, which together constitute 95 per cent of cases. Eight hundred sixty-two patients with pectus excavatum and 94 patients with pectus carinatum were operated upon at Children's Hospital Medical Center, Boston, during the period from 1952 to 1981. Thirty-two additional patients were operated upon for Poland's syndrome, vertebral and rib anomalies, and various clefts.

Pectus Excavatum

Complications of pectus excavatum repair have been few and relatively unimportant except for major recurrence in 16 patients, necessitating reoperation in 12 (Table 14–1). Full-thickness wound separation with obligatory mediastinitis occurred in four patients. All four cases occurred early and

TABLE 14–1 COMPLICATIONS OF PECTUS EXCAVATUM REPAIR*

Complication	Number of Patients
Segmental left lower lobe atelectasis	86
Recurrence necessitating reoperation	16
Pneumothorax requiring tube	14
Migration of Steinmann pin	12
Seroma	10
Excessive bleeding	8
Hypertrophic scar revision	6
Wound infection	6
Wound separation (dehiscence)	4
Necrosis of skin flap	4
Deaths	0
Total	166 (20%)

*Operations performed on 862 patients with pectus excavatum at Children's Hospital Medical Center, Boston, 1952 to 1981.

were due to inaccurate development of the pectoral and rectus muscle layers, making them unsuitable for watertight closure.

SEGMENTAL LEFT LOWER LOBE ATELECTASIS

The most frequent postoperative complication was segmental left lower lobe atelectasis. Diagnosis is made on the basis of x-ray films showing collapse or reduced volume of the anterior and medial basal segments of the left lower lobe. Preoperative xenon-133 lung scans show diminished ventilation and perfusion in the corresponding area (Fig. 14–1). There is compacting of lower lobe bronchi and airless intervening parenchyma due to compression of these segments between the depressed chest wall and the flattened (cor planum) heart (Fig. 14–2). The condition is self-limited and clinically unimportant. No patient required bronchoscopy to expand these segments. Postoperative xenon studies in 20 patients showed substantial improvement in ventilation and perfusion in this area of suspected collapse. Left lower lobe atelectasis is seen postoperatively in many patients undergoing thoracic surgery, including cardiovascular procedures. If this diagnosis is to be made at all in the pectus patient, anteroposterior (AP) and lateral films of the chest are required. Hazy density on the AP film corresponds to the area of the operation and the distribution of "segmental atelectasis." Our radiologists no longer make this diagnosis from the routine AP portable upright film taken in the recovery room.

RECURRENT PECTUS EXCAVATUM

The result of surgery for pectus excavatum has been uneven at best. Gall et al. reported 214 patients, 50 per cent of whom

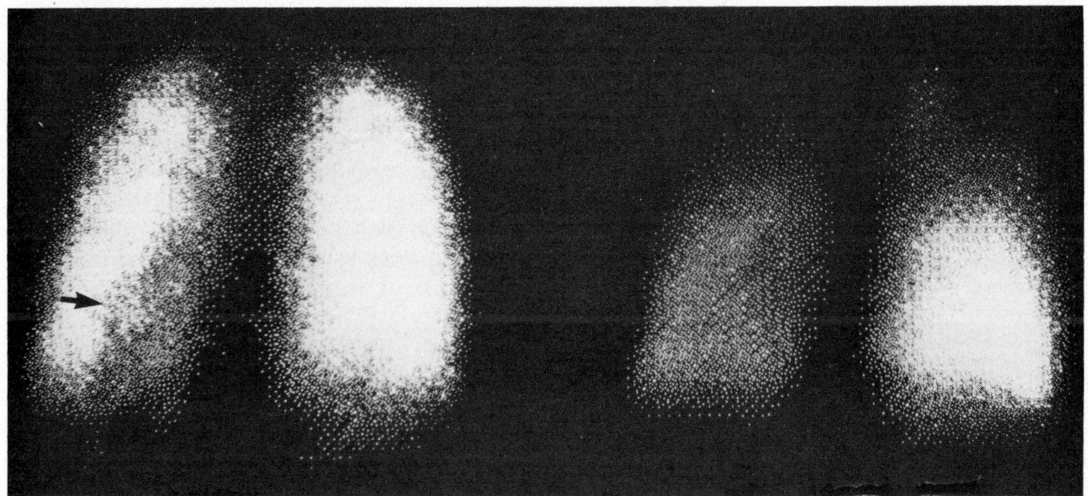

Figure 14–1 Xenon-133 lung scan of a 12-year-old girl 1 month before surgical correction of pectus excavatum. The area of diminished ventilatory function corresponding to the anterior medial and basal segments of the left lower lobe is indicated by the arrow. Total ventilatory function of the left lung is normal, while perfusion is diminished.

had ideal repair; Haller et al., 108 patients, 60 per cent of whom had excellent repair; and Wada et al., 199 patients, with 63 per cent excellent results.[3, 5, 11] Robicsek et al. reported 458 patients, with 353 (77 per cent) good, 44 acceptable, and 61 unsatisfactory repairs.[9] Personal results, reported as author's series (Table 14–2), are based on systematic follow-up of 531 consecutive patients for more than 2 years postoperatively. Eighty-four per cent of results were excellent or good, i.e., quality grade 1 or 2. In other series, follow-up has been inadequate to assess long-term results. Recommended follow-up is 1 week and 6 weeks after operation, then 6 months, 1 year, and every 2 years until full height is achieved (in girls, age 16 years; in boys, age 18 years). On each

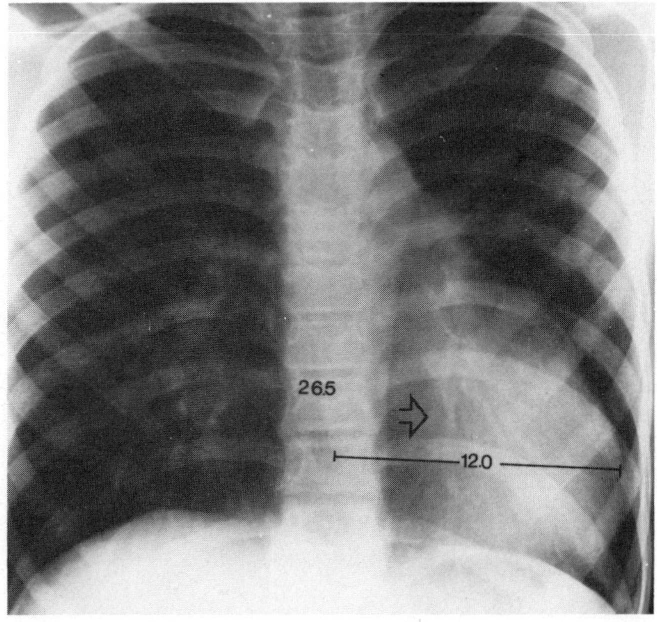

Figure 14–2 Anteroposterior preoperative radiograph of the patient in Figure 14–1, showing left cardiac displacement and compression of the underlying basal segments of the left lower lobe. There is compacting of bronchi supplying these segments and airless intervening parenchyma. Postoperatively, both ventilation and perfusion of the left lung were normal, i.e., 50 per cent contribution of each lung to total pulmonary function.

TABLE 14–2 LONG-TERM RESULTS OF
SURGICAL REPAIR OF PECTUS EXCAVATUM*

	Per Cent	Number of Patients
Normal chest (grade 1 or 2)	84	446
Mild recurrence or asymmetry (grade 3 or 4)	8	42
Moderate recurrence	5	27
Recurrence necessitating reoperation	3	16

*Author's series of 531 consecutive patients, followed up for more than 2 years after operation, to age 18 years.

return visit the repair is assessed (standing AP, lateral, and supine) and assigned a quality grade on a scale of 1 to 10. Major recurrences are never encountered early when substernal bars or traction devices are in place. Most repairs are satisfactory for as long as 2 years following surgery. Recurrences develop during the period of active growth.

The most distressing complication of surgical correction of pectus excavatum is major and total recurrence of the deformity 2 to 16 years after the original repair (Fig. 14–3). Most but not all patients seem to have a broad connective tissue disorder with hypotonia, poor posture and muscular development, and a tall, asthenic build. A few have marfanoid features. It is impossible for

me to predict accurately which patient will have a major recurrence necessitating reoperation. Fortunately, this occurs in only 3 per cent of patients. The single most important factor in achieving excellent long-term results is referral of the patient for surgical correction at the time of election, at age 2 to 5 years. Average age at referral of the last 300 patients was, unfortunately, 9.7 years; 35 per cent were older than 10 years, and some were adults (Table 14–3).

Sanger and coworkers reported on surgical correction of recurrent pectus excavatum.[10] They resected the regenerated fibrocartilage plate, repeated the osteotomy, and closed the pectoral muscles behind the sternum. Ten patients had an early good result. My experience is limited to 12 patients. Though recurrences appear to be symmetric, they are in fact right-sided with a deep right parasternal gutter and sternal obliquity. The third, fourth, and fifth rib ends have migrated medially and are in contact with the right edge of the sternum. Resection of segments of the third through fifth ribs is necessary to unlock the deformity. After clearing the tip of the sternum, resection of the left fibrocartilage plate to the level of the fourth perichondrial sheath allows the sternum to be brought anteriorly and rotated to an acceptable horizontal plane. Ten of 12 corrective operations were performed without entering the pleural cav-

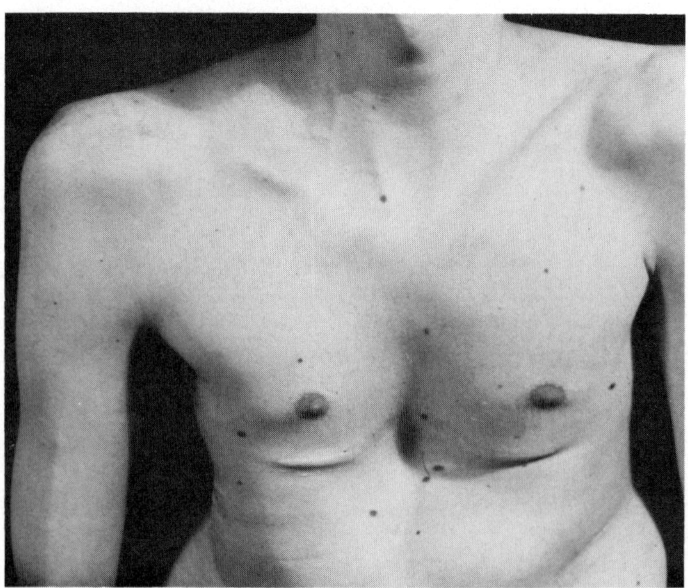

Figure 14–3 Severe recurrent pectus excavatum in an 18-year-old boy. Operation was performed at age 13 years in another city. The repair was satisfactory for nearly 2 years and then rapidly returned to the original deformity.

TABLE 14–3 AGE AT REFERRAL OF 300 PECTUS EXCAVATUM PATIENTS, 1976–1981

Age (yr)*	Number of Patients	Per Cent
2–5	116	39
5–10	78	26
10–15	66	22
15–20	34	11
>20	6	2

*Average age, 9.7 yr; oldest, age 41 yr.

ity. Because of lack of confidence in a second operation, all patients had internal fixation with a Steinmann pin. Follow-up of patients who underwent reoperation ranged from 3 to 12 years. Eight patients had acceptable thoracic contour, two had a broad, shallow depression with cartilage angularity, and two had frank recurrence.

PNEUMOTHORAX

Pneumothorax, very often bilateral, was frequently encountered in the early part of the series. With the adoption of a standard operative technique,[12] pneumothorax is currently found in 5 per cent of postoperative patients. Most have a small, 10 per cent pneumothorax on the right side. Pneumothorax requiring aspiration, 10 to 30 per cent, is next most common. Pneumothorax requiring tube thoracostomy is extremely rare (Fig. 14–4*A*, *B*). Of 14 cases, only five occurred during the past decade, when most of the operations were performed. The secret of avoiding pleural cavity entry is accurate establishment of tissue planes and preservation of the perichondrial sheaths. Entry through the base of the perichondrial sheath implies violation of the endothoracic fascia and the parietal pleura. More commonly, pneumothorax occurs because of failure to establish the sheath with accuracy. Entry is made through the intercostal bed above or below the cartilage to be resected. Another factor leading to pneumothorax is inexpert use of a mechanical breathing device. If volume or pressure is too high, the lungs are intermittently hyperinflated and the pleural envelopes are forcibly distended. To correct this situation, the patient is taken off the machine. The anesthetist returns to hand-compression of an inflatable bag, and the likelihood of pleural entry is vastly diminished. The right pleura often extends well beyond the tip of the xyphoid to the left subcostal area. The most common point of entry is at the level of or medial to the right costal arch. Occasionally the surgeon will create a pinhole-sized entry or tear, usually on the right side, after sternotomy has been performed and the sternum

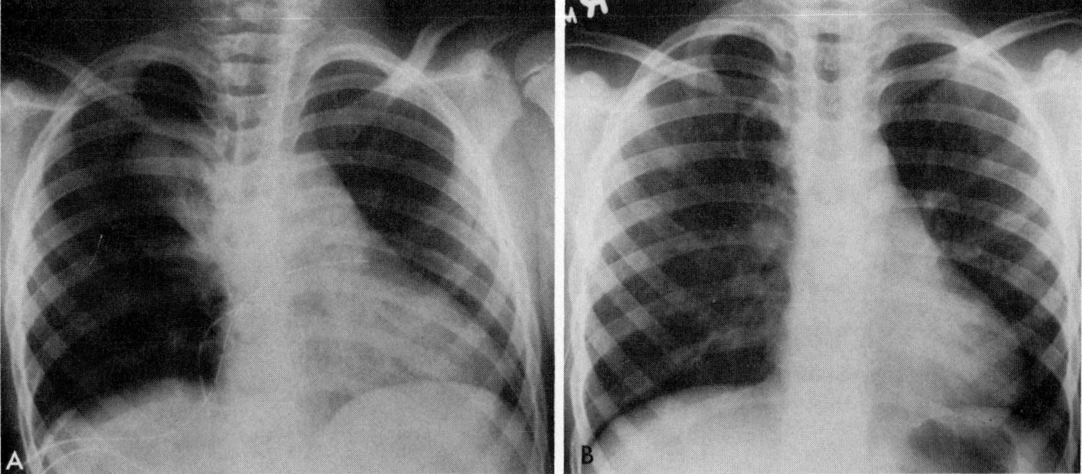

Figure 14–4 *A*, Massive right pneumothorax with atelectasis of the right lung discovered on portable upright anteroposterior recovery-room radiograph. Auscultation of the right lung was thought to be normal during the 3-hour operative procedure. *B*, Anteroposterior radiograph of the same patient taken 48 hours later shows complete expansion of the right lung and no residual pneumothorax. The intercostal drainage catheter enters the chest in the midaxillary line in the fifth interspace.

drawn forward to correct the deformity. We test each patient for air leak by flooding the operative field with warm Ringer's solution containing cephalothin (Keflin). Air bubbles seen on manual hyperinflation indicate pleural entry. Air seldom re-enters through the pinhole tract. With a larger leak, the anesthetist is asked to hyperinflate and hold the lung while a single mattress suture of 4-0 silk is placed and tied. If the pneumothorax recurs after aspiration or if the pleural rent cannot be closed, intercostal tube drainage is required. Continuing air leak in three patients resulted from injury to the subjacent pulmonary parenchyma. In two, a transient bronchopleural fistula was caused by overzealous hyperinflation of the lung.

PROSTHESES, EXTERNAL TRACTION, AND INTERNAL FIXATION

Fortunately, at our institution we have a very limited experience with contoured Silastic implants as a mode of therapy for pectus excavatum. Even if the implant provided a satisfactory external contour, it would not deal with the underlying thoracic deformity and the cardiopulmonary handicap. With an increasing number of patients presenting with pectus excavatum and scoliosis, we are even more reluctant to use this approach. Ravitch observed that one would not use a prosthesis for a depressed skull fracture.[7]

During the past decade, two patients were treated by insertion of a preformed gel prosthesis. There was delayed wound healing in both, with extrusion of the prosthesis in one and removal in the other because of infection within a pseudocystic capsule surrounding the prosthesis.

External traction was recommended by Garnier in 1934[4] and was used extensively at our institution in the 1950's. Heavy nonabsorbable sutures were passed through the sternal table, brought out through the skin below the incision, and anchored to a preformed malleable metal arch. These sutures were left in place for 10 days to 2 weeks. Initially, traction was used to treat flail chest. External traction sutures violate a principle of surgery in that they serve as routes of entry for skin organisms into the considerable retrosternal space. No patient in recent

years, when external traction has been seldom used, has had any problem with postoperative flail chest. Children with excessive tonsillar and adenoidal tissue may require a nasopharyngeal airway in the recovery room, but once awake they breathe normally. If retraction is observed in an older patient, the problem is in the upper airway and larynx. Urgent medical intervention is required. No patient has required bronchoscopy and none has required tracheostomy for airway obstruction in this series. Overnight ventilatory assistance has been required by a few obtunded patients.

Various methods of internal fixation have been recommended. Overholt used a Steinmann pin.[12] Adkins and Blades[1] and Rehbein and Wernicke[8] used a flat, stainless steel bar much like a malleable retractor. Currently, no type of brace, bar, or internal fixation is used routinely. Thirty of 816 patients have had internal fixation; this form of treatment is limited to patients with Marfan's disease who have the worst deformities, those reoperated upon for major recurrence, and adults with combined se-

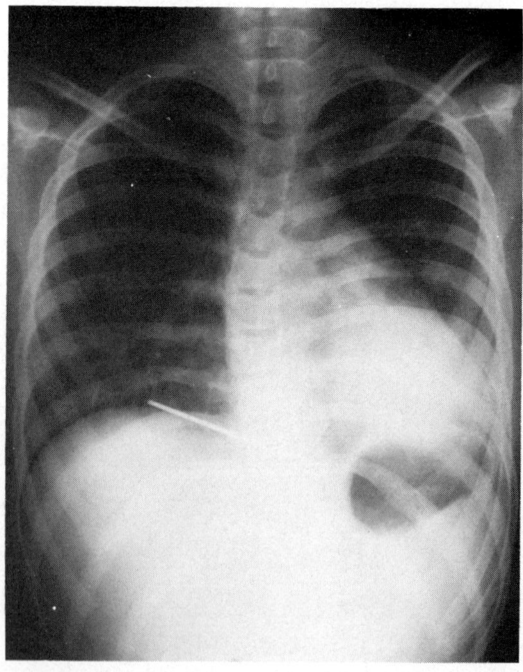

Figure 14–5　This 9-year-old patient had severe asymmetric pectus excavatum and scoliosis. The short segment of Steinmann pin is seen in proper position entering the intramedullary cavity of the fourth rib.

vere asymmetric deformity and scoliosis. A short (8 to 10 cm) segment of 5/32-inch Steinmann pin has been used. This is drilled transsternally, then through a longitudinal segment of resected cartilage, and on into the intramedullary cavity of the right fourth or fifth rib, picking out the highest point (Fig. 14–5). Eighteen patients are asymptomatic with the pin having been in place as long as 12 years. In 10 patients the pin migrated superficially 6 months to 5 years after operation and was removed without anesthesia when it presented as a subcutaneous cyst, right or left. In one patient the pin migrated into the left thorax, caused pericardial effusion, and was removed by anterior thoracotomy. In one other patient the pin was fractured in an automobile accident; one segment was removed. In another accident the right side of the pin was driven through the posterior cortex of the fifth rib. The pin was removed by vertical sternotomy, using the original incision.

There appears to be no completely satisfactory method of internal fixation. The deaths of two patients (elsewhere) resulted from use of the retrosternal metal bar (usually left in place for 6 months to 1 year) through erosion of the left ventricle.[13] Undoubtedly, other cases remain unreported.

SEROMA FORMATION

Seroma formation occurred in 10 patients. Suction drainage is routinely employed. A short segment of one limb of a Hemovac system is placed beneath the left pectoral muscle, then brought to the right of the sternum through the retrosternal space, exiting 2 inches below the end of the incision (Fig. 14–6). The apparatus is left in place for 48 hours. By the end of the second day, drainage has virtually ceased. When the patient is discharged on the sixth postoperative day, he is examined for evidence of a retrosternal ballotable fluid accumulation. If such is present, the retrosternal space must again be evacuated by mediastinal aspiration (Fig. 14–7). About 5 per cent of patients may require a second mediastinocentesis at the time of the first postoperative visit. In a few patients, fluid will continue to form in the retrosternal space, now lined by a pseudocapsule with an oncotic pressure effect. At this stage the patient should be readmitted to the hospital and a slip drain placed through the center of the incision into the retrosternal space. Drainage decreases rapidly. The wound heals satisfactorily and completely, and the end result is not compromised.

Frank wound dehiscence occurred in four patients in the early part of the series. Insufficient attention was given to development of adequate flaps of pectoral and rectus muscle to effect primary watertight closure without tension at the muscular level. In three patients with severe deformity I was not able to accomplish primary closure and was left with an arrowhead muscular defect. The flaring edges of the pectoral muscles and the advanced rectus apex flap could not be approximated. Marlex was used successfully in each patient.

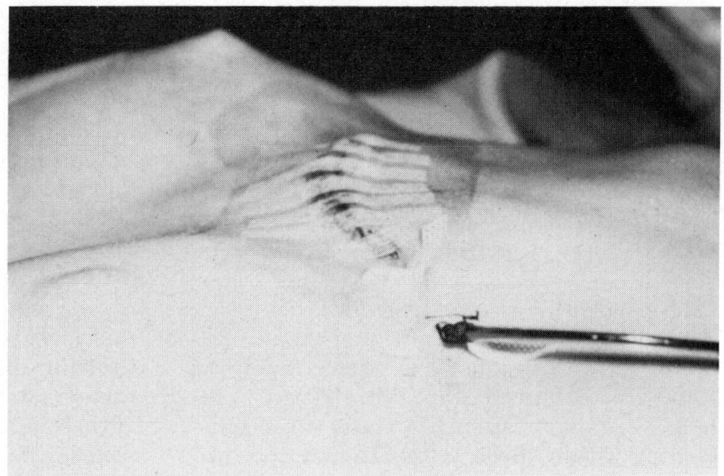

Figure 14–6 Postoperative photograph of a 15-year-old girl following surgical correction of pectus excavatum. The Hemovac catheter is brought out well below and to the right of the incision in the inframammary crease. Only one limb of the Hemovac catheter is used.

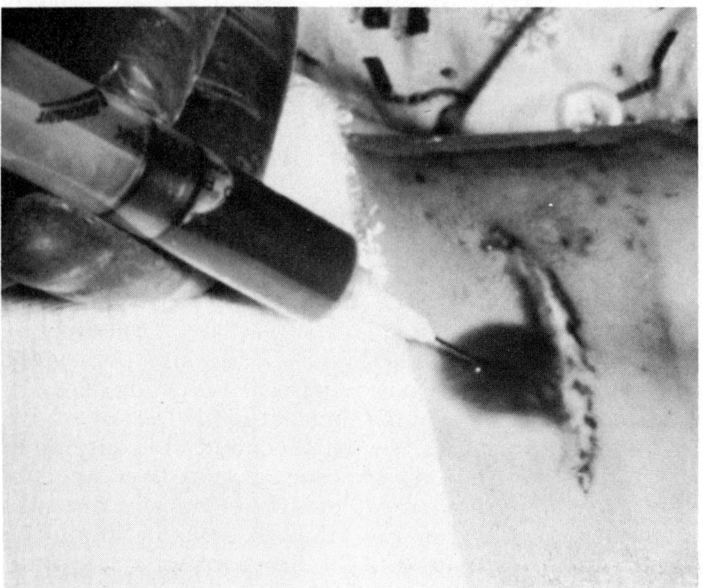

Figure 14–7 Mediastinocentesis produced 35 ml of thin, clear, purplish fluid in this 5-year-old boy on the sixth postoperative day. The 18 French angiocatheter has been introduced beneath the midpoint of the incision identifying the tip of the sternum and then sliding into the retrosternal space. No further aspirations were required.

EXCESSIVE BLEEDING

Excessive bleeding was encountered in eight patients — in four intraoperatively and in four postoperatively. One patient had a right hemopneumothorax with loss of 1700 ml of whole blood. In three patients there was excessive Hemovac drainage with a fall in hematocrit level necessitating blood transfusion. In four patients there was a history of recent aspirin intake with abnormal platelet function. One patient was deficient in factor V. In three patients the bleeding was unexplained and presumed to be from the internal mammary or intercostal arteries. Intraoperative bleeding is largely controlled by proper setting of the Bovie electrosurgical unit: mode 2 adequate coagulating current and cutting current set to complete control of bleeding from perforating vessels. Establishment of the proper submuscular planes (in areolar tissue) further reduces blood loss.

MISCELLANEOUS COMPLICATIONS

Hypertrophic scar requiring revision occurred in six patients, although many patients have transient scar hypertrophy in some area of the incision. With patient waiting, 90 per cent of such scars become satisfactory within three years. In patients undergoing revision, the new scar was not much of an improvement over the original. Scars on the anterior chest are less satisfactory in appearance than scars on any other part of the body, and they are worst following vertical incisions for sternal split. We use a transverse skin incision well within the nipple lines at the level of the fifth interspace. The patient should be carefully inspected for evidence of hypertrophic scar formation (old lacerations, previous surgical incisions, and so forth). The family should be warned in advance about this potential. Injection of triamcinolone into the edges of the wound at 1-month intervals has been recommended but has not been rewarding in my experience. Local steroids produce a very thin scar with telangiectasia and do not prevent widening.

Necrosis of the skin flap occurred in four patients. Every time the incision veers off horizontal, this possibility exists. Attempts to contour the incision to breast configuration or to make the upper part of the operation easier place the apex of the inferior flap in jeopardy. Superficial necrosis heals spontaneously; no patient in whom it has occurred has required a graft. At the time of closure the wound edges should be carefully examined for local injury by retractors or by inadvertent contact with the Bovie blade. The inferior margin of the superior flap is often trimmed back to fresh bleeding. Failure to do so results in some delay of wound healing and a wet wound at 10 to 12 days, when healing should be complete at the skin level.

The incidence of wound infections (0.6 per cent) has been far below the acceptable level for clean surgery for all other conditions in our institution. Factors in cartilage, bone, marrow, and muscle must play a protective role. Five wound infections were superficial, involving skin and subcutaneous tissues. One patient with deep infection presented with high fever and a positive blood culture (*Staphylococcus aureus*). Hospital readmission, antibiotic therapy, and drainage of the wound resulted in prompt control and spontaneous healing.

Completing the list of miscellaneous complications, one patient had right bronchial intubation with airway anoxia. The tube was replaced and operation was uneventful. Intravenous lines became disconnected in two patients. In each instance the anesthetist was administering intravenous morphine sulfate and a relaxant (succinylcholine); both failed to reach the patient. All functioning intravenous lines being used to administer anesthetic agents should be in clear view of the anesthetist and not under drapes. In two patients the Hemovac catheter was severed at skin level. The catheters were extruded 1 week and 6 weeks later, respectively.

Pectus Carinatum

Pectus carinatum is one tenth as common as pectus excavatum. It may be that patients with moderate to severe carinate deformities are not being referred for surgical treatment because cardiopulmonary handicap has not been identified in male adolescents with this deformity. Congenital heart disease has been reported in females and in younger patients.[2] Most patients have minor deformity until the period of most active growth. The protrusion increases in severity each subsequent year from age 13 to 18 years. The operation for pectus carinatum described by Lam and Taber[6] has been in use for approximately 15 years and is essentially a mirror image of the operation I described for pectus excavatum, employing the same techniques and surgical principles.[12, 15] To date, 94 patients have been operated upon, and no deaths have occurred.

Five patients experienced transient lobar atelectasis. Postoperative segmental left lower lobe atelectasis is seldom diagnosed. Atelectasis is not limited to the anterior and medial basal segments of the left lower lobe; rather, a total lobe is involved and represents a complication of anesthesia. With upper lobe involvement, aspiration is suspected. Pneumothorax occurred in five (5.5

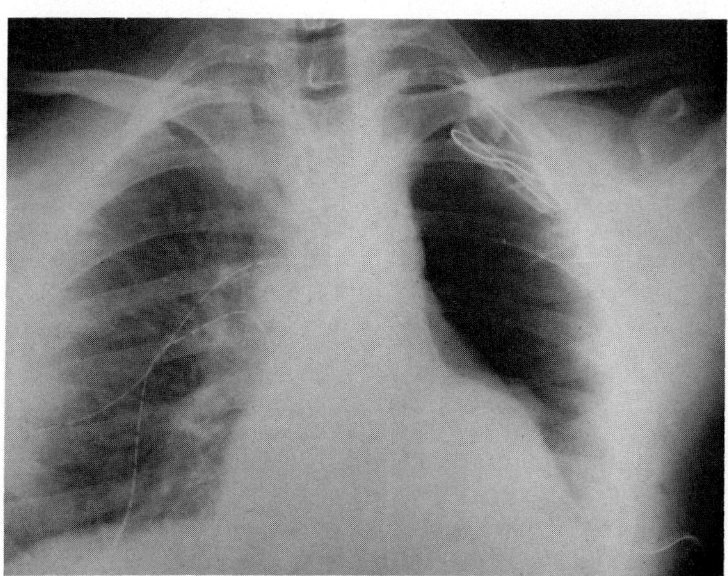

Figure 14–8 Pectus carinatum. Total left pneumothorax and atelectasis are identified in the upright portable anteroposterior recovery-room radiograph. The mediastinal structures are in normal position. An intercostal catheter has been inserted in the second interspace anteriorly in the midclavicular line and placed on waterseal suction drainage. The left lung rapidly re-expanded, and the pneumothorax did not recur.

per cent) patients. None had a recurrence following aspiration, and one required an intercostal tube (Fig. 14–8). No form of internal fixation is used or required. Flail chest has not been observed. Because the sternum is displaced posteriorly, closure of the muscle layers is relatively easy even though the pectoral muscles are widely separated from the midline. There is no retrosternal space; consequently, seromas do not form. Superficial necrosis of the lower skin flap was observed once after an attempt to contour the incision. Excessive intraoperative blood loss occurred once, and Hemovac loss necessitating transfusion occurred twice. Postoperative wound hematoma presenting as extensive ecchymosis occurred twice and was thought to be due to aspirin sensitivity; drainage was required. Operative correction of pectus carinatum is in many ways easier than correction of pectus excavatum, taking less time and causing less blood loss. The postoperative course is usually benign. Patients are ambulatory after the first postoperative day. Time in hospital averaged 5.8 days. Fortunately, no patient experienced a recurrence. Early in the series, patients with mostly one-sided deformity had unilateral cartilage resection limited to the area of maximal protrusion. Most patients have some degree of sternal obliquity and concavity of the corresponding cartilages on the opposite side. We recommend symmetric and adequate removal of the involved cartilages (usually the fourth through seventh and occasionally the third on each side).[14]

DIAPHRAGMATIC HERNIA

The most serious complication of surgical treatment of diaphragmatic hernia in newborns is death. More than 50 per cent of infants born with diaphragmatic hernia are stillborn or die immediately after delivery in spite of every resuscitative effort.[30] Of the hypoxic infants who reach a hospital alive and undergo surgical treatment, 50 per cent survive.[19, 30] There has been no improvement in mortality in this group of patients in the past decade. Of the infants born alive, most (70 to 80 per cent) are full term and have no associated anomalies except patent ductus, colonic malrotation, and duodenal obstruction.[20, 22, 29, 31] The often large patent ductus may, according to circumstances, be preserved pharmacologically, closed pharmacologically, or closed surgically.

Persistence of Fetal Circulation

The immediate complications of untreated diaphragmatic hernia are anoxia, hypocarbia, and acidosis with hypothermia; all adversely affect pulmonary artery pressure. The most serious complication that follows surgical repair and is beyond the surgeon's control is persistence of fetal circulation. Obstruction in the pulmonary vascular bed as a result of persisting muscularity of small arteries or vasospasm in resistance vessels occurs in 50 per cent of patients; few survive. Low birth weight, high Apgar score, a left-sided lesion, and unrelieved cyanosis necessitating intubation provide clues to the diagnosis. Pre- and postductal P_{CO_2} and Pa_{O_2} measurements define the degree of right-to-left shunt and are obtained from a low-positioned umbilical artery catheter and a radial artery catheter. A falling Pa_{CO_2}, a rising Pa_{O_2}, and reduction of pulmonary artery pressure to below systemic pressure in response to treatment are considered omens of success.

The pharmacologic treatment of persistent fetal circulation is still in the experimental stage. Results vary, as do treatment protocols. Our cardiologists[32] prefer an inlying open-end pulmonary artery catheter for monitoring pressures in the pulmonary artery bed whether intervention is pharmacologic, surgical by closure of the ductus, or both, as advocated by Collins et al.,[22] Boix-Ochoa et al.,[17] and Raphaely and Downes.[33] The ductus can be kept open by administering prostaglandin E_1 (0.1 mg/kg/hr), which reduces arteriolar musculature, and can be closed by administering indomethacin (Indocin), 1 mg/ml, which blocks prostaglandin. Tolazoline HCl (Priscoline) may be injected peripherally (2 mg/kg/hr) or directly into the pulmonary artery to relieve vasospasm in resistance vessels, thus lowering pulmonary artery pressure and allowing left-to-right shunt through the diminishing ductus lumen (Fig. 14–9). Chlorpromazine HCl (Thorazine), 1 mg/kg/hr, acts in a similar way. Dopamine (Intropin), 5 to 20

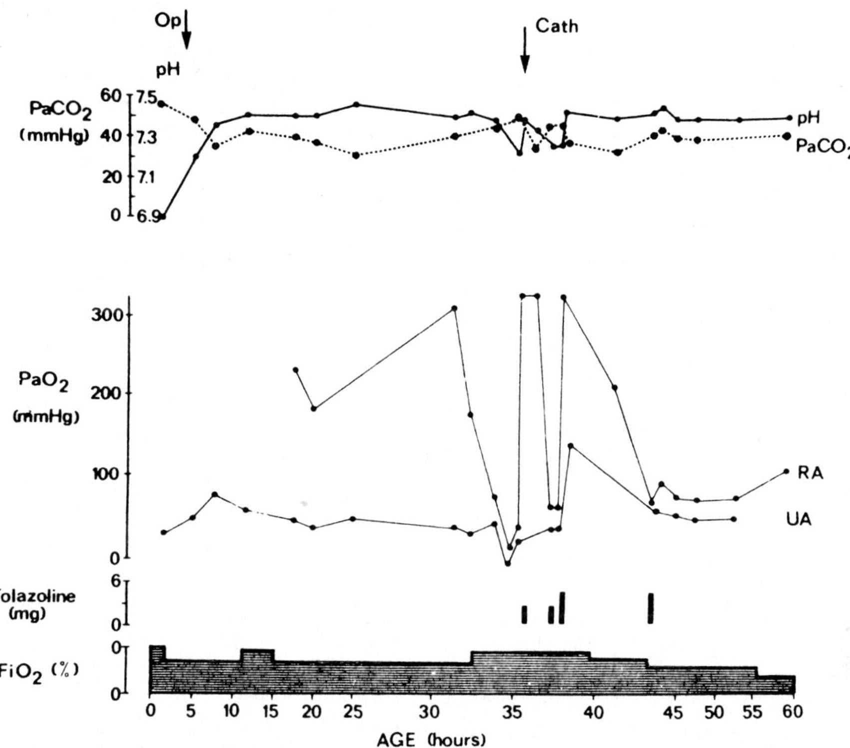

Figure 14–9 Clinical course and effects of tolazoline therapy on oxygenation and acid-base balance in neonate with congenital diaphragmatic hernia and persistent fetal circulation (PFC). Op = repair of diaphragmatic hernia; Cath = cardiac catheterization; RA = radial artery; UA = umbilical artery. (From Levey, R. J., Rosenthal, A., Freed, M. O., et al.: Persistent pulmonary hypertension in a newborn with congenital diaphragmatic hernia. Successful management with tolazoline. Pediatrics 60:740, 1977.)

μg/kg/min, is an ionotropic agent that raises systemic arterial pressure by increasing peripheral resistance; it has no effect on the pulmonary vascular bed. Acetylcholine (no longer available), nitroprusside, and phenothiazine have been used with inconsistent success. Approval is being sought for a protocol involving Priscoline, prostaglandin E_1, a pulmonary arterial hypertension index, and a lung maturity index.[24]

These drugs can and do cause complications. Indocin may cause blindness through a simultaneous obliterative effect on ophthalmic vessels. Blindness and cerebral air embolism have occurred as a result of misuse of a temporal artery catheter to measure preductal blood gases. Gangrene of extremities and midgut ischemic infarction have been reported with use of dopamine.[36]

Two of our patients with persistent fetal circulation have been treated with tolazoline and have survived. Of five patients reported by Collins et al. who underwent ligation of a patent ductus and reduction of pulmonary artery pressure using tolazoline, three survived.[21] Although tolazoline reduced pulmonary artery pressure and improved Pa_{O_2} in four patients reported by Boles and Anderson, it did not improve mortality.[19] Improvement in Pa_{CO_2} is not directly related to the degree of lung expansion as determined by radiographs or xenon lung scans. Nor has improvement in Pa_{O_2} increased survival consistently in the small and uncontrolled groups of patients reported.[18, 19, 21, 23, 29] Extracorporeal membrane oxygenation (ECMO) may provide the time necessary to advance pulmonary function to a level compatible with survival.[25, 26] Hardesty et al., using ECMO for periods ranging from 48 to 216 hours, saved three of five infants whose conditions were deteriorating after repair of diaphragmatic hernia.[28] All patients were adequately monitored and had pharmacologic manipulation without improvement.

True bilateral lung hypoplasia has been documented in only three of our more than 200 patients. In most, the number of lung units is appropriate to the size and gestational age of the infant; most are full term. Hypoplastic lung has been the cover term for clinical failures; it has been vastly overused and poorly documented. Nevertheless, diminished function of the ipsilateral lung has been proved by xenon lung scans in long-term follow-up of patients operated on for diaphragmatic hernia during the first 2 days of life.

Iatrogenic Surgical Complications

A most avoidable complication is operation on the wrong side of the abdomen or chest because of reliance on outside radiographs with absent or incorrect left and right markers. In patients with right-sided diaphragmatic hernia (10 to 15 per cent) the liver is usually intrathoracic and there is at best subtle distinction between hepatic and gastric outlines to guide the surgeon to the appropriate side of the lesion. An error in diagnosis may lead to thoracotomy for a lesion thought to be a pulmonary cyst or laparotomy for a pulmonary cyst thought to be a foramen of Bochdalek hernia. One patient had three incisions before proper identification and treatment of a right Bochdalek hernia. Every effort should be made and enough time taken to diagnose diaphragmatic hernia with certainty and to establish its laterality. Hepatic scintiscan can be helpful. Patients with bilateral diaphragmatic hernia are extremely rare, and none have survived.[30]

Postoperative pneumothorax on the ipsilateral side is uncommon. A tube thoracostomy is established prior to closure of the diaphragmatic defect and placed on −10 cm waterseal drainage. Pleurovac and three-bottle systems should not be used.[21] Low ventilatory pressures (20 to 30 cm H_2O) and positive end-expiratory pressure of less than 5 cm H_2O will diminish the chance of contralateral pneumothorax.[21]

The key to successful postoperative management of diaphragmatic hernia (once normal pulmonary artery flow has been established) is full and gradual expansion of the ipsilateral lung over a period of 7 to 10 days, during which time pancuronium bromide (Pavulon) paralysis and assisted ventilation are required.

There are few direct surgical complications of this relatively simple neonatal surgical procedure, which is most often accomplished through a subcostal incision. Injury to the spleen occurs with left-sided lesions. Direct splenic repair should be carried out rather than splenectomy, which has the attendant problem of postsplenectomy overwhelming infection. Injury to the adrenal gland has occurred in patients with right-sided lesions, leading to an addisonian state in one.[30] Injury to the right colon necessitating resection has been reported.[19]

Recurrence of diaphragmatic hernia following proper closure through imbrication using interrupted nonabsorbable sutures is uncommon today. Marlex or Teflon mesh may be required in closing the largest defects. Recurrence of right-sided lesions is uncommon because the liver buttresses the phrenic repair.

Postoperative duodenal obstruction as a complication of diaphragmatic hernia repair implies failure to deal fully and directly with the nearly always associated colonic malrotation. Infants with orthorotation do well, presumably because of improved lung maturity. Noting absence of the ligament of Treitz, one must pursue the duodenum from the pyloric vein, down the right side of the abdomen, and into the iliac gutter. External freeing up of this segment is followed by passage of a catheter through the gastrotomy site and on through the now vertical duodenal segment. The right kidney often resides in a thoracic position. To our knowledge, obstructive uropathy has not been associated with repair of diaphragmatic hernia.

Most patients requiring ventral hernia formation following closure of the diaphragmatic defect died, a testimony to their poor pulmonary circulation and function. Stress anoxia, sepsis, midgut volvulus, and hemorrhage from disseminated intravascular coagulopathy have accounted for other deaths not directly related to surgical repair or persistent fetal circulation.[19]

Among our miscellaneous complications,

splenic laceration unsuspected at the time of operation was diagnosed at autopsy following exsanguinating blood loss through a left thoracostomy tube. Gangrene of the right foot followed pharmacologic intervention in one patient.[36]

In a few patients the diaphragmatic defect has been very large, with only a rim of muscular tissue available posteriorly. In two such patients primary closure using Teflon or Marlex mesh was successful. Marlex was used for recurrence in two patients. In the first a pseudosac was excised and Marlex was sutured to the exposed muscular rim. In the second (left Bochdalek hernia) conventional repair was carried out twice, with recurrence followed by the insertion of mesh and a satisfactory outcome.

DIAPHRAGMATIC PARALYSIS

A high diaphragm in the postoperative patient with initially low and comparable diaphragmatic outlines is occasionally seen after various thoracic neonatal surgical procedures. It also occurs as a complication of obstetric delivery. The injury lies somewhere between the third and fifth cervical nerve origins and their final course and distribution to the right and left diaphragmatic leaves. The phrenic nerve is readily identified and spared in the upper chest (except in the case of malignant neoplasia). In the region of the diaphragm it is very difficult to identify and trace. The diaphragm can be safely incised peripherally, as in the Waterston procedure, or radially, as in full thoracoabdominal incision for right hepatic lobectomy. Anterior and midmediastinal tumors are most likely to be associated with direct and at times unavoidable injury to the phrenic nerve. If the nerve is anatomically divided or a segment is removed, immediate neurorrhaphy should be performed with magnification. If a sufficient segment is missing, interposition of a segment of intercostal nerve using microsurgical technique is recommended.[37] Direct intermittent stimulation of the injured nerve has been unsatisfactory even with modern techniques. Surgical intervention is recommended when a high diaphragm is associated with severe respiratory symptoms for more than 2 weeks and the patient cannot be weaned from the respirator.[22, 27, 34] Temporary diaphragmatic paralysis in patients

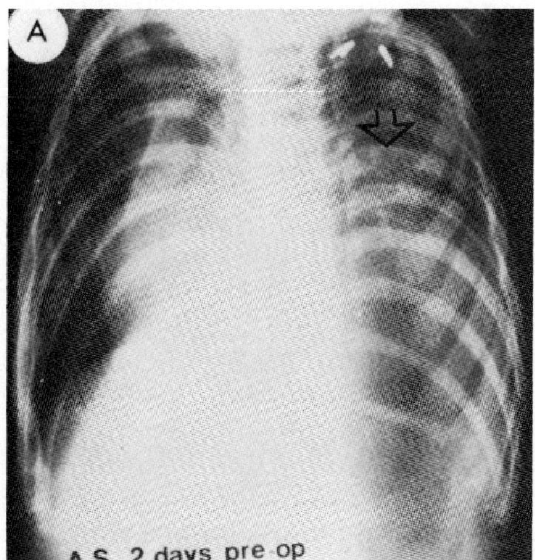

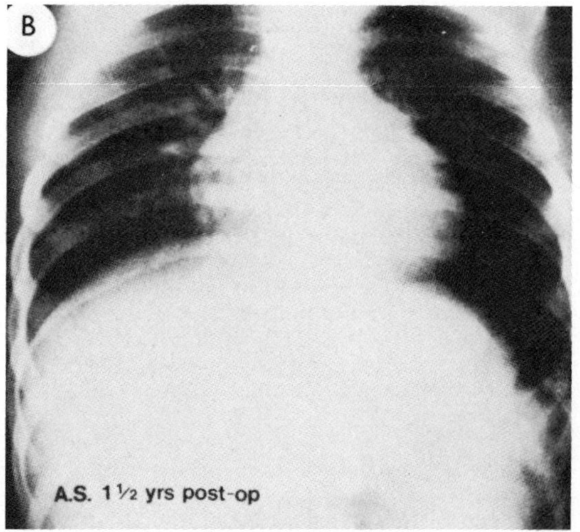

Figure 14–10 *A,* Complete paralysis of left diaphragm following removal of a left cervical neuroblastoma in a 5-month-old boy. Diaphragmatic apex is indicated by arrow. *B,* Anteroposterior radiograph obtained 18 months after transabdominal plication of the left diaphragm using multiple reefing sutures. A subcostal incision was used. Ventilatory function of the left lung is now normal. As with most iatrogenic injuries of the phrenic nerve, there was no return of diaphragmatic function. The plicated diaphragm remains in a fixed low position with a stable mediastinum. (From Schwartz, M. Z., and Filler, R. M.: Plication of the diaphragm for symptomatic phrenic nerve paralysis. J. Pediatr. Surg. 13:259, 1978.)

ventilated for respiratory distress syndrome is common and unexplained. Fortunately, the condition is self-limited. Later intervention is required in symptomatic patients when no improvement in diaphramatic position or function is noted for several months. Some authors recommend radial incision between the anterior and median phrenic branches at the diaphragmatic level and closure by imbrication.[30] Others have used a series of reefing sutures, hoping to miss substantial components of phrenic nerve distribution.[16, 34]

Iatrogenic diaphragmatic paralysis occurred once following removal of a cervical neuroblastoma and once following removal of a malignant epithelial thymoma (Fig. 14–10*A, B*). Plication was also required in three patients who had repair of esophageal atresia and in two patients operated upon for congenital heart disease. Our total experience now consists of nine patients; six were reported by Schwartz and Filler.[34] Patients with left-sided and bilateral cases were operated upon through a subcostal incision. Right diaphragmatic palsy is more common and requires a thoracic incision. Ventilatory function was improved in all but one patient. Diaphragmatic function returned after plication in two patients.

References

Anterior Thoracic Deformities

1. Adkins, P. C., and Blades, B.: A stainless steel strut for correction of pectus excavatum. Surg. Gynecol. Obstet. 113:111, 1961.
2. Currarino, G., and Silverman, F. N.: Premature obliteration of the sternal sutures and pigeon breast deformities. Radiology 70:532, 1958.
3. Gall, F. P., Hegemann, G., Köllermann, M. W., et al.: Surgical treatment of funnel chest. Dis. Chest 52:10, 1967.
4. Garnier, C.: Traitement chirurgical du thorax en entonnoir. Rev. Orthopéd. 21:385, 1934.
5. Haller, J. A., Jr., Peters, G. N., Mazur, D., et al.: Pectus excavatum. A 20 year surgical experience. J. Thorac. Cardiovasc. Surg. 60:375, 1970.
6. Lam, C. R., and Taber, R. E.: Surgical treatment of pectus carinatum. Arch. Surg. 103:191, 1971.
7. Ravitch, M. M.: Congenital Deformities of the Chest Wall and Their Operative Correction. Philadelphia, W. B. Saunders Co., 1977.
8. Rehbein, F., and Wernicke, H. M.: The operative treatment of the funnel chest. Arch. Dis. Child. 32:5, 1957.
9. Robicsek, F., Daugherty, H. K., Mullen, D. C., et al.: Technical considerations in the surgical management of pectus excavatum and carinatum. Ann. Thorac. Surg. 18:549, 1974.
10. Sanger, P. W., Taylor, F. H., and Robicsek, F.: Deformities of the anterior wall of the chest. Surg. Gynecol. Obstet. 116:515, 1963.
11. Wada, J., Ikeda, K., Ishida, T., et al.: Results of 271 funnel chest operations. Ann. Thorac. Surg. 10:526, 1970.
12. Welch, K. J.: Satisfactory surgical correction of pectus excavatum deformity in childhood. J. Thorac. Surg. 36:697, 1958.
13. Welch, K. J.: Pectus excavatum: Complications and longterm results in 734 patients. *In* W. B. Kiesewetter (ed.): Longterm Follow-up in Congenital Anomalies. Pittsburgh, Mellon Foundation, 1980.
14. Welch, K. J.: Chest wall deformities. *In* Holder, T. M., and Ashcraft, K. W. (eds.): Pediatric Surgery. Philadelphia, W. B. Saunders Co., 1980, pp. 162–182.
15. Welch, K. J., and Vos, A.: Surgical correction of pectus carinatum (pigeon breast). J. Pediatr. Surg. 5:659, 1973.

Diaphragm

16. Bishop, H. C., and Koop, C. E.: Acquired eventration of the diaphragm in infancy. Pediatrics 22:1088, 1958.
17. Boix-Ochoa, J., Natal, A., Canal, J., et al.: The important influence of arterial blood gases on the prognosis of congenital diaphragmatic hernia. World J. Surg. 1:783, 1977.
18. Boix-Ochoa, J., Peguero, G., Seijo, G., et al.: Acid-base balance and blood gases in prognosis and therapy of congenital diaphragmatic hernia. J. Pediatr. Surg. 9:49, 1974.
19. Boles, E. T., and Anderson, G.: Diaphragmatic Hernia in the Newborn in Long Term Follow-up in Congenital Anomalies. Children's Hospital Surgical Symposium, Pittsburgh, 1979.
20. Boles, E. T., Schiller, M., and Weinberger, M.: Improved management of neonates with congenital diaphragmatic hernias. Arch. Surg. 103:344, 1971.
21. Collins, D. L.: Diaphragmatic hernia. *In* Holder, T. M., and Ashcraft, K. W.: Pediatric Surgery. Philadelphia, W. B. Saunders Co., 1980, pp. 227–240.
22. Collins, D. L., Pomerance, J. J., Travis, K. W., et al.: A new approach to congenital posterolateral diaphragmatic hernia. J. Pediatr. Surg. 12:149, 1977.
23. Dibbins, A. W., and Wiener, E. S.: Mortality from neonatal diaphragmatic hernia. J. Pediatr. Surg. 9:653, 1974.
24. Freed, M., and Reed, L.: Personal communication.
25. German, J. C., Bartlett, R. H., Gazzaniga, A. B., et al.: Pulmonary artery pressure monitoring in persistent fetal circulation (PFC). J. Pediatr. Surg. 12:913, 1977.
26. German, J. C., Gazzaniga, A. B., Amlie, R., et al.: Management of pulmonary insufficiency in congenital diaphragmatic hernia using extracorporeal circulation with a membrane oxygenator (ECMO). J. Pediatr. Surg. 12:905, 1977.

27. Greene, W., L'Heureux, P., and Hunt, C. E.: Paralysis of diaphragm. Am. J. Dis. Child. 129:1402, 1975.

28. Hardesty, R. L., Griffith, B. P., and Debski, R. F.: Extracorporeal membrane oxygenation: Successful treatment of persistent fetal circulation following repair of congenital diaphragmatic hernia. J. Thorac. Cardiovasc. Surg. *81*:556, 1981.

29. Harrison, M. R., Bjordal, R. J., Langmork, F., et al.: Congenital diaphragmatic hernia: The hidden mortality. J. Pediatr. Surg. 13:227, 1978.

30. Holder, T. M., and Ashcraft, K. W.: Diaphragmatic hernia. *In* Ravitch, M. M., Welch, K. J., Benson, C. D., et al. (eds.): Pediatric Surgery, 3rd edition. Chicago, Year Book Medical Publishers, 1979, pp. 432–445.

31. Johnson, D. G., Deaner, R. M., and Koop, C. E.: Diaphragmatic hernia in infancy: Factors affecting the mortality rate. Surgery 62:1082, 1967.

32. Levey, R. J., Rosenthal, A., Freed, M. O., et al.: Persistent pulmonary hypertension in a newborn with congenital diaphragmatic hernia. Successful management with tolazoline. Pediatrics 60:740, 1977.

33. Raphaely, R. C., and Downes, J. J., Jr.: Congenital diaphragmatic hernia: Prediction of survival. J. Pediatr. Surg. 8:815, 1973.

34. Schwartz, M. Z., and Filler, R. M.: Plication of the diaphragm for symptomatic phrenic nerve paralysis. J. Pediatr. Surg. 13:259, 1978.

35. Stauffer, U. G., and Rickham, P. P.: Acquired eventration of the diaphragm in the newborn. J. Pediatr. Surg. 7:635, 1972.

36. Welch, K. J.: Gangrene of the extremities. *In* Ravitch, M. M., Welch, K. J., Benson, C. D., et al. (eds.): Pediatric Surgery, 3rd edition. Chicago, Year Book Medical Publishers, 1979.

37. Welch, K. J., Tapper, D., and Vawter, G. P.: Surgical treatment of thymic cysts and neoplasms in children. J. Pediatr. Surg. 14:691, 1979.

TRACHEA, LUNGS, AND PLEURAL CAVITY

15

H. Biemann Othersen, Jr., M.D.

TRACHEA

Iatrogenic complications are common in the child's airway, which is strikingly different, both anatomically and physiologically, from that of the adult. The child has a large head and a short neck, and the larynx is more anterior and cephalad. The child's tongue is large, and the epiglottis is longer, stiffer, and V-shaped. The trachea descends through the chest at a 30-degree angle to the long axis of the body, and the narrowest point of the airway in a child is at the cricoid, not at the glottis (Fig. 15–1). Size itself is a major consideration. One millimeter of edema of the vocal cords in an adult may cause only hoarseness, but in an infant the same millimeter will reduce the glottic airway by 65 per cent.[20] Air flow depends upon the fourth power of the radius of the airway. Slight congenital narrowing in the subglottic area of a child may, with the edema resulting from subglottic croup, further reduce the internal diameter of the airway to a critical point. For example, a 20 per cent decrease in internal diameter of the trachea from 6 mm to 4.8 mm would result in reduction of the cross-sectional area from 28 sq mm to 19 sq mm, a 36 per cent constriction of the airway (Fig. 15–2).

Physiologically, respiration in children differs from that in adults. The infant is an obligate nose-breather with a fragile airway and may die from obstructed nares alone.[22] The neonate breathes almost exclusively with his diaphragm and receives little help from the intercostal muscles. To complicate matters further, physicians who treat children must make diagnoses without help, and sometimes with resistance, from their patients. A serious or even fatal iatrogenic complication may be the price of eliminating a medical problem. Disastrous results occur when the qualitative and quantitative differences between children and adults are unknown, unrecognized, or unheeded.

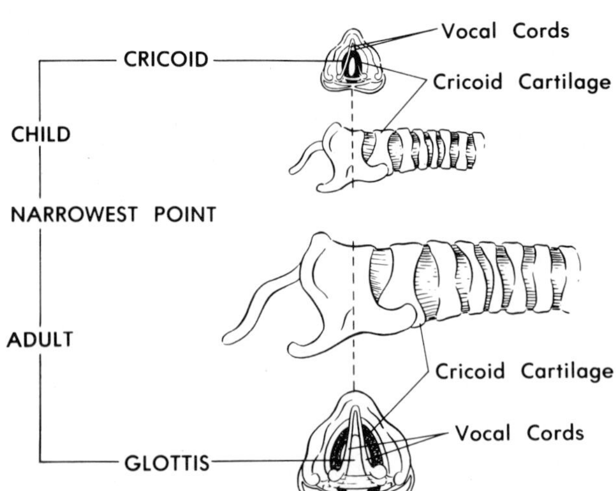

Figure 15–1 Anatomic differences between the upper airway of a child and that of an adult. The major difference is that the smallest diameter in the child is at the cricoid ring, not at the glottis. (From Othersen, R. B., Jr.: Intubation injuries of the trachea in children. Management and prevention. Ann. Surg. 189:601, 1979.)

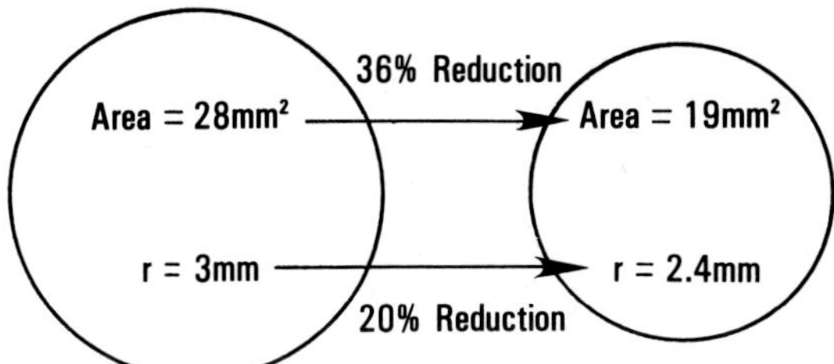

Figure 15–2 Diagrammatic representation of the almost twofold reduction in cross-sectional area that accompanies reduction in the radius.

Etiology

Complications involving the trachea and bronchi of infants and children usually result from infection or trauma; both reduce the airway lumen.

INFECTION

The most serious offender in this category is virus-induced subglottic croup, sometimes called laryngotracheitis.[6] It is important to distinguish this variety from spasmodic croup, which is self-limited and responds well to inhalations of moist air, and from epiglottitis, a bacterial infection usually due to *Hemophilus influenzae*. Laryngotracheobronchitis, now rarely seen, is a viral laryngotracheitis with bacterial superinfection progressing from the trachea to the lungs. This condition, now called "bacterial tracheitis,"[12] responds to endotracheal intubation with aspiration of pus and administration of systemic antibiotics.

Spasmodic croup is less likely to lead to complications. It typically begins at night with sudden dyspnea, croupy cough, and inspiratory stridor without fever. Reassurance, moist air, and possibly ipecac are rapidly beneficial. In other types of croup severe enough to warrant hospital admission, the child is taken directly to the operating room if the airway obstruction is severe but incomplete. Endotracheal intubation or tracheostomy should not be performed in the emergency room unless respiratory tract obstruction is complete. The mother accompanies her child to the operating table, since crying may precipitate complete airway obstruction. With the patient under sedation or light anesthesia, direct laryngoscopy is

performed, which may reveal the typical cherry-red inflammation of epiglottitis without glottic involvement. With this diagnosis, an endotracheal tube is immediately inserted. The child is treated with antibiotics for 24 to 48 hours and then extubated. Bronchoscopy and tracheostomy are unnecessary and impose a great risk of complications. If the inflammatory process is observed to involve the glottis and trachea, particularly with edema in the area of the cricoid cartilage, an endotracheal tube is placed for temporary airway control. A tracheostomy is then performed, since even short-term endotracheal intubation invites pressure necrosis when swelling occurs around the tube. The tracheostomy tube should remain in place for 5 to 7 days or until the inflammatory process has subsided and the airway is patent. Recent evidence suggests the value of steroids.[14] Our treatment consists of steroids and antibiotics (ampicillin 50 to 100 mg/kg/day and dexamethasone 0.8 mg/kg/day divided into four doses and given intravenously every 6 hours). Prompt administration may prevent the need for tracheal intubation.

Complications following treatment involve the subglottic region or the tracheostomy stoma. An endotracheal tube that fits through the glottis may be too tight at the cricoid, where inflammatory edema and the complete ring of unyielding cartilage produce pressure necrosis and ulceration. In addition, the reciprocating motion imparted to an endotracheal tube by a ventilator or by alternate flexion and extension of an unrestrained head adds a shearing force to the tracheal mucosa. Following extubation, obstruction may result from edema or granulation tissue; a constricting scar follows.[17]

Cuffed endotracheal or tracheostomy tubes should not be used in children maintained by mechanical ventilators. With inadequate ventilation, inspiratory volume can be increased to attain adequate tidal volume in spite of leak. Damage to the trachea at the cuff site is common and serious because of the low location of the injury.

Prevention. Prevention of complications requires an awareness of the possibility of their presence and meticulous attention to details of treatment. The size and composition of endotracheal tubes are critical con-

TABLE 15–1 ENDOTRACHEAL TUBE SIZE
BASED ON PATIENT'S AGE*

Patient's Age	Internal Diameter of Tube
3 mo	3.0 mm
3–6 mo	3.5 mm
6–12 mo	4.0 mm
1–2 yr	4.5 mm
Older than 2 yr	$\dfrac{\text{Age in years}}{4} + 4.5$ mm

*Data from Webster.[24]

siderations. A rough guide to the proper size of an endotracheal tube is the diameter of the external nares or the tip of the patient's little finger.[17] Another guideline, based on the patient's age, is described in Table 15–1.[24]

Only soft polyvinyl tubes, such as the Portex variety, should be used — never rubber or rigid tubes. Cole tubes are easier to insert in small infants but can produce vocal cord and laryngeal injury if advanced too far (Fig. 15–3). A straight laryngoscope blade (we prefer Miller #1 or #2) is best for intubation of newborns and small infants. For older children the Wis-Hipple blade allows insertion of an endotracheal tube through the blade itself. A small air leak is desirable. Once an adequate airway has been established, a decision must be made between persisting with endotracheal intubation or proceeding to tracheostomy. The guidelines listed in Table 15–2 are helpful.

The following protocol is used for removal of an endotracheal tube that has been in place for 3 to 4 days[19]:

1. To avoid edema from overhydration, intravenous fluids are limited to 1200 ml/M²/24 hr for the 12 hours just prior to extubation.

2. The head of the patient's bed is elevated 30 degrees to enlist the help of gravity in preventing edema in the airway.

3. The child should be well sedated (2 mg/kg secobarbital) 1 hour prior to extubation.

4. Approximately 30 to 60 minutes before extubation, the following medications are given: dexamethasone 0.2 mg/kg intra-

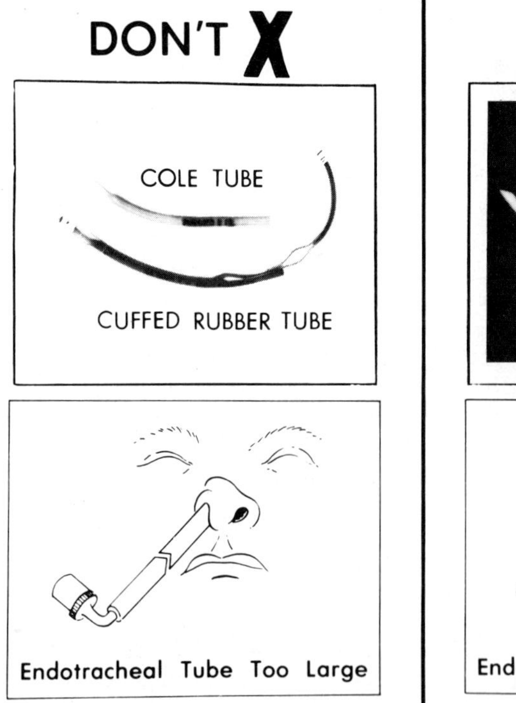

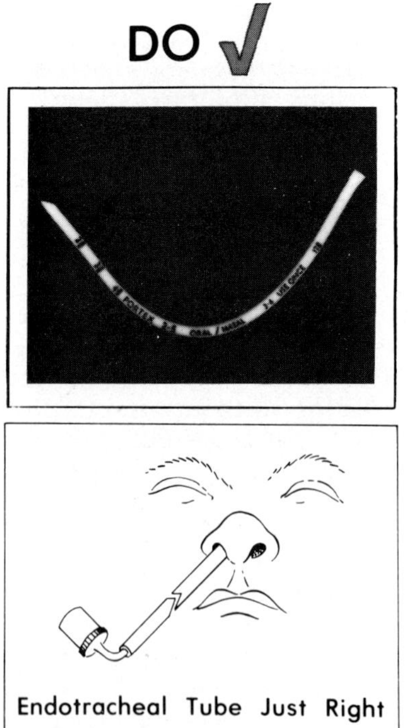

Figure 15–3 Endotracheal tubes that should no longer be used in children. The preferred tube is made of soft polyvinyl. Tubes should fit through the external naris without deforming it. (From Othersen, R. B., Jr.: Intubation injuries of the trachea in children. Management and prevention. Ann. Surg. 189:601, 1979.)

TABLE 15–2   INDICATIONS FOR ENDOTRACHEAL INTUBATION AND FOR TRACHEOSTOMY

Endotracheal Intubation	Tracheostomy
Patient less than 6 months old or, if more than 6 months old, intubation for less than 72 hours	Patient more than 6 months old and intubation for more than 72 hours
Respiratory support required for less than 48 hours	Respiratory support required for more than 48 hours
Inflammatory disease involving the epiglottis or supraglottic structures	Inflammatory diseases involving the glottis and trachea
To serve as a temporary airway until tracheostomy can be established	Long-term respirator support and/or tracheal toilet

venously, furosemide (Lasix) 1 mg/kg intravenously, and albumin 0.5 gm/kg intravenously.

An anesthesiologist skilled in endotracheal intubation must be present when the tube is removed. Racemic epinephrine (0.125 cc to 0.25 cc diluted in 2 ml of saline solution) is administered by nebulization immediately after extubation. Extubation can usually be accomplished safely and complications avoided using this technique. If respiratory distress occurs and does not respond to the racemic epinephrine, an endotracheal tube is reinserted and the child is scheduled for bronchoscopy and direct visualization of the trachea.

Tracheostomy Complications. Tracheostomy produces additional problems when the tube is too large and causes necrosis of the superior and lateral cartilaginous rings with subsequent anterior tracheomalacia. Granuloma at the stoma or at the tip of a rigid metal tube may also produce obstruction. Supervening infection in the trachea predisposes to scarring and stenosis at the tracheostomy stoma.[3] If the skin is closed during performance of a tracheostomy, air escaping from the trachea may pass down into the mediastinum and thence into the pleural cavities, producing pneumothorax (Fig. 15–4). A tube may become dislodged or occluded, causing complete obstruction. Other complications include false passage, erosions, perforation of the posterior wall, and recurrent laryngeal nerve injury (Fig. 15–5).

If the decision is made to perform tracheostomy in a small child, complications can be prevented by proper technique, proper equipment (tubes), and meticulous care. The technique is as follows:

1. An endotracheal tube or bronchoscope is inserted, if possible, to allow the procedure to be done without haste. When intubation is impossible, a cricothyroidotomy with a scalpel or a plastic cannula needle may be necessary (Fig. 15–6). These maneuvers will allow a small airway to be established until tracheostomy can be performed. A 14- or 16-gauge needle may be inserted through the cricothyroid membrane or just below the cricoid cartilage.[21]

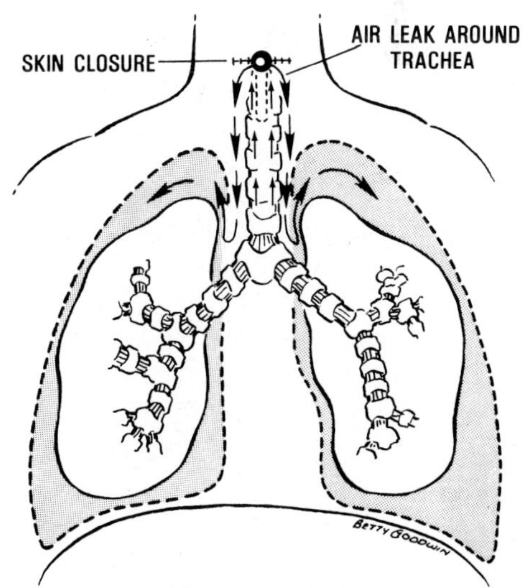

Figure 15–4 Mechanism of pneumothorax after tracheostomy. When the skin is closed around the tracheostomy tube, the air that leaks from the trachea cannot escape, passes down into the mediastinum, and may rupture into the pleural cavity.

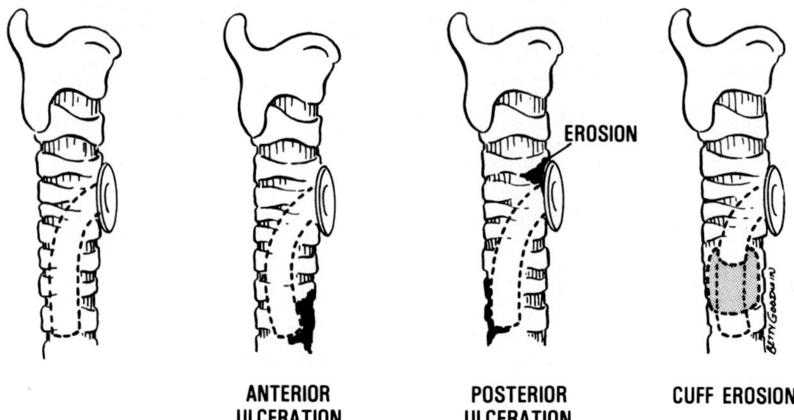

Figure 15–5   Tubes that are rigid and nonpliable may produce either anterior or posterior ulcerations in the trachea. The cartilage superior to the tracheostomy stoma may also be eroded. Cuff pressure may erode the trachea and produce stenosis below the tracheostomy.

2. A transverse incision is made in the neck between the larynx and the suprasternal notch, and the strap muscles are separated in the midline.

3. The trachea is identified by repeated palpation so that dissection proceeds directly down to the anterior tracheal wall.

4. The pretracheal fascia is incised and dissected only slightly laterally to allow insertion of a small retractor on either side. Retract the thyroid isthmus superiorly or divide it if necessary.

5. A linear incision is made through tracheal rings two and three (and through

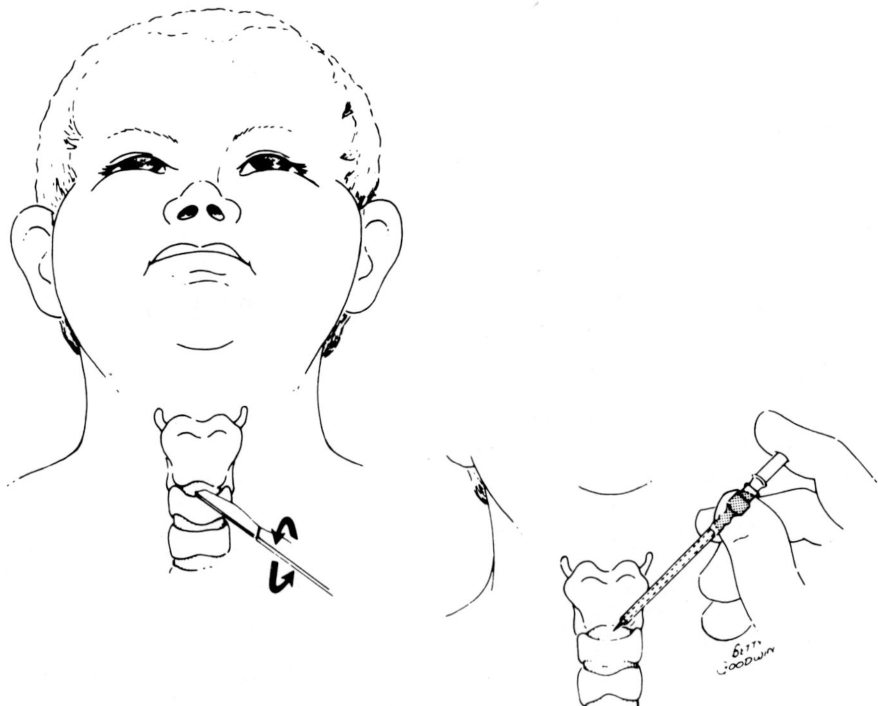

Figure 15–6   Technique of cricothyroidotomy with knife or needle. (From Touloukian, R. J., ed.: Pediatric Trauma. New York, John Wiley & Sons, 1978, p. 339.)

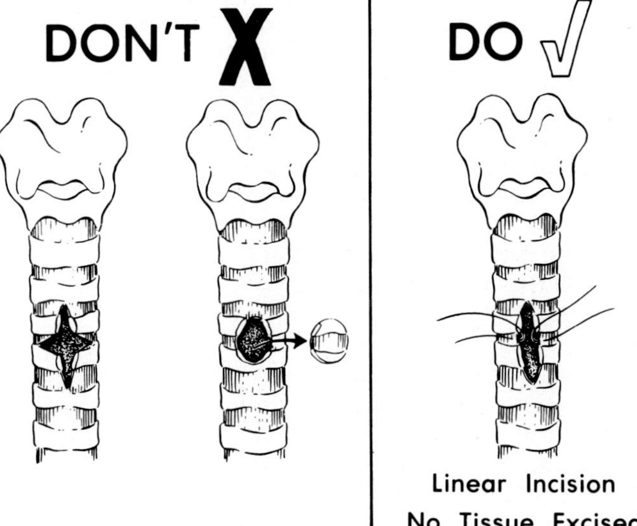

Figure 15–7 The preferred tracheal incision is linear with no excision of tissue. (From Othersen, R. B., Jr.: Intubation injuries of the trachea in children. Management and prevention. Ann. Surg. 189:601, 1979.)

four if necessary). No tracheal tissue is excised. Palpate the cricoid to maintain orientation (Fig. 15–7).

6. Hemostasis, especially of the small tracheal vessels, is carefully secured with electrocautery.

7. A suture is placed on either side of the tracheal incision.

8. Retraction of the sutures allows insertion of the tracheostomy tube without inverting any tissue. The tube should not fit too tightly.

9. A Shiley (polyvinyl) or Dow-Corning (Silastic) tube of the Aberdeen design is used. These tubes are not rigid and will flex slightly to avoid injury at the tip.

10. The skin incision is not closed. Air escapes from the trachea around the tube and must be allowed to exit through the wound. Otherwise, the air passes into the mediastinum and ruptures the pleura, producing pneumothorax.

Controversies still exist concerning the best type of tracheal incision — button excision, vertical slit, or transverse slit.[4] We prefer the simple longitudinal slit, but if the opening in a small trachea appears tight and if retraction of the edges produces buckling, a simple maneuver of pinching out a small piece of cartilage (leaving the perichondrium intact) will often be effective (Fig. 15–8).

When a tracheostomy tube has been in place for longer than 2 weeks, extubation is usually done under general anesthesia and bronchoscopic visualization. At that time excessive granulations or infolded tissue can be removed through the bronchoscope. If tracheal inflammation or early scar forma-

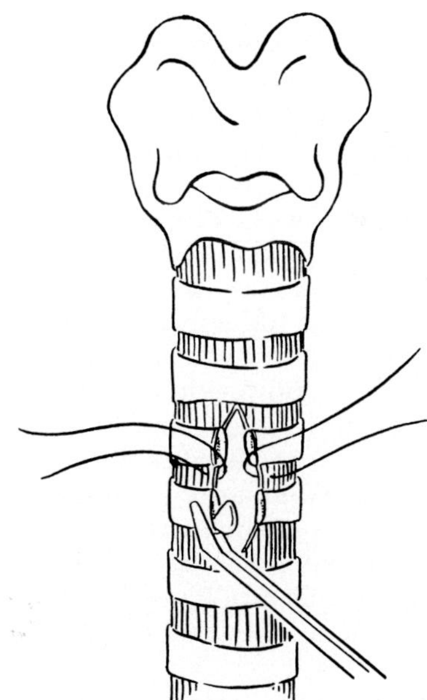

Figure 15–8 If the opening, when retracted, produces buckling of the tracheal wall and pressure around the tracheostomy tube, a small amount of cartilage can be extruded, leaving the perichondrium intact for regeneration. (From Othersen, R. B., Jr.: Intubation injuries of the trachea in children. Management and prevention. Ann. Surg. 189:601, 1979.

tion is present, intralesional injection of triamcinolone is done. If the edema or induration is sufficient to produce airway compromise, the area is injected with triamcinolone (10 mg/ml) and the stenotic segment is carefully stretched with Jackson laryngeal dilators. An appropriate Portex endotracheal tube is then inserted to act as a stent. The child is kept sedated and quiet with the head restrained and elevated while dexamethasone 0.8 mg/kg/day is given in four divided doses for a total of 48 to 72 hours. Extubation without bronchoscopy is then accomplished using the preceding protocol. Acute and subacute ulcerations and scars respond well to this regimen. The earlier the problem is detected, the easier it is to correct. On the other hand, chronic scars and strictures often require long-term tracheostomy and attempted removal by dilation and steroids combined with an endotracheal stent. This technique was originally described by Birck and modified by us.[16] With earlier detection of tracheal injury and prompt therapy the long-term stent has been used less frequently.

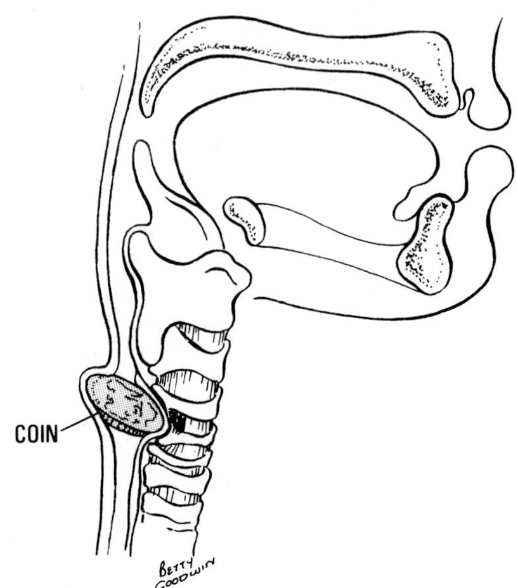

Figure 15–9 A foreign body lodged in the esophagus may produce edema and encroachment on the membranous portion of the airway.

TRAUMA

Tracheal problems producing airway obstruction can result from trauma and are similar to those caused by infection. Extrinsic trauma is often impressive and life-threatening, but intrinsic trauma occurs more frequently. Children may ingest or inhale foreign bodies, which can produce obstruction, ulceration, or perforation. Foreign bodies lodged in the esophagus excite inflammatory edema, which may encroach on the posterior membranous tracheal wall and cause airway compromise (Fig. 15–9). Large nasogastric tubes passing through the esophagus combined with an endotracheal or tracheostomy tube may produce pressure necrosis of the intervening tracheal and esophageal walls, with resultant tracheoesophageal fistula. Fiberoptic endoscopy has been extended to children, and general anesthesia is often required. When a large endoscope is passed down the esophagus with an endotracheal tube in place, enough damage may be done to the larynx and trachea to cause severe edema and obstruction when the endotracheal tube is removed postoperatively. Suction catheters passed too far in neonates may perforate the bronchi or lung (Fig. 15–10). Vigorous resuscitation can produce pneumatic perforations of the trachea or lungs. Rigid Jackson laryngeal dilators have been passed through the vocal cords and trachea and have also been observed by us to slide from the larynx into the esophagus and produce esophageal perforation.

Other unusual complications are mediastinal displacement after pneumonectomy[2] and pulmonary consolidation resembling atelectasis after repair of a tracheoesophageal fistula.[11]

Prevention. Anticipation is the key to effecting a reduction in these iatrogenic complications. Suction catheters and endotracheal tubes should be carefully measured before insertion, and the position of inlying tubes should be checked by x-ray examination. Infants who require frequent suctioning should have a reference tape prominently displayed so that nursing personnel do not introduce the catheters too far. When an endotracheal or tracheostomy tube is in place, a spare tube of the same size and type

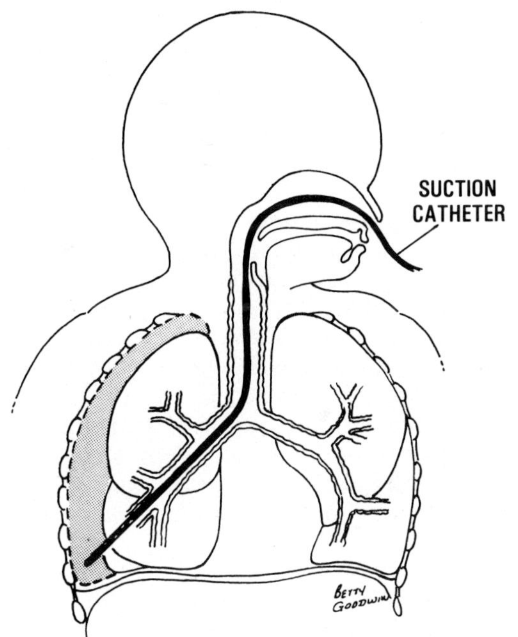

Figure 15–10   A rigid suction catheter passed into the trachea of an infant may perforate the lung and produce pneumothorax.

should be kept taped to the child's bed. A tube one size smaller should also be available in case reinsertion is difficult. Before the child is discharged, the parents are instructed and observed in changing the tracheostomy tube and are urged to do so weekly or monthly unless there is great difficulty. If the parents are confident in changing the tube, they will not hesitate to remove a tube occluded by a plug and replace it with a new one rather than dash to the hospital emergency room. Parents can be taught to care for a tracheostomy tube as effectively as hospital personnel.

The design and construction of tracheostomy tubes is more important in children than it is in adults. Most studies in adults concern the comparison of cuffed tubes,[9] whereas in children the flexibility, curve, and tissue reactivity are most important.[1] We prefer the Shiley and Silastic tubes (Fig. 15–11).

Remember: **Tubes in the trachea should be "just right" — not too large, not too rigid, and not left too long.**

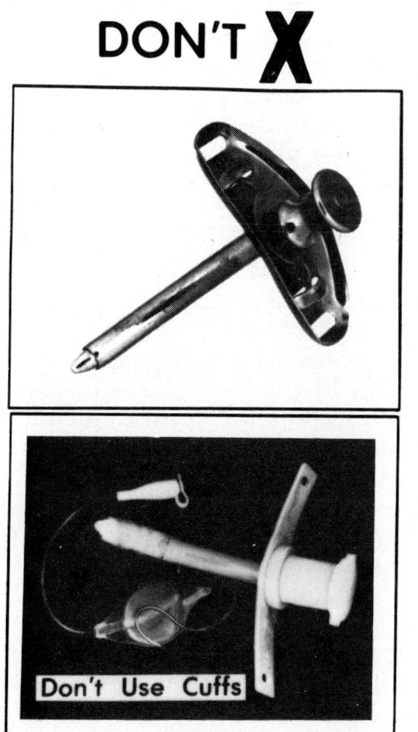

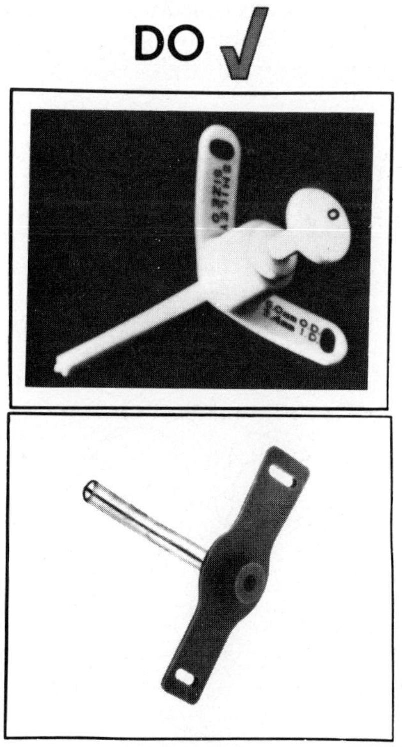

Figure 15–11   Rigid or cuffed tubes are unnecessary in children. The soft polyvinyl or Silastic tubes are preferred. (From Othersen, R. B., Jr.: Intubation injuries of the trachea in children. Management and prevention. Ann. Surg. 189:601, 1979.)

LUNGS

Complications affecting the pulmonary parenchyma include collapse, compression, congestion, infection, and embolization.[26]

Collapse, or atelectasis, is a result of bronchial obstruction or inadequate expansion and aeration of alveoli. Insufficient insufflation during operation or postoperative splinting may produce collapse with shunting of blood and hypoxemia. Major consolidation and infection may follow. The aspiration of harmful material may lead to collapse and superimposed infection. External compression of the resilient chest wall of the child may produce pulmonic parenchymal injury with edema, congestion, and roentgenographic evidence of "lung contusion," a prominent part of the syndrome of "traumatic asphyxia." The lung also acts as a filter, trapping particles of fat that have been released into the blood stream from bony fractures. The clinical and radiographic findings of pulmonic consolidation are similar with "traumatic wet lung," "fat embolism," and "shock lung."[19]

Laceration of the lung may occur from attempts to treat atelectasis by positive pressure insufflation. Staphylococcal abscesses of the lung may rupture into the pleural cavity, producing pneumothorax and empyema (Fig. 15–12).

Prevention

The life-threatening pulmonic consolidation found in "traumatic wet lung" or other forms of pulmonic parenchymal injury such as smoke inhalation can be prevented or ameliorated by the following measures: elevation of the head and chest to allow drainage by gravity; restriction of intravenous fluids; and administration of steroids. Experiments in animals have shown that in a lung damaged by external compression, consolidation and "wet lung" will develop when even usual maintenance amounts of fluids are given intravenously. When fluids are restricted, the full picture of pulmonic consolidation does not occur. Diuretics may be helpful in removing excess fluids. Steroids, to be effective, must be given early and usually in pharmacologic doses (prednisolone 20 to 30 mg/kg).[19]

Postoperative pulmonary physiotherapy with measures such as deep breathing and coughing and postural drainage may help prevent mucous plugs and atelectasis.[8] An empty stomach decompressed by a functioning nasogastric tube helps to prevent aspiration of gastric contents. Lobar pneumonia, which may be due to Staphylococcus, should be treated vigorously with intravenous antibiotics to prevent lung abscess. If a lung abscess is enlarging and compressing adjacent lung or threatening to rupture into the pleural cavity, drainage may be attempted. Bronchoscopic drainage is not as successful in children as it is in adults. If the abscess abuts the pleura and pleural symphysis has occurred, a tube can be safely introduced through the chest wall into the abscess for external drainage. When pleural adhesion has not occurred because the abscess is deep, trocar puncture can be dangerous. Air and pus will spill into the pleural cavity, producing tension pneumothorax and empyema (Fig. 15–13). To prevent this complication, a Monaldi procedure may be employed, i.e., the resection of a small portion of rib overlying the abscess and incision down to the parietal pleura. A sponge soaked with an irritant such as merbromin

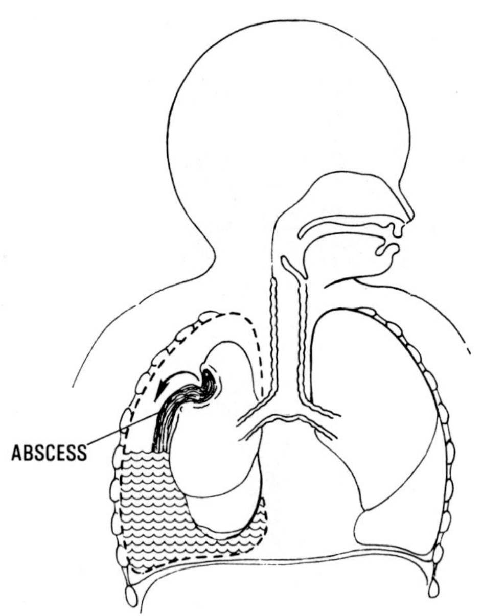

Figure 15–12 A pulmonary parenchymal abscess (usually of staphylococcal origin) may rupture, producing a pyopneumothorax.

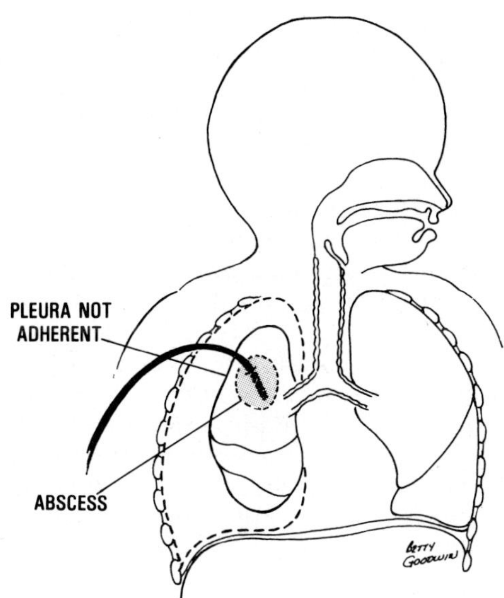

Figure 15–13 If the pulmonary abscess is not peripheral and the pleura is not adherent, a catheter passed into the abscess for drainage may produce pneumothorax and occasionally a collection of air and pus under tension.

(Mercurochrome) is placed against the pleura to allow adhesions to occur. External drainage can then be safely performed.

Fat embolism is insidious but can be recognized through a combination of signs including fever, tachycardia, anemia, thrombocytopenia, and coagulopathy. Retinal embolization of fat is diagnostic.[25]

In all the conditions producing pulmonic consolidation from trauma, infection, or fat embolism, blood gas abnormalities are usually the harbinger of complications. Roentgenographic changes follow the aberrations in blood gases.

Remember: **Anticipate problems when arterial blood gas changes occur.**

PLEURAL CAVITY

Complications in the pleural cavity consist primarily of abnormal collections of air (pneumothorax) or fluid (hydrothorax, chylothorax, or hemothorax) and are usually due to infection, trauma, or congestion from overhydration.

Infection. Empyema, or pus in the pleural cavity, may develop postoperatively, following pneumonia, or as a result of rupture of a pulmonic abscess into the pleural

cavity. The mechanism of this complication was described in the preceding section.

Trauma. Tracheal or esophageal rupture will usually produce a combination of fluid and air in the pleural cavity. Perforations of the esophagus, bronchi, and lung are not uncommonly produced by suction catheters and endotracheal tubes. External injury or operative injury of the lymphatics constituting the thoracic duct produces troublesome and persistent collections of chyle in the pleural cavity (chylothorax).[5] Large volumes of lymph are lost, causing pulmonary compression and severe nutritional depletion. A simple procedure such as internal jugular puncture on the left side may lacerate the thoracic duct and cause chylothorax (Fig. 15–14).

Remember: **Know the anatomic location of major lymphatics** (Fig. 15–15).

Hemothorax is usually the result of injury to the lung or chest wall. The color of the blood (its state of oxygenation) usually indicates its source. Blood from the lung and pulmonary artery is dark, whereas blood from the systemic circulation of the chest wall is bright red. Inadequately drained pus or blood in the pleural cavity may lead to fibrothorax with disturbance of growth of the lung and the chest wall; scoliosis may

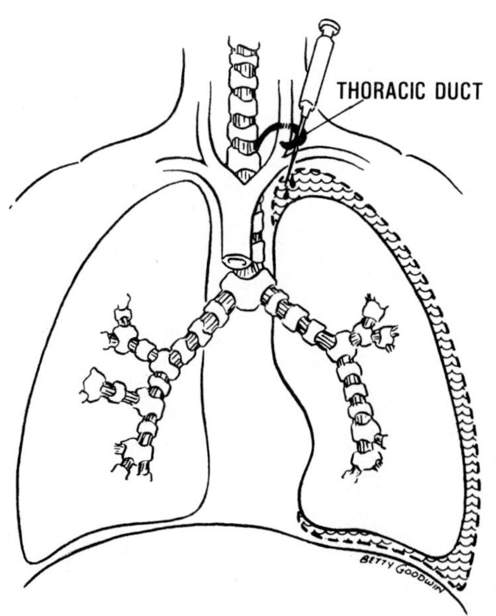

Figure 15–14 Avoid needle aspiration of the jugular vein on the left, since the thoracic duct may be lacerated, producing chylothorax.

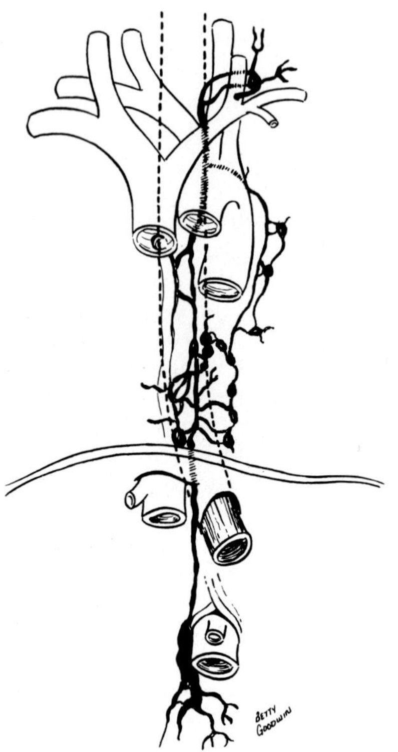

Figure 15–15 Anatomic representation of the lymphatic system indicates the sites of possible injury during operation on the esophagus and great vessels.

result. Emphysematous bullae or the abnormal lungs of patients with cystic fibrosis may lead to recurrent pneumothorax necessitating repeated tube thoracostomies or even intrapleural instillations to produce pleural adhesions.[13]

Unusual Complications. Remember that any possible complications will inevitably occur, and most have been reported. Reduced lung volume resulting from pulmonary artery obstruction[7] and diminished blood flow is seen after repair of diaphragmatic hernia.[27] Ventriculoperitoneal shunts have caused pleural effusions and coagulopathy.[15] Transposition of the spleen into the chest for the treatment of portal hypertension has resulted in increased left atrial flow simulating mitral stenosis.

Prevention

Most complications of the pleural cavity can be prevented by prompt and adequate drainage. The technique of thoracentesis (Fig. 15–16) and tube thoracostomy is extremely important. Chest tubes should not be introduced anteriorly in infants. The chest wall is so thin that leakage of air

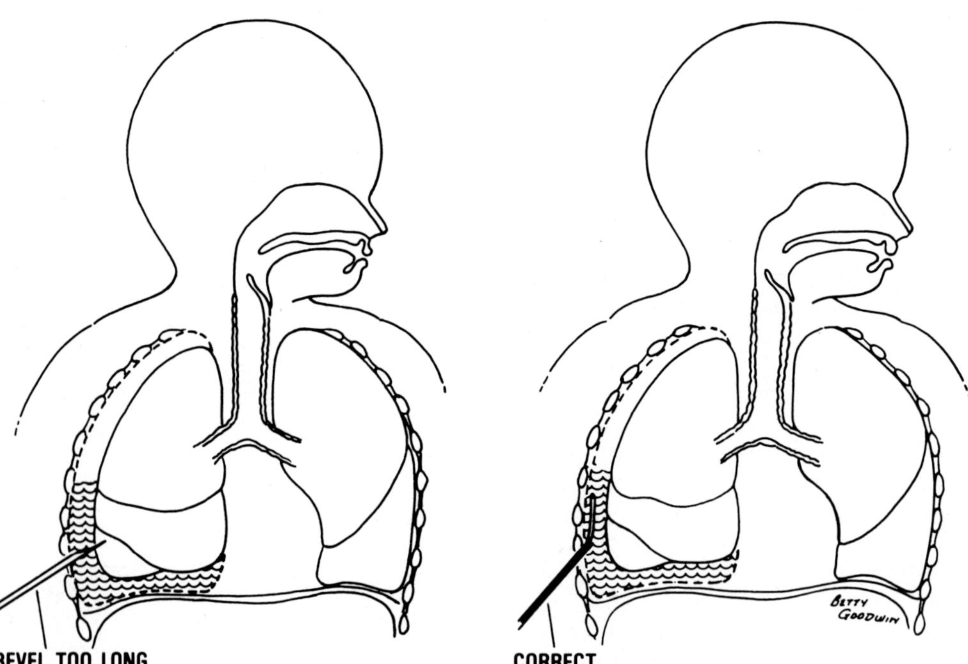

Figure 15–16 Thoracentesis with a rigid needle and a long bevel may produce pneumothorax as a complication. A plastic cannula needle with a short bevel is preferable.

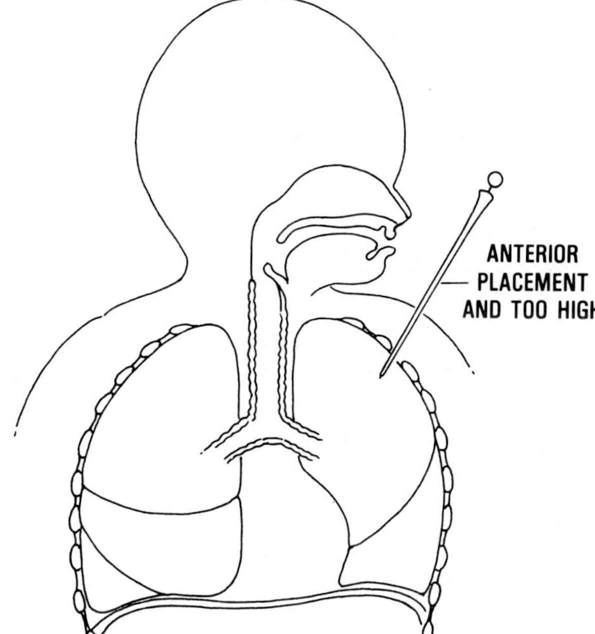

Figure 15–17 Tube thoracostomy anteriorly may allow air leaks around the tube, since the anterior chest wall of infants is very thin.

around the tube is common (Fig. 15–17) and the axillary vein may be lacerated (Fig. 15–18). Low, lateral insertion of the tube through an oblique, subcutaneous, and muscular tunnel to the apex of the pleural cavity is preferred.

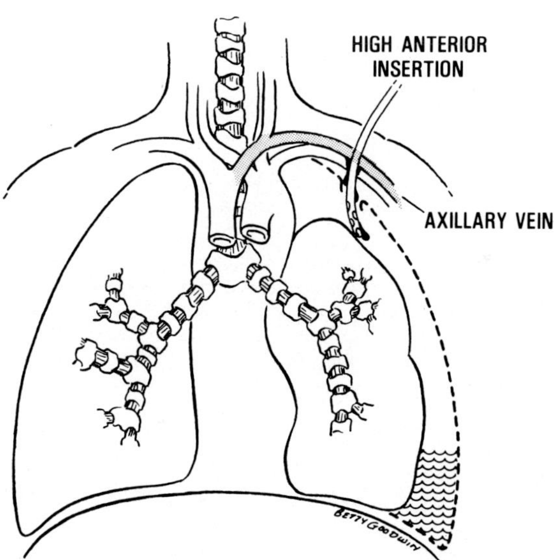

Figure 15–18 High insertion of the tube may lacerate the axillary vein, producing traumatic hemothorax.

TECHNIQUE OF INTERCOSTAL TUBE PLACEMENT (Fig. 15–19)

A small incision is made in the midaxillary line just over the eleventh or twelfth rib. The incision is only large enough to admit the tip of the selected catheter. The catheter should be of a size that will just fit between two ribs. The polyvinyl catheters with a self-contained stylet are convenient to use. The tip of the stylet is bent slightly, and the catheter and stylet are inserted with the tip directed outward. After subcutaneous tunneling for 3 to 4 cm, the proper interspace is selected so that the catheter is introduced into the lower limits of the pleural cavity. The tip of the catheter is then rotated so that the stylet can be inserted into the interspace, care being taken to hug the top of the rib below the interspace in order to avoid the intercostal vessels. As soon as the pleural cavity has been entered, the tip is again rotated so that the point faces the parietal pleura. The stylet is removed as the catheter is introduced to the apex along the lateral chest wall (Fig. 15–20). The catheter should then be connected to underwater drainage with 3 to 5 cm of negative pressure. Figure 15–21 shows improper placement of chest tubes bilaterally.

One final word of caution: Don't be

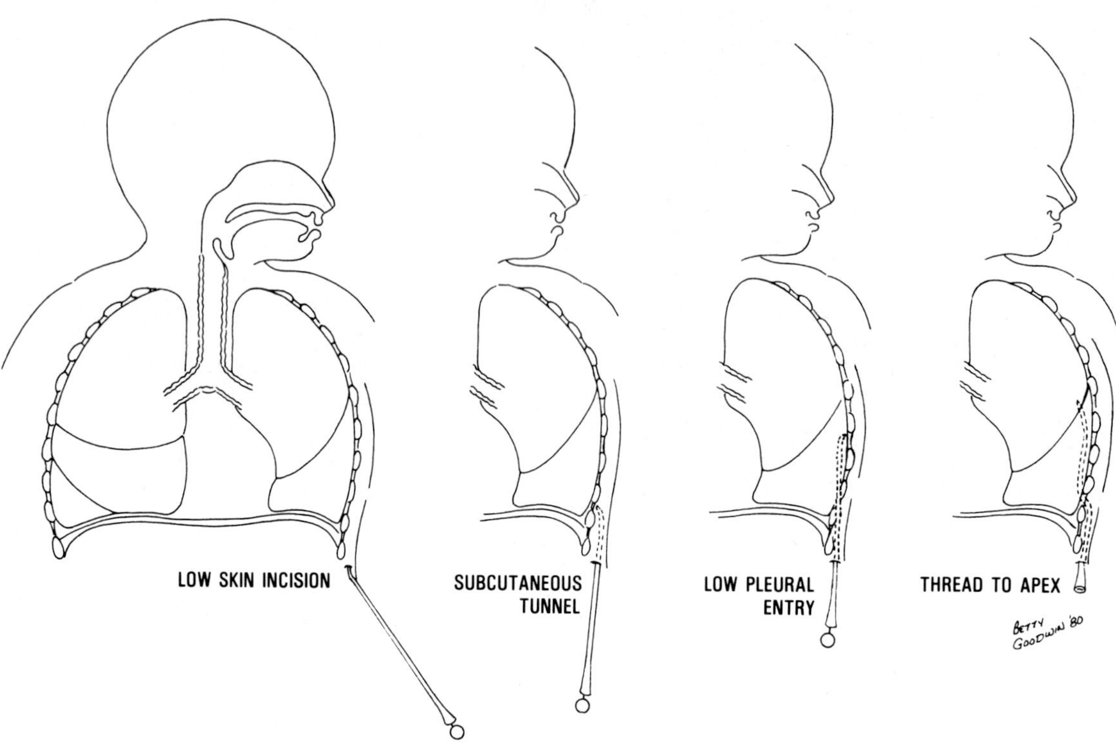

Figure 15–19 Using correct technique for chest tube insertion may prevent complications.

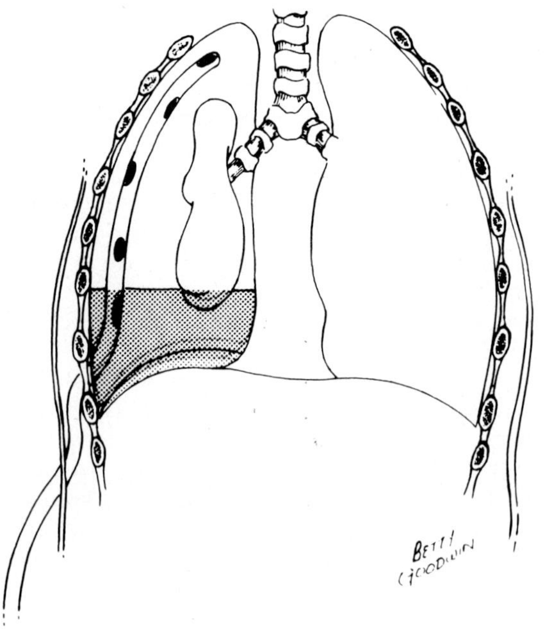

Figure 15–20 Correct position of the chest tube with holes placed so that it drains both fluid and air. Note oblique path through chest wall. (From Touloukian, R. J., ed.: Pediatric Trauma, New York, John Wiley & Sons, 1978, p. 314.

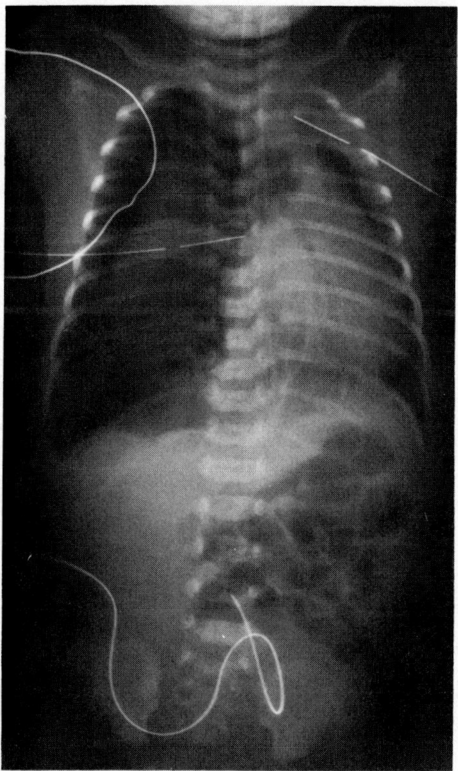

Figure 15–21   The tube on the patient's right is lateral but too high and not positioned along the chest wall. The tube in the left chest is dangerously high and anterior. Note the undrained air on the right.

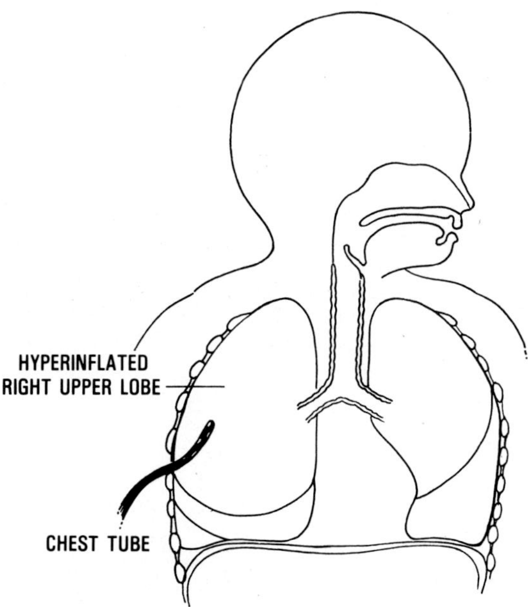

Figure 15–22   Chest tubes are occasionally inserted when lobar emphysema is mistaken for pneumothorax. Look for lung markings and compressed lung in the bases and costal angles.

misled by lobar emphysema resembling pneumothorax (Fig. 15–22). With pneumothorax the costophrenic angles are clear and sharp, whereas in lobar emphysema of the upper or middle lobes, the remaining lung is compressed inferiorly.

EXPERIENCE

Our personal experience at the Medical University of South Carolina includes 60 children treated for tracheal stenosis severe enough to produce respiratory distress. Of this number, 31 required tracheostomy and the remainder were treated by repeated bronchoscopy, dilation, and temporary internal stents. Ten of 31 patients with tracheostomy have been successfully extubated, are asymptomatic, and have been discharged. Nineteen additional children have been extubated but are returning periodically for endoscopic evaluation and occasional dilations. Thirty-three children have been discharged as cured. Four died during therapy — two from complications of the procedure and two from underlying disease. Follow-up information could not be obtained on four patients.

The children who died of complications are worthy of mention. One child, 2 months of age, was in a convalescent home and died suddenly. The tracheostomy tube was neither obstructed nor dislodged. Perhaps the child turned his head and occluded the tube orifice. This very young infant probably should have been hospitalized until the tracheostomy tube was removed.

The other lethal complication was also unusual. A 5-year-old girl with longstanding tracheal stenosis had dilation of the stricture with Jackson laryngeal dilators. She was discharged but admitted to a hospital by her family physician when fever and "pneumonia" developed. A small amount of air was seen in the mediastinum on chest roentgenogram. The child was being prepared for transfer back to us because of bleeding from a "stress ulcer" with hematemesis. Just prior to transfer, exsanguination with massive hematemesis occurred. An autopsy showed a 2-mm esophageal fistula with a small mediastinal abscess that had eroded into the aorta. We surmise that one of the rigid dilators had been passed into the esophagus rather than the trachea and had perforated the esophagus. The resulting mediastinal abscess eroded into the aorta. The presence of the mediastinal air and fever were indications of this serious complication.

Remember: **Anticipation and prevention are the best treatments for complications.**

References

1. Aberdeen, E., and Downes, J. J.: Artificial airways in children. Surg. Clin. North Am. 54:1155, 1974.
2. Adams, H. D., Junod, F. L., Aberdeen, E., et al.: Severe airway obstruction caused by mediastinal displacement after right pneumonectomy in a child. J. Thorac. Cardiovasc. Surg. 63:534, 1972.
3. Andrews, M. J.: The incidence and pathogenesis of tracheal injury following tracheostomy with cuffed tube and assisted ventilation. Analysis of a 3-year prospective study. Br. J. Surg. 60:129, 1973.
4. Bryant, L. R., Mujia, D., Greenberg, S., et al.: Evaluation of tracheal incisions for tracheostomy. Am. J. Surg. 135:675, 1978.
5. Cevese, P. G., Vecchioni, R., D'Amico, D. F., et al.: Postoperative chylothorax: Six cases in 2,500 operations, with a survey of the world literature. J. Thorac. Cardiovasc. Surg. 69:966, 1975.
6. Cherry, J. D.: The treatment of croup: Continued controversy due to failure of recognition of historic, ecologic, etiologic, and clinical perspectives. J. Pediatr. 94:352, 1979.
7. Fletcher, B. D., Garcia, E. J., Colenda, C., et al.: Reduced lung volume associated with acquired pulmonary artery obstruction in children. Am. J. Roentgenol. 133:47, 1979.
8. Fonkalsrud, E. W.: Inhalation therapy in infants and children. Pediatr. Clin. North Am. 16:613, 1969.
9. Galoob, H. D., and Toledo, P. S.: Comparison of five types of tracheostomy tubes in the intubated trachea. Ann. Otol. 87:99, 1978.
10. Greeway, R. E.: Tracheostomy: Surgical problems and complications. Int. Anesthesiol. Clin. 10:151, 1972.
11. Haddadin, A. J., and Emery, J. L.: Pulmonary retention simulating pneumonia as a cause of death in children with tracheoesophageal fistula. Surgery 70:311, 1971.
12. Jones, R., Santos, J. E., and Overal, J. C.: Bacterial tracheitis. JAMA 242:721, 1979.
13. Larrieu, A. J., Tyers, G. F. O., Williams, E. H., et al.: Intrapleural instillation of quinacrine for treatment of recurrent spontaneous pneumothorax. Ann. Thorac. Surg. 28:146, 1979.
14. Leipzig, B., Oski, F. A., Cummings, C. W., et al.: A prospective randomized study to determine the efficacy of steroids in the treatment of croup. J. Pediatr. 94:194, 1976.
15. Obrador, S., and Villarego, F.: Hydrothorax: Unusual complications of ventriculoperitoneal shunts. Acta Neurochir. 39:167, 1977.
16. Othersen, H. B., Jr.: The technique of intraluminal stenting and steroid administration in the treatment of tracheal stenosis in children. J. Pediatr. Surg. 9:683, 1974.
17. Othersen, H. B., Jr.: Prevention and treatment of tracheal injuries in children. Am. Surg. 43:108, 1977.
18. Othersen, H. B., Jr.: Cardiothoracic injuries. *In* Touloukian, R. J. (ed.): Pediatric Trauma. New York, John Wiley & Sons, 1978, pp. 315–320.
19. Othersen, H. B., Jr.: Intubation injuries of the trachea in children. Management and prevention. Ann. Surg. 189:601, 1979.
20. Pelton, D. A., and Whalen, J. S.: Airway obstruction in infants and children. Int. Anesthesiol. Clin. 10:123, 1972.
21. Spoerel, W. E., Narayanan, P. S., and Singh, N. P.: Transtracheal ventilation. Br. J. Anaesth. 43:932, 1971.
22. Stark, A. R., and Thach, B. T.: Mechanisms of airway obstruction leading to apnea in newborn infants. J. Pediatr. 89:982, 1976.
23. Sztaba, R., and Pikiel, L.: Serious complications after splenopneumopexy in portal hypertension in children. Ann. Chir. Gynaecol. Fenn. 63:395, 1974.
24. Webster, A. C.: Anesthesia for operations on the upper airway. Int. Anesthesiol. Clin. 10:61, 1972.
25. Weisz, G. M., Schramek, A., Abrahamson, J., et al.: Fat embolism in children: Tests for its early detection. J. Pediatr. Surg. 9:163, 1974.
26. Williams, M. C., and Galvis, A. G.: Pulmonary complications in infants. Surg. Clin. North Am. 54:1137, 1974.
27. Wohl, M. E. B., Griscom, N. T., Strieder, D. J., et al.: The lung following repair of congenital diaphragmatic hernia. J. Pediatr. 90:405, 1977.

16

ESOPHAGUS

Thomas M. Holder, M.D.
Keith W. Ashcraft, M.D.

Lesions necessitating esophageal operation in infants and children are all benign. Gentle handling of tissues and surgical skill prevent most complications of esophageal surgery, which can be exceedingly difficult to manage and may be fatal. The major conditions with which we shall be concerned are listed in Table 16–1.

ANATOMY

The esophagus is a muscular tube connecting the pharynx with the stomach. It extends without redundancy from the neck through the posterior mediastinum and the esophageal hiatus, where it joins with the fundus of the stomach. The upper third of the esophagus is composed of two layers of striated muscle, which blend with the two layers of smooth muscle that constitute the lower two thirds of the esophagus. Swallowing is initiated voluntarily, but once the peristaltic wave reaches the juncture of the upper and middle thirds of the esophagus, it is carried on involuntarily to the stomach.

The blood supply to the upper portion of the esophagus is axial, coming from the vessels of the neck. This permits mobilization without risk of devascularization. The blood supply to the middle third of the esophagus is segmental, being provided by small branches from the aorta. Extensive surgical mobilization of the middle third of the esophagus is fraught with the hazard of devascularization and its attendant complications. The lower portion of the esophagus is supplied, again, from axial vessels arising from the phrenic arteries.

There are three natural areas of narrowing in the esophagus — the thoracic inlet or cricopharyngeus, the region of the aortic arch, and the distal esophagus at the diaphragm.

The esophagus is a muscular organ fixed at either end. It is capable of being stretched to allow approximation for anastomosis, but it also has intrinsic muscular elasticity that causes some tension on an anastomosis. Extensive mobilization of the esophagus to reduce anastomotic tension runs the risk of displacing the distal end of the esophagus through the esophageal hiatus, producing an incompetent gastroesophageal junction. The esophagus lacks a serosal covering; therefore, anastomotic strength is wholly dependent upon the submucosa.

SPECIFIC COMPLICATIONS OF ESOPHAGEAL OPERATIONS

Esophageal Anastomotic Stricture

Esophageal anastomosis in pediatric surgical practice is done most frequently for congenital atresia of the esophagus associated with tracheoesophageal fistula. Esophagoesophageal anastomosis may be carried out in the older child for a very localized stenotic injury to the esophagus such as might be produced by the ingestion of a

TABLE 16–1 ESOPHAGEAL CONDITIONS NECESSITATING SURGERY IN INFANTS AND CHILDREN

Esophageal atresia/tracheoesophageal fistula
Achalasia and chalasia
Corrosive strictures
Gastroesophageal reflux
Esophageal substitution
Esophageal perforations

Clinitest tablet. Anastomosis of the esophagus to interposed colon or gastric tube is necessary in esophageal replacement procedures.

Several factors are believed to be important in the development of anastomotic stricture. These include tension on the suture line, tenuous blood supply at the point of anastomosis, the type of anastomosis performed,[7] and localized inflammation produced by anastomotic leak[7] or by gastroesophageal reflux of acid.[2, 16] Inadequate removal of esophageal cicatrix is certainly a factor in the development of anastomotic stricture after resection for caustic or other esophageal strictures. Gastroesophageal reflux may also cause anastomotic strictures.

Although the variants of esophageal atresia with tracheoesophageal fistula are many, most patients will have a blind upper pouch with the distal esophagus attached as a fistula to the posterior wall of the trachea. Extensive mobilization of the lower esophagus after division of the fistula is unnecessary and undesirable. Small vagal nerve branches as well as the small blood vessels that supply this portion of the esophagus are interrupted by this maneuver.[14] The upper pouch, however, with its longitudinal blood supply, may be safely mobilized well into the neck and even lengthened by circular myotomy to provide a tension-free anastomosis in the mediastinum.[10] This anastomosis should be made under as little tension as possible in hope of preventing anastomotic leak and subsequent stricture.

The type of esophageal anastomosis done for esophageal atresia has been implicated in the development of anastomotic stricture. A survey of members of the Surgical Section of the American Academy of Pediatrics assessed the incidence of stricture with the Haight double-layer "vested" anastomosis, the two-layer end-to-end anastomosis, and the single-layer end-to-end anastomosis.[7] The incidence of stricture, defined as an anastomosis requiring four or more dilatations, was 25 per cent with the Haight anastomosis, 14 per cent with the two-layer end-to-end anastomosis, and 18 per cent with the single-layer end-to-end anastomosis. Interestingly, the incidence of esophageal anastomotic leak was inversely related to the incidence of stricture following these three types of anastomoses. In our personal

TABLE 16–2 ANASTOMOTIC COMPLICATIONS IN ESOPHAGEAL ATRESIA PATIENTS (AUTHORS' EXPERIENCE 1965–1979)

Anastomosis	Stricture*	Leak
Haight	10/39 (26%)	4/39 (10%)
Single-layer	7/29 (24%)	4/29 (14%)

*Anastomoses requiring one or more dilatations.

experience, at least one dilatation was required in 26 per cent of patients having a Haight anastomosis and in 24 per cent of those having a single-layer anastomosis. Esophageal anastomotic leak occurred in 10 per cent of patients with a Haight anastomosis and in 14 per cent of patients with a single-layer anastomosis (Table 16–2). In only three of eight patients who had anastomotic leak did stricture subsequently develop.

Pieretti and coworkers first brought attention to the fact that anastomotic stricture following repair of esophageal atresia might be related to the presence of gastroesophageal reflux.[16] The presumed mechanism for this stricture development is the esophagitis produced by acid reflux in the presence of the healing anastomosis. They found (as have we) that the prevention of reflux by fundoplication has been associated with a significant reduction in anastomotic stricture.[2, 15, 16] Following repair of esophageal atresia by direct anastomosis, the presence of gastroesophageal reflux should be actively sought before the development of anastomotic stricture. Should a stricture develop, fundoplication may be necessary in conjunction with the treatment of the stricture.

TREATMENT OF ESOPHAGEAL ANASTOMOTIC STRICTURE

The patient with esophageal anastomotic stricture should be investigated for gastroesophageal reflux (Fig. 16–1). If present, this condition should be treated, since it often prevents satisfactory treatment of the stricture by dilatation or even by resection.

Esophageal dilatation is usually all that is needed for most anastomotic strictures. This is either carried out endoscopically with the patient under general anesthesia, using one of the many types of esophageal bougies, or is done with Tucker retrograde dilators in the sedated or fully anesthetized patient. Our preference is for the use of filiforms and followers introduced endoscopically while the patient is under general anesthesia. Anastomotic dilatation should be done gently until small amounts of blood begin to appear on the dilator as it is removed. Further dilatation runs a significant risk of lacerating the esophagus, with subsequent development of mediastinitis. (See section on esophageal perforation later.) Short anastomotic strictures may benefit

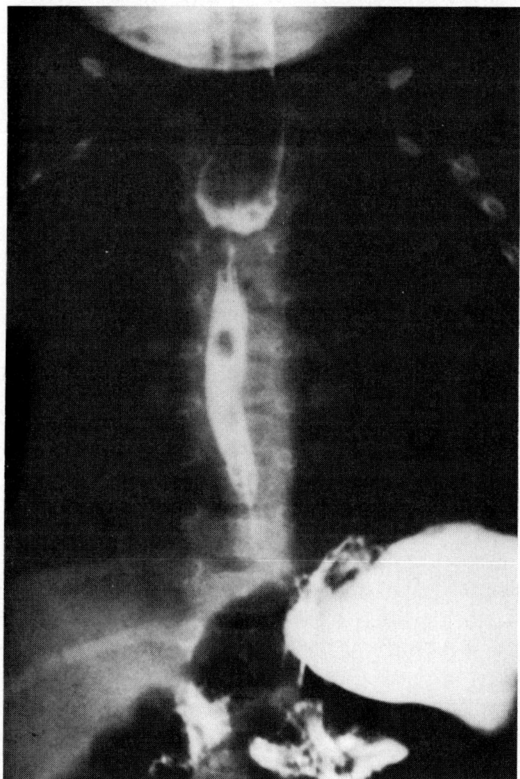

Figure 16–1 Esophageal anastomotic stricture associated with gastroesophageal reflux. Barium contrast study shows the anastomotic stricture. Considerable dilatation of the upper esophagus implies that the stricture is functionally significant. The presence or absence of gastroesophageal reflux should be determined when studying patients with esophageal anastomotic stricture. This may be difficult if very little barium passes the anastomotic stricture site. Instillation of barium into the stomach of the postoperative patient with esophageal atresia will sometimes demonstrate massive reflux. If the gastrostomy has been removed, it may be necessary to dilate the stricture and then repeat the barium study, looking specifically for gastroesophageal reflux.

from injection of triamcinolone coupled with dilatation.[6] The steroids presumably prevent recurrence of the stricture by dissolving collagen within the scar.[8]

Recalcitrant strictures occasionally require resection and end-to-end anastomosis. Usually by the time this has occurred the esophagus has grown with the child and there is enough mobility to provide a tension-free anastomosis (provided that gastroesophageal reflux has been eliminated). Results from a second anastomosis are often very gratifying, and stricture seldom recurs.

Esophageal Leak Following Anastomosis

Most anastomotic suture-line leaks are due to excessive tension, impaired blood supply, or an improperly constructed anastomosis. Anastomotic tension is usually a problem only in repair of esophageal atresia. Stretching the blind ends of the esophagus before anastomosis may allow approximation of the esophageal ends but may still result in tension leading to an esophageal leak. Of the patients reported from the Children's Hospital of Los Angeles, a leak developed in 11 of 12 treated in this manner by direct anastomosis, but most healed spontaneously.[13] Elongation of the upper esophageal pouch by circular myotomy is a means of reducing anastomotic tension in the repair of esophageal atresia with distal tracheoesophageal fistula.[10] Still, leaks occur even in anastomoses performed by the most experienced surgeons. Anastomotic leak in esophageal substitution procedures usually is due to poor suture technique or diminished blood supply rather than to tension. Careful preservation of blood supply and approximation of tissues is the best prevention for anastomotic leak.

A presumption of possible leak should accompany each esophageal anastomosis. Adequate drainage of the region in anticipation of a leak is important in preventing serious complications resulting from anastomotic leak. Use of the extrapleural approach in esophageal anastomosis is one means of preventing empyema after a leak. Failure to drain the area adequately may result in abscess formation, which can produce complete anastomotic disruption. We

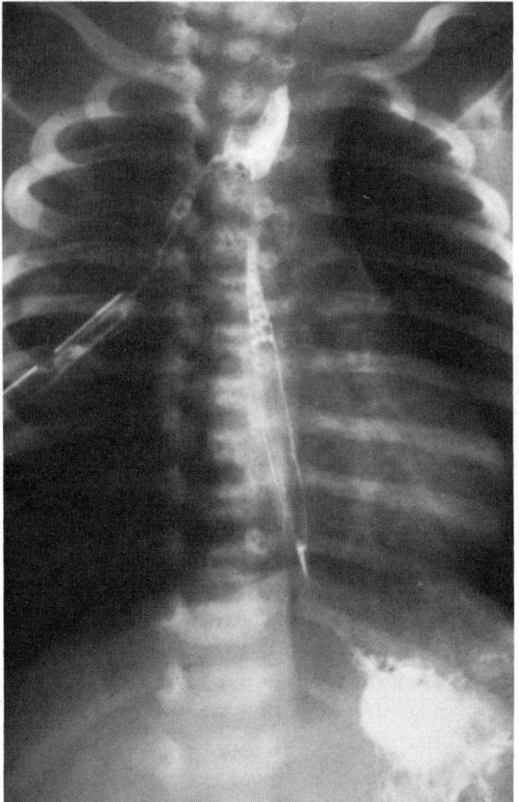

Figure 16–2 Esophageal anastomotic leak. A leak is seen after the extrapleural repair of esophageal atresia and distal tracheoesophageal fistula. The extrapleural chest tube allows the leaking saliva (or contrast material) to exit without producing significant mediastinal infection or abscess formation.

place and maintain anastomotic area drains for a minimum of 10 days postoperatively (Fig. 16–2).

Care in performing the anastomosis is probably the most important factor in prevention of esophageal anastomotic leak. Careful approximation of tissues, inverting the mucosal edges, is paramount in achieving this goal. Sutures must not be tied too tightly, and trauma to the ends of the esophagus must be avoided at all cost. We most often use a nerve hook to manipulate the ends of the esophagus for esophageal anastomosis in esophageal atresia rather than using tissue forceps, because it is impossible to crush the ends of the esophagus if one does not have tissue forceps in hand.

TREATMENT OF ESOPHAGEAL ANASTOMOTIC LEAK

Once an anastomotic leak is established, a variety of approaches to treatment are possible. If the child has undergone extrapleural repair of esophageal atresia, the anastomotic leak will most often heal on its own, provided that nutrition is maintained. In the presence of a normal gastroesophageal junction the child is fed by gastrostomy. If there is gastroesophageal reflux a central venous line is placed to provide total parenteral nutrition while the anastomotic leak heals.

An alternative to this approach, particularly when the leak occurs early and the repair has been done transpleurally, is to attempt resuture of the anastomosis. We have accomplished this on two occasions with very satisfactory results.

It is exceedingly rare that the anastomotic leak indicates complete disruption of the anastomosis or that it will not heal given sufficient time. The problem then becomes one of waiting for closure of the leak. A leak may be followed by anastomotic stricture,[7] although in our experience only three of 17 patients with anastomotic stricture had a leak.

ESOPHAGEAL PERFORATIONS

Esophageal perforation occurs most frequently during instrumentation, either for dilatation of a stricture or for removal of a foreign body. The potential for perforation must always be kept in mind during instrumentation and foreign-body removal. Blind passage of instruments or dilators is especially hazardous. Gentle technique is the best preventive measure. In spite of gentleness and experience, however, an occasional perforation of the esophagus will occur at the time of dilatation or foreign-body removal. Recognition and prompt treatment of esophageal leak are exceedingly important.[11]

Three signs that occur after esophageal perforation should alert the surgeon to this complication. These are mediastinal pain, subcutaneous emphysema or pneumothorax, and evidence of acute inflammation, fever, and tachycardia. Fascial planes surrounding the esophagus will allow air to present in the subcutaneous tissues of the neck from a lower esophageal perforation and will allow a rapid extension of mediastinitis or extravasated fluid collection down into the mediastinum from a cervical esophageal laceration. Radiographic demonstration of esophageal leak should probably be done with contrast material even though air may be present in the tissues of the neck or mediastinum.[11] Localization of the area of perforation is important in selecting the approach to be used for surgical drainage or closure. Occasionally, air will be present to indicate esophageal perforation, but contrast material will not demonstrate any extravasation (Fig. 16–3). In these instances it is probably safe to wait and watch the patient, treating him with antibiotics and intravenous fluids and hoping that the leak has sealed and that further surgical treatment will be unnecessary.[11]

When the esophagus is reasonably normal and the perforation is acute, surgical closure of the laceration is probably indicated through a right or left thoracotomy, depending upon the level of perforation. The upper esophagus is often best reached through a right thoracotomy and the lower esophagus through a left thoracotomy. Direct suture closure of the esophagus, using permanent suture material, should be carried out and the area drained.[11] If the laceration is recognized late and the edges are not amenable to primary repair, local drainage coupled with feeding gastrostomy or insertion of a total parenteral nutrition line may be necessary, forgoing primary suture repair.

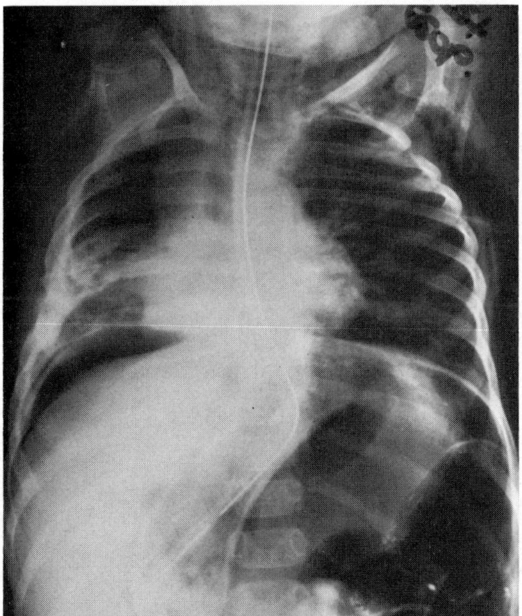

RECURRENT TRACHEOESOPHAGEAL FISTULA

Following repair of esophageal atresia and tracheoesophageal fistula, the incidence of recurrent tracheoesophageal fistula is exceedingly difficult to assess. It probably comes about as a result of anastomotic suture-line leak with local infection, abscess formation, and erosion through the previous site of tracheoesophageal fistula.[17] Recognition of this fistula may be difficult and may require repeated contrast studies of the esophagus. Endoscopic examination of both the esophagus and the trachea with instillation of methylene blue dye into the trachea during esophagoscopy may be required.[15] The recurrent fistula must be surgically divided and some precautions taken to prevent another recurrence. This may include the interposition of a pleural flap, pericardial flap, or intercostal muscle.

Recurrent tracheoesophageal fistula seems most common after ligation, in continuity, of the fistula with end-to-side esophagoesophagostomy.[4, 12, 19]

Demonstration of a fistula after repair of esophageal atresia and tracheoesophageal fistula may indicate either a second fistula missed during the initial operation or a recurrent fistula. Usually the second (missed) fistula is located in the upper me-

Figure 16–3 Esophageal perforation after dilatation. This patient had repair of esophageal atresia with subsequent stricture and fundoplication. Continued anastomotic structure necessitated dilatation. After one of these dilations, subcutaneous emphysema with abdominal distension was noted several hours postoperatively. In spite of several contrast studies to demonstrate a leak, none was found. The patient was treated with intravenous fluids, systemic antibiotics, and nasogastric suction, resulting in complete healing of the perforation.

diastinum, and its surgical division is best done from a cervical approach. Patients with a proximal pouch fistula often have more severe pneumonitis before initial repair and continue to have symptoms of isolated tracheoesophageal fistula postoperatively.

A fistula located below the level of the second thoracic vertebra is best approached through the thorax rather than through the neck.

MEDIASTINAL INFECTION

Infection of the mediastinum, once considered life-threatening, is now much less of a problem. The availability of antibiotics and adequate surgical drainage make mediastinitis a treatable lesion today. Mediastinal abscesses may go undiscovered for weeks or months following injury to the esophagus and may then present as a necessitating posterior intercostal abscess.

NERVE INJURY

Injury to the vagus nerve or to its primary thoracic branches, the right and left recurrent laryngeal nerves, is a potential complication of esophageal surgery. The position of these nerves in the mediastinum is familiar to all thoracic surgeons, and preservation is simply a matter of being careful in most circumstances. Nerve injury may occur as a result of crushing with the tissue forceps, electrical injury from cautery, or actual transection. Cognizance on the part of the surgeon that these nerves are important is usually all that is required to avoid injury to them. Complete transection of the recurrent laryngeal nerve warrants careful reapproximation with microscope because regeneration may be possible.

The most difficult place to avoid injury to the recurrent laryngeal nerve is in the cervical region during dissection for caustic injury to the esophagus or resection of an anastomotic cervical esophageal stricture. It is not easy to locate the nerve under these circumstances, making both preservation of the nerve and recognition of an injury sometimes exceedingly difficult.

VASCULAR AND OTHER RELATED INJURIES

The most common vascular structure injured in esophageal surgery is the thoracic duct or one of its major branches. This can occur on either the right or the left side and results in the development of chylothorax, which can be as minor as "troublesome" or as major as "life-threatening." Reoperation may be required to control the lymph leak, although if ingested fats are limited to medium-chain triglycerides and if drainage is adequate, spontaneous closure of a thoracic duct fistula will usually result.

Hard and fast rules regarding the length of time one should try chest tube drainage anticipating spontaneous closure of a thoracic duct fistula are difficult to establish. With appropriate dietary measures (e.g., avoiding a great deal of fat, which produces large amounts of chyle) a steady decrease in the daily drainage should be noted if this approach is going to be successful. Should the drainage volume continue unabated for 14 to 21 days, it is likely that surgical intervention will be needed. Localization of the fistula at thoracotomy is often not easy. It may be aided by the administration of several ounces of cream into the stomach by nasogastric tube after the patient is anesthetized and intubated. The milky chyle will thus be easily recognized, and the leak can then be oversewn. Particularly likely points of injury include the mediastinum low on the right side of the chest and the area of the highest intercostal vein on the left side. If a specific leak is not found, ligation of the thoracic duct at the diaphragm may be successful in stopping the leak.

Other vascular injuries reported have included injuries to intercostal vessels, to major branches of the aorta, and to the aorta itself. The azygos vein and the highest intercostal vein obviously are easily seen and ligated during the operative approach to the esophagus and therefore do not usually pose much threat of an intraoperative complication.

Perhaps the most significant vascular injury to the esophagus is one that is never recognizable by bleeding. It is the stripping of the small feeding vessels to the middle esophagus during repair of esophageal atresia with distal tracheoesophageal fistula. This vascular injury may result in anastomotic stricture or leak, as discussed previously in this chapter.

COMPLICATIONS OF ESOPHAGEAL REPLACEMENT

Replacement of the esophagus with gastric tube or colon interposition is fraught with dangers of anastomotic leak, anastomotic stricture, and slough of the interposed segment. Minor leaks of the cervical anastomosis are not uncommon. The cervical anastomosis should always be drained prophylactically. If there is not an associated slough of the interposed segment, the leak will almost certainly close spontaneously.

Interposition of gastric tube to replace the esophagus sometimes results in development of an area of peptic ulceration in the esophageal mucosa just above the anastomosis. This is usually an acute process that presents as bleeding, although pain of perforation may be the initial sign. Chronic ulceration with anemia, pain, and dysphagia has also been reported following gastric tube and colon interposition procedures.[1] Administration of cimetidine may allow healing of the ulcers, although more definitive long-term measures to reduce acid production, such as vagotomy, pyloroplasty, and ensuring that the interposed segment itself is not obstructed at the diaphragm, may be necessary. Total or partial necrosis of the interposed colon or gastric tube does occur. Although many anastomotic problems are thought to be due to venous obstruction, necrosis is probably a result of damaged or obstructed arterial supply. We have seen complete necrosis of two transthoracic left colon interpositions as well as the upper half of a substernal gastric tube. Very meticulous dissection and ensuring an adequate diaphragmatic hiatus to prevent vascular pedicle constriction may be the best preventatives.

Early recognition of necrosis of an interposition is difficult but is almost tantamount to successful management. A leak at the proximal anastomosis, fever, and leukocytosis are early findings. An esophagram may demonstrate the leak, but more important, it will show the absence of a normal mucosal pattern within the interposed segment. Endoscopy is not likely to be of help in the diagnosis of this disastrous complication. Cervical esophageal drainage, removal of the interposed segment with drainage of the mediastinum or chest, and a feeding gastrostomy are necessary until another interposition can be done.

Colon interposition may present more long-term complications than does a gastric tube. In addition to having two anastomoses that may leak or become constricted, the lower end of the interposed colon is subject to peptic ulceration and stricture. Frequently, no matter how short the interposed segment of colon is at the time of its interposition, elongation will occur much more rapidly than does elongation of the body. Redundancy that produces functional obstruction of this interposed colon may occur as a result of differential growth in length. Since the kinks usually occur just above the diaphragm, straightening of the interposed colon is easiest through an upper abdominal approach. While the blood supply to the entire colon is carefully protected, the lower portion of the colon is dissected free and pulled down into the abdominal cavity. The redundant segment is resected carefully while the mesenteric blood supply is preserved, and another anastomosis to the stomach is done.

COMPLICATIONS OF OPERATIONS TO STOP GASTROESOPHAGEAL REFLUX

Patients who have had surgical procedures intended to relieve the symptoms of gastroesophageal reflux may have had one of many forms of fundoplication or a gastropexy to hold the lower end of the esophagus within the abdominal cavity. Fundoplication is the most effective and most common procedure for stopping gastroesophageal reflux. The Nissen fundoplication is most frequently employed. It is occasionally associated with esophageal obstruction because the fundic wrap is made too tight. Placement of a large nasogastric tube or bougie alongside the esophagus during construction of the fundoplication will usually prevent this complication. The most frequent problem following the Nissen procedure is gas bloat syndrome, which occurs when the gastroesophageal valve mechanism is made too competent.[9] The looser wrap is less likely to be associated with gastric dilatation.

An uncommon but serious complication occurs when the fundal wrap slips down from about the esophagus to produce a midgastric narrowing (Fig. 16–4). Obstruction usually results and reoperation is required. Prevention is best accomplished by firmly anchoring the gastric wrap to the lower end of the esophagus.

Lesser degrees of fundoplication such as those described by Thal, Hill, and Belsey have fewer problems in regard to both obstruction and gas bloats. Since the repair involves suturing the stomach to the esophagus, the likelihood of esophageal perforation and paraesophageal abscess formation is increased. We have not seen this complication in our series of more than 350 fundoplications of the Thal variety.

A recent report from Switzerland indicated that fatal air embolism can occur as a result of mobilization of the liver from the underside of the diaphragm during operations for gastroesophageal reflux.[3] In our experience it has been unnecessary to mobilize the liver this extensively to expose the hiatus. Since these procedures are all done through the abdominal cavity, the gamut of complications that can occur after laparotomy are also possible. In our experience, when nothing other than fundoplication is done, the incidence of complications such as wound disruption and intestinal obstruction due to adhesive bands is zero.

Failure of fundoplication to prevent reflux is probably an indication for another surgical procedure. The reasons for failure, in our experience, have been two. One is that the fundoplication comes loose from the esophagus, and the other is that the fundoplication and esophagus are herniated up through a large hiatus into the mediastinum and the reflux recurs. The former complication is prevented by using permanent suture material and taking adequate bites in the esophagus, the latter by placing a limiting stitch in the two limbs of the crura behind the esophagus. Paraesophageal abscess formed from penetration of the esophageal or gastric mucosa should be drained through a transabdominal approach if diagnosed, in hope that the fundoplication will remain intact.

ACHALASIA

Achalasia, or poor esophageal motility associated with the failure of relaxation of the distal end of the esophagus, results from an unknown cause, with hypertrophy of the esophageal muscle in its lower portion being accentuated at the gastroesophageal junction. Perhaps the best treatment for this is an anterior myotomy of the lower esophageal muscle and upper gastric muscle to relieve the obstruction. Occasionally, the mucosa will be entered or bleeding will be troublesome. Since the esophagus is hypertrophied, a simple mucosal closure alone may be difficult and is likely to be weak. It is

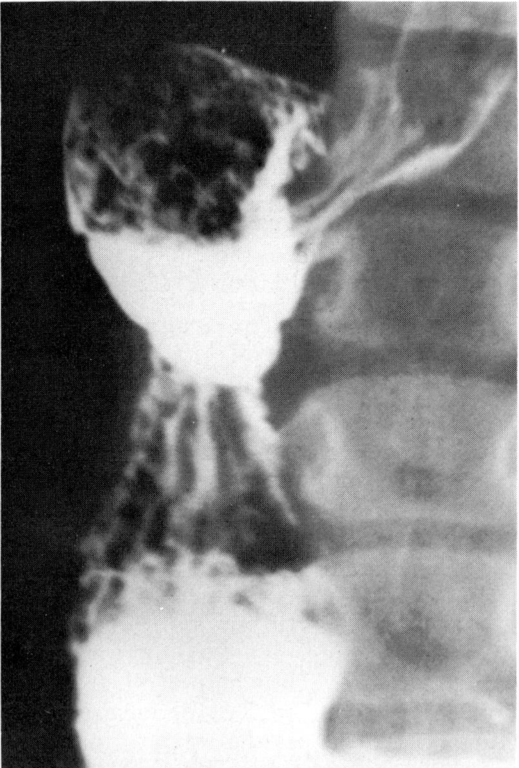

Figure 16–4 Barium swallow showing partial gastric obstruction due to a "slipped" Nissen fundoplication. There is an hourglass deformity of the stomach as a result of the constriction of the midportion of the body of the stomach.

probably best in this situation to bring a patch of gastric fundus, using the serosa as a covering for the submucosal esophageal repair.[18] Because gastroesophageal reflux is a common occurrence following the esophageal myotomy, a Thal fundoplication as part of the initial surgical therapy of all patients seems warranted.

References

1. Anderson, K. D.: Esophageal substitution. *In* Holder, T. M., and Ashcraft, K. W. (eds.): Pediatric Surgery. Philadelphia, W. B. Saunders Co., 1980.
2. Ashcraft, K. W., Goodwin, C., Amoury, R. A., and Holder, T. M.: Early recognition and aggressive treatment of gastroesophageal reflux following repair of esophageal atresia. J. Pediatr. Surg. 12:317, 1977.
3. Bettex, M., Oesch-Amrein, I., and Kuffer, F.: Mortality after operation for hiatus hernia. *In* Rickham, P. P., Hecker, W. C., and Prevot, J. (eds.): Causes of Postoperative Death in Children. Baltimore, Urban & Schwarzenberg, 1979, pp. 245–252.
4. Ein, S. H., and Theman, T. E.: A comparison of the results of primary repair of esophageal atresia with tracheoesophageal fistulas using end-to-side and end-to-end anastomoses. J. Pediatr. Surg. 8:641, 1973.
5. Gans, S. L., and Berci, G.: Inside tracheoesophageal fistula: New endoscopic approaches. J. Pediatr. Surg. 8:205, 1973.
6. Holder, T. M., Ashcraft, K. W., and Leape, L.: The treatment of patients with esophageal strictures by local steroid injections. J. Pediatr. Surg. 4:646, 1969.
7. Holder, T. M., Cloud, D. T., Lewis, J. E., Jr., and Pilling, G. P., IV: Esophageal atresia and tracheoesophageal fistula: A survey of its members by the Surgical Section of the American Academy of Pediatrics. Pediatrics 34:542, 1964.
8. Ketchum, L. D., Smith, J., Robinson, D. W., and Masters, F. W.: The treatment of hypertrophic scar, keloid and scar contracture by triamcinolone acetonide. Plast. Reconstr. Surg. 38:209, 1966.
9. Leape, L. L.: Gastroesophageal reflux. *In* Holder, T. M., and Ashcraft, K. W. (eds.): Pediatric Surgery. Philadelphia, W. B. Saunders Co., 1980.
10. Livaditis, A., Radberg, L., and Odensjo, G.: Esophageal end-to-end anastomosis. Reduction of anastomotic tension by circular myotomy. Scand. J. Thorac. Cardiovasc. Surg. 6:206, 1972.
11. Loop, F. D., and Groves, L. K.: Esophageal perforations. Ann. Thorac. Surg. 10:571, 1970.
12. Lopez-Perez, G. A.: A modified method for the repair of esophageal atresia with tracheoesophageal fistula. Surgery 79:499, 1976.
13. Mahour, G. H., Woolley, M. M., and Gwinn, J. L.: Elongation of the upper pouch and delayed anatomic reconstruction in esophageal atresia. J. Pediatr. Surg. 9:373, 1974.
14. Othersen, H. B.: Esophageal lesions. *In* Holder, T. M., and Ashcraft, K. W. (eds.): Pediatric Surgery. Philadelphia, W. B. Saunders Co., 1980.
15. Parker, A. F., Christie, D. L., and Cahill, J. L.: Incidence and significance of gastroesophageal reflux following repair of esophageal atresia and tracheoesophageal fistula and the need for antireflux procedures. J. Pediatr. Surg. 14:5, 1979.
16. Pieretti, R., Shandling, B., and Stephens, C. A.: Resistant esophageal stenosis associated with reflux after repair of esophageal atresia: A therapeutic approach. J. Pediatr. Surg. 9:355, 1974.
17. Stanford, W., Armstrong, R. G., Cline, R. E., and Williams, M. J.: Recurrent tracheoesophageal fistula. Ann. Thorac. Surg. 15:452, 1973.
18. Thal, A. P.: A unified approach to surgical problems of the esophagogastric junction. Ann. Surg. 168:542, 1968.
19. Touloukian, R. J., Pickett, L. K., Spackman, T., and Biancani, P.: Repair of esophageal atresia by end-to-side anastomosis and ligation of the tracheoesophageal fistula: A critical review of 18 cases. J. Pediatr. Surg. 9:305, 1974.

ABDOMEN | 4

17

THE ABDOMINAL PARIETES

C. D. Smith

COMPLICATIONS OF OMPHALOCELE AND GASTROSCHISIS

A surgical aphorism states, "In massive insults to the organism, treat the patient for the insult, without waiting for the response to the insult."[23] Omphalocele and gastroschisis constitute two of the most massive neonatal insults a pediatric surgeon is called on to treat. Prior to this century, survival was rare, although the first survivor following primary closure was reported in 1803.[15] The modern era of treatment began with the report by Gross in 1948 of skin flap closure of giant omphaloceles.[12] Grob[10] in 1957 reintroduced the concept of conservative management of the large intact omphalocele, originally reported by Ahlfeld.[2] Schuster first employed prosthetic material in closure in 1959 and reported his early results in 1967.[26] In the past decade, improved results have been reported by adherents of primary closure,[22] skin flap closure,[33] conservative management,[8] and staged prosthetic closure.[28] Despite major advances due to improved surgical techniques and improved medical management, serious complications still occur. Schuster et al. classified complications under three headings: inadequate perinatal resuscitation, associated anomalies, and surgical management.[28]

Etiology

Moore has summarized the major clinical differences between patients with gastroschisis and those with omphalocele.[18] For the clinician, however, the major problems are a large mass of eviscerated intestine and a small abdominal cavity. Pulmonary and circulatory compromise results from closure under too much tension. Sepsis is the major

risk if skin closure is not accomplished. In both conditions, the baby is frequently of low birth weight and is susceptible to hypothermia, hypovolemia, hypoxia, and acidosis because of the large evaporative surface in the form of eviscerated intestine. As with any low-birth-weight infant, there is an increased incidence of central nervous system hemorrhage secondary to stress.

Patients with ruptured omphalocele and gastroschisis have decreased levels of serum immunoglobulins and albumin,[13] apparent

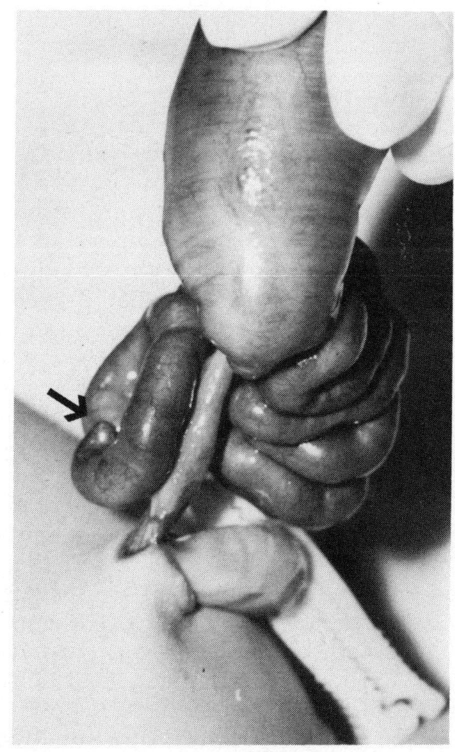

Figure 17–1 Gastroschisis with small abdominal wall defect admitting only vascular supply to eviscerated bowel. Contraction of the umbilical ring in utero produced jejunal and colonic atresia. *Arrow* points to blind beginning of ileum.

shortening of the bowel,[9, 30] and altered gastrointestinal function.[14, 19, 25, 34] These babies have an increased susceptibility to infection and to prolonged ileus.

The most common associated anomaly in patients with omphalocele or gastroschisis is malrotation, which may be complicated by midgut volvulus. Jejunoileal atresia, secondary to pressure necrosis caused by impingement of the contracting umbilical ring on the small bowel, is frequently encountered in infants with gastroschisis (Fig. 17–1). Major anomalies involving the heart, diaphragm, urinary tract, and spinal cord are not uncommon in patients with omphalocele, and they complicate management. The Beckwith-Weidemann syndrome, which includes omphalocele as one of its features, is often complicated by severe hypoglycemia.

Prevention

Response to the insult of omphalocele and gastroschisis can be significantly reduced by optimal preoperative and intraoperative management.

PERINATAL STRESS

Prevention of hypothermia is one of the most difficult aspects of pre- and intraoperative management. Wrapping the bowel in warm, saline-soaked sponges before operation, a procedure that is often advised, can increase heat loss rather than prevent it. We recommend dry sponges and an impermeable plastic dressing. If exposed bowel appears ischemic, the fascial defect is enlarged as rapidly as possible by simple incision under local anesthesia. Further preoperative manipulation resulting in exposure of the baby is to be avoided. A chest x-ray film to rule out associated diaphragmatic hernia and a heel stick for hematocrit and blood glucose determinations are sufficient. Blood for typing and crossmatching need not be obtained until cutdowns are performed in the operating room or, if delay is unavoidable, under a radiant heater. We have seen the temperature of a small baby with a large intact omphalocele drop to 92°F over a 10-minute period in the emergency room while attempts were made to establish an intravenous line and draw blood.

The operating room, preparatory solutions, anesthetic gases, and blood for transfusion should all be warm. Thompson and Fonkalsrud stress the need to protect the bowel during surgery by having the assistant hold the eviscerated bowel in his hands during the procedure.[33]

Hypotension can be avoided only by careful monitoring of the patient. Conflicting data regarding the fluid requirements of these babies have been reported.[17, 21, 22] For the individual patient, however, administration of fluid should be varied to maintain central venous pressure, arterial pressure, blood pH, and urine output within normal limits. When a major portion of the liver is eviscerated, the hepatic veins are elongated (Fig. 17–2). If the liver is retracted to one side, the venous return from the liver can be cut off, causing hypovolemia. This complication can be avoided by keeping the liver in the midline throughout surgery. Obstruction of the inferior vena cava with resultant Budd-Chiari syndrome after giant omphalocele repair has been reported.[5]

The first step in avoiding sepsis is the administration of broad-spectrum antibiot-

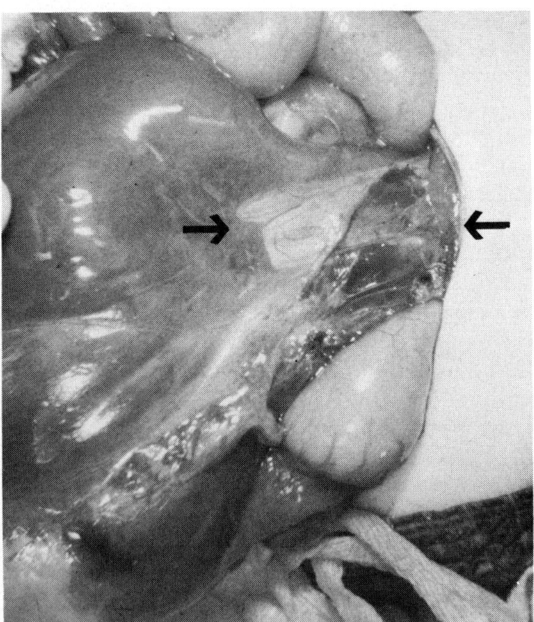

Figure 17–2 Omphalocele with herniation of liver through abdominal wall defect. Note elongated hepatic veins *(arrows)*. Baby became hypotensive whenever the liver was displaced away from the midline during the operation.

ics as soon as intravenous access is established. Colloid should be administered in the form of fresh frozen plasma, since this contains both immunoglobulin G and immunoglobulin M. If fresh frozen plasma is unavailable, gamma globulin (IgG) should be given.

SURGICAL COMPLICATIONS

There is general agreement that primary all-layer closure of the abdominal defect is the procedure of choice, but achievement of this goal depends on a number of factors, including the experience of the surgeon. In a baby whose condition is stable, extensive manipulations, including antegrade and retrograde decompression of the bowel and stretching of the abdominal wall, are justified, because these measures facilitate all-layer closure or at least partial fascial closure with skin flap coverage.[1, 22, 33] Postoperative respirator support is often needed to maintain adequate ventilation for the first few days after surgery while the abdomen enlarges to accommodate the large visceral mass.

Insistence on primary closure at the expense of excessive stress to the baby is unjustified. Increased intra-abdominal pressure causes hypovolemia due to vena caval obstruction and respiratory compromise due to elevation of the diaphragms. When this occurs, the excess pressure must be relieved by removal of fascial sutures and skin closure or creation of a ventral hernia with prosthetic material. In patients with an intact sac, conservative management with application of biologic dressings[29] or escharotics offers an alternative that does not increase intra-abdominal pressure. Unfortunately, this form of treatment has a number of drawbacks, including long hospitalization, mercury intoxication, unrecognized intra-abdominal catastrophe, and inevitable ventral hernia.[8, 11, 31] As a primary mode of treatment, it is usually reserved for the small intact omphalocele in babies with severe associated anomalies or for larger defects in very small premature infants. As an escharotic, merbromin, (Mercurochrome) is used in 0.5 per cent concentration with frequent monitoring of serum mercury levels.[7]

Postoperative sepsis is the main complication of the use of prosthetic materials in the closure of large defects. Rubin and Ein have reported a 65 per cent incidence of sepsis in 31 patients with omphalocele and gastroschisis in whom a Silon pouch was used. Half

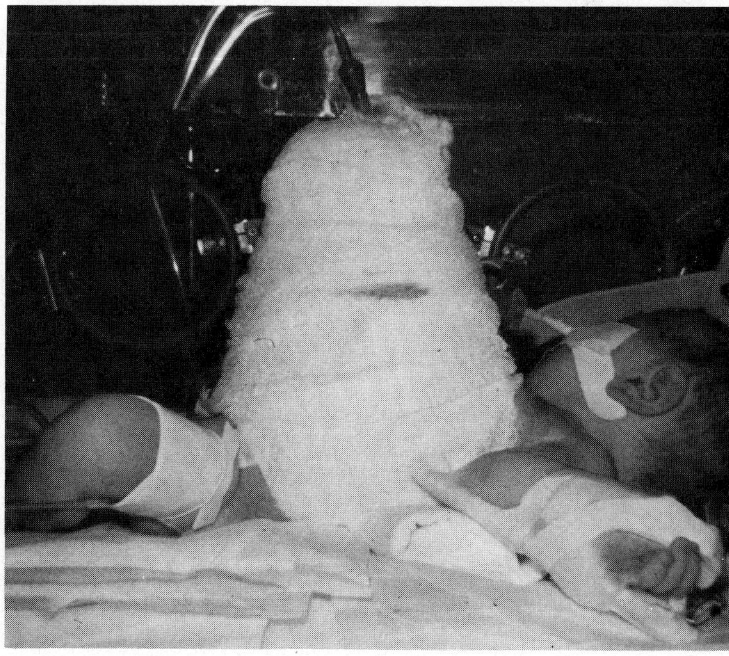

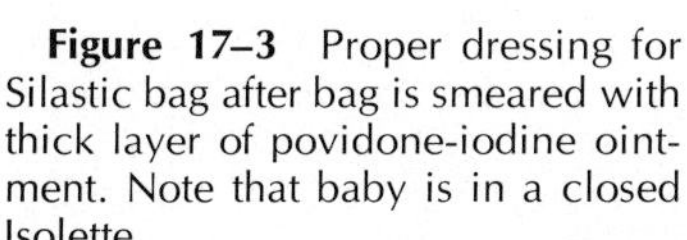

Figure 17–3 Proper dressing for Silastic bag after bag is smeared with thick layer of povidone-iodine ointment. Note that baby is in a closed Isolette.

of the septic patients died.[24] The incidence was much lower at Children's Hospital Medical Center in Boston, where sepsis was not responsible for any deaths during the last 7 years.[28] This experience and that of others[3, 16] suggest that life-threatening septic complications can be prevented if certain principles are followed with regard to choice of material, use of sterile technique, and timing of abdominal closure.

Schuster has described the use of Teflon mesh with or without an underlying layer of polyethylene film, depending on whether an intact membrane is present.[27] The advantage of this material is that it allows ingrowth of fibroblasts through its interstices. It is less likely to become infected and can be safely left in place longer than nonporous materials such as Silon. When nonporous materials are used, wound infection with

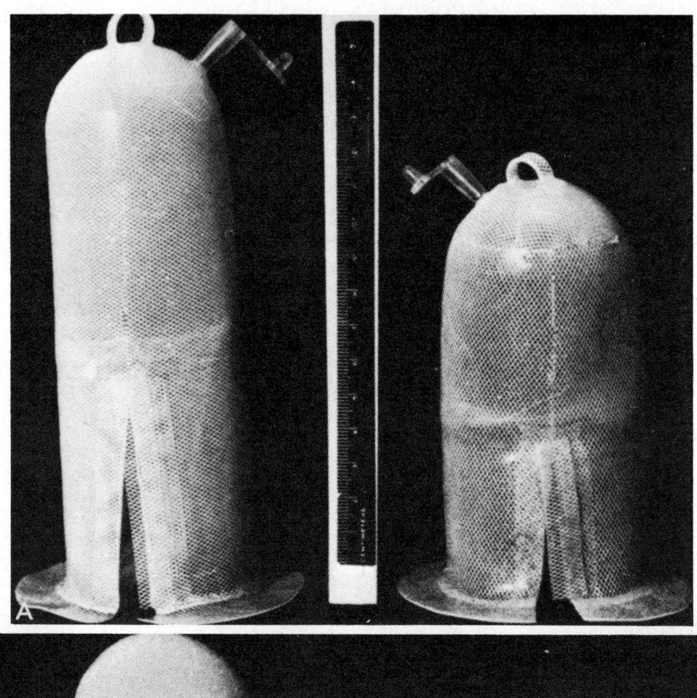
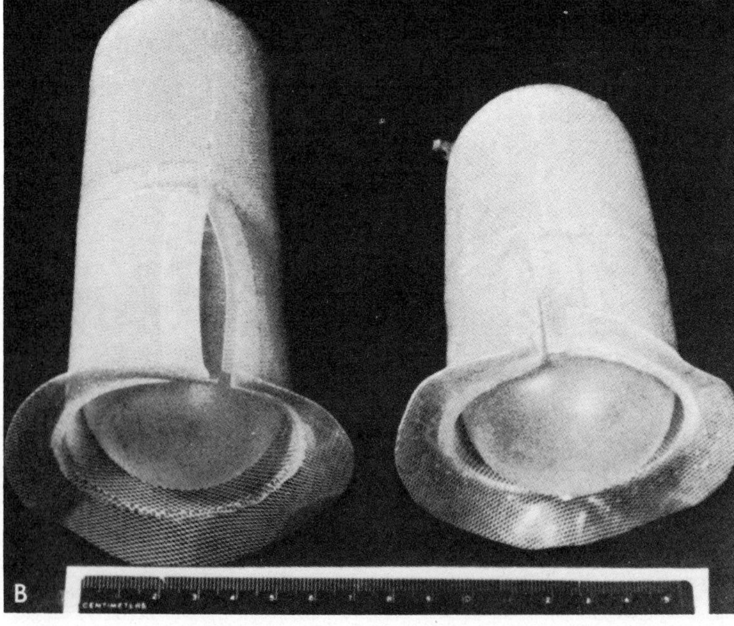

Figure 17–4   *A,* Two sizes of bag made from Dacron-reinforced Silastic. *B,* Bottom view of the pneumatic chamber inflated with air. (From Othersen, H. B., Jr., and Hargest, T. S.: A pneumatic reduction device for gastroschisis and omphalocele. Surg. Gynecol. Obstet. 144:244, 1977, by permission of Surgery, Gynecology & Obstetrics.)

sloughing of the prosthesis is likely if abdominal closure is not accomplished within 7 to 10 days.

Strict sterile technique in handling of the prosthetic sac is mandatory. At the time of surgery the sac should be smeared with a thick layer of povidone-iodine ointment and wrapped with an occlusive dry gauze dressing. If his condition permits, the baby is transferred to a closed Isolette (Fig. 17–3). Sterile gloves are used for all manipulations of the baby. The dressing is changed once or twice a day as needed to remove exudate-soaked sponges and to reduce the size of the prosthetic sac through staged closure. Broad-spectrum antibiotics are administered until the prosthetic material has been removed. Nystatin (Mycostatin) is also given by nasogastric tube or gastrostomy to prevent *Candida* colonization. Opinion varies with regard to the increased risk of infection associated with placement of a gastrostomy tube. In general it is probably best not to use one, but if one is employed, it should be placed in an extreme lateral position beyond the level of skin flap dissection.

At the Medical University of South Carolina we have achieved closure of the abdominal wall within 7 to 10 days in all patients since the introduction by Othersen and Hargest of a preformed Silastic bag with a built-in pneumatic chamber (Fig. 17–4). Sequential reduction of the contents of the bag is performed in the Isolette one or more times a day by manually squeezing the sac, then maintaining the bowel in the reduced position by insufflation of the balloon (Fig. 17–5). Further details of this procedure are reported elsewhere.[20] We think that when a nonporous material such as Silastic is used, early removal is even more critical than when Teflon mesh is used. Antibiotic impregnation of Silastic is currently undergoing evaluation.[4]

Fistula formation is the result of pressure necrosis due to contact of the bowel with a fold of noncompliant prosthetic material, apposition of an anastomosis to the prosthetic sac, or inadvertent needle puncture of the bowel at the time of prosthetic sac plication or fascial closure. Schuster et al. recommend avoiding bowel anastomosis when

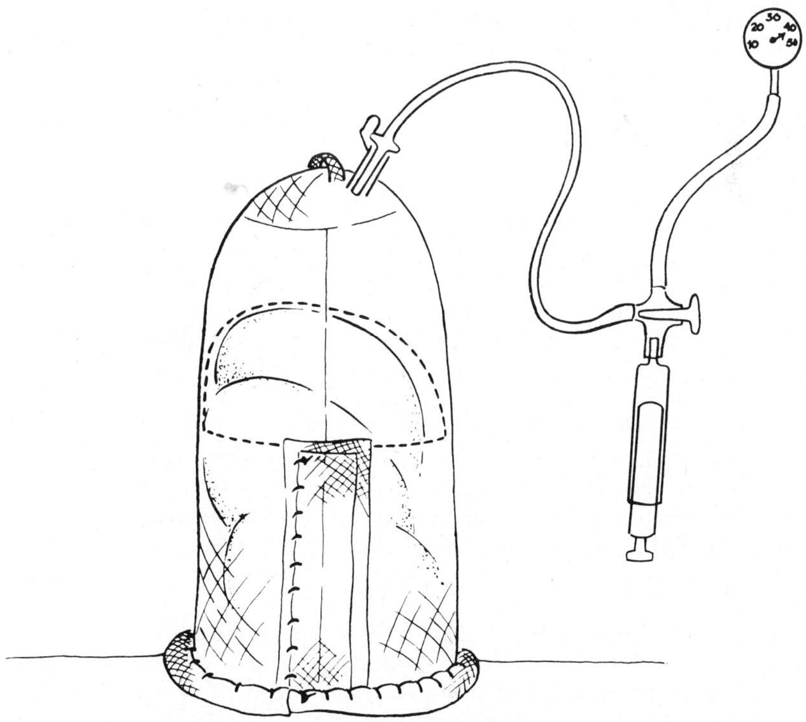

Figure 17–5 Intestines have been partially displaced from the bag by squeezing. Air is injected into the pneumatic chamber to maintain the reduction. (From Othersen, H. B., Jr., and Hargest, T. S.: A pneumatic reduction device for gastroschisis and omphalocele. Surg. Gynecol. Obstet. 144:244, 1977, by permission of Surgery, Gynecology & Obstetrics.)

prosthetic material is used and, if anastomosis is unavoidable, taking precautions to prevent contact of the anastomosis with the foreign material.[28] Ideally, repair of an atresia is delayed until the abdominal wound has healed.

One of the major lessons learned since the institution of hyperalimentation is that bowel obstruction in patients with omphalocele and gastroschisis usually results from prolonged inhibition of bowel motility (paralytic ileus) rather than from mechanical causes. Unless there are indications of bowel compromise, laparotomy for lysis of adhesions is delayed as long as 2 to 4 months. In most cases the "obstruction" resolves spontaneously. One should not forget, however, that mechanical obstruction due to unrecognized atresia or midgut volvulus can occur. Obstruction due to meconium plug has also been reported.[6] Manual decompression of the bowel during initial surgery should avoid this complication. If obstruction is recognized later, water-soluble contrast enema should be curative.

COMPLICATIONS OF REPAIR OF INGUINAL, FEMORAL, AND UMBILICAL HERNIAS

Inguinal Hernia

Repair of inguinal hernia is the most common general surgical procedure performed in the child. The complication rate is fortunately low, but when errors are made, the result can be catastrophic. In 1964 a study of deaths from anesthesia in infants and children reported an overall mortality of 3.3 per 10,000 anesthetizations, and more than half of these deaths occurred in apparently healthy children, many undergoing herniorrhaphy.[45] Insensitive handling of children undergoing even relatively straightforward procedures such as hernia repair have long-term adverse effects.[40] Testicular atrophy as a result of injury to spermatic vessels, division of the vas deferens, inadvertent bladder entry, gonad excision, iatrogenic cryptorchidism, and recurrent or missed hernia are major surgical complications of inguinal herniorrhaphy in children.

ETIOLOGY

The most common sources of error in pediatric inguinal hernia repair are inexperience in dealing with diminutive structures, unfamiliarity with special anatomic variations, and application of adult concepts of hernia and hydrocele repair to the child. The high incidence of hernias in the premature infant[48] and of incarceration during the first year of life[76] has led to the recommendation that such hernias be repaired as soon as diagnosed, provided there are no medical contraindications to surgery. The high incidence of a patent processus vaginalis on the contralateral side in the infant has influenced most pediatric surgeons to perform bilateral exploration.[37] Under optimal conditions (surgeon and anesthesiologist skilled and experienced, patient without serious underlying condition, operation smooth and lasting less than 1 hour), repair by high ligation of the sac and contralateral exploration are done with minimal risk to the patient. However, Chamberlain made the following comment many years ago:

> Only rarely is this procedure as easy to carry out as it sounds, sometimes because the neck of the sack is large and sometimes because the sac is firmly adherent to the spermatic cord, but most often because of the extreme thinness and fragility of the wall of the sac.[36]

Injury to the vas deferens, testicular vessels, and ilioinguinal nerve is more likely during negative groin exploration, when all the cord structures must be dissected to verify the absence of a patent processus vaginalis, than when a definite sac is present.[78] Reports of long-term follow-up after pediatric inguinal herniorrhaphy are few and have usually been compiled at institutions where there is great expertise in pediatric surgery. It is most likely that the incidence of surgical complications following pediatric hernia repair is much higher than the literature suggests.

Important anatomic variations in the inguinal region of the small child include the proximity of the bladder to the inguinal ring (Fig. 17–6) emphasized by Shaw and Santulli,[69] occasional ureteral prolapse through the internal ring,[60] and the high incidence of sliding hernias in the female child. Patients with Hurler-Hunter or

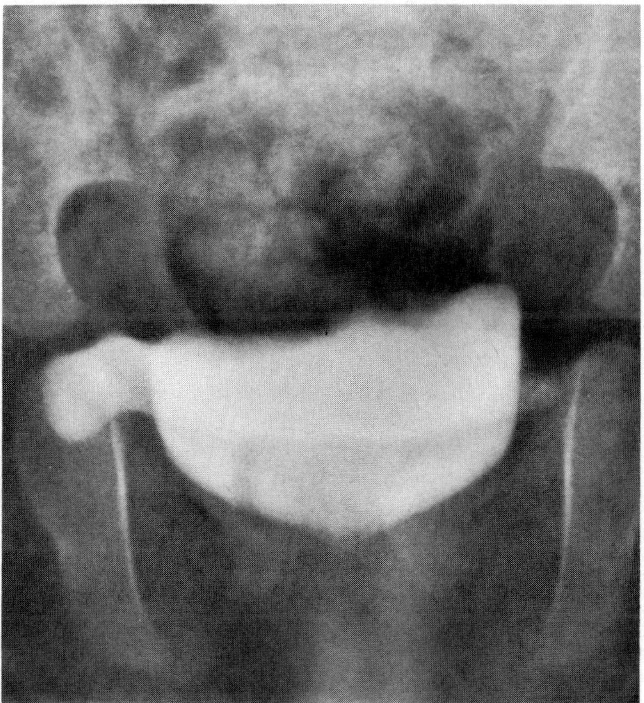

Figure 17–6 "Bladder ear" projecting through internal inguinal ring in an infant undergoing excretory urogram. With decompression of bladder this sliding hernia is reduced. (Courtesy of Robert L. Lorenzo, M.D.)

Ehlers-Danlos syndrome frequently have inguinal hernias that are prone to recur unless an inguinal floor repair is added to the usual high ligation of the sac.[38, 59, 83] The same is true of patients with congenital infections due to cytomegalovirus (CMV) and those with congenital pelvic defects such as exstrophy of the bladder and vesicointestinal fissure. There is an increased incidence of inguinal hernia in children with ventriculoperitoneal shunts for hydrocephalus.[46] The surgeon operating on one of these patients should preoperatively diagnose — and be prepared to deal with — the presence of shunt tubing in the hernial sac. Splenogonadal fusion, with extension of splenic tissue into the scrotum inside the hernial sac, is a surgical curiosity in children.[81] The surgeon must recognize that this "tumor" can be excised without sacrificing the testis. Finally, the informed surgeon has the opportunity to diagnose certain major underlying condi-

TABLE 17–1 SERIOUS UNDERLYING CONDITIONS IN PEDIATRIC HERNIA PATIENTS

Diagnosis	Surgical Findings	Indicated Work-up
Hurler-Hunter syndrome	Recurrent hernia[38, 83]	Urine mucopolysaccharide screen
Ehlers-Danlos syndrome	Recurrent hernia, extreme skin laxity, extreme blood vessel fragility[51, 59, 83]	Clinical observation,* coagulation work-up
Testicular feminization syndrome	Abnormal-appearing gonad, absence of fallopian tube[61]	Biopsy of gonad, buccal smear, vaginal endoscopy
Cystic fibrosis	Absent or abnormal vas deferens[57]	Sweat chloride determination
Unilateral renal agenesis	Absent vas deferens[57]	Intravenous pyelogram
Congenital rubella infection	Absent vas deferens[64]	Rubella titers, history of maternal rubella infection

*Characteristic clinical features may not be present in the infant.

tions and prevent delay in appropriate therapy (Table 17–1).

In 1899 Ferguson stated the following:

Tearing the cord out of its bed is without anatomic reason to recommend it, a physiologic act to suggest it, an etiologic factor in hernia, congenital or acquired, to indicate it, nor [does it give] brilliant surgical results to justify its continuance. Leave the cord alone, for it is the sacred highway along which travel vital elements indispensable to the perpetuity of our race.[42]

It has been shown repeatedly that the rate of recurrence is less than 1 per cent in large series of children with hernias treated by high ligation alone.[39, 47, 54, 55, 63, 79] Dissection and attempted repair of the inguinal floor has often been implicated as a cause of development of direct hernia in patients undergoing indirect inguinal herniorrhaphy. Therefore, except in the special circumstances mentioned above or when there is a very large internal ring or an obvious direct hernia, simple high ligation of the indirect sac without disturbance of the inguinal floor is recommended.

Similarly, hydrocele repair differs for adults and children. In adults, there is usually no associated hernia. The hydrocele is approached through the scrotum, most of the sac is removed, and the remainder is sutured behind the testis. In children, however, an associated indirect hernia is uniformly present. For this reason, operation is performed through an inguinal approach, the hernia is repaired, and a portion of the wall of the hydrocele sac is excised. Use of the "bottle" technique in children has been reported to have a high complication rate.[41]

PREVENTION

Adequate exposure, good lighting, and meticulous technique should prevent most surgical complications of inguinal herniorrhaphy. Because of the extreme friability of the sac at the time of incarceration and the increased incidence of recurrence following emergency surgery for this condition, most pediatric surgeons attempt nonoperative reduction, a technique that has recently been reviewed in detail.[81] This technique, applied to infants and children who show no signs of

strangulation or frank peritonitis, should be successful in 80 per cent of patients with incarcerated hernias.[67] Although very rare, reduction of nonviable bowel in children has been reported.[58] For this reason, any child whose incarcerated hernia has been reduced nonoperatively should be admitted to the hospital and observed carefully for development of signs of peritonitis. Elective repair is performed 24 to 48 hours later, when tissue edema has largely resolved.

Opening the hernial sac before high ligation should prevent inadvertent injury to an unsuspected sliding component such as bladder, ureter, ovary, or fallopian tube. In girls, traction on the round ligament will enable the surgeon to bring the ipsilateral fallopian tube into view and thereby rule out testicular feminization syndrome.[77] In some institutions, buccal smears are obtained in all girls undergoing herniorrhaphy.[62]

Loss of control of the proximal hernial sac, particularly in the small infant, can lead to an increased chance of injuring the vas and vessels and to possible recurrence. We have found the technique routinely employed in dissecting the hernial sac from the cord structures during orchiopexy to be useful in regaining control of the sac when it becomes torn or retracts (Fig. 17–7).

A final precaution to prevent unintended injury to the vas or vessels is to be sure that these structures are not included at the base of the twisted sac at the time of high ligation. *Positive identification of the vas and vessels is mandatory before division or ligation of the sac.* Silber strongly recommends use of ocular loupes when performing herniorrhaphy in infants to prevent injury to the vas.[73]

COMPLICATIONS

Division of the Vas. Until recently, reconstruction of the divided vas deferens in a child was regarded as a technical impossibility.[66] Development of microsurgical techniques has now changed this dismal outlook. Following extensive work in the laboratory, Silber has reported outstanding results in vasovasostomy in adults.[74] The technique is illustrated in Figure 17–8. Experience with this operation in children is at present small.[73] The main question seems no longer

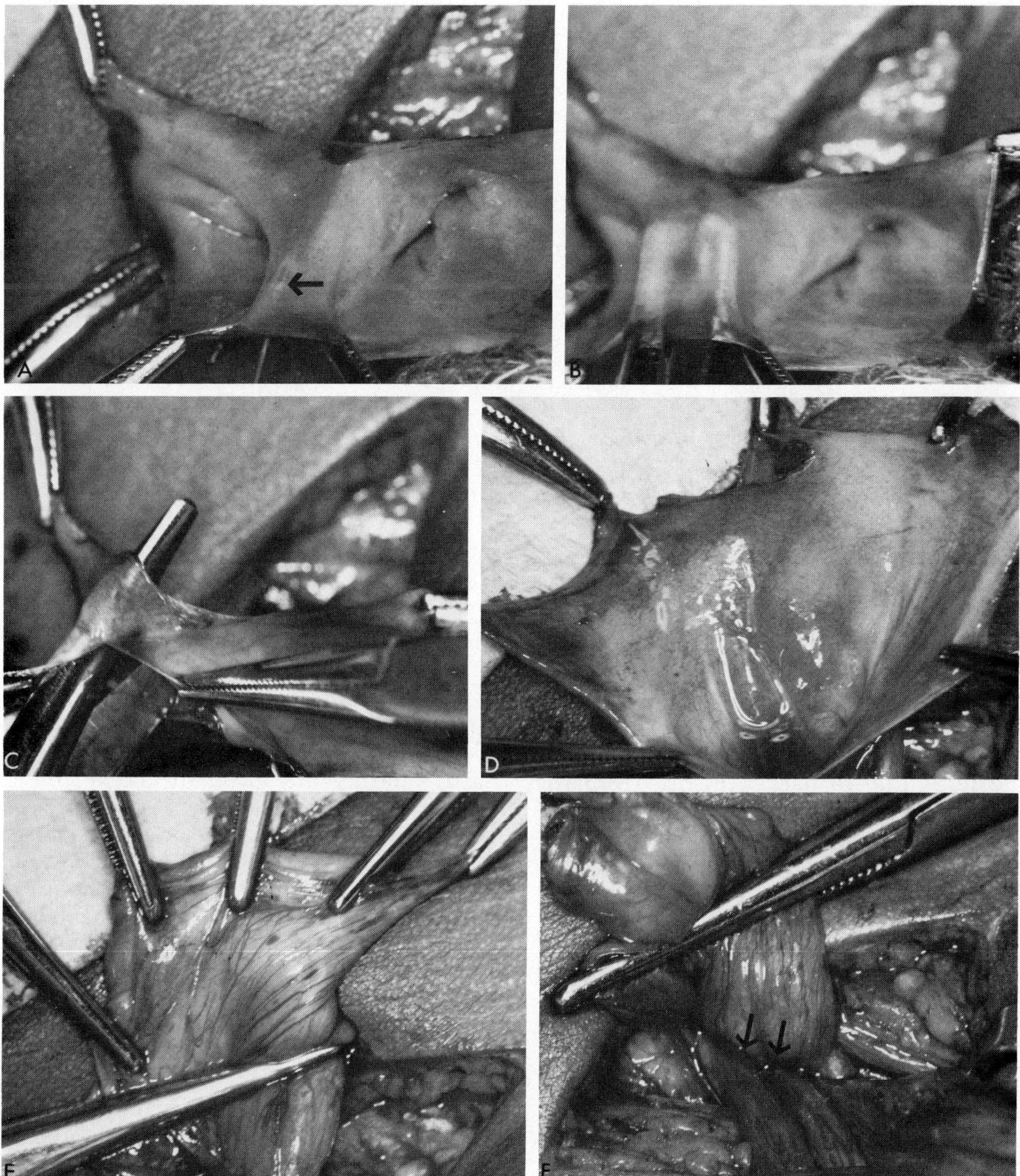

Figure 17–7 Technique used to regain control of torn sac or to dissect densely adherent cord structures from sac. *A,* Anterior wall of sac has been divided. Plane between sac and cord structures is being injected with saline solution *(arrow)* to facilitate dissection. *B,* Fine, round-tipped scissors are used to develop plane between sac and cord structures. Note that scissors are kept parallel to plane between sac and vessels, and scissors points are always kept in view through sac. *C,* Dissection completed. Spreading scissors further opens plane. *D,* Straight clamps are now placed around perimeter of proximal sac opening. *E,* Anterior and posterior walls of sac are now grasped by clamps, and dissection is continued proximally until a single straight clamp can be placed across the sac. *F,* Dissection has now been carried to internal ring. Note vas and vessels below sac *(arrows)*. If additional exposure is needed, the internal oblique muscle is divided laterally to expose the retroperitoneum. High ligation under direct vision is now possible.

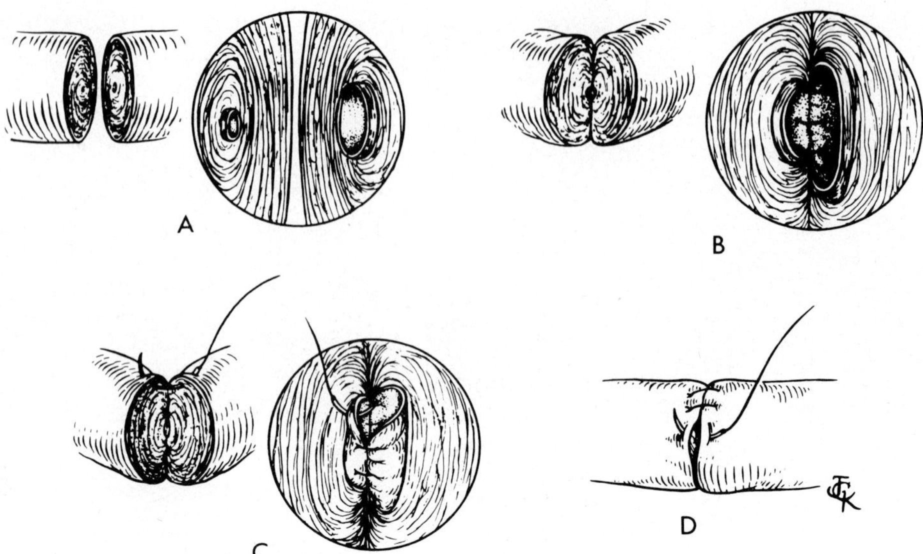

Figure 17–8 Steps in microscopic technique of vasovasostomy. *A,* The lumen is inspected for patency. *B* and *C,* Mucosal anastomosis. *D,* Separate anastomosis of muscularis. (Reproduced from Silber, S. J.: Microscopic technique for reversal of vasectomy. Surg. Gynecol. Obstet. 143:630, 1976, by permission of Surgery, Gynecology & Obstetrics.)

one of technical feasibility but one of optimal timing. There are two reasons to defer repair until early puberty: First, damage to the testis due to back pressure from the obstructed vas is unlikely before that time because of the lack of seminal fluid production in the younger child. Second, as with a vascular anastomosis, patency of a vasovasostomy is more likely when there is a normal flow of fluid in the vessel.[72]

Atrophy of the Testis. Primary repair of inadvertently transected spermatic vessels has not been reported, although microsurgical anastomoses have been used successfully in orchiopexy.[75] At the time of operative reduction of incarceration or strangulation, the testis sometimes appears nonviable. Replacement of the testis after capsulotomy rather than excision is recommended.[50] In this situation and when inadvertent injury to the spermatic vessels occurs during elective herniorrhaphy, atrophy of the testis is common. Replacement of the atrophic testis with a prosthetic testis at puberty should be considered.[65]

Recurrence. In some cases, clinical examination does not provide certain evidence that a recurrence is present. Herniography can both settle the question and define the nature of the recurrence, if present. Repair depends on the cause of the recurrence, i.e., missed direct or femoral hernia, insufficiently high ligation of the indirect sac, or iatrogenically produced direct hernia. A preperitoneal approach by a surgeon experienced in this technique should be considered in a patient who has had more than one recurrence.[35, 44, 68] Use of prosthetic material for repair of recurrent inguinal hernia is rarely, if ever, indicated in children.

Iatrogenic Cryptorchidism. This complication occurs when the surgeon fails to place the testis in normal position at the conclusion of herniorrhaphy.[53] If the testis has been dissected out of the scrotum during herniorrhaphy or hydrocelectomy and the surgeon is not certain that the testis will remain in the correct position, fixation in the scrotum by dartos pouch[82] or window septopexy technique[80] should be carried out. When iatrogenic cryptorchidism is diagnosed postoperatively, formal orchiopexy is required.

Femoral Hernia

Femoral hernias are so rare in childhood that no one surgeon has a significant experience. There is no consensus regarding optimal repair of such hernias, although it is agreed that simple ligation of the sac is associated with an excessively high recurrence rate. Closure of the femoral defect from either above or below the inguinal ligament has been recommended.[56] Others favor a suprainguinal or preperitoneal Cooper's ligament repair.[44, 52] Better exposure is obtained than in the infrainguinal approach; therefore, damage to the femoral vein should be less likely.[43]

Umbilical Hernia

Dissection of the umbilical sac and the fascial rim is carried out through a small curvilinear incision made within the umbilicus superiorly or inferiorly. The defect is closed with interrupted, nonabsorbable sutures after the sac has been either excised or invaginated. Complications include hematoma or seroma, wound infection, recurrence, and bowel perforation.

Hematoma and seroma formation can be prevented by attention to several details. Limiting dissection of the fascia to the fascial rim avoids injury to the perforating vessels of the anterior rectus sheath, which can retract beneath the fascia and be difficult to control. The operative field should be dry at the time of closure. When the dissection has been extensive and significant serous drainage is anticipated, a closed-system, suction catheter should be left in the wound overnight. Most surgeons leave a pressure dressing in place for a minimum of 3 days.

Recurrent hernia most commonly follows wound infection or emergency repair at the time of incarceration, which is rare. Repair should be delayed for a year, if possible. Patients with a history of wound infection should be given antibiotics preoperatively.

Personal observation of complications of umbilical herniorrhaphy has included two instances of bowel injury. The first (recognized postoperatively when pneumoperitoneum developed) was perforation of the small intestine that occurred during placement of a fascial suture. The second was perforation of the sac and the transverse colon that occurred during blunt dissection of the superior wall of a large, redundant hernial sac.

COMPLICATIONS OF ABDOMINAL WOUND HEALING

Complications of abdominal wound healing encompass three entities of vastly different clinical significance: superficial wound dehiscence, in which the fascia remains intact; ventral hernia, in which the fascia separates but the superficial tissues remain closed; and complete dehiscence, in which all layers of the abdominal wall separate, often allowing protrusion of the abdominal viscera (evisceration). The true incidence of these wound complications is difficult to quantify. There are only two large studies of pediatric surgical patients with complete wound dehiscence; both are retrospective and uncontrolled.[88, 93]

Ultimately, wound disruption is the result of failure of the suture or failure of the tissue. Since the unsuitability of chromic suture for fascial closure was recognized,[92] premature dissolution of suture material has become less common. Spontaneous unraveling of surgical knots is a problem of the neophyte. Failure of the tissue results from an imbalance between collagen synthesis and collagen lysis (Table 17–2).[96, 100] Experimental and clinical evidence of factors

TABLE 17–2 FACTORS THAT DECREASE COLLAGEN SYNTHESIS AND INCREASE COLLAGEN LYSIS*

Preoperative
  Starvation (protein depletion)
  Steroids
  Infection
  Associated injuries
  Hypoxia
  Radiation injury
  Uremia
  Diabetes

Operative
  Tissue injury
  Poor blood supply

Postoperative
  Starvation
  Hypovolemia
  Hypoxia
  Drugs (e.g., actinomycin, 5-fluorouracil, methotrexate)

*Adapted from Hunt, T. K.: Disorders of repair and their management. *In* Hunt, T. K., and Dunphy, J. E. (eds.): Fundamentals of Wound Management. New York, Appleton-Century-Crofts, 1979, p. 120.

interfering with wound healing is presented by Hunt and Dunphy.[100]

Prevention

With current availability of parenteral and enteral techniques of nutritional support, few patients should come to surgery in a debilitated state. Vitamin and trace element supplementation is an integral part of such a program. The administration of vitamin C and zinc is particularly important to wound healing. The pediatric surgical patient most likely to be deficient in zinc is probably the infant receiving long-term hyperalimentation, who has been deprived of trace elements.

It has long been known that steroids have potent anti-inflammatory effects and that patients receiving steroids are at risk for wound complications. Less generally appreciated is the fact that vitamin A selectively reverses the antagonistic effect of cortisone on wound healing.[89] Currently, Hunt treats selected patients receiving steroids with five times the daily recommended dose of vitamin A for 6 days, 2 days preoperatively and 4 days postoperatively.[99] He urges caution in using systemic vitamin A when there is a vital need for steroid suppression of inflammation, e.g., in the patient with a kidney transplant in jeopardy of rejection, and notes that topical vitamin A has been helpful in such cases.[97]

Control of intercurrent infection, uremia, and diabetes is obviously desirable preoperatively. In uremic patients, nutritional supplementation may be as important as dialysis to wound healing. In patients with coagulopathy, it has been shown that prophylactic treatment of coagulation disorders lowers the rate of wound-healing complications.[114]

Operation is best avoided shortly before and after treatment with radiation, because inhibition of differentiation of "stem" cells into fibroblasts and of endothelial cells into new vessels is maximal within the first week after this kind of therapy. When possible, surgery should be delayed until 4 to 8 weeks after radiation therapy is completed. Months to years later, wound healing is again impaired by the microvascular insufficiency that radiation therapy produces in treated tissues.[98] Because the risk of wound

complications is then much greater, fascial closure of abdominal incisions should be performed with nonabsorbable, monofilament suture material. Similarly, in other patients in whom poor wound healing can be expected, such as those with severe trauma, jaundice, or diabetes and those receiving antineoplastic drug therapy, absorbable suture material should be avoided.

Since oxygen tension in the wound affects the rate of healing,[105] it is particularly important for the surgeon to prevent hypovolemia and hypoxia and to avoid strangulation of tissue by sutures tied too tightly or placed under too much tension by excess intra-abdominal pressure. Careful management of the airway by the anesthesiologist during extubation will minimize paroxysmal coughing and straining at that time.[101] Intestinal decompression by either nasogastric or gastrostomy tube is recommended to prevent postoperative vomiting and distention whenever postoperative ileus is anticipated.

Prosthetic material to avoid excess suture-line tension is rarely needed in pediatric surgical patients, but it can be lifesaving in special situations.[102]

The choice of suture material, incision, and suture technique can be critical in the patient at risk for wound complications. The lowest rate of dehiscence in the Children's Memorial Hospital series was found in transverse and gridiron-type incisions.[88] Experimental data support this clinical experience.[111] These incisions, which are well suited to the broad abdomen of the infant and child, are therefore recommended when feasible. The weakest of all incisions, the muscle-splitting paramedian incision, is mentioned only to be condemned.

Relative merits of the various types of sutures have recently been reviewed.[90, 113] Despite the disadvantage of a requirement for multiple knots, thin-gauge monofilament synthetic suture (polypropylene) is thought to be best in the contaminated or otherwise at-risk wound because it resists infection, produces minimal tissue reaction, infrequently causes sinus formation, and maintains its strength.[94] Chromic catgut has been shown to be unsatisfactory in such wounds because its integrity is affected by local vascularity and infection and because, even under ideal conditions, 50 per cent of its tensile strength is lost by 14 days. Unlike chromic catgut, polyglycolic acid suture is hydrolyzed and is therefore not as subject to premature absorption, but it loses its tensile strength almost as rapidly as chromic. In adult series, closure with this suture has been shown to compare favorably in terms of incidence of wound dehiscence, sinus formation, and incisional hernia with other reported series.[85] However, it is doubtful whether polyglycolic acid suture will retain adequate strength to support an abdominal incision when healing is grossly impaired.

The halstedian concept of placing many sutures close to the wound edge has been challenged as the best technique for closure of the tenuous wound on the basis of experimental evidence of collagen dissolution near the fascial edge[84] and the clinical results obtained with nonabsorbable ligatures placed more than 5 mm from the fascial edge to approximate the fascial edges in a near-far figure-of-eight fashion.[103] *The main drawback of this technique is the tendency of the inexperienced surgeon to make the sutures too tight and strangulate the tissue.* Retention sutures are preferred by some surgeons despite the disadvantages of pain, difficulty in adjusting tension, scarring, and lack of guarantee against dehiscence. It is not clear whether these sutures offer any advantage over the "internal retention" sutures described earlier.

Since infection interferes with healing, prevention of wound infection is a priority. Burke recommends preoperative administration of antibiotics if there is a high probability that a patient's natural resistance to bacterial invasion will not overcome the combined bacterial and physiologic challenge of a surgical procedure.[86]

Normovolemic, mild to moderate anemia in otherwise healthy individuals does not impair delivery of oxygen to the wound and is of no consequence in wound healing.[95] In a patient with severe anemia or in a compromised patient with limited cardiac reserve, hypovolemia, or malnutrition, preoperative correction of anemia is indicated.

Complications

COMPLETE WOUND DEHISCENCE

This dread complication typically occurs by the fifth to eighth postoperative day in patients in whom a healing ridge has not developed.[107] In many patients a sudden serosanguineous drainage is noted. In others whose superficial tissues have remained intact, there may be unexplained prolongation of ileus. When dehiscence is suspected, one or two sutures should be removed to confirm the diagnosis. If dehiscence is present, the patient should be taken to the operating room for removal of the remaining sutures, débridement and irrigation of the wound, and formal all-layer closure of the incision using either far-near figure-of-eight monofilament synthetic sutures or retention sutures. If wound infection is present, the soft tissues should be packed open and an occlusive dressing applied. The dressing should not be removed until the fourth or fifth day, when delayed primary closure is performed.[87, 91] If infection is still evident, frequent dressing changes are begun. If retention sutures are used, tension must be readjusted as needed to prevent excessive tightness or laxity. They can be removed after 14 to 21 days, depending on when a healing ridge is well established.

INCISIONAL OR VENTRAL HERNIA

The incidence of incisional hernia is 10 per cent after wound infection and greater than 30 per cent after dehiscence. The basic principles of management are as follows:

1. Repair is delayed for at least 1 year following resolution of all infection.

2. Antibiotics specific for the original infection are begun preoperatively.

3. For large hernias, preoperative intestinal decompression is carried out. For very large hernias, preoperative progressive pneumoperitoneum has its adherents.[108, 112]

4. At surgery, the hernia ring is excised and a search is made for associated defects.

5. Primary closure with all-layer, nonabsorbable, monofilament synthetic sutures is performed. If closure cannot be achieved in this manner without excessive tension on the suture line, relaxing incisions in the rectus fascia can be made. Rarely, fascia lata or prosthetic material has to be used in the closure. Moazam et al. have reported leaving Teflon mesh in for long periods.[104] In

most cases it would seem preferable to employ the staged closure advocated by Schuster in which the prosthetic sac is sequentially excised. This procedure was required in five of the 18 patients with ventral hernia described in the Children's Hospital Medical Center, Boston, review of anterior abdominal wall defects.[110] A layer of polyethylene film is placed between viscera and the Teflon mesh.[109]

Long-term implantation of prosthetic material in children may be carcinogenic.[106]

References

Omphalocele and Gastroschisis

1. Aaronson, I. A., and Eckstein, H. B.: The role of Silastic prosthesis in the management of gastroschisis. Arch. Surg. 112:297, 1977.
2. Ahlfeld, F.: Alkohol bei der Behandlund inoperabeler Bauchbruchen. Monatsschr. Geburtshilfe Gynakol. 10:124, 1899.
3. Allen, R. G., and Wrenn, E. L.: Silon as a sac in the treatment of omphalocele and gastroschisis. J. Pediatr. Surg. 4:3, 1969.
4. Bayston, R.: The antibacterial effects of impregnated Silastic and its possible applications in surgery. J. Pediatr. Surg. 12:55, 1977.
5. Carlton, G. R., Towne, B. H., Bryan, R. W., and Chang, J. H. T.: Obstruction of the suprahepatic inferior vena cava as a complication of giant omphalocele repair. J. Pediatr. Surg. 14:733, 1979.
6. Coupland, G. A. E.: Gastroschisis and colonic obstruction. Med. J. Aust. 1:344, 1969.
7. Fagan, D. G., Pritchard, J. S., Clarkson, T. W., and Greenwood, M. R.: Organic mercury levels in infants with omphalocele treated with organic mercurial antiseptic. Arch. Dis. Child. 52:962, 1977.
8. Firor, H. V.: Omphalocele — an appraisal of therapeutic approaches. Surgery 69:208, 1971.
9. Gilbert, M. G., Mencia, L. F., Puranik, S. R., et al.: Management of gastroschisis and short bowel: A report of 17 cases. J. Pediatr. Surg. 7:598, 1972.
10. Grob, M.: Lehrbuch der Kinderchirurgie. Stuttgart, Georg Thieme, 1957, p. 311.
11. Grob, M.: Conservative treatment of exomphalos. Arch. Dis. Child. 38:148, 1963.
12. Gross, R. E.: A new method for surgical treatment of large omphaloceles. Surgery 24:277, 1948.
13. Gutenberger, J. E., Miller, D. L., Dibbins, A. W., and Gitlin, D.: Hypogammaglobulinemia and hypoalbuminemia in neonates with ruptured omphaloceles and gastroschisis. J. Pediatr. Surg. 8:353, 1973.
14. Haller, J. A., Beat, H. K., Shaker, I. J., et al.: Studies of the pathophysiology of gastroschisis in fetal sheep. J. Pediatr. Surg. 9:627, 1974.
15. Hey, W.: Practical Observations in Surgery. London, Cadell and Davies, 1803, p. 266.
16. Hollabaugh, R. S., and Boles, E. T.: The management of gastroschisis. J. Pediatr. Surg. 8:263, 1973.
17. Mollitt, D. L., Ballantine, T. V. N., Grosfeld, J. L., and Quinter, P.: Critical assessment of fluid requirements in gastroschisis. J. Pediatr. Surg. 13:217, 1978.
18. Moore, T. C.: Gastroschisis and omphalocele: Clinical differences. Surgery 82:561, 1977.
19. O'Neill, J. A., and Grosfeld, J. L.: Intestinal malfunction after antenatal exposure of the viscera. Am. J. Surg. 127:129, 1974.
20. Othersen, H. B., Jr., and Hargest, T. S.: A pneumatic reduction device for gastroschisis and omphalocele. Surg. Gynecol. Obstet. 144:243, 1977.
21. Phillipart, A. R., Canty, T. G., and Filler, R. M.: Acute fluid volume requirements in infants and children with anterior abdominal wall defects. J. Pediatr. Surg., 7:553, 1972.
22. Raffensperger, J. G., and Jona, J. Z.: Gastroschisis. Surg. Gynecol. Obstet. 138:230, 1974.
23. Ravitch, M. M.: Surgical aphorisms. Res. Staff Phys. June 1972, p. 55.
24. Rubin, S. Z., and Ein, S. H.: Experience with 55 Silon pouches. J. Pediatr. Surg. 11:803, 1976.
25. Sang, K., Dorst, J. P., Dominguez, R., and Girdany, B. R.: Abnormal intestinal motility in gastroschisis. Radiology 127:457, 1978.
26. Schuster, S. R.: A new method for the staged repair of large omphaloceles. Surg. Gynecol. Obstet. 125:837, 1967.
27. Schuster, S. R.: Omphalocele, hernia of the umbilical cord and gastroschisis. In Ravitch, M. M., Welch, K. J., Benson, C. D., et al. (eds.): Pediatric Surgery. Chicago, Year Book Medical Publishers, 1979.
28. Schuster, S. R., Ballantine, T. V. N., and Smith, C. D.: Staged prosthetic closure of congenital abdominal wall defects: A twenty year review (in preparation).
29. Seashore, J. H., MacNaughton, R. J., and Talbert, J. T.: Treatment of gastroschisis and omphalocele with biologic dressings. J. Pediatr. Surg. 10:9, 1975.
30. Sherman, N. J., Asch, M. J., Isaacs, H., Jr., and Rosenkrantz, J. G.: Experimental gastroschisis in the fetal rabbit. J. Pediatr. Surg. 8:165, 1973.
31. Soave, F.: Treatment of giant omphalocele. Arch. Dis. Child. 38:130, 1963.
32. Talbert, J. L., Rodgers, B. M., and Moazam, F.: Surgical management of massive ventral hernias in children. J. Pediatr. Surg. 12:63, 1977.
33. Thompson, J., and Fonkalsrud, E. W.: Reappraisal of skin flap closure for neonatal gastroschisis. Arch. Surg. 111:684, 1976.
34. Touloukian, R. J., and Spackman, T. J.: Gastrointestinal function and radiologic appearance following gastroschisis repair. J. Pediatr. Surg. 6:427, 1971.

Inguinal Femoral and Umbilical Hernias

35. Boley, S. J., and Kleinhaus, S.: A place for the Cheatle-Henry approach in pediatric surgery? J. Pediatr. Surg. 1:394, 1966.

36. Chamberlain, J. W.: Anomalies and accidents complicating repair of inguinal hernias in infancy and childhood. Boston Med. Q. 7:23, 1956.

37. Clatworthy, H. W.: Special comment: Routine bilateral herniorrhaphy for infants and children. *In* Nyhus, L. M., and Condon, R. E. (eds.): Hernia. Philadelphia, J. B. Lippincott Co., 1978, p. 132.

38. Coran, A. G., and Eraklis, A. J.: Inguinal hernia in the Hurler-Hunter syndrome. Surgery 61:302, 1967.

39. DeBoer, A.: Inguinal hernia in infants and children. AMA Arch. Surg. 75:920, 1957.

40. Dombro, R. H.: The surgically ill child and his family. Surg. Clin. North Am. 50:759, 1970.

41. Fahlstrom, G., Holmberg, L., and Johannson, H.: Atrophy of the testis following operation upon the inguinal region in infants and children. Acta Chir. Scand. 126:221, 1963.

42. Ferguson, A.: Oblique inguinal hernia — typic operation for its radical cure. JAMA 33:6, 1899.

43. Fonkalsrud, E. W., deLorimier, A. A., and Clatworthy, H. W., Jr.: Femoral and direct hernias in infants and children. JAMA 192:597, 1965.

44. Fowler, R.: Special comment: Preperitoneal approach in childhood. *In* Nyhus, L. M., and Condon, R. E. (eds.): Hernia. Philadelphia, J. B. Lippincott Co., 1978.

45. Graff, T. D., Phillips, O. C., Benson, D. W., and Kelly, E.: Baltimore Anesthesia Study Committee: Factors in pediatric anesthesia mortality. Anesth. Analg. 43:407, 1964.

46. Grosfeld, J. L., and Cooney, D. R.: Inguinal hernia after ventriculoperitoneal shunt for hydrocephalus. J. Pediatr. Surg. 9:311, 1974.

47. Gross, R. E.: The Surgery of Infancy and Childhood. Philadelphia, W. B. Saunders Co., 1953, p. 461.

48. Harper, R. G., Garcia, A., and Sia, C.: Inguinal hernia: A common problem of premature infants weighing 1000 grams or less at birth. Pediatrics 56:112, 1975.

49. Heifetz, C. J., Bilsel, Z. T., and Gaus, W. W.: Observations on the disappearance of umbilical hernia in infancy and childhood. Surg. Gynecol. Obstet. 116:469, 1963.

50. Hill, M. R., Pollock, W. F., and Sprong, D. R.: Testicular infarction and incarcerated inguinal herniae. Arch. Surg. 85:351, 1962.

51. Hunt, T. K.: Disorders of repair and their management. *In* Hunt, T. K., and Dunphy, J. E. (eds.): Fundamentals of Wound Management. New York, Appleton-Century-Crofts, 1979, pp. 125–128.

52. Immordino, P. A.: Femoral hernia in infancy and childhood. J. Pediatr. Surg. 7:40, 1972.

53. Kaplan, G. W.: Iatrogenic cryptorchidism resulting from hernia repair. Surg. Gynecol. Obstet. 142:671, 1976.

54. Kiesewetter, W. B.: Hernias and hydroceles. Pediatr. Clin. North Am. 6:1129, 1959.

55. Kurlan, M. Z., Wels, P. B., and Piedad, O. H.: Inguinal herniorrhaphy by the Mitchell Banks technique. J. Pediatr. Surg. 7:427, 1972.

56. Lickley, H. L. A., and Trusler, G. A.: Femoral hernia in children. J. Pediatr. Surg. 1:338, 1966.

57. Lukash, F., Zwiren, G. T., and Andrews, H. G.: Significance of absent vas deferens at hernia repair in infants and children. J. Pediatr. Surg. 10:765, 1975.

58. Lynn, H. B., and Johnson, W. W.: Inguinal herniorrhaphy in children. Arch. Surg. 83:573, 1961.

59. McEntyre, R. L., and Raffensperger, J. G.: Surgical complications of Ehlers-Danlos syndrome in children. J. Pediatr. Surg. 12:531, 1977.

60. Morris, L. L., Caldicott, W. J., and Savage, J. P.: Inguinal herniation of the ureter. Pediatr. Radiol. 6:107, 1977.

61. Nielsen, D. F., and Bulow, S.: The incidence of male hermaphroditism in girls with inguinal hernia. Surg. Gynecol. Obstet. 142:875, 1976.

62. Pergament, E., Heimler, A., and Shah, P.: Testicular feminization and inguinal hernia. Lancet 2:740, 1973.

63. Potts, W. J., Riker, W. L., and Lewis, J. E.: The treatment of inguinal hernias in infants and children. Ann. Surg. 132:566, 1950.

64. Priebe, C. J., Holahan, J. A., and Ziring, P. R.: Abnormalities of the vas deferens and epididymis in cryptorchid boys with congenital rubella. J. Pediatr. Surg. 14:834, 1979.

65. Puranik, S. R., Mencia, L. F., and Gilbert, M. G.: Artificial testicles in children: A new Silastic gel testicular prosthesis. J. Urol. 109:735, 1973.

66. Ravitch, M. M.: Repair of Hernias. Chicago, Year Book Medical Publishers, 1969, p. 83.

67. Rowe, M. I., and Clatworthy, H. W.: Incarcerated and strangulated hernias in children: A statistical study of high risk factors. Arch. Surg. 101:136, 1970.

68. Shandling, B., and Thomson, S.: The Cheatle-Henry approach for inguinal herniotomy in infants and children: The Hospital for Sick Children, Toronto. Can. J. Surg. 6:484, 1963.

69. Shaw, A., and Santulli, T. V.: Management of sliding hernias of the urinary bladder in infants. Surg. Gynecol. Obstet. 124:1314, 1967.

70. Sibley, W. L., III, Lynn, H. B., and Harris, L. E.: A twenty-five year study of infantile umbilical hernia. Surgery 55:462, 1964.

71. Silber, S. J.: Microscopic technique for reversal of vasectomy. Surg. Gynecol. Obstet. 143:630, 1976.

72. Silber, S. J.: Perfect anatomic reconstruction of vas deferens with microscopic surgical technique. Fertil. Steril. 28:72, 1977.

73. Silber, S. J.: Microsurgery of the male genitalia: Non-vascular. *In* Silber, S. J. (ed.): Microsurgery. Baltimore, Williams & Wilkins Co., 1979, p. 367.

74. Silber, S. J., Galle, J., and Friend, D.: Microscopic vasovasostomy and spermatogenesis. J. Urol. 117:299, 1977.

75. Silber, S. J., and Kelly, J.: Successful autotransplantation of an intra-abdominal testis to the scrotum by microvascular technique. J. Urol. 115:452, 1976.

76. Snyder, W. H., Jr., and Greaney, E. M., Jr.: Inguinal hernias. *In* Mustard, W. T., Ravitch, M. M., Snyder, W. H., Jr., et al. (eds.): Pediatric Surgery. Chicago, Year Book Medical Publishers, 1969, p. 704.

77. Soper, R. T., Hendren, W. H., III, Johnson, D. G., and Randolph, J. G.: Hernia management in newborns and children. Contemp. Surg. 3:102, 1973.

78. Sparkman, R. S.: Bilateral exploration in inguinal hernia in juvenile patients. Surgery 51:393, 1962.

79. Stevenson, J. K., and Johnson, L. P.: Groin hernias in infants and children. *In* Nyhus, L. M., and Harkins, H. N. (eds.): Hernia. Philadelphia, J. B. Lippincott Co., 1964.

80. Welch, K. J.: Orchiopexy: A new anchoring technique, window septopexy. J. Pediatr. Surg. 7:163, 1972.

81. White, J. J., and Haller, J. A.: Groin hernia in infants and children. *In* Nyhus, L. M., and Condon, R. E. (eds.): Hernia. Philadelphia, J. B. Lippincott Co., 1978, p. 111.

82. Woolley, M. M.: Cryptorchidism. *In* Ravitch, M. M., Welch, K. J., Benson, C. D., et al. (eds.): Pediatric Surgery. Chicago, Year Book Medical Publishers, 1979, pp. 1406–1407.

83. Woolley, M. M., Morgan, S., and Hays, D. M.: Heritable disorders of connective tissue; surgical and anesthetic problems. J. Pediatr. Surg. 2:325, 1967.

Abdominal Wound Healing

84. Adamsons, R. J., Musco, F., and Enquist, I. F.: The chemical dimensions of a healing incision. Surg. Gynecol. Obstet. 23:515, 1966.

85. Bentley, P. G., Owen, W. G., Girolami, P. L., and Dawson, J. L.: Wound closure with Dexon (polyglycolic acid). Ann. R. Coll. Surg. 60:125, 1978.

86. Burke, J. F.: Infection. *In* Hunt, T. K., and Dunphy, J. E. (eds.): Fundamentals of Wound Management. New York, Appleton-Century-Crofts, 1979, p. 202.

87. Burke, J. F.: Infection. *In* Hunt, T. K., and Dunphy, J. E. (eds.): Fundamentals of Wound Management. New York, Appleton-Century-Crofts, 1979, pp. 214–216.

88. Campbell, D. P., and Swenson, O.: Wound dehiscence in infants and children. J. Pediatr. Surg. 7:123, 1972.

89. Ehrlich, H. P., Tarver, H., and Hunt, T. K.: The effects of vitamin A and glucocorticoids upon repair and collagen synthesis. Ann. Surg. 177:22, 1973.

90. Everett, W. G.: Sutures, incisions and anastomoses. Ann. R. Coll. Surg. 55:31, 1974.

91. Ferguson, C. C.: The abdominal parietes. *In* Ravitch, M. M., Welch, K. J., Benson, C. D., et al. (eds.): Pediatric Surgery. Chicago, Year Book Medical Publishers, 1979, p. 770.

92. Goligher, J. C., Irvin, T. T., Johnston, D., et al.: A controlled clinical trial of three methods of closure of laparotomy wounds. Br. J. Surg. 62:823, 1975.

93. Gross, R. E., and Ferguson, C. C.: Abdominal incisions in infants and children: A study of evisceration. Ann. Surg. 137:349, 1953.

94. Hermann, R. E.: Abdominal wall closure using a new polypropylene monofilament suture. Surg. Gynecol. Obstet. 138:84, 1974.

95. Heughan, C., Grislis, G., and Hunt, T. K.: The effect of anemia on wound healing. Ann. Surg. 179:163, 1974.

96. Hunt, T. K.: Disorders of repair and their management. *In* Hunt, T. K., and Dunphy, J. E. (eds.): Fundamentals of Wound Management. New York, Appleton-Century-Crofts, 1979, pp. 36–37.

97. Hunt, T. K.: Disorders of repair and their management. *In* Hunt, T. K., and Dunphy, J. E. (eds.): Fundamentals of Wound Management. New York, Appleton-Century-Crofts, 1979, pp. 77, 79.

98. Hunt, T. K.: Disorders of repair and their management. *In* Hunt, T. K., and Dunphy, J. E. (eds.): Fundamentals of Wound Management. New York, Appleton-Century-Crofts, 1979, pp. 92–94.

99. Hunt, T. K.: Personal communication.

100. Hunt, T. K., and Van Winkle, W., Jr.: Normal repair. *In* Hunt, T. K., and Dunphy, J. E. (eds.): Fundamentals of Wound Management. New York, Appleton-Century-Crofts, 1979, pp. 36–37.

101. Kewenter, J., Koch, N. G., and Lundberg, H.: Wound separation and intra-abdominal pressure. Acta Anesthesiol. Scand. 13:97, 1969.

102. Mathes, S. J., and Stone, H. H.: Acute traumatic losses of abdominal wall substance. J. Trauma 15:386, 1975.

103. McCallum, G. T., and Link, R. F.: The effect of closure techniques on abdominal disruption. Surg. Gynecol. Obstet. 119:75, 1964.

104. Moazam, F., Rodgers, B. M., and Talbert, J. L.: Use of Teflon mesh for repair of abdominal wall defects in neonates. J. Pediatr. Surg. 14:347, 1979.

105. Niinikoski, J.: Oxygen and wound healing. Clin. Plast. Surg. 4:361, 1977.

106. O'Connell, T. X., Fee, H. J., and Golding, A.: Sarcoma associated with Dacron prosthesis material — case report and review of the literature. J. Thorac. Cardiovasc. Surg. 72:94, 1976.

107. Pareira, M. D., and Serkes, K. D.: Prediction of wound disruption by use of the healing ridge. Surg. Gynecol. Obstet. 115:72, 1962.

108. Ravitch, M. M.: Omphalocele: Secondary repair with the aid of pneumoperitoneum. Arch. Surg. 99:166, 1969.

109. Schuster, S. R.: Omphalocele, hernia of the umbilical cord and gastroschisis. *In* Ravitch, M. M., Welch, K. J., Benson, C. D., et al. (eds.): Pediatric Surgery. Chicago, Year Book Medical Publishers, 1979, pp. 789–793.

110. Schuster, S. R., Ballentine, T. V. N., and Smith, C. D.: Staged prosthetic closure of congenital

abdominal wall defects: A twenty year review (in preparation).

111. Seidel, W., Tauber, R., and Hoffschulte, K. H.: Messungen zur Festigkeit der Bauchdeckennaht. (Measurements of tensile strength of sutured abdominal incisions.) Chirurg 45:266, 1974.

112. Talbert, J. L., Rodgers, B. M., and Moazam, F.: Surgical management of massive ventral her-nias in children. J. Pediatr. Surg. 12:63, 1977.

113. Van Winkle, W., Jr., and Hastings, J. C.: Choice of suture materials for various tissues. Surg. Gynecol. Obstet. 135:113, 1972.

114. Warnig, P., and Fischer, M.: Postoperative de-fects of wound healing and blood coagula-tion in pediatric surgery. Acta Chir. Aust. 6:S1, 1974.

PERITONEAL CAVITY

Bradley M. Rodgers, M.D.

Intraperitoneal complications of abdominal surgery in children continue to cause significant morbidity and mortality despite increased awareness of the importance of peritoneal toilet and use of antibiotics. Indeed, postoperative peritonitis in infants is associated with a greater mortality than that encountered in adults.[20] A thorough understanding of the pertinent anatomy and pathophysiology as well as early recognition and therapy of these catastrophes is essential to achieve a successful outcome.

ANATOMY

The peritoneal cavity is divided into three major anatomic regions: In the upper abdomen the lesser sac occupies the major proportion; the midabdomen is considered the "general" peritoneal cavity; and in the lower abdomen the pelvis is considered as a separate anatomic area. The peritoneum itself is composed of a single layer of flat mesothelial cells resting on a layer of highly vascular, loose areolar tissue. The entire peritoneal cavity is lined by the parietal peritoneum, while the extension of this layer over the abdominal viscera and mesentery is termed the visceral peritoneum. The total surface area of the peritoneal layer approximates that of the skin[11] and, thus, plays the role of an extremely important membrane in the fluid shifts encountered in peritonitis. Innervation is most rich to the parietal peritoneum, permitting localization of areas of irritation. The visceral peritoneum receives innervation only from the autonomic nervous system. Visceral pain is poorly localized and often perceived only as a midabdominal ache or colic. The peritoneal cavity usually contains a small amount of clear fluid, serving to lubricate abdominal viscera. The peritoneal membrane allows bidirectional trans-

port of fluid; therefore, the peritoneal cavity should be considered a component of the extracellular fluid compartment. Larger molecules such as albumin are freely transported across the peritoneal membrane.[7] This movement of fluid and chemicals across the peritoneal membrane assumes great importance in the absorption of endogenous and exogenous toxins and intraperitoneally administered antibiotics.

The peritoneum is uniquely capable of regeneration. Large defects in the peritoneum are renewed by transformation of the underlying mesothelial cells in addition to ingrowth of cells from the perimeter of the injury.[9] Rapid healing of peritoneal defects is a major preventative of adhesion formation. Fibrinous exudate on the peritoneal surface, stimulated either by peritonitis or operative insult, leads to the ingrowth of collagenous tissue and the formation of fibrous adhesions.

PHYSIOLOGY

The peritoneum responds to most types of injury in a predictable fashion. The initial alteration is vasodilatation and hyperemia of the vascular connective tissue beneath the mesothelial layer, followed by a transudation of fluid and leukocytes onto the peritoneal surface. The edema formed in the region of acute inflammation impairs, but does not completely interrupt, the absorption of peritoneal fluid and toxins. Continued inflammation permits loss of protein-rich fluid into the peritoneal cavity.[13] The fibrin contained within this exudate causes agglutination of the intraperitoneal structures in the region of inflammation and, in most cases, helps to limit the spread of this inflammation. These primary peritoneal responses to injury, if sufficiently severe and prolonged, lead to secondary systemic responses to peritonitis. The principal mechanism of these secondary responses appears to be a decrease in extracellular volume as a consequence of accumulation of edema and free peritoneal fluid. Although systemic responses to severe peritonitis in children have not been thoroughly evaluated, they appear to be aimed at maintenance of extracellular volume and adequate tissue perfusion. An adrenal medullary response, with release of catecholamines, causes peripheral vasoconstriction and maintenance of systemic blood pressure. The adrenal cortex responds by secretion of aldosterone in an attempt to preserve extracellular volume. The increased metabolic demands associated with peritoneal inflammation occur at a time when the cardiopulmonary system may be sufficiently compromised as to be unable to provide for increase in tissue oxygen demands. The resultant shift to anaerobic metabolism permits accumulation of lactic acid and the development of metabolic acidosis.[7]

CLINICAL PRESENTATION

The clinical manifestations of peritonitis vary considerably, depending upon the etiology and the location of the peritoneal inflammation. In the postoperative state, many of the clinical and laboratory manifestions may be masked by changes resulting from operation. Abdominal pain, which almost always accompanies acute peritonitis, is usually more severe than that experienced from the surgical incision alone and may be referred to areas distant from the operative field. The pain of peritonitis is usually maximal in the area most severely involved, but it may be quite diffuse. Ileus associated with peritonitis often exceeds the expected duration of postoperative ileus and leads to anorexia and abdominal distention. The onset of peritonitis in children is usually accompanied by a spiking fever. Laboratory evaluation of a child with postoperative peritonitis will usually show an increase in the leukocyte count, with a left shift in the differential, suggesting an acute inflammation. Serum electrolyte determinations may reveal a hypernatremia due to loss of sodium-poor fluids into the peritoneal cavity.

The radiologic changes in early peritonitis may be subtle, often limited to mild intestinal distention suggesting a paralytic ileus. In more advanced states, evidence of free peritoneal fluid with separation of bowel loops (Fig. 18–1), air-fluid levels (Fig. 18–2), or excessive free intraperitoneal air (Fig. 18–3) may be observed. Following surgery, all of the findings must be interpreted in light of expected postoperative radiographic changes, including the normal postoperative pneumoperitoneum, which may persist for 5 to 7 days in children. Barium contrast radiographs may assist in the localization of abscess accumulations in the upper abdomen or pelvis (Figs. 18–2 and 18–4). Recently abdominal ultrasound and computed tomography have been used to identify abnormal intra-abdominal fluid collections.[15, 16]

Usually diagnosis of an early postoperative peritoneal complication may be made on the basis of a high index of clinical suspicion and physical findings; laboratory evidence may be quite delayed. Any interruption of the expected postoperative recovery, any deterioration of the child's clinical condition, and any delay in resumption of normal intestinal function should raise the suspicion of intraperitoneal complications.

ACUTE GENERALIZED POSTOPERATIVE PERITONITIS

The peritoneal cavity usually recovers rapidly from routine operative trauma. Gentle handling of the abdominal viscera during laparotomy minimizes the injury to the peritoneal membrane and results in a relatively short period of postoperative ileus. Generalized peritonitis is occasionally seen as a postoperative complication in children, as a consequence of either inadequate peritoneal toilet at the time of surgery or anastomotic breakdown. The bacterial organisms encountered in postoperative peritonitis will vary, depending upon the level of the contaminating source. Bell and associates evaluated the contaminating organisms encountered in infants with necrotizing enterocolitis and recovered *Escherichia coli* and *Klebsiella pneumoniae* from both gastric and fecal cultures,[5] a somewhat different

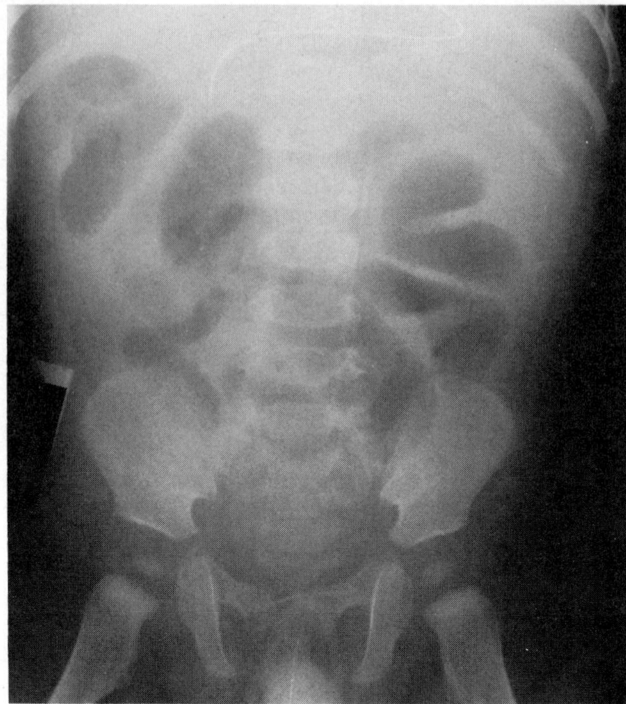

Figure 18–1   Flat abdominal radiograph of a 7-month-old boy suffering intestinal infarction and perforation 24 hours after operative reduction of an ileocolic intussusception. Separation of air-filled loops of bowel indicates intraperitoneal fluid.

bacterial spectrum from that usually encountered in the adult patient. These findings emphasize the importance of obtaining both aerobic and anaerobic cultures at the time of the initial surgery. The results of inadequately treated bacterial contamination of the peritoneal cavity vary under different circumstances and clearly depend upon more than the size of the bacterial inoculum. The presence of intraperitoneal adjuvants such as hemoglobin, bile, and fibrin significantly increases the virulence of these bacteria.[2, 12] In addition, simultaneous contamination with both anaerobic and aerobic organisms appears to enhance the virulence of anaerobic organisms.[3, 18, 23]

The probability of developing complications and mortality from postoperative generalized peritonitis increases with the duration of peritoneal contamination. It therefore becomes paramount to detect this catastrophe at the earliest possible moment and to institute appropriate therapy. Generalized peritonitis is most commonly seen between the third and seventh postoperative days. In the small infant, unable to complain of peritoneal pain, this complication is manifested by an interruption of the normal postoperative recovery with fever, increasing abdominal tenderness, and distention. The older patient may complain of inordinate abdominal pain, usually poorly localized and unlike incisional pain. The presence of fever and mounting leukocytosis should increase the suspicion. On physical examination generalized abdominal tenderness and guarding are found.

The therapy of generalized peritonitis depends upon the etiology. Mild forms, not associated with continued intraperitoneal contamination, may respond to the administration of intravenous antibiotics. The appropriate choice of antibiotics depends upon the source of peritoneal contamination and the results of intraoperative cultures. Contamination from the proximal gastrointestinal tract or biliary system will involve organisms generally sensitive to penicillin and the aminoglycosides. We prefer to use ampicillin and gentamycin. Contamination from the distal gastrointestinal tract usually results in heavier contamination with penicillin-resistant anaerobic organisms, particularly *Bacteroides fragilis,* and requires the addition of clindamycin or a cephalosporin.

More severe postoperative peritonitis, particularly that associated with continued

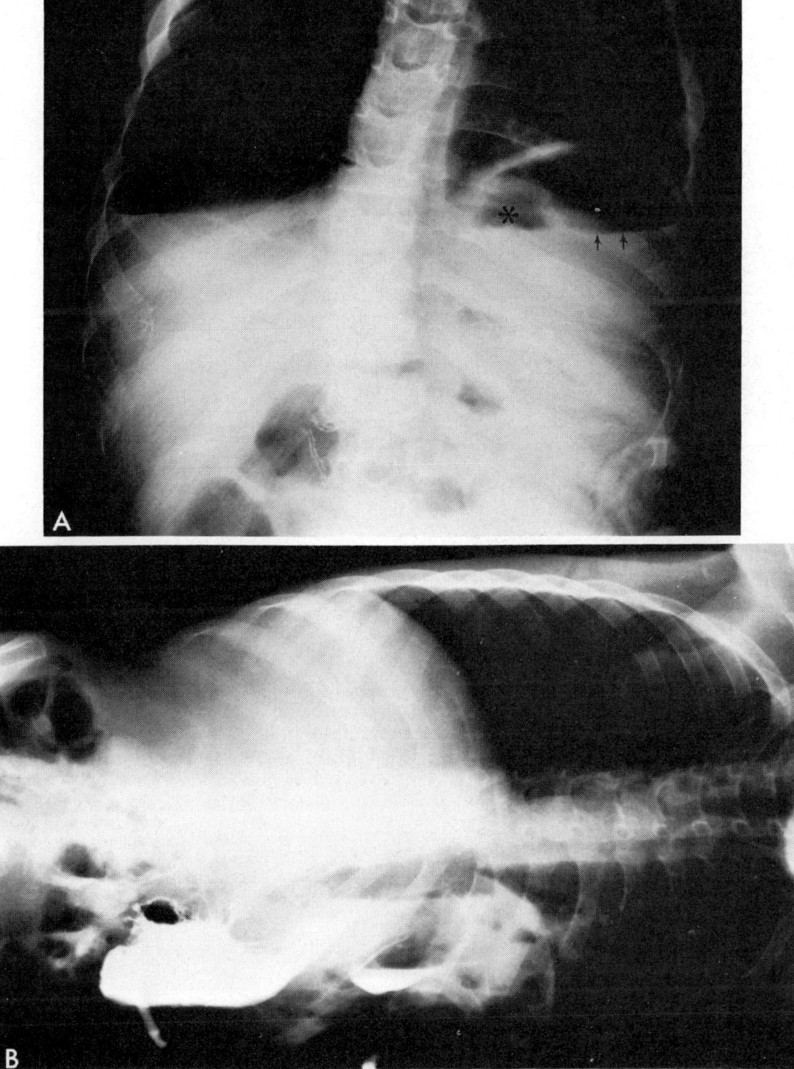

Figure 18–2 *A,* Upright abdominal radiograph of a 17-year-old retarded girl with fever and ileus 4 days following a duodenojejunostomy and gastrostomy performed for superior mesenteric artery syndrome. A large air-fluid level is evident in the left upper quadrant (arrows) lateral to the stomach bubble (asterisk). *B,* In the decubitus position, instillation of barium through the gastrostomy identifies a perforation at the esophagogastric junction and a large left subphrenic abscess. Control of the perforation and drainage of the abscess were accomplished by a transperitoneal approach.

contamination from anastomotic leakage, demands immediate surgical intervention. Once the source of contamination has been controlled, the peritoneal cavity should be irrigated copiously with warmed saline solution. Recently, irrigating solutions containing various antimicrobial agents have been used.[8, 10, 21] Some authors have recommended using povidone-iodine solution for peritoneal irrigation. Most evidence suggests that this agent is minimally effective and may even increase peritoneal irritation.[17]

Meticulous surgical debridement of all fibrinous exudate within the peritoneal cavity has been recommended as important in controlling postoperative peritonitis in adults.[14] Recent evidence, however, suggests that this difficult and prolonged dissection does not increase survival.[19]

Postoperative drains should be reserved for complications associated with abscess formation. Postoperative abdominal cavity irrigation with antibiotic solution in cases of generalized peritonitis has been recom-

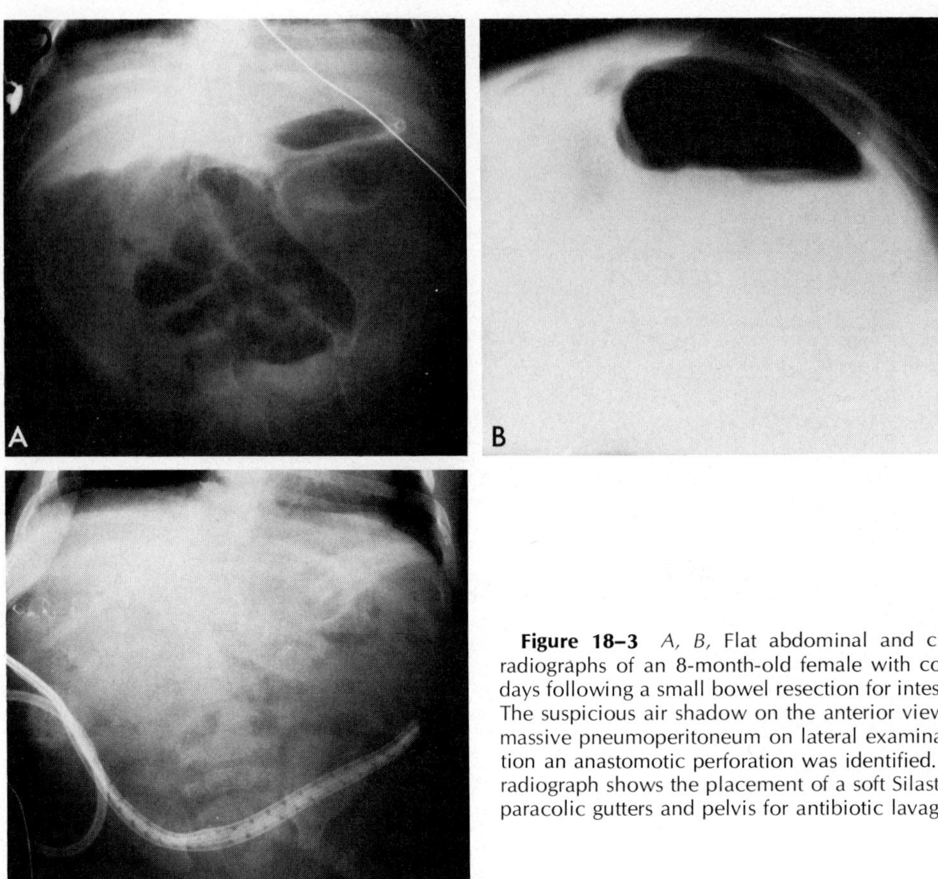

Figure 18–3 *A, B,* Flat abdominal and cross-table lateral radiographs of an 8-month-old female with continued sepsis 5 days following a small bowel resection for intestinal obstruction. The suspicious air shadow on the anterior view is confirmed as massive pneumoperitoneum on lateral examination. At exploration an anastomotic perforation was identified. *C,* Postoperative radiograph shows the placement of a soft Silastic catheter in the paracolic gutters and pelvis for antibiotic lavage.

mended by many authors and should be considered in selected patients with severe contamination.[22] Soft Silastic drains placed in the lateral abdominal gutters or pelvis allow thorough irrigation of the peritoneal cavity for 1 to 2 days postoperatively (Fig. 18–3*C*). Later the drain tracts become relatively isolated by fibrinous exudate and irrigations are less efficacious.

A special type of postoperative generalized peritonitis is the chemical peritonitis associated with contamination from secretions of the stomach, biliary tract, or pancreas. Contamination by these secretions is usually not associated with bacterial organisms. The initial injury is due to chemical irritation with an inflammatory response. Management of this type of peritonitis is similar to that of other forms except that early operative intervention with control of the site of leakage and drainage is more urgent. Antibiotics are administered to avoid secondary infection in the contaminated peritoneal compartments of the upper abdomen.

INTRA-ABDOMINAL ABSCESSES

Postoperative peritonitis, when successfully contained by host defense mechanisms, may resolve into an intra-abdominal abscess. Loculations of purulent fluid generally occur in areas anatomically most dependent, such as the pelvis and the subphrenic, subhepatic, or paracolic space.[4] The development of an intraperitoneal abscess often occurs after a brief period of

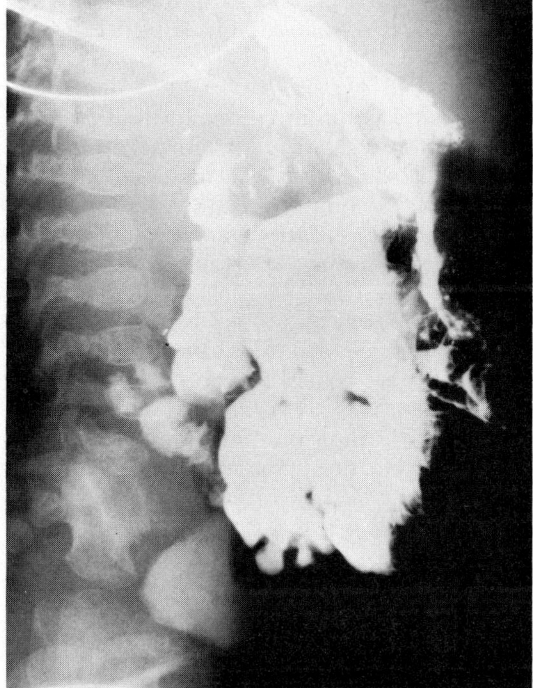

Figure 18–4 Lateral radiograph of an upper intestinal barium study of a 2-month-old male with fever 4 weeks following a near-total pancreatectomy for nesidioblastosis. An abscess in the lesser peritoneal sac is evident with displacement of the stomach anteriorly.

clinical improvement, and this complication is detected somewhat later than is generalized peritonitis. The anatomy of the peritoneal cavity is such that inflammation or leakage from certain organs tends to produce intra-abdominal abscesses in characteristic locations. Understanding of the pathology of upper abdominal abscesses has changed considerably in the past decade owing to more precise knowledge concerning the suspensory ligaments of the right lobe of the liver. Recognition that the triangular and coronary ligaments of the liver attach posteriorly rather than superiorly permits identification of a single right subphrenic space and a right subhepatic space.[6]

Gastric Operations

Postoperative complications from gastric procedures usually result in abscesses in the right subphrenic, right subhepatic, or left subphrenic space (Fig. 18–2). The most common cause of such abscesses in pediatric patients is leakage from a gastric suture line. Inadvertent perforation of the distal esophagus or fundus of the stomach during the performance of a fundoplication may lead to fluid accumulation and abscess formation in the left subphrenic space. Undetected mucosal perforations following pyloromyotomy usually result in abscesses of the right subhepatic space. Because of their etiology, most of these abscesses are associated with continued contamination and require early surgical intervention for successful management. Although the empty stomach of a child normally contains scant microorganisms, the abscesses are quickly invaded by oral microflora, particularly staphylococci and aerobic and anaerobic streptococci. The clinical manifestations of these abscesses in the upper abdomen may be minimal, and their detection is often difficult. Abdominal x-rays may reveal an air-fluid level or a sympathetic pleural effusion (Fig. 18–2). Fluoroscopy may reveal paresis of the involved hemidiaphragm. The expanded use of abdominal ultrasound and computed tomography has significantly enhanced the ability to diagnose abscesses in the abdominal cavity, and these studies should be performed at the time of earliest suspicion. Drainage of abscesses in the left subphrenic space may be accomplished through a retroperitoneal approach, resecting the twelfth rib. This approach may be quite successfully employed for isolated left subphrenic abscesses, such as might be encountered following a splenectomy. On the other hand, with gastric contamination, left subphrenic abscesses may frequently be accompanied by an abscess within the lesser sac, which cannot be adequately drained extraperitoneally. In this situation, an upper abdominal, transperitoneal incision should be employed.

Right subhepatic and subphrenic abscesses may also be drained following a retroperitoneal approach, resecting the eleventh or twelfth rib. However, their frequent association with multiple intra-abdominal abscesses makes the transperitoneal approach preferable.

Biliary Tract

Complications following operations upon the biliary tract and liver usually involve the right subhepatic space. In small children, abscesses in this area most commonly are encountered following operations for biliary atresia or choledochal cysts. In older children, they may be encountered after liver resection for trauma or tumors. Although bile is usually sterile initially, the peritoneal irritation caused by bile leakage results in considerable fluid accumulation, which quickly becomes secondarily infected with upper intestinal organisms. The bacteria most commonly isolated from these right subhepatic abscesses are *E. coli* and *Klebsiella*. Anaerobic organisms are encountered less frequently. The clinical signs of a right subhepatic abscess include upper abdominal tenderness and fullness. Laboratory tests may reveal an elevated serum bilirubin level and, with partial or complete biliary obstruction, elevation of alkaline phosphatase level. Plain abdominal radiographs may demonstrate displacement of air-filled abdominal viscera and a upper intestinal barium contrast study may show inferior displacement of the stomach and duodenum. Abscesses in the right subhepatic space can usually be well delineated by abdominal ultrasound. Intraperitoneal abscesses developing from bile leakage are associated with a very high mortality in children. Early transperitoneal drainage

and control of the source of contamination are mandatory.

Pancreas

Abscesses seen following pancreatic operations or pancreatic trauma usually involve the lesser peritoneal sac. These abscesses are polymicrobial and fecal flora, particularly *E. coli,* are found. There may be very few physical findings. In addition to fever and leukocytosis there may be an elevation of serum and urinary amylase levels. Abscesses within the lesser peritoneal sac are best diagnosed by abdominal ultrasound. Upper intestinal barium radiographs, particularly with lateral projections, may demonstrate displacement of the stomach anteriorly (Fig. 18–4). As with biliary abscesses, pancreatic abscesses are associated with a high mortality in children and require early surgical intervention. Transperitoneal drainage with thorough debridement and irrigation of the lesser sac is indicated. An attempt should be made to control the area of pancreatic leakage, although this is frequently unsuccessful. Obstructions of the pancreatic duct are unusual in children. Drainage of the lesser peritoneal sac with soft Silastic catheters is usually sufficient to allow spontaneous closure of these fistulae.

Small Intestine

Complications subsequent to operations on the small intestine are usually associated with generalized peritonitis. In the later phase, interloop abscesses may form as the contamination is localized by fibrinous adhesions. These abscesses usually contain both aerobic and anaerobic organisms. Abdominal symptoms are usually quite vague and are of little help in localizing the areas of abscess formation. Abdominal radiographs may show displacement of air-filled viscera. Computed tomography is most helpful in localizing these abscesses. Once an interloop abscess has been identified, transperitoneal evacuation is necessary. Often these abscesses are multiple and thorough abdominal exploration is required. In the absence of continued contamination from the small intestine, external drains are not indicated.

Appendix

Postoperative abscesses following appendectomy are almost always associated with preoperative rupture and generalized peritoneal contamination. These abscesses may be insidious and may present in almost any abdominal location, yet they most commonly are found in the paracecal region or pelvis. These abscesses contain aerobic organisms (*E. coli* and enterococci) as well as anaerobes (*Bacteroides* and anaerobic streptococci). Clinical symptoms may include lower abdominal pain, dysuria, and tenesmus. Once mature, these abscesses can be palpated by careful rectal examination. Abdominal radiographs may demonstrate displacement of the viscera from the right lower quadrant or pelvis. Abdominal and pelvic ultrasound and computed tomography have been very successful in locating and defining the extent of these abscesses (Fig. 18–5). Mature and well-contained pelvic abscesses can be conveniently drained through the rectum or vagina in children. The placement of a small Foley catheter into the abscess cavity aids in continued evacuation and irrigation. Compound and complicated pelvic and right lower quadrant abscesses due to appendicitis require transabdominal evacuation and drainage.

Colon

Postoperative abscesses resulting from colonic procedures in children are most common following operations for Hirschsprung's disease. Leakage from the long suture line of a Duhamel operation or contamination along the muscular cuff following a Soave procedure usually leads to pelvic, muscular sleeve, or pericolic abscesses. These abscesses are heavily contaminated with fecal flora and contain both aerobic and anaerobic organisms. The physical

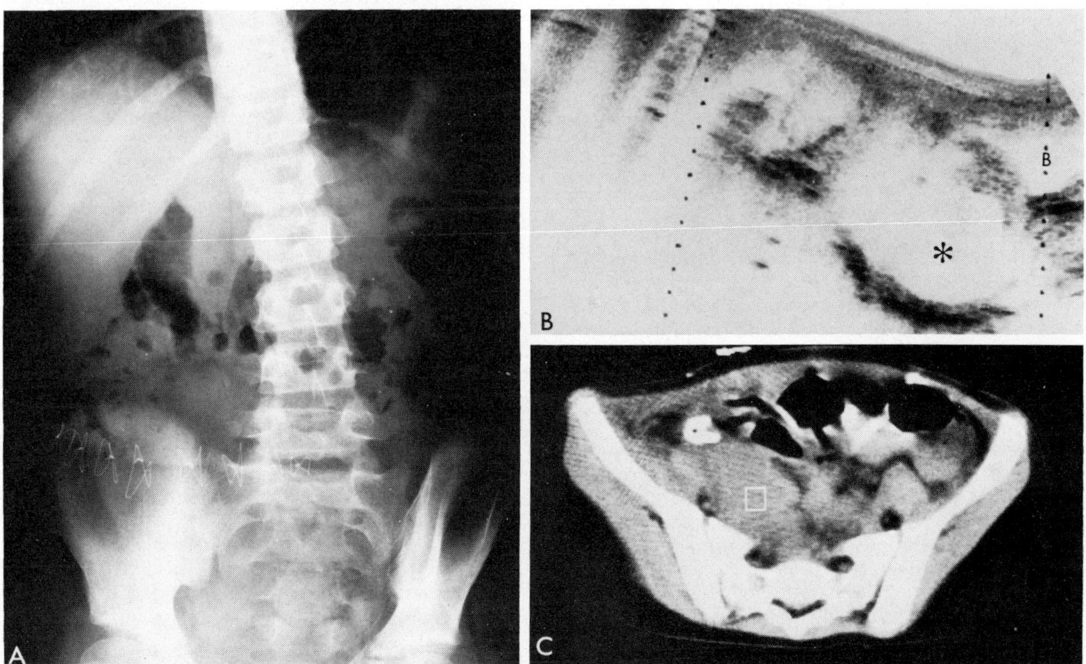

Figure 18–5   *A,* Flat abdominal radiograph of a 9-year-old female with fever and ileus 9 days following appendectomy for a ruptured appendix. A soft tissue density is noted in the right lower quadrant with right lumbar scoliosis. *B,* Longitudinal ultrasound study showing a large right paracecal and pelvic abscess (asterisk). (B, bladder). *C,* Computed tomography confirms a large paracecal abscess. Because of the extent of this lesion, transabdominal drainage was employed.

signs include lower abdominal pain and tenderness as well as tenesmus. Often there is an inordinate amount of pain on rectal examination and a mass may be palpated. Localization of these lesions is best achieved with abdominal ultrasound or computed tomography. Abscesses associated with continued colonic contamination carry a very high mortality and demand early operative intervention. Occasionally these lesions may be drained transrectally or through the perineum; however, most require transperitoneal exploration and drainage. Attempts at identification and control of the area of leakage are usually unsuccessful, and a proximal diverting colostomy should be performed. Pelvic drains should be placed to evacuate any residual space.

References

1. Ahrenholz, D. H., and Simmons, R. L.: Povidone-iodine in peritonitis. I. Adverse effect of local instillation in experimental *E. coli* peritonitis. J. Surg. Res. *26*:458, 1979.
2. Ahrenholz, D. H., and Simmons, R. L.: Fibrin in peritonitis: I. Beneficial and adverse effects of fibrin in experimental *E. coli* peritonitis. Surgery *88*:41, 1980.
3. Altemeier, W. A.: Bacterial flora of acute perforated appendicitis with peritonitis: Bacteriologic study based upon 100 cases. Ann. Surg. *107*:517, 1938.
4. Altemeier, W. A., Culbertson, W. R., and Fullen, W. D.: Intra-abdominal sepsis. Adv. Surg. *5*:281, 1971.
5. Bell, M. J., Shackelford, P., Feigin, R. D., et al.: Epidemiologic and bacteriologic evaluation of neonatal necrotizing enterocolitis. J. Pediatr. Surg. *14*:1, 1979.
6. Boyd, D. P.: The subphrenic spaces and the emperor's new robes. N. Engl. J. Med. *275*:911, 1966.
7. Condon, R. E.: Peritonitis and intraabdominal abscesses. *In* Schwartz, S. I., Shires, G. T., Spencer, F. C., and Storer, E. H. (eds): Principles of Surgery, 3rd edition. New York, McGraw-Hill Book Co., 1979, p. 1397.
8. DiVincenti, F. C., and Cohn, I., Jr.: Intraperitoneal kanamycin in advanced peritonitis. Am. J. Surg. *111*:147, 1966.
9. Eskeland, G.: Regeneration of parietal peritoneum in rats. I. A light microscopical study. Acta Pathol. Microbiol. Scand. *68*:353, 1966.
10. Fowler, R.: A controlled trial of intraperitoneal cephaloridine administration in peritonitis. J. Pediatr. Surg. *10*:43, 1975.
11. Hau, T., Ahrenholz, D. H., and Simmons, R. L.: Secondary bacterial peritonitis. The biological basis of treatment. Curr. Probl. Surg., *16*:1, 1979.
12. Hau, T., and Simmons, R. L.: Mechanisms of the adjuvant effect of hemoglobin in experimental peritonitis. III. The influence of hemoglobin on phagocytosis and intracellular killing by human granulocytes. Surgery *87*:588, 1980.
13. Hedberg, S., and Welch, E.: Suppurative peritonitis with major abscesses. *In* Hardy, J. D. (ed.): Critical Surgical Illness, 2nd edition. Philadelphia, W. B. Saunders Co., 1980, p. 423.
14. Hudspeth, A. S.: Radical surgical debridement in the treatment of advanced generalized bacterial peritonitis. Arch. Surg. *110*:1233, 1975.
15. Koehler, P. R., and Moss, A. A.: Diagnosis of intra-abdominal and pelvic abscesses by computerized tomography. J.A.M.A. *244*:49, 1980.
16. Korobkin, M., Callen, P. W., Filly, R. A., et al.: Comparison of computed tomography, ultrasonography and gallium-67 scanning in the evaluation of suspected abdominal abscess. Radiology *129*:89, 1978.
17. LaGarde, M. C., Bolton, J. S., and Cohn, I., Jr.: Intraperitoneal povidone-iodine in experimental peritonitis. Ann. Surg. *187*:613, 1978.
18. MacKowiak, P. A.: Microbial synergism in human infections. N. Engl. J. Med. *298*:21, 83, 1978.
19. Polk, H. C., Jr., and Fry, D. E.: Radical peritoneal debridement for established peritonitis. Ann. Surg. *192*:350, 1980.
20. Prevot, J., Grosdidier, G., and Schmitt, M.: Fatal peritonitis. Progr. Pediatr. Surg. *13*:257, 1979.
21. Sindelar, W. F., Mason, G. R.: Intraperitoneal irrigation with povidone-iodine solution for the prevention of intra-abdominal abscesses in the bacterially contaminated abdomen. Surg. Gynecol. Obstet. *148*:409, 1979.
22. Stephen, M., Lowenthal, J.: Continuing peritoneal lavage in high-risk peritonitis. Surgery *85*:603, 1979.
23. Stone, H. H., Kolb, L. D., and Geheber, C. E.: Incidence and significance of intraperitoneal anaerobic bacteria. Ann. Surg. *181*:705, 1975.

LIVER, GALLBLADDER, AND EXTRAHEPATIC BILE DUCTS

John R. Lilly, M.D.
Thomas E. Starzl, M.D., Ph.D.

Most operations upon the biliary tract in infants and children are done for congenital malformations rather than for acquired disease. Surgical complications, consequently, are often different and sometimes quite distinct from those encountered in adult patients. In contrast, the majority of liver operations in children are done for the same indications as in older patients, e.g., trauma, tumor. Complications are similar.

THE BILIARY SYSTEM

The principal malformations of the biliary system requiring surgical correction are biliary atresia, biliary hypoplasia, choledochal cyst (and Caroli's disease), and spontaneous perforation of the extrahepatic bile ducts. Landing has presented evidence indicating that the first three entities are simply different manifestations of a single disease.[17] Nevertheless, the operations for the individual conditions are so disparate that each is considered separately.

Biliary Atresia

Traditionally, biliary atresia has been separated into "correctable" and "noncorrectable" types. In the former, the extrahepatic bile duct is grossly patent in its proximal portion but atretic distally. Bile flow is blocked outside the liver. Operative relief of biliary obstruction is relatively straightforward. Biliary drainage is provided by Roux-en-Y choledochojejunostomy (in which the jejunum is anastomosed to the patent proximal bile duct) or by choledochoduodenostomy. In "noncorrectable" biliary atresia, the lumen of the proximal, and often the entire, extraphepatic bile duct is obliterated, and thus biliary obstruction is intrahepatic. Surgical correction is more complicated.

CORRECTABLE BILIARY ATRESIA

The distal extrahepatic bile duct is obliterated in patients with correctable biliary atresia. Contrary to what would be anticipated with longstanding obstruction, the intrahepatic biliary system is not dilated but is, in fact, hypoplastic (Fig. 19–1). Histologically and morphologically, the hepatic parenchymal changes are indistinguishable from those of noncorrectable biliary atresia. Because of intrahepatic disease, the postoperative course generally parallels that observed in patients with noncorrectable biliary atresia. The severity of complications is attested to in a survey conducted by the Surgical Section of the American Academy of Pediat-

This work was supported in part by research grants from the Veterans Administration, by grants AM-17260 and AM-07772 from the National Institutes of Health, and by grants RR-00051 and RR-00069 from the General Clinical Research Centers Program of the Division of Research Resources, National Institutes of Health.

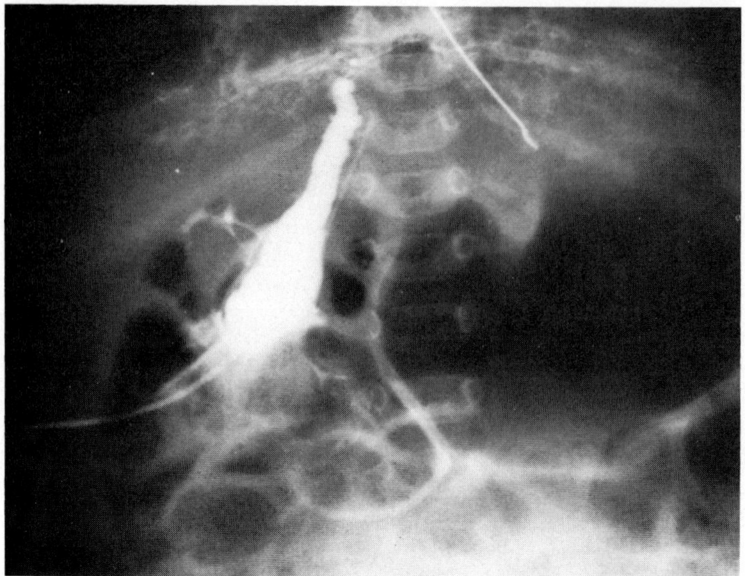

Figure 19–1 Operative cholecystogram in an infant with "correctable" biliary atresia. The gallbladder, cystic duct, and common hepatic ducts are open and communicate with the intrahepatic biliary system. The common bile duct is nonpatent. Note that the intrahepatic bile ducts (and common hepatic duct) are hypoplastic despite prolonged biliary obstruction. The patient was treated by cholecystojejunostomy (Roux-en-Y) by Dr. Dennis Shermeta and was well when last seen (6 months).

rics. Half of the patients with correctable biliary atresia were dead at the time of the report.[13]

One complication, anastomotic stricture, may be preventable. The distal end of the patent portion of the extrahepatic bile duct is almost always structurally abnormal and often lacks a mucosal surface. Intestinal anastomosis to this end may result in late anastomotic stricture. To avoid this complication, the intestinal anastomosis should be done not to the end of the patent bile duct, but to its proximal portion, at the liver hilus. In this location the duct is usually normal. In addition to anastomotic stricture, all the complications of noncorrectable biliary atresia described in the following section are encountered in patients with correctable biliary atresia, albeit usually in a less severe form.

NONCORRECTABLE BILIARY ATRESIA

Despite the connotation of atresia, the extrahepatic bile ducts are patent in most infants less than 2 months of age who have biliary atresia. The common hepatic duct contains a minute bile duct that communicates with the intrahepatic biliary tree. Sometime between the third and fourth months of life, patency of the residual duct is lost. The reason for the ongoing obliteration of the ductal system is that biliary atresia is not a true error of bile duct development but is instead a dynamic obliterative disease of the biliary tract. The concept of a progressive disease process is essential to understanding and treating the complications following corrective surgery for biliary atresia.

Corrective surgery is considered to be the operation described by Kasai and coworkers in which the fibrotic extrahepatic biliary tree is totally excised and bile drainage is established by anastomosis of an intestinal conduit to the liver hilus.[15] If the residual bile duct is still patent, bile drains from the intrahepatic biliary system into the interposed bowel. In time, an autoanastomosis presumably occurs between the transected bile duct and the intestinal mucosa. The diminutive caliber of this anastomosis is most likely responsible for the main complication of Kasai's operation, cholangitis. The operation is a major undertaking requiring extensive dissection of the portal triad. Operative technical intricacies are compounded in 10 to 20 per cent of patients by the presence of associated perihepatic intestinal and vascular anomalies such as a preduodenal portal vein (Fig. 19–2) and intestinal malrotation.[25] Incorporation of portal vein or hepatic artery adventitia or both is often required for the hilar anastomosis. The operation is hazardous, and intraoperative complications include injury to the hepatic arterial or portal venous system. Late problems include subphrenic abscess, biliary fistula, and intestinal anastomotic breakdown.

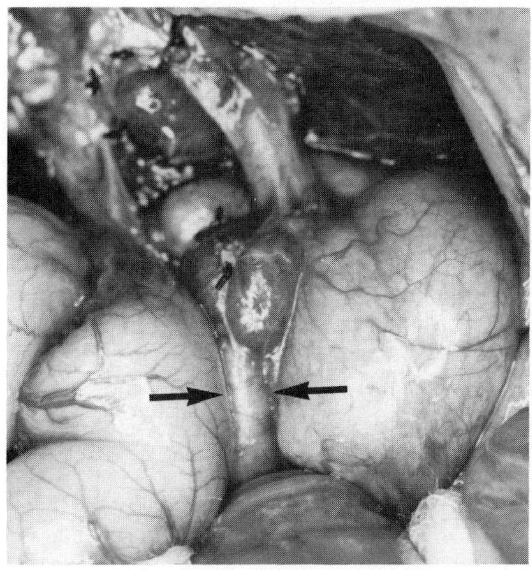

Figure 19–2 Operative photograph in an infant with biliary atresia and associated preduodenal portal vein *(arrows)*. The patient had no clinical signs of duodenal obstruction. A standard hepatic portoenterostomy procedure was done.

Early in our experience, a subphrenic abscess occurred in a patient secondary to a hilar bile leak. Because the abdominal bilioenteric exteriorization site was too small, bile drainage was impeded, causing a disruption of the hilar anastomosis. A deliberate effort is now made to make the intestinal conduit exteriorization site adequate in caliber. Other complications specific to Kasai's hepatic portoenterostomy operation are listed in Table 19–1 and described below.

Absence of Bile Flow. Failure of biliary drainage after operation indicates that the intrahepatic ductal system has not been surgically opened at the porta hepatis. The complication may stem from pre-existing total obliteration of the residual extrahepatic bile duct or from obstruction of the intrahepatic bile ducts. In either case, surgery has nothing to offer. However, postoperative absence of bile flow may be a consequence of too distal transection of the

TABLE 19–1 COMPLICATIONS OF HEPATIC PORTOENTEROSTOMY FOR BILIARY ATRESIA

Absence of bile drainage
Recurrent cholangitis
Progressive cirrhosis
Fat-soluble vitamin deficiency
Portal hypertension

common hepatic bile duct. Histologic verification of a microscopic bile duct in the most proximal portion of the surgical specimen is an essential requirement of the operation. Moreover, it is crucial that the residual bile duct (Fig. 19–3*A*) be distinguished from biliary glands (Fig. 19–3*B*) and collecting ductules of biliary glands (Fig. 19–3*C*) at the time of intraoperative histologic evaluation.[30] These glands and ductules do not communicate with the intrahepatic biliary system. In the absence of a true bile duct, operative exploration should be extended deeper into the porta hepatis.

Postoperative Cholangitis. In the Denver series, every patient in whom biliary obstruction was relieved and bile drainage was achieved by means of an intestinal conduit experienced recurrent cholangitis during the first postoperative year. The pathogenesis of the complication is unknown. Absence of cholangitis in patients who have undergone hepatic portocholecystostomy using the gallbladder, cystic duct, and common bile duct for the biliary conduit (Fig. 19–4) incriminates an "ascending" bacterial infection from the intestinal conduit.[20] If either a lymphatic[11] or a portal venous[6] mechanism were responsible, the incidence of cholangitis would be the same irrespective of the type of biliary reconstruction.

Cholangitis is characterized by an otherwise unexplained fever followed by decreased quality and quantity of bile drainage, leukocytosis, and finally a rise in serum bilirubin level. The keystone of treatment is the parenteral administration of aminoglycoside antibiotics. In recalcitrant cases, carbenicillin may also be required. Systemic steroid therapy is used if fever persists despite antibiotic administration.

Modification of Kasai's original operation (simple Roux-en-Y hepatic portoenterostomy) by exteriorization of the biliointestinal conduit lessens the severity and facilitates control of individual attacks of cholangitis. Most types of biliary reconstruction currently in use are designed to isolate the hilar anastomosis from the gastrointestinal tract (Fig. 19–4). Since the predisposition to cholangitis appears to be a consequence of a contaminated intestinal conduit[12] in immediate proximity to a partially obstructed intrahepatic biliary system, even trivial aggravation of bile flow from intestinal stasis triggers attacks of cholangitis.

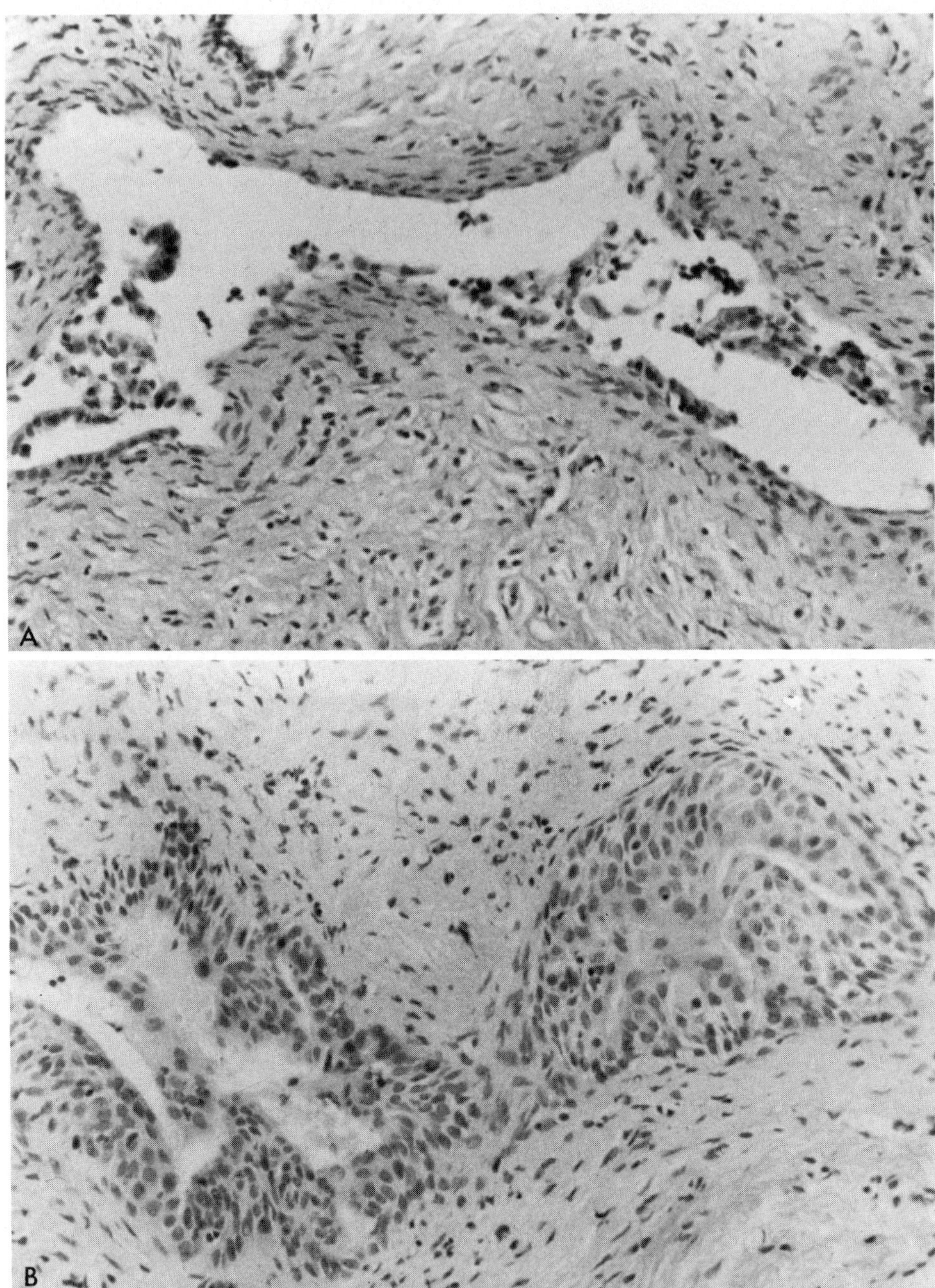

Figure 19–3 Biliary atresia. Histology of three different specimens of bile duct remnants at the porta hepatis. *A,* Bile duct: The lining cells are of flat columnar epithelium. There is partial epithelial ulceration and no evidence of cellular proliferation. An inflammatory reaction is present in the surrounding concentric layers of fibrous tissue. Bile is not present in the lumen in this case, but it is occasionally noted in other specimens containing a true bile duct. *B,* Biliary glands: Biliary glands are randomly distributed in the fibrous tissue. The glandular walls are exclusively lined by cuboidal epithelium. The lumen never contains bile.

Illustration continued on opposite page

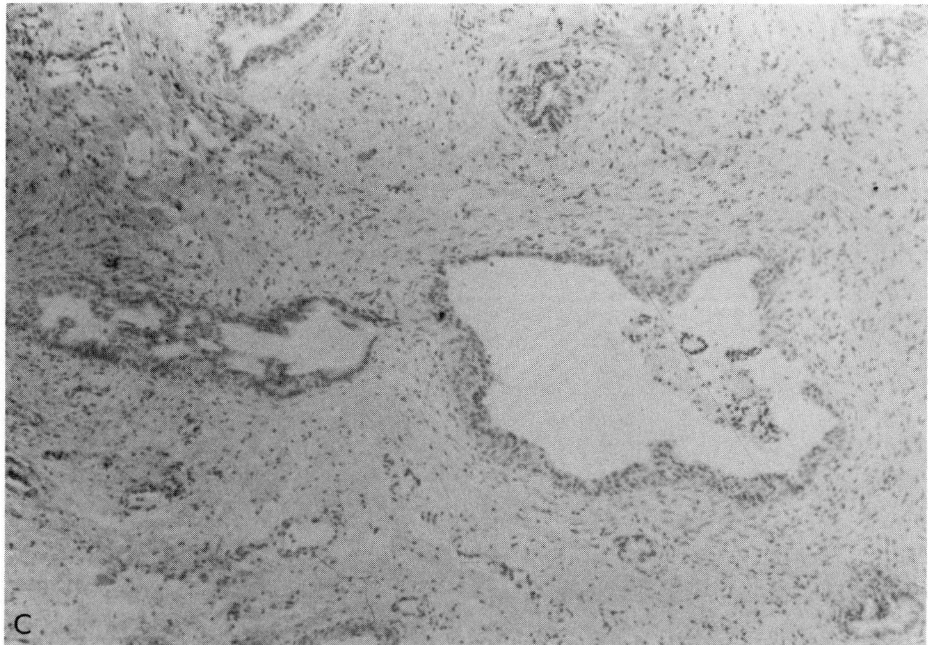

Figure 19–3 *Continued*   *C,* Collecting ductules of biliary glands: The basic morphologic characteristic is that of a biliary gland. The walls are perfectly lined by high cuboidal epithelium, which sometimes shows cellular proliferation. As is true in biliary glands, bile is never found in the lumen. Occasionally a dilated lumen may be filled with an epithelial cluster or amorphous material.

In the early postoperative period, severe cholangitis may result in cessation of bile flow. Operation and ductal re-excision at the liver hilus may cause a resumption of bile drainage and should be attempted (Fig. 19–5). A short course of systemic steroid therapy, in this situation, may be helpful in maintaining a patent bilioenteric anastomosis.

About 12 to 18 months after operation, bile flow becomes normal and susceptibility to cholangitis resolves. Thereafter, cholangitis is usually a consequence of mechanical factors such as partial obstruction of the intestinal conduit at the stoma or by adhesive bands across the defunctionalized intestinal limb. Secondary surgical procedures to alleviate the partial obstruction may be required.

Progressive Cirrhosis. All children with biliary atresia have some degree of liver disease at the time of operative intervention. Pre-existing hepatic damage is rarely reversed and, indeed, is often progressive during the first postoperative year.[2] At least two mechanisms may be responsible. First, serum bile acid studies have shown that bile flow, although sufficient to eliminate jaundice, is inadequate for many months after operation.[24] Second, as alluded to earlier, biliary atresia is a panductular disease involving intrahepatic as well as extrahepatic bile ducts. Inflammation of the intrahepatic bile ducts continues for some time after operation, even with surgical relief of extrahepatic biliary obstruction.[4] In the majority of patients having successful surgery, the intrahepatic disease appears to be self-limited. After several years, first stabilization and then improvement of liver histology is noted.[16] In a significant subgroup, however, hepatobiliary disease continues despite biliary drainage. Though anicteric, these patients frequently have evidence of progressive hepatic disease. Unless saved by liver transplantation, most die of liver failure within the first postoperative year.

Fat-soluble Vitamin Deficiency. Fat-soluble vitamins require bile salts for absorption. Since bile salt flow does not reach normal for many months, impairment in fat-soluble vitamin absorption is to be anticipated. Low serum levels of vitamins A and E have been documented in all the pa-

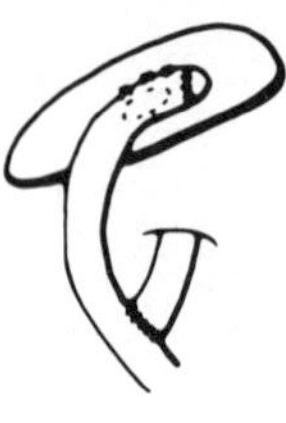
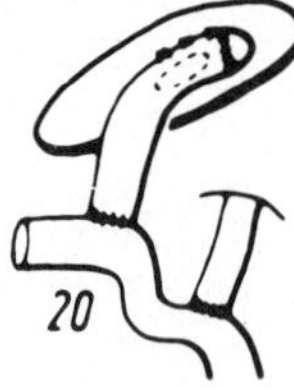
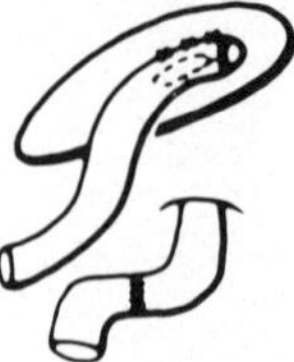

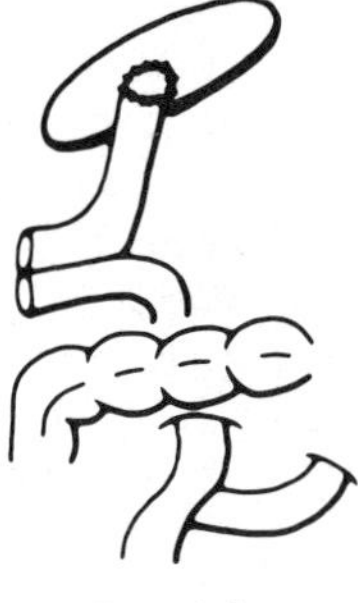
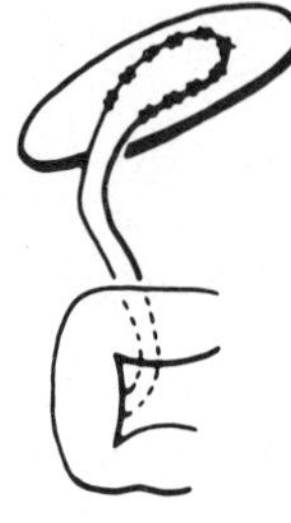

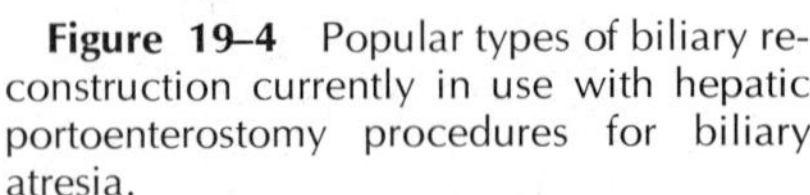

Figure 19–4 Popular types of biliary reconstruction currently in use with hepatic portoenterostomy procedures for biliary atresia.

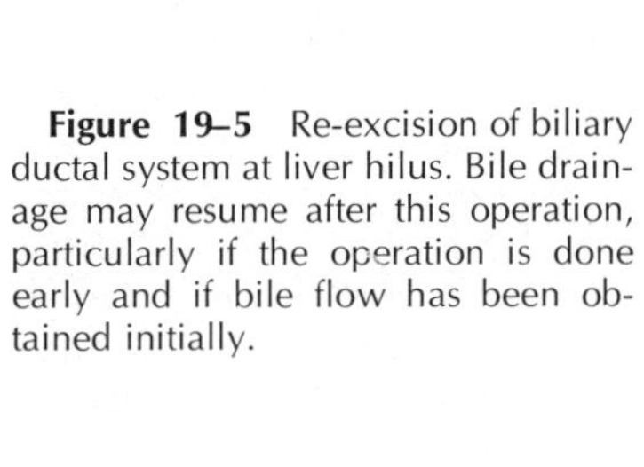

Figure 19–5 Re-excision of biliary ductal system at liver hilus. Bile drainage may resume after this operation, particularly if the operation is done early and if bile flow has been obtained initially.

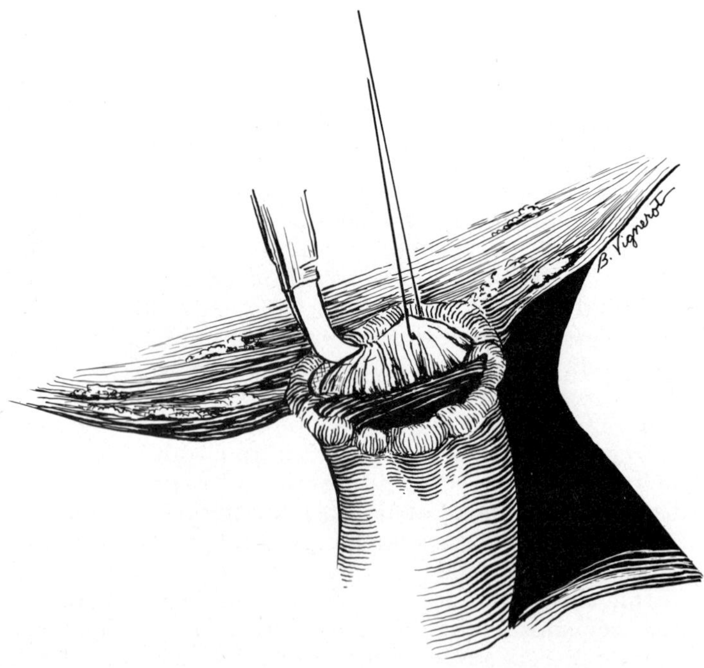

tients we have tested thus far. Radiographic evidence of vitamin D deficiency is routinely observed. In most patients in whom bile flow was re-established surgically, radiographic improvement and cure of rickets was noted within 2 to 3 years without vitamin D supplementation. A recent patient, however, sustained bilateral rachitic femoral fractures. Vitamin D metabolite treatment in this exceptional patient resulted in healing of the fractures.

Delay in gross motor development may be secondary to vitamin E deficiency.[3] Susceptibility to infection (cholangitis) may be aggravated by vitamin A deficiency. Postoperative supplementation of vitamins A and E is currently being evaluated.

Portal Hypertension. Because of pre-existing liver damage, most infants with biliary atresia have elevated portal pressure at the time of initial surgery.[42] Esophageal varices frequently develop despite gradual return of serologic liver functions toward normal. Variceal hemorrhage, however, is unusual following successful operations. Moreover, long-term studies demonstrate that in many patients, varices spontaneously disappear.[1] This disappearance may reflect decreased portal hypertension subsequent to improvement of hepatic parenchymal disease. Because of the rarity of significant variceal hemorrhage and the background of

spontaneous improvement, we have shied away from portal diversion operations. Instead, the few Denver patients with variceal hemorrhage have been treated by endosclerosis of the esophageal varices.[23, 26] Although experience with this new technique is limited, variceal bleeding has not recurred to date.

Biliary Hypoplasia

Biliary hypoplasia describes a morphologic state of the biliary system. Usually demonstrated by operative cholangiography, the extrahepatic bile ducts appear exceptionally small although patent throughout (Fig. 19–6). Biliary hypoplasia is not a specific disease entity but is a consequence of a variety of hepatobiliary disorders, both structural and functional (Table 19–2). Examples of the latter are neonatal hepatitis, alpha$_1$-antitrypsin deficiency, and intrahepatic biliary atresia. The diminutive caliber of the biliary system in this group of patients is most likely a result of "disease atrophy" secondary to severely impaired bile flow.

Biliary hypoplasia may also occur secondary to structural damage of the ductal system. The predisposing disease is probably a variant, or a milder form, of classic biliary

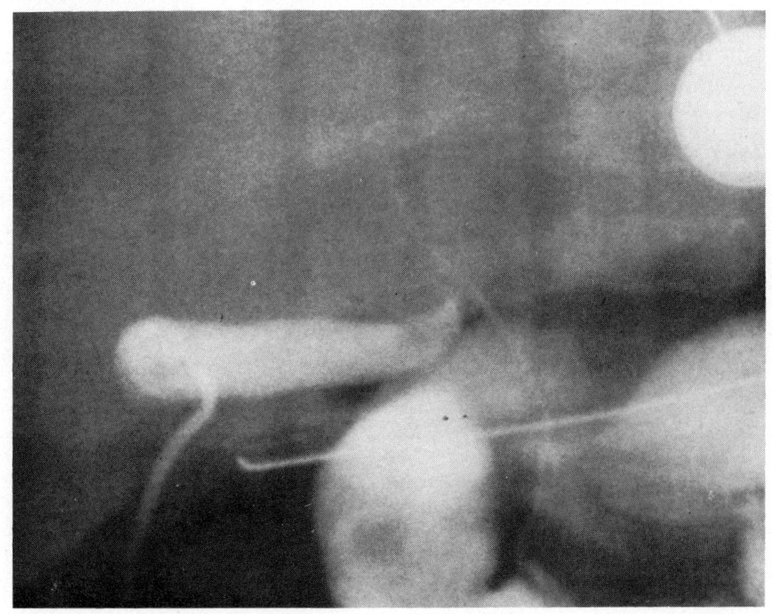

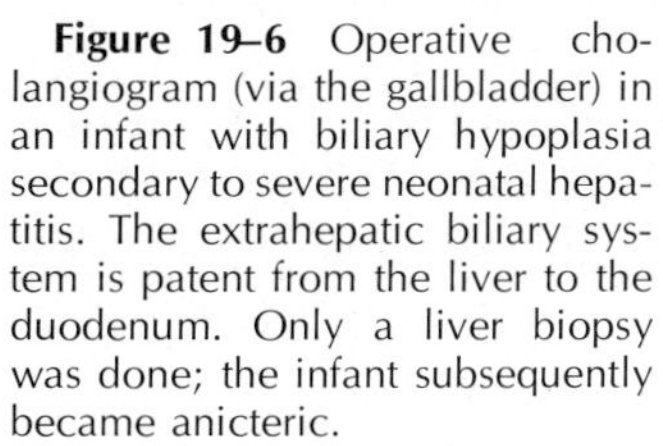

Figure 19–6 Operative cholangiogram (via the gallbladder) in an infant with biliary hypoplasia secondary to severe neonatal hepatitis. The extrahepatic biliary system is patent from the liver to the duodenum. Only a liver biopsy was done; the infant subsequently became anicteric.

TABLE 19–2 ETIOLOGIC FACTORS IN
BILIARY HYPOPLASIA

Functional	Structural
Neonatal hepatitis	Choledochal cyst
Alpha$_1$-antitrypsin deficiency	Extrahepatic biliary atresia
Intrahepatic biliary atresia	

atresia.[31] Prolonged survival has been reported in some patients,[29] presumably because patency of the extrahepatic biliary system persists. However, we have encountered three of 62 infants with biliary atresia and one of nine patients with a choledochal cyst in whom patency of the initially hypoplastic biliary system was subsequently lost. A Kasai hepatic portoenterostomy procedure was ultimately required in all four patients.[18] At the time of operation, the extrahepatic bile ducts were totally obliterated. Biliary hypoplasia in these patients simply represents a way station in the disease process of biliary atresia.

Complications of operations for biliary hypoplasia may be due to misinterpretation of low flow syndromes as structural malformations. We have observed two infants with biliary hypoplasia, one secondary to homozygous ZZ alpha$_1$-antitrypsin deficiency and one secondary to intrahepatic biliary atresia, both of whom were treated by Kasai hepatoportoenterostomy procedure without improvement. It is unlikely that bypassing the hypoplastic extrahepatic ductal system will relieve intrahepatic cholestasis. Procrastination in the converse situation, i.e., structural disease misinterpreted as a functional syndrome, is even more dangerous. Infants in whom biliary hypoplasia is secondary to an underlying ductal sclerotic process may lose ductal patency and require total extirpation of the extrahepatic biliary system and replacement with an intestinal conduit. The operation should be done promptly under these circumstances, since protracted biliary obstruction will result in irreversible biliary cirrhosis.

Choledochal Cyst

Internal drainage and primary excision are the operative procedures generally employed for treatment of congenital choledochal cyst in infants and children. Traditionally, the former has been performed by most surgeons in the United States, whereas the latter is preferred by many pediatric surgeons in Japan, France, and Australia. The specific complications of internal intestinal drainage, either by choledochocystoduodenostomy or choledochocystojejunostomy, consist of anastomotic stricture, biliary stasis, recurrent cholangitis, biliary lithiasis, and pancreatitis (Table 19–3). The incidence of such complications was recently reviewed by Flanigan and found to be from 34 per cent to 58 per cent.[7]

The fundamental reason for the high rate of complications is that diseased tissue is employed for the biliary reconstruction. Choledochal cysts are composed essentially of scar tissue (Fig. 19–7A, B). Consequently, the cyst rarely shrinks to a normal caliber, biliary stasis persists, and the stage is set for recurrent cholangitis and biliary lithiasis. Furthermore, the absence of a normal cyst epithelial lining in most cases prevents a mucosa-to-mucosa anastomosis with the intestine, thus predisposing to subsequent anastomotic stricture.

Two recent reviews have also reported that the incidence of malignancy of the extrahepatic biliary tract is about 20 times greater in patients with choledochal cysts than in the population at large.[8, 41] The susceptibility to malignancy was not eliminated by internal drainage of the cyst. In fact, in about half the patients, carcinoma

TABLE 19–3 COMPLICATIONS FOLLOWING CORRECTION OF CHOLEDOCHAL CYST

Internal Drainage	Primary Excision
Anastomotic stricture (12%)	Anastomotic stricture (5%)
Recurrent cholangitis (50%)	Recurrent cholangitis (8%)
Biliary malignancy (2.5%)	Biliary malignancy (<1%?)
Biliary lithiasis	Pancreatic fistula (<1%)
Pancreatitis (1%?)	

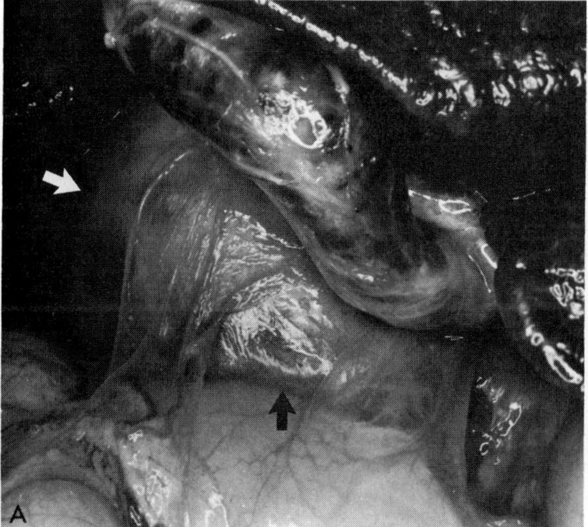

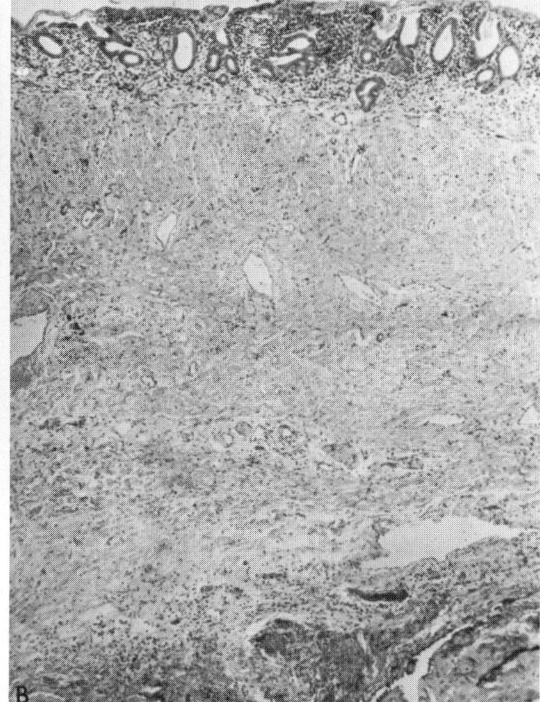

Figure 19–7   *A,* Operative photograph of a choledochal cyst *(arrows)* in a 3-month-old infant. There is obvious liver disease as a consequence of complete biliary obstruction, but the intrahepatic bile ducts were grossly dilated, unlike those of the infant described in Figure 19–1. Hepatic histology was normal 1 year later. *B,* The cyst wall is partially lined by epithelium and contains scattered distorted glands. The mucosa is infiltrated with chronic inflammatory cells. In some areas the mucosal epithelium is replaced by fibrin. A muscle layer is not present. Most of the wall consists of dense fibrous connective tissue containing scattered blood vessels. (Magnification ×30. Courtesy of Dr. Robert H. Shikes.)

developed a mean of 4 years after an internal drainage procedure.

The mortality resulting from excision of choledochal cyst was long thought to be greater than that from internal drainage operations. This belief has not been confirmed by contemporary reviews, which report operative mortality to be about 7 per cent for both operations.[7, 33] The dissection of the cyst from the adjacent portal vein and hepatic artery does, however, present a hazard in resectional operations that is not encountered in internal drainage procedures. Injury to neighboring vascular structures may be avoided by excising the cyst except for the outer shell of its posterior wall overlying the vascular structures.[21] A plane of dissection is developed in the posterior wall by opening the cyst and carrying out the dissection from the inside (Fig. 19–8*A, B*).

Complications specific to resection of choledochal cyst consist of intraoperative hemorrhage, anastomotic stricture, recurrent cholangitis, and pancreatic fistula (Table 19–3). Stricture of the choledochojejunostomy occurs in about 5 per cent of patients after excisional operations.[33] Anastomotic stricture is almost always a consequence of failure to excise the cyst completely. Hence, the defunctionalized Roux-en-Y jejunostomy is anastomosed to a diseased, scarred portion of the common hepatic duct. To avoid this complication, care must be taken to excise all of the choledochal cyst to the normal hepatic duct. Although attractive technically, leaving a rim of the choledochal cyst behind to facilitate the intestinal anastomosis is actually counterproductive. When the choledochal cyst disease process extends into the primary branches of the intrahepatic bile ducts, anastomotic stricture may be inescapable because intestinal anastomosis to a normal duct is not possible. Under these circumstances, the anastomosis should be made as large as feasible. This may necessitate laying open a portion of the main right or left hepatic duct.[22]

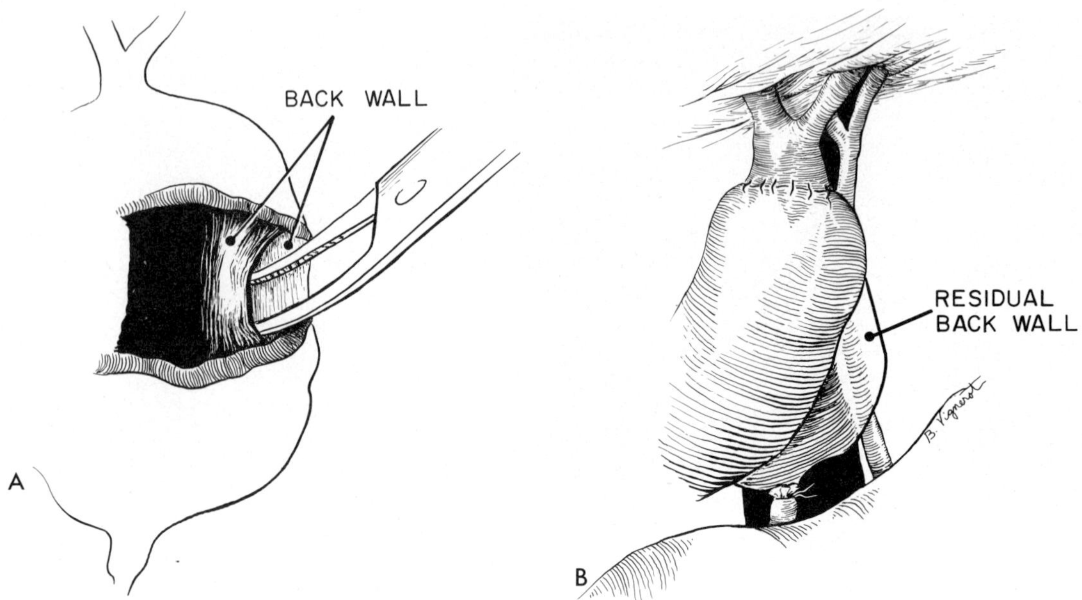

Figure 19–8 *A,* Excision of choledochal cyst. After the cyst is opened, dissection is begun in the posterior wall, separating it into two layers. The inner layer is completely transected and the cyst is excised except for the outer layer of the back wall. *B,* The operation is completed by end-to-end choledochojejunostomy (Roux-en-Y). The distal common bile duct has been suture ligated. The residual back wall of the choledochal cyst overlies the portal vein and hepatic artery. (From Lilly, J. R.: Total excision of choledochal cyst. Surg. Gynecol. Obstet. 146:254, 1978, by permission.)

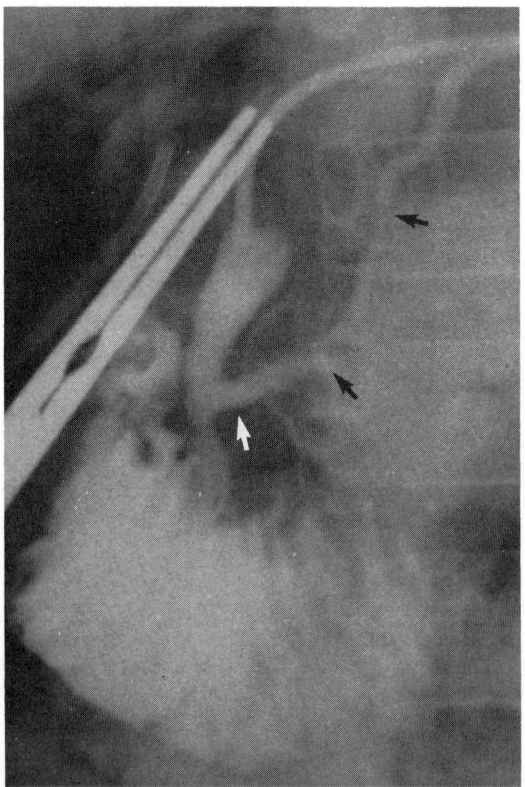

Figure 19–9 Operative cholangiogram in a patient with a choledochal cyst demonstrating the aberration of the junction of the common bile duct and the pancreatic duct *(arrows).* Note that the union of the two ducts is almost at a right angle and is much farther from the ampulla of Vater than is normal, creating a long "common channel." The cholangiogram was obtained by dividing the choledochal cyst, excising the proximal cyst, and placing a vascular clamp across the distal cyst before injection of the contrast medium. (Courtesy of Dr. David C. Hitch.)

Recurrent cholangitis after cyst excision may be secondary to anastomotic stricture or to associated intrahepatic cystic disease. Coexisting intrahepatic biliary cysts are more common than was previously appreciated (nine of 16 patients reported by Tsuchida and Ishida[40] and four of 11 patients in Denver). Excision of the choledochal cyst is not curative in this situation. Biliary stasis and the likelihood of cholangitis persist despite provision of normal extrahepatic bile drainage.

Finally, in most, if not all, patients with choledochal cyst, the pancreatic duct joins the common bile duct at a point considerably more proximal than normal. Unwary surgery during the distal dissection of the cyst may lead to inadvertent transection of the pancreatic duct.[14] The complication is preventable by visualizing the common bile duct–pancreatic duct junction either by operative cholangiogram (Fig. 19–9) or by direct inspection before resecting the choledochal cyst.

Caroli's Disease

In true Caroli's disease the secondary and tertiary branches of the bile ducts are grossly distorted with multiple cysts. There is no, or only limited, disease of the extrahepatic bile ducts. In most patients with intrahepatic cystic disease, however, a choledochal cyst is also present (Fig. 19–10). Because of biliary stasis, afflicted persons are subject to recurrent cholangitis, biliary lithiasis, and biliary cancer. Excision of a coexisting choledochal cyst, when present, may aid in the control of the complications but is not curative. Hepatic lobectomy or segmentectomy should be considered for patients in whom the intrahepatic disease is localized.

Perforation of the Common Bile Duct

Spontaneous perforation of the extrahepatic bile duct is a rare but highly specific lesion in infants. It probably originates from a localized mural malformation of the common bile duct, since the site of the perforation is almost always at the union of the cystic and common ducts. The operative cholecystogram frequently demonstrates a biliary pseudocyst (Fig. 19–11). Slow escape of bile from the tiny perforation permits its temporary encapsulization. Because of sludge in the partially defunctionalized distal common bile duct, there may be a mistaken impression of distal obstruction.

Surgical dissection of the inflamed portal triad should not be undertaken. Multiple soft rubber drains are placed in the area of

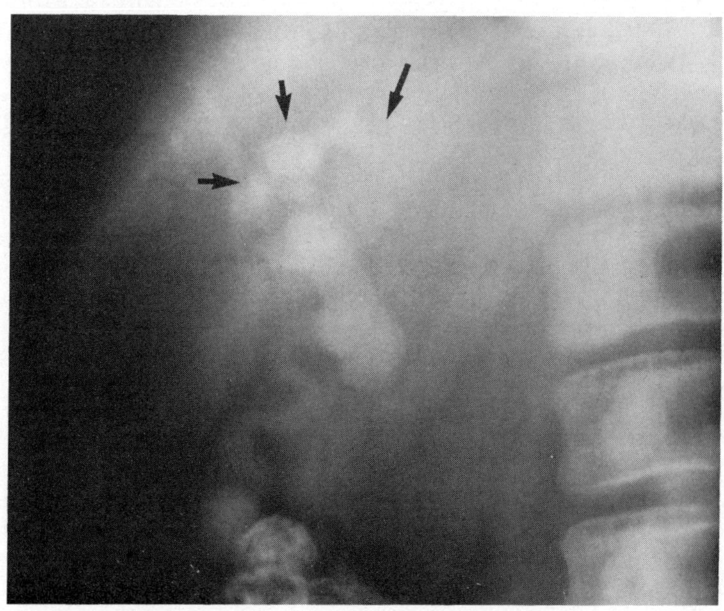

Figure 19–10 Oral cholecystogram in a child with "Caroli's disease." The intrahepatic cystic disease *(arrows)* is associated with a choledochal cyst. The choledochal cyst was excised and a choledochojejunostomy (Roux-en-Y) was performed for biliary drainage. The child has improved but is not cured. The intrahepatic cysts are unchanged 1 year later.

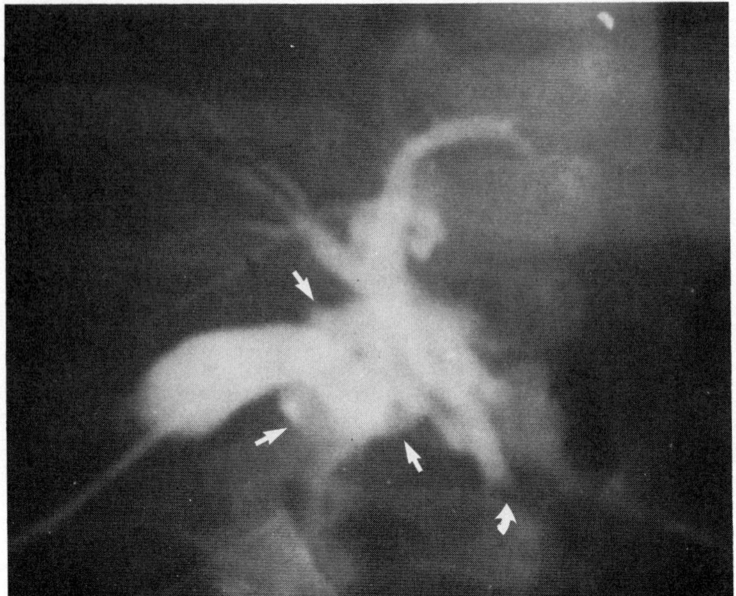

Figure 19–11 Operative cholangiogram in an infant with perforation of the common bile duct. Contrast medium injected into the gallbladder spills out into a biliary pseudocyst *(straight arrows)*. A meniscus sign *(curved arrow)* in the distal common bile duct suggests a choledocholith. Resolution of the perforation, biliary pseudocyst, and "choledocholith" followed simple peritoneal drainage adjacent to the site of perforation.

the perforation, and the abdomen is closed. A cholecystostomy catheter is left in place so that healing of the perforation may be assessed postoperatively. Premature removal of the drains will lead to reaccumulation of bilious ascites.[27] Spontaneous closure of the ductal leak may take several weeks.

Surgical complications of perforation of the common bile duct are primarily due to overzealous surgery. In most cases, spontaneous closure of the leak and subsequent cure have followed simple drainage of the perforation.[32] Attempts to close the perforation, drain the common bile duct, remove the ductal sludge, or bypass a mistakenly interpreted distal obstruction may lead to major biliary complications. An even more serious complication results from the misinterpretation of the biliary pseudocyst as a choledochal cyst. An intestinal anastomosis to the pseudocyst is usually lethal.

The overall experience with spontaneous perforation of the extrahepatic ducts in infants indicates that the lesion is self-limited and the sole error in ductal development. Thus, residual biliary tract disease or other sequelae would not be anticipated.

THE LIVER

There are few congenital malformations of the liver that necessitate surgical intervention. The bulk of hepatic surgery in infants and children consists of resectional operations, usually for tumor and occasionally for trauma. The complications of resectional operations have a common pathogenesis irrespective of the original condition for which the surgery was performed.

Hepatic surgery in infants and children is not often indicated. When required, the operation most commonly consists of partial resection. In the most extreme case, complete removal and replacement of the liver with a cadaveric organ (orthotopic transplantation) may be performed.

Partial Hepatic Resections

Removal of part of the liver is done usually for tumors and occasionally for trauma. The basis for orderly subtotal resection of the liver is found in anatomic studies, which have been summarized.[35] For practical purposes, only four surgical units lend themselves to controlled excision (Fig. 19–12), including the right and left true lobes, which consist of two segments each. The third possibility is removal of the complete right lobe plus the medial segment of the left lobe. This operation (Fig. 19–12) is most correctly called right trisegmentectomy, although the term "extended right hepatic lobectomy" has frequently been used. The

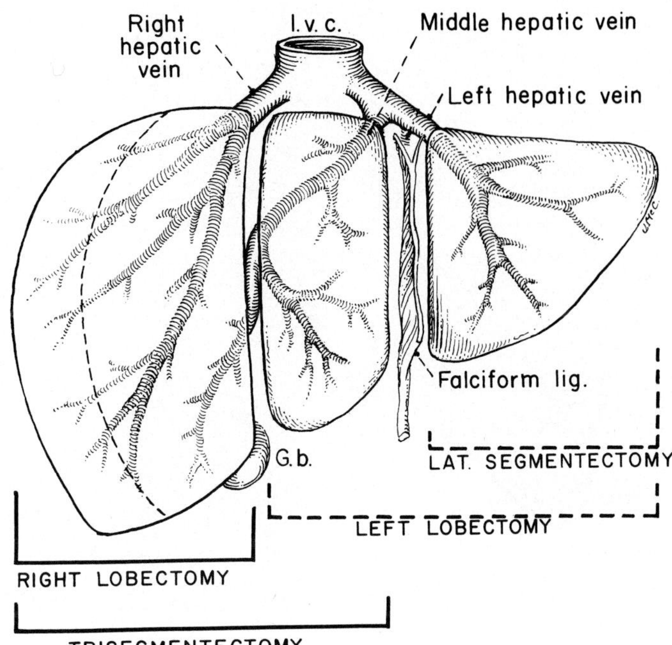

Figure 19–12 The usual kinds of partial hepatectomy. Note that there are only four common resections. (From Starzl, T. E., Bell, R. H., Beart, R. W., et al.: Hepatic trisegmentectomy or extended right lobectomy: Relation to other liver resections. Surg. Gynecol. Obstet. 141:429, 1975, by permission.)

fourth possibility is excision of the liver to the left of the falciform ligament. The removal of this single segment (Fig. 19–12) should be known as lateral segmentectomy instead of left lobectomy.

In infants and children, any of the four resections can be done through an abdominal incision (Fig. 19–13). The principles of the operations are simple.[34, 37] They consist of preliminary ligation of the hilar structures going to the planned specimen (Fig. 19–14), early control of the drainage hepatic veins when possible, and transection of the hepatic parenchyma along exact intersegmental or interlobar planes (Fig. 19–15). Sometimes the huge size of right lobar tumors or invasion of the diaphragm by these tumors makes it impossible to obtain preliminary control of the right hepatic vein. In such cases, we have approached the right hepatic vein from within the right hepatic parenchyma (Fig. 19–15).[38]

There are five complications after hepatic resections in children.[9, 10, 28, 35, 38, 43] The most avoidable is injury to the triad structures that pass to the retained fragment. When the right three segments (trisegmentectomy) (Fig. 19–15) or the left lateral segment (Fig. 19–16) is removed, the anatomy in and around the plane of the falciform ligament (Fig. 19–16) must be understood

precisely. In the first instance, an injury to the hilar structures passing to the residual lateral segment would almost immediately be lethal (see Fig. 19–15). In the second instance, an injury to the medial segmental ("feedback") hilar structures during lateral segmentectomy (see Fig. 19–16) would cause a regional infarction. Sometimes only one structure is damaged, most commonly the hepatic duct to the liver remnant. We have performed liver transplantation 5 years after such an injury in a teenage girl who had been kicked by a horse, because repeated efforts to repair the severed duct had failed.

Even in modern times, hemorrhage has been the most common cause of death during and just after partial hepatic resection. That such a complication is unnecessary has been shown in our experience with 87 consecutive hepatic resections in adults and children. Although brisk bleeding was always encountered at the time of parenchymal transection, this promptly came under control after removal of the specimen. No matter how alarming the hemorrhage as the parenchyma was split, hemostasis was easily achieved because the plane of resection was anatomically correct. Secondary postoperative hemorrhage necessitating re-exploration was seen only once.

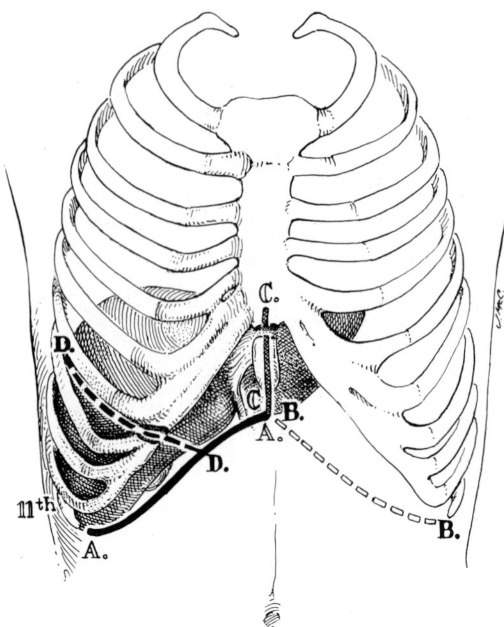

Figure 19–13 Approaches for trisegmentectomy and true right lobectomy. Note that several extensions may be made from the basic right subcostal incision, A to A, that is always used. More than one of the depicted extensions may be required in a given patient. For left hepatic lobectomy or lateral segmentectomy, mirror images of the extensions shown can be added to the basic left subcostal incision. In infants and children, it is almost never necessary to have a thoracic component, since the mobility of the costal margin permits effective retraction. (From Starzl, J. E., Bell, R. H., Beart, R. W., et al.: Hepatic trisegmentectomy or extended right lobectomy: Relation to other liver resections. Surg. Gynecol. Obstet. 141:429, 1975, by permission.)

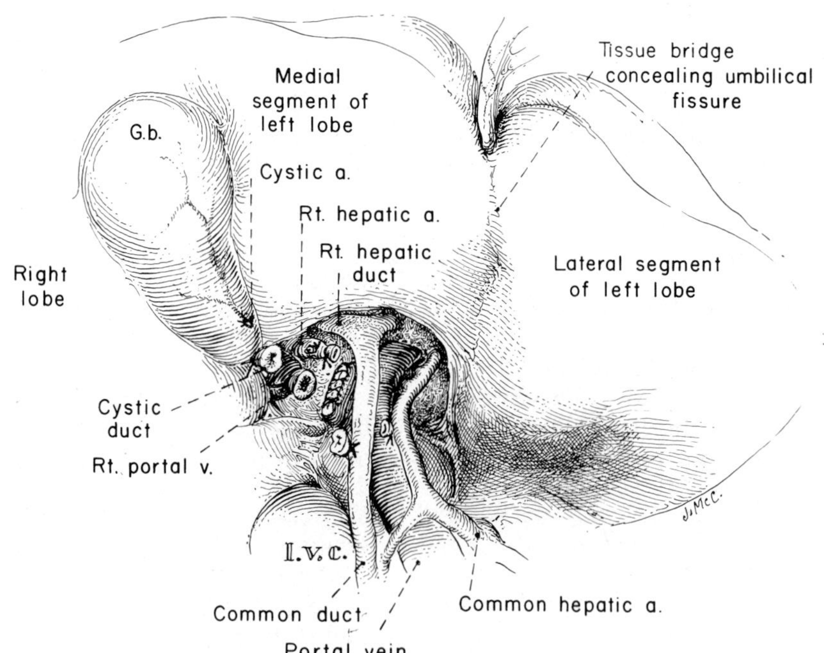

Figure 19–14 Devascularization of the true right lobe. The cystic artery and cystic duct are ligated and divided to aid in the dissection. Of the structures constituting the portal triad, the bifurcation of the common duct is almost always the most superior, the portal vein is intermediate, and the hepatic artery is most inferior. The lateral suture closure of the portal vein is at the site of detachment of the right portal branch. The tissue bridge conceals the umbilical fissure, behind which a finger can be inserted. The bridge is present in about half of all patients. (From Starzl, T. E., Bell, R. H., Beart, R. W., et al.: Hepatic trisegmentectomy or extended right lobectomy: Relation to other liver resections. Surg. Gynecol. Obstet. 141:429, 1975, by permission.)

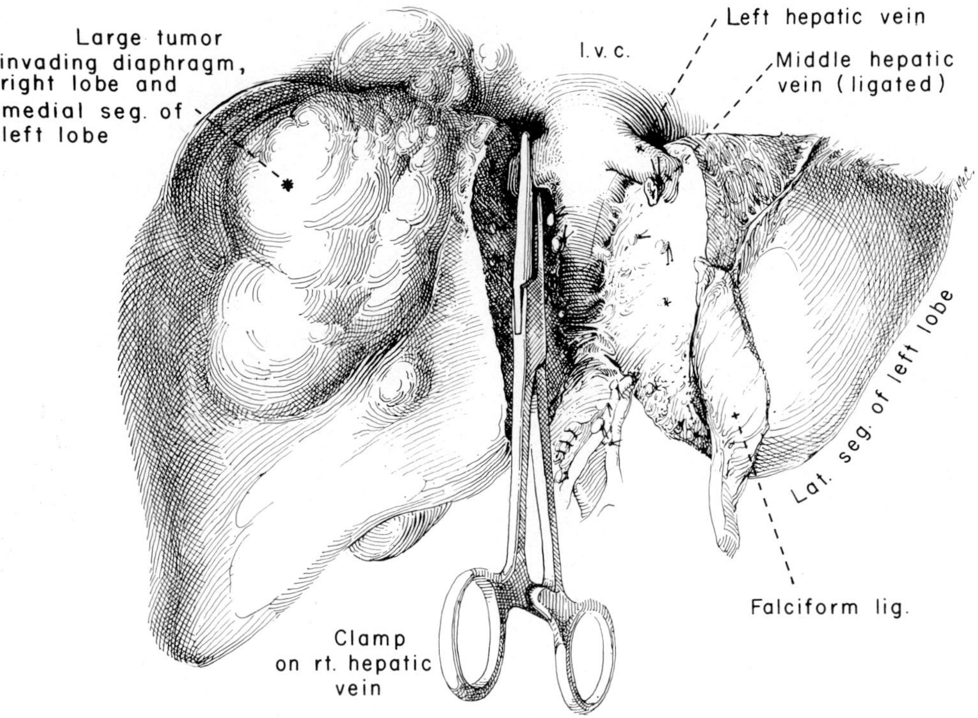

Figure 19–15　Control of right hepatic vein from within the liver. The technique may be required when large tumors prevent preliminary dissection and clamping of this vein. (From Starzl, T. E., Koep, L. J., Weil, R., et al.: Right trisegmentectomy for hepatic neoplasms. Surg. Gynecol. Obstet. 150:208, 1980, by permission.)

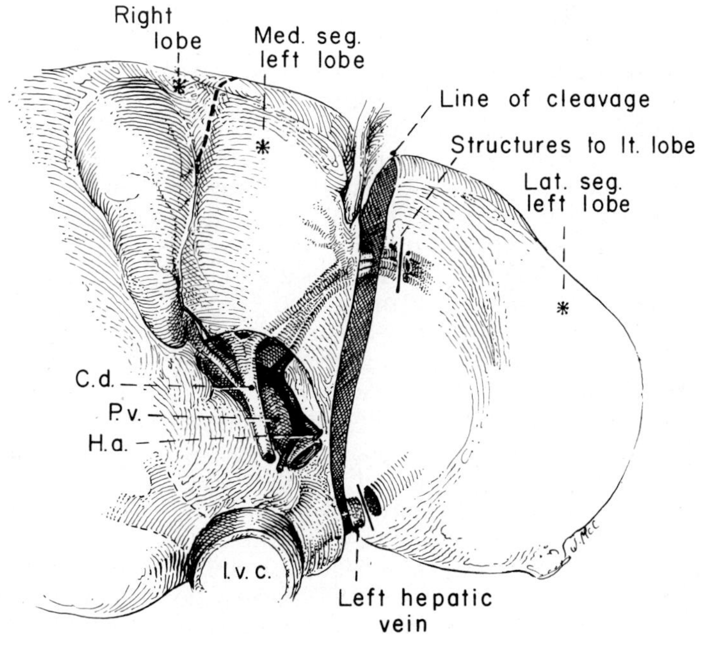

Figure 19–16　Site of ligation of portal structures for lateral segmentectomy. The dissection is kept to the left of the umbilical fissure to prevent injury to the structures feeding back from the fissure to the medial segment. (From Starzl, T. E., Bell, R. H., Beart, R. W., et al.: Hepatic trisegmentectomy or extended right lobectomy: Relation to other liver resections. Surg. Gynecol. Obstet. 141:129, 1975, by permission.)

Two historically important causes of death, air embolism and hypothermia, have essentially been eliminated by improvements in anesthesia. The air emboli originated from cut hepatic veins and were sucked into the circulation in patients whose diaphragm was intact and whose anesthesia was light enough to permit respiratory efforts. The combination of adequate depth of anesthesia and end-expiratory positive pressure ventilation has prevented air embolism in our experience. Intraoperative temperature control is important because infants and children may be poikilothermic.

Aside from hemorrhage, the most frequently fatal complication in modern times has been regional infection. To avoid this, the cavities caused by major resections must be adequately drained. We often achieve this by leaving open a portion of the wound through which eight to 12 1-inch Penrose drains are inserted (Fig. 19–17). Two or 3 days after operation the drains are removed and daily irrigations of the cavity are begun. The cavity is allowed to close in from the bottom over several weeks. In spite of these precautions, abscesses in residual subphrenic cavities have required later drainage in about 10 per cent of our patients following right lobectomy or right trisegmentectomy. Occasionally, partial evisceration through the drain tracts may require control by packing. In one of our patients it was necessary to carry out formal repair of an incisional hernia at this site.

With right and left true lobectomy and with lateral segmentectomy, jaundice should not occur postoperatively, nor should there be any major disturbances of liver function, provided that the retained liver tissue is normal. In contrast, all patients become jaundiced after right trisegmentectomy (Fig. 19–18). The residual 10 to 30 per cent of liver represented by the lateral segment begins prompt regeneration, and completely normal liver function can be expected within a few days.

There should be no later functional sequelae following successful hepatic resection. The special question of late morbidity following trisegmentectomy was recently examined in 30 patients.[38] Only one death (3 per cent) occurred in the hospital or within the first 2 postoperative months. Those who survived for longer periods, including four

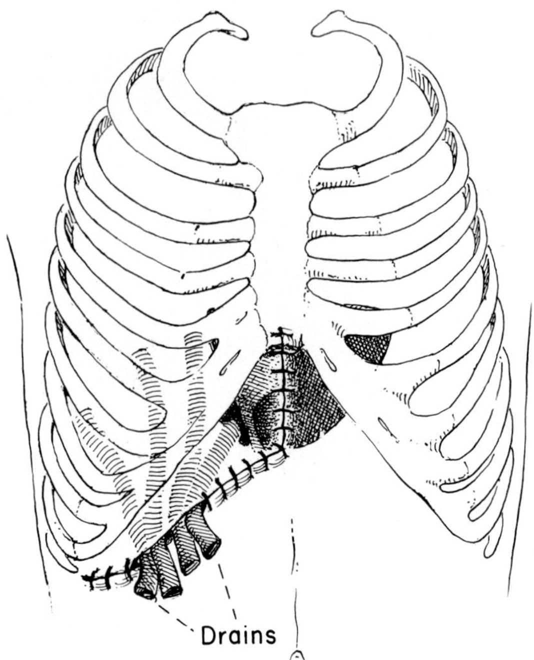

Figure 19–17　Wound drainage after trisegmentectomy. Usually either the medial or the lateral portion of the wound is kept open 3 or 4 inches. (From Starzl, T. E., Bell, R. H., Beart, R. W., et al.: Hepatic trisegmentectomy or extended right lobectomy: Relation to other liver resections. Surg. Gynecol. Obstet. 141:129, 1975, by permission.)

who had benign lesions, had completely normal results of liver function tests when followed up as long as 9 years after resection.

Pediatric patients with malignant neoplasms should be strongly considered for adjuvant chemotherapy. Although postoperative treatment with drugs and irradiation has been said to be worthless, we have made a case for using these modalities.[38] Eight of our children with very advanced neoplasms were treated after trisegmentectomy with cyclophosphamide, vincristine, and 5-fluorouracil to which doxorubicin (Adriamycin) was frequently added. Seven of these eight patients are still alive 1 to 6½ years after operation, a record of survival hard to envision with treatment of such unfavorable lesions by surgery alone.

The safety of major hepatic resections has increased our willingness to perform such procedures, which at one time were viewed as heroic. Only one death, that of an elderly woman, has occurred among the last 90

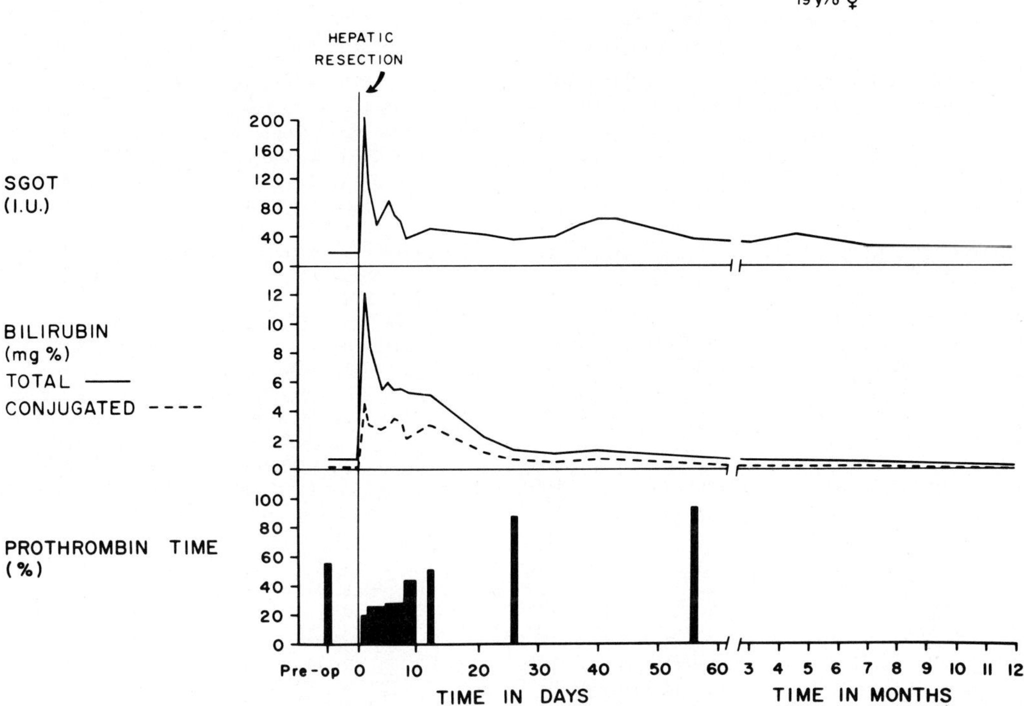

Figure 19–18   Postoperative course after trisegmentectomy. The elevated bilirubin level and the depressed prothrombin time returned to normal in about 1 month. (From Starzl, T. E., Putnam, C. W., Groth, C. G., et al.: Alopecia, ascites, and incomplete regeneration after 85 to 90 per cent liver resection. Am. J. Surg. 129:587, 1975.)

patients treated by resection, 37 of whom were given right trisegmentectomies. Exceptionally low mortality has been reported by other surgeons as well.[9, 10, 28, 43]

Liver Transplantation

The ultimate extirpative procedure is orthotopic liver transplantation, an approach now rarely used to treat otherwise nonresectable malignant tumors. The tumors have recurred with such regularity after liver replacement that the potential value of transplantation has been vitiated.[36, 37] Interestingly, the tumors have reappeared in the graft itself.

In a recent summary of the indications for liver replacement in children, the leading indication was biliary atresia.[37] This diagnosis accounted for 48 of the first 74 pediatric liver replacements. Chronic aggressive hepatitis was a distant second. An especially interesting group of patients had

inborn errors of metabolism (Wilson's disease, alpha$_1$-antitrypsin deficiency, Type IV glycogen storage disease, and tyrosinemia) that were cured by the provision of phenotypically normal livers.[36, 37]

Although much progress has been made in liver transplantation, the procedure has not yet provided predictable and reliable results. In our own experience and that of Calne and Williams,[5] the results have improved during the last few years, but at best we have been able to achieve only a 50 per cent 1-year patient survival.[36, 37]

Many of the lethal complications of liver transplantation have derived directly from or have been made worse by immunosuppression, which is necessary for any kind of homotransplantation. However, an extensive list of nonimmunologic complications has been recorded.[5, 36, 37] These have included biliary tract obstruction and/or fistulae, enteric fistulae, thrombosis of the homograft and host vessels, unknowing use of irreversibly damaged organs, air embolization from the large veins of the homograft, crushing and paralysis of the recipient right phrenic nerve, venous infarction of the right adrenal gland, postoperative gastrointestinal hemorrhage, and pancreatitis, to provide a very incomplete listing. In addition, hepatitis caused by hepatitis B surface antigen, adenovirus, cytomegalovirus, and herpesvirus have been shown to cause postoperative homograft dysfunction that has sometimes been so severe and acute as to cause death.

The avoidance of these many problems and their treatment when they occur have been discussed extensively elsewhere.[5, 34, 36, 37] The management principles are much the same as for immunologically normal patients, but the margin of permissible error is much smaller or may be nonexistent in recipients under immunosuppression. The interested reader should refer to specialty publications[5, 34, 36, 37] to obtain insight into the complex problems that can result from such a massive surgical procedure in metabolically and immunologically depleted patients.

References

1. Alagille, D.: Long-term results of hepatic portoenterostomy. *In* Javitt, N. B. (ed.): Neonatal Hepatitis and Biliary Atresia. DHEW Publication No. (NIH) 79–1296. Washington, D.C., U.S. Government Printing Office, 1979.
2. Altman, R. P., Chandra, R., and Lilly, J. R.: Ongoing cirrhosis after successful porticoenterostomy in infants with biliary atresia. J. Pediatr. Surg. 10:685, 1975.
3. Barkin, R. M., and Lilly, J. R.: Biliary atresia and the Kasai operation: Continuing care. J. Pediatr. 96:1015, 1980.
4. Bill, A. H., Haas, J. E., and Foster, G. L.: Biliary atresia: Histopathologic observations and reflections upon its natural history. J. Pediatr. Surg. 12:977, 1977.
5. Calne, R. Y., and Williams, R.: Liver transplantation. Curr. Prob. Surg. 16:1, 1979.
6. Danks, D. M., Campbell, P. E., Clarke, A. M., et al.: Extrahepatic biliary atresia. The frequency of potentially operable cases. Am. J. Dis. Child. 128:684, 1974.
7. Flanigan, D. P.: Biliary cysts. Ann. Surg. 182:635, 1975.
8. Flanigan, D. P.: Biliary carcinoma associated with biliary cysts. Cancer 40:880, 1976.
9. Fortner, J. G., Dong, K. K., MacClean, B. J., et al.: Major hepatic resection for neoplasia. Ann. Surg. 188:363, 1978.
10. Foster, J. H.: Survival after liver resection for cancer. Cancer 26:493, 1970.
11. Hirsig, J., Kara, O., and Rickham, P. P.: Experimental investigations into the etiology of cholangitis following operation for biliary atresia. J. Pediatr. Surg. 13:55, 1978.
12. Hitch, D. C., and Lilly, J. R.: Identification, quantification, and significance of bacterial growth within the biliary tract after Kasai's operation. J. Pediatr. Surg. 13:563, 1978.
13. Izant, R. J., Jr., Akers, D. R., Hays, D. M., et al.: Biliary atresia survey. Surgical Section, American Academy of Pediatrics, 1965.
14. Kasai, M., Asakura, Y., and Taira, Y.: Surgical treatment of choledochal cyst. Ann. Surg. 182:844, 1970.
15. Kasai, M., Kimura, S., Asakura, Y., et al.: Surgical treatment of biliary atresia. J. Pediatr. Surg. 3:665, 1968.
16. Kasai, M., Watanabe, I., and Ohi, R.: Follow-up studies of long-term survivors after hepatic portoenterostomy for "noncorrectable" biliary atresia. J. Pediatr. Surg. 10:173, 1975.
17. Landing, B. H.: Considerations of the pathogenesis of neonatal hepatitis, biliary atresia, and choledochal cyst. The concept of infantile obstructive cholangiography. *In* Bill, A. H., and Kasai, M. (eds.): Progress in Pediatric Surgery. Vol. 6. Baltimore, University Park Press, 1974, p. 113.
18. Lilly, J. R.: The surgery of biliary hypoplasia. J. Pediatr. Surg. 11:815, 1976.
19. Lilly, J. R.: Total excision of choledochal cyst. Surg. Gynecol. Obstet. 146:254, 1978.
20. Lilly, J. R.: Hepatic portocholecystostomy for biliary atresia. J. Pediatr. Surg. 14:301, 1979.
21. Lilly, J. R.: The surgical treatment of choledochal cyst. Surg. Gynecol. Obstet. 149:36, 1979.
22. Lilly, J. R.: Surgery of coexisting biliary malformations in choledochal cyst. J. Pediatr. Surg. 14:643, 1979.
23. Lilly, J. R.: Treatment of esophageal variceal hemorrhage by endosclerosis. Surg. Gynecol. Obstet. (in press).
24. Lilly, J. R., and Javitt, N. B.: Biliary lipid excretion after hepatic portoenterostomy. Ann. Surg. 184:369, 1976.
25. Lilly, J. R., and Starzl, T. E.: Liver transplantation in children with biliary atresia and vascular anomalies. J. Pediatr. Surg. 9:707, 1974.
26. Lilly, J. R., Terblanche, J., and Silverman, A.: Sclerotherapy of esophageal varices in children. Gastroenterology 75:974, 1978.
27. Lilly, J. R., Weintraub, W. H., and Altman, R. P.: Spontaneous perforation of the extrahepatic bile ducts and bile peritonitis in infancy. Surgery 75:664, 1974.
28. Lin, T.: Recent advances in technique of hepatic lobectomy and results of surgical treatment for primary carcinoma of the liver. Prog. Liver Dis. 5:668, 1976.
29. Longmire, W. P.: Congenital biliary hypoplasia. Ann. Surg. 159:335, 1964.
30. Ohi, R., Shikes, R. H., and Lilly, J. R.: Bile duct remnants in biliary atresia. Ann. Surg. (in press).
31. Popper, H., and Schaffner, F.: Liver: Structure and Function. New York, McGraw-Hill Book Co., The Blakiston Division, 1957, Chap. 20.
32. Prevot, J., and Babut, J. M.: Spontaneous perfora-

tions of the biliary tract in infancy. Prog. Pediatr. Surg. 3:187, 1971.

33. Saito, S., and Ishida, M.: Congenital cyst (cystic dilatation of the common bile duct). *In* Bill, A. H., and Kasai, M. (eds.): Progress in Pediatric Surgery. Vol. 6. Baltimore, University Park Press, 1974, p. 63.

34. Starzl, T. E. (with the assistance of Putnam, C. W.): Experience in Hepatic Transplantation. Philadelphia, W. B. Saunders Co., 1969.

35. Starzl, T. E., Bell, R. H., Beart, R. W., et al.: Hepatic trisegmentectomy or extended right lobectomy: Relation to other liver resections. Surg. Gynecol. Obstet. 141:429, 1975.

36. Starzl, T. E., Koep, L. J., Halgrimson, C. G., et al.: Fifteen years of clinical liver transplantation. Gastroenterology 77:375, 1979.

37. Starzl, T. E., Koep, L. J., Schroter, G. P. J., et al.: Liver replacement for pediatric patients. Pediatrics 63:825, 1979.

38. Starzl, T. E., Koep, L. J., Weil, R., et al.: Right trisegmentectomy for hepatic neoplasms. Surg. Gynecol. Obstet. 150:208, 1980.

39. Starzl, T. E., Putnam, C. W., Groth, C. G., et al.: Alopecia, ascites, and incomplete regeneration after 85 to 90 per cent liver resection. Am. J. Surg. 129:587, 1975.

40. Tsuchida, Y., and Ishida, M.: Dilatation of the intrahepatic bile ducts in congenital cystic dilatation of the common bile duct. Surgery 69:776, 1971.

41. Tsuchiya, R., Harada, N., Ito, T., et al.: Malignant tumors in choledochal cysts. Ann. Surg. 186:22, 1977.

42. Valayer, J.: Hepatic porto-enterostomy. Surgical problems and results. *In* Berenberg, S. R. (ed.): Liver Diseases in Infancy and Childhood. The Hague, Martinus Nijhoff Medical Division, 1976.

43. Wilson, S. M., and Adson, M. A.: Surgical treatment of hepatic metastases from colorectal cancers. Arch. Surg. 111:330, 1976.

PANCREAS

Robert M. Filler, M.D.

20

The problems for which pancreatic surgery is needed in childhood are relatively uncommon. Of more than 25,000 general surgical operations performed from 1969 to 1980 at The Hospital for Sick Children, Toronto, only 21 were for lesions involving the pancreas. The pancreatic operations performed are listed in Table 20–1. This chapter will concentrate on the complications related to the surgical treatment of pancreatic pseudocyst and hypoglycemia in infancy, the main reasons for pancreatic surgery in the young.

COMPLICATIONS OF TREATING PANCREATIC PSEUDOCYST

About 60 per cent of pancreatic pseudocysts in children are secondary to pancreatic injury following blunt abdominal trauma. The remainder are presumably from pancreatitis, although data confirming this etiology are absent in most cases.[6] A major difference between adults and children with pseudocysts is that in the latter group, the pancreas and its ducts are less likely to be abnormal, because most of the pseudocysts are due to trauma or nonprogressive pancreatitis. In contrast, almost 80 per cent of pseudocysts seen in adults are secondary to alcoholic pancreatitis.[19] As a result, complications are less frequently encountered in the management of pseudocysts in children.

Some pseudocysts are small and do not require surgical drainage. They often disappear spontaneously during several weeks of observation. Surgical drainage is usually necessary if the mass persists or enlarges, especially when it is responsible for pain, fever, or vomiting and the inability to maintain normal nutrition. Both external and internal drainage procedures have been successful in treating these lesions.

External Drainage

When drainage of a pseudocyst becomes necessary during the first month after its formation, the wall of the cyst is usually so thin that it is impossible to anastomose it to the intestinal tract. In this case, external drainage is the procedure of choice. Several well-recognized complications may occur because of the "controlled" pancreatic fistula, which is produced by such a procedure.

PROLONGED LOSS OF FLUID, ELECTROLYTES, AND PANCREATIC ENZYMES

Because some pseudocyts have a direct communication with the main pancreatic duct, the pancreatic fistula can drain as much as 1500 ml of pancreatic juice each day. By virtue of its sodium content (140

TABLE 20–1 PANCREATIC SURGERY PERFORMED AT THE HOSPITAL FOR SICK CHILDREN, TORONTO, 1969–1980

Procedure	Number of Patients
Treatment of pancreatic pseudocyst*	
Cystogastrostomy	3
Roux-en-Y cystojejunostomy	1
External drainage	2
Peustow procedure	2
Treatment of hypoglycemia	
90% Pancreatectomy	9
70% Pancreatectomy for insulinemia	1
Treatment of miscellaneous conditions	
Partial pancreatectomy	3

*Pseudocyst caused by trauma in five patients, pancreatitis in three.

mEq/l), potassium content (5.0 mEq/l), and alkalinity (pH 8.0 to 8.3), persistent unreplaced drainage will result in hyponatremia, hypokalemia, and metabolic acidosis. In addition, nutrition is adversely affected by a high-output fistula because of the high protein content of the pancreatic juice (1 to 3 per cent) and the fact that diversion of all pancreatic enzymes from the intestines causes serious malabsorption. Depending on the volume of drainage and the function of the intestinal tract, some patients can keep pace with losses by increasing oral intake. However, when fistula outputs are high, most individuals require intravenous alimentation to replace losses and to ensure adequate nutrition. By supplying all nutrients by vein and eliminating oral feedings, fistula output usually can be significantly decreased because secretin stimulation of the pancreas is markedly reduced.

In most children, pancreatic fistula persists for 2 to 8 weeks after the institution of external drainage.[6] By comparison, the mean duration of drainage reported for adults is about 6 months.[1, 20]

INFECTION

One of the most frequent complications of external drainage is infection in the residual pseudocyst. Infection generally implies inadequate drainage. Although bacteria can always gain entrance to the cyst cavity through or around the drainage tube, significant clinical infection occurs only when the cyst cavity does not collapse after drainage. Its undrained contents support the growth of microorganisms, which can multiply when protected from the host defenses. When signs of intra-abdominal abscess are noted after external drainage of a pseudocyst, a search for undrained portions of the cyst is necessary. Ultrasonography and x-ray examination of the pseudocyst after injection of the drainage tract with radiocontrast material are useful diagnostic maneuvers. Establishment of satisfactory drainage by repositioning the drainage tube or inserting additional drains is usually necessary. Antibiotics effective against the organisms cultured should be administered to the septic patient.

EROSION INTO ADJACENT VISCERA

Fresh pancreatic juice is not proteolytic until it is activated. Activation may occur by trypsin itself or by enterokinase present in the succus entericus. Consequently, stagnation of pancreatic juice due to inadequate drainage of a pseudocyst may activate proteolytic enzymes, which can erode into adjacent viscera, especially those whose walls have been injured. However, erosion into an adjacent viscus after external drainage is more likely to be due to pressure necrosis from a hard drainage catheter than from pancreatic enzymes. If sump tubes are used to apply continuous suction to the cyst cavity, they must be soft and pliable and placed so that they will not rest against the stomach, colon, small bowel, or duodenum. To avoid the possibility of this complication, many surgeons do not use sump tubes, relying instead on soft Penrose drains. If a Penrose drain is used, an ileostomy stoma appliance can be fitted around the drain at its exit from the skin. A karaya seal on the appliance serves to protect the skin. If the device is applied properly, all drainage should remain contained in its pouch.

Fistulae from the stomach, duodenum, or small or large intestine can be disastrous in the presence of pancreatic fistula. Initial treatment should include removal of the offending catheter, adequate drainage, and institution of intravenous alimentation. Most cases can be managed successfully by these measures, and the gastric or intestinal fistula will close spontaneously. Some, especially a side duodenal fistula, may require operative intervention as described later.

HEMORRHAGE

Although serious hemorrhage is a major complication of untreated pseudocyst, it is much less common after adequate external drainage. We have not seen this problem in our small series, and Cooney and Grosfeld did not report it in their review.[6] When significant bleeding occurs, it usually arises from an extrapancreatic blood vessel rather than from the gland itself. Normal blood vessels are not usually digested by pancreatic juice. However, vessels that have been damaged, transected and sealed by clot, or sutured are particularly vulnerable to the action of pancreatic enzymes, especially in the presence of bacterial infection. Hemorrhage also implies that the cyst has not been adequately drained. When excessive bleeding occurs, localization of the bleeding site by angiography is an extremely valuable maneuver. Some bleeding sites can be controlled by embolization, others by the infusion of vasopressin. However, if these measures fail, exploration is necessary. Simple ligation of the bleeding vessel is often not feasible, and pancreatic resection with splenectomy is usually necessary.

RECURRENCE OF PSEUDOCYST

The incidence of recurrent pseudocyst following external drainage ranges from 22 to 24 per cent in large adult series.[1, 20] However, we have observed no recurrences, and Cooney and Grosfeld noted only one recurrence after external drainage in 25 children.[6] The low incidence of recurrence after external drainage in pediatric patients is probably related to the fact that the cysts are most often caused by trauma and the pancreas and its duct are otherwise normal.

Internal Drainage

Because of the possibility that the pancreatic fistula that is produced by external drainage will not close for many months, internal drainage is preferable to external drainage when a choice is available. Either cystogastrostomy or Roux-en-Y cystojejunostomy is employed, depending on the location of the pseudocyst.[4, 7, 12]

HEMORRHAGE

Hemorrhage is the most serious complication encountered after an internal drainage procedure. The problem has been reported to be more frequent after cystogastrostomy than after Roux-en-Y cystojejunostomy.[2, 16] Hutson et al., for example, noted a 50 per cent hemorrhage rate after cystogastrostomy.[13]

The most common site of hemorrhage after cystogastrostomy is at the anastomosis of the posterior gastric wall to the cyst. In these cases the bleeding is usually from submucosal vessels in the stomach wall. One of the factors that may predispose to bleeding is the use of a running catgut suture to oversew the edge of the cystogastrostomy anastomosis. When the catgut dissolves, the cut ends of the vessels in the stomach wall are exposed to activated pancreatic enzymes and bleeding becomes likely. Therefore, to eliminate this possibility, individual vessels in the stomach wall should be ligated with nonabsorbable sutures before the anastomosis is completed.

Less commonly, bleeding is from a blood vessel in the lesser sac that is in direct contact with the cyst fluid. The likeliest cause of bleeding in these cases is inadequate cyst drainage, because of a small anastomosis, or the inadvertent creation of a one-way valve mechanism at the anastomotic site. Since a running suture tends to produce an anastomosis with a rigid stoma, some suggest that the use of interrupted sutures for the anastomosis will ensure better cyst drainage.[15] In fact, when careful attention has been given to the techniques of vascular control and suture approximation of the stomach and cyst, the incidence of serious hemorrhage from cystogastrostomy is markedly reduced. Schumer et al.[18] and Warshaw[21] report only a 3 per cent incidence of hemorrhage after cystogastrostomy in a large number of patients. In Cooney and Grosfeld's review of pseudocysts in 75 children, only one of 21 patients who had cystogastrostomy had significant postoperative hemorrhage.[6]

The treatment depends on the site of bleeding. Bleeding from the wall of the stomach or intestine is usually best handled by immediate re-exploration and suture ligation of the bleeder. Bleeding from the lesser sac may necessitate pancreatectomy. If the rate of bleeding is such that immediate laparotomy is not necessary, gastroscopy and angiography can be useful in determining the exact site of bleeding.

RECURRENCE

Experience indicates that recurrence of pseudocyst is as frequent after internal drainage as after external drainage. In a review of 1020 patients (mostly adults), Becher et al.[3] noted a recurrence rate of 2.3 per cent after cystogastrostomy, 4.5 per cent after cystojejunostomy, and 5.2 per cent after cystoduodenostomy. No recurrences were noted in our own series, and only one recurrence was noted after internal drainage in 34 patients in a large pediatric review.[6]

DEATH

Death in children with pancreatic pseudocyst is unusual, regardless of the type of drainage procedure performed. Among 96 patients studied by Welch, only three deaths occurred.[22] Two patients had not been treated surgically, and the other died on the operating table of "cardiac arrest."

COMPLICATIONS OF TREATING HYPOGLYCEMIA OF INFANCY

In most infants with hyperinsulinemic hypoglycemia, dietary therapy is sufficient to control blood sugar and allow the disorder to resolve spontaneously. In others, administration of diazoxide or other nonoperative measures have led to remission. However, a small group of patients remain refractory to medical therapy, and a portion or all of the pancreas must be removed to achieve control of blood sugar.[9-11] Except for the rare insulinoma, the precise etiology of the hyperinsulinemic state in these patients is still not established. Nesidioblastosis, adenomatosis, islet cell hyperplasia, and, more recently, "endocrine cell dysplasia" have been used to describe the pathologic findings in the pancreas.[14] Several types of complications can occur when pancreatectomy is used to control hypoglycemia in these children.

Failure to Control Hypoglycemia

Graham and Hartmann first reported the value of subtotal pancreatectomy in 1934.[8] In a review of subtotal pancreatectomy for hypoglycemia in 101 children, Welch noted that only 64 patients were normoglycemic without medication following surgery, although glycemia in 23 others could be controlled medically.[22]

One of the reasons for failure appears to be the extent of pancreatectomy. For example, the study of Harken et al. indicated that the failure rate was 50 per cent when a traditional two-thirds pancreatectomy was performed.[11] In this series, near-total pancreatectomy eventually controlled the hypoglycemia of those patients whose initial surgery failed. On the basis of similar experiences, most pediatric surgeons now choose to remove about 85 per cent of the pancreas during the first operation. This more extensive pancreatectomy appears to lower the failure rate but still does not cause diabetes and intestinal malabsorption from pancreatic enzyme insufficiency. The extended subtotal pancreatectomy requires resection of the pancreas from its tail to the right of the superior mesenteric vessels, removing about half the head of the pancreas. In a personal series of seven patients treated by 85 per cent pancreatectomy, hypoglycemia was permanently eliminated in six. In the other child, recurrent hypoglycemia was successfully treated by a second operation in which half the remaining pancreas was resected.

It remains difficult to predict which patients will not be cured by 85 per cent pancreatectomy. A recent study by Jaffe et al. suggests that persons with isolated rather than diffuse "endocrine cell dysplasia" are likely to respond more favorably.[14] However, information of this type, which might be used as a guide to the extent of resection, is not available to the surgeon because of the time required to perform the histochemical and immunostaining techniques used in the analysis. Similarly, immediate blood sugar response to pancreatectomy is an unreliable predictor of the success of surgery. In all patients there is an immediate increase in blood glucose after subtotal pancreatectomy (Figs. 20–1 and 20–2). In those in whom surgery eventually fails, hypoglycemia usually does not recur until 2 days to 2 weeks later. Blood sugar levels and glucose intake in a child in whom pancreatectomy controlled hypoglycemia are shown in Figure 20–1, and similar data from a child in whom operation failed are shown in Figure 20–2. Failures of surgery will continue to occur until a test is developed that

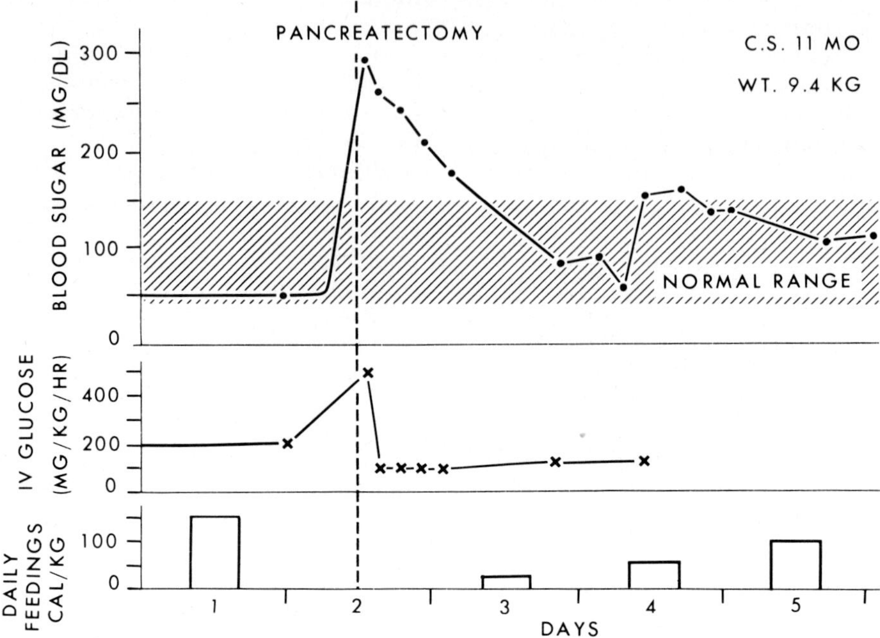

Figure 20–1   Blood glucose levels, intravenous glucose intake, and oral intake before and after 85 per cent pancreatectomy in a 1-month-old child with nesidioblastosis. Elevations in blood sugar persisted for 1 day despite low glucose intake. Insulin was not required. Blood sugars remained in the normal range thereafter. Hypoglycemia never recurred.

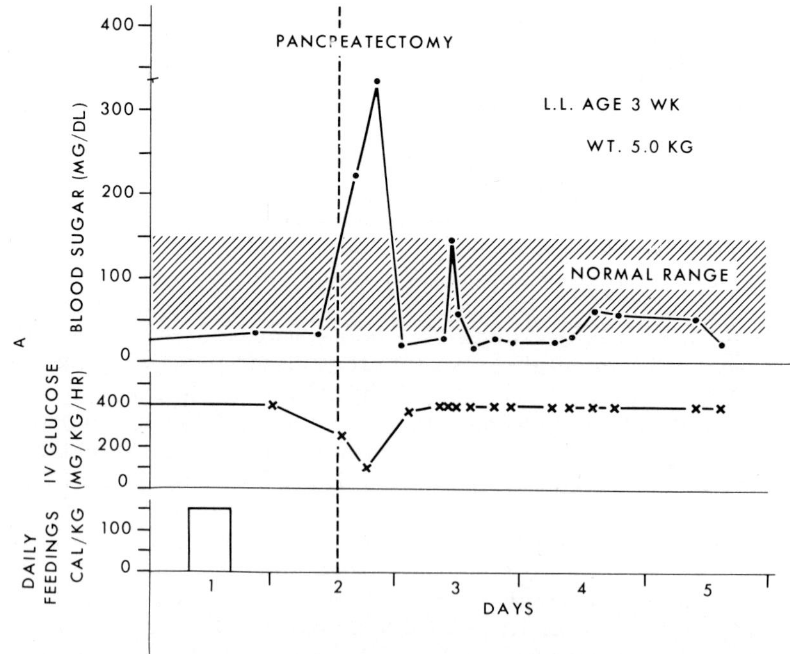

Figure 20–2   Blood glucose levels, intravenous glucose intake, and oral intake before and after 85 per cent pancreatectomy in a 3-week-old child with nesidioblastosis. Elevations in blood sugar persisted for 18 hours. By the first postoperative day, hypoglycemia recurred despite infusion of large quantities of intravenous glucose. Hypoglycemia was unremitting, and a more extensive pancreatectomy was required 1 week later.

will accurately predict whether an immediate favorable response to pancreatectomy will persist.

Postoperative Hyperglycemia

Blood sugar increases dramatically immediately after removal of more than 50 per cent of the pancreas (Figs. 20–1 and 20–2). We have observed blood sugar levels as high as 800 mg/dl within 12 hours after surgery. This extreme hyperglycemia can usually be avoided by decreasing the rate of glucose administration as soon as the pancreas is resected. Infusion of 2.5 per cent glucose solution at a rate (4 ml/kg/hr) that provides approximately 100 mg glucose/kg/hr will usually prevent this complication. Insulin usually is not needed to control postoperative hyperglycemia. However, insulin should be given when a decrease in glucose administration does not lower blood sugar levels sufficiently to avoid an osmotic diuresis or when significant ketosis develops.

Splenic Injury

In the initial descriptions of pancreatectomy for hypoglycemia, concomitant splenectomy was suggested because the splenic artery and vein must be ligated during removal of the body and tail of the pancreas.[9] As evidence accumulated to show that splenectomy subjected these infants to a high risk of sepsis and death, attempts were made to preserve the spleen during pancreatectomy. It is now recognized that in most patients the splenic artery and vein can be divided and the spleen will subsist on the short gastric vessels.[22] Therefore, splenectomy should not be performed during resection of the tail of the pancreas, and every precaution should be taken to preserve the short gastric vessels during dissection near the hilum of the spleen. Since it is still possible that a portion or all of the splenic blood supply will be permanently disrupted, it is wise to obtain a spleen scan 2 to 3 weeks after pancreatectomy. A scan at this time will usually show some decrease in blood flow, but the size of the functioning splenic tissue should be normal. If splenic function is not present, appropriate prophylactic

measures to prevent postsplenectomy sepsis must be taken (see Chapter 21).

Pancreatic Fistula

Although fistula formation is a significant problem after pancreatic resection in adults with carcinoma and pancreatitis, it rarely occurs after pancreatectomy for neonatal hypoglycemia. This complication was not seen in any of the infants treated at this hospital, nor has it been reported in any other large series. Drainage of the lesser sac following pancreatectomy, as advocated by some, has not been used in my last seven patients, and no complications have occurred.

Complications of "Total" Pancreatectomy

Near-total pancreatectomy has been employed in those infants with hypoglycemia that cannot be controlled by medication after 85 per cent or greater pancreatectomy. The technique of "total" pancreatectomy for hypoglycemia has been described by Harken et al.[11] The residual pancreas is peeled off the duodenum and common bile duct, leaving small nests of pancreatic tissue on the duodenal blood vessels to avoid devascularization of the duodenum, Injuries to the duodenum and common bile duct are the most serious potential complications of total pancreatectomy, although none of these problems occurred in the only reported large series of "total" pancreatectomies in children.

A small inadvertent opening into the duodenum should be closed transversely and the area drained. A more serious problem arises when a significant length of duodenum is devascularized during pancreatic resection. Ortiz et al. noted this complication in one child in whom the duodenum appeared dusky at the completion of total pancreatectomy.[17] At a "second look" operation performed the next day, the descending duodenum was necrotic, but the common bile duct was viable. The necrotic duodenum was resected except for a 7-mm patch of full-thickness duodenum around the ampulla. After the viable ends of the duodenum were united by duodenoduodenostomy, the patch of duodenum containing the common bile duct was implanted into the lateral wall of the third portion of the duodenum. This child was reported to be asymptomatic with a normal biliary tract 6 months later.

If an opening into the duodenum is not recognized, if the duodenal closure breaks down, or if the blood supply to the duodenum is disrupted, a side duodenal fistula will result. In the past, mortality as high as 50 per cent has followed this complication. However, with the use of hyperalimentation and suture closure of the pylorus when indicated, mortality can be reduced markedly. The initial treatment of duodenal fistula requires nasogastric suction and total parenteral nutrition. The area around the fistula must be drained adequately, which often requires suction drainage through a sump tube. Most fistulae will show signs of closing in 1 or 2 weeks with this type of treatment. However, when loss of large quantities of gastrointestinal secretions persists, operative intervention is necessary. The surgical technique employed depends on the pathologic condition. In some cases the fistula can be closed and the repair reinforced with omentum. If the defect is large, a loop of proximal jejunum can be anastomosed to it. Alternatively, the serosal surface of the jejunal loop can be used as a patch to cover the fistula. When these procedures are not feasible, the side jejunal fistula should be converted to an end fistula by closing the pylorus with sutures and draining the stomach by the creation of a gastrojejunostomy. A Witzel jejunostomy can be used in combination with this procedure for enteral feedings.[20]

Whenever more than 90 per cent of the pancreas is removed, injury to the common bile duct is a definite hazard. Intubation of the bile duct can aid in its localization, but this is not wise in the infant because intubation of the normal small bile duct is likely to result in stricture. Injury to the common bile duct can be avoided only by very careful dissection. Although common duct injury was not noted in the series of "total" pancreatectomies reported by Harken et al.,[11] Child and coworkers[5] reported a 6 per cent incidence of common duct injury after 95 per cent pancreatectomy in a much larger series of adults. If a small opening is made

in the duct, it should be sutured. As noted, a T tube usually cannot be used safely as a stent in these small patients. If the entire duct is transected, primary end-to-end anastomosis should be attempted. When a significant length of duct is destroyed or devascularized, Roux-en-Y choledochojejunostomy will be necessary.

Diabetes and pancreatic insufficiency are the late sequelae of "total" pancreatectomy. Diabetes in these children is usually much easier to control than ordinary juvenile-onset diabetes. Some children require low doses of insulin, but others need no insulin because the nests of pancreatic tissue left in situ or ectopic pancreas will produce sufficient quantities. All children have malabsorption due to loss of pancreatic enzymes. However, normal growth and nutrition can be maintained by the administration of pancreatic enzymes in regimens similar to those used for children with cystic fibrosis.

References

1. Attard, J.: Pseudocyst of the pancreas in a child. Br. J. Surg. 56:235, 1969.
2. Balfour, J. F.: Pancreatic pseudocysts: Complications and their relations to the timing of treatment. Surg. Clin. North Am. 50:395, 1970.
3. Becher, W. F., Pratt, H. S., and Ganji, H.: Pseudocysts of the pancreas. Surg. Gynecol. Obstet. 127:744, 1968.
4. Blumenthal, H. T., and Probstein, J. G.: Acute pancreatitis in the newborn, infancy and childhood. Ann. Surg. 27:533, 1961.
5. Child, C. G., III, Frey, C. F., and Fry, W. J.: A reappraisal of removal of 95 per cent of the distal portion of the pancreas. Surg. Gynecol. Obstet. 129:49, 1969.
6. Cooney, D. R., and Grosfeld, J. L.: Operative management of pancreatic pseudocysts in infants and children. A review of 75 cases. Ann. Surg. 182:590, 1975.
7. Gibson, L. E., and Haller, J. A.: Acute pancreatitis associated with congenital cyst of the common bile duct. J. Pediatr. 55:650, 1959.
8. Graham, E. A., and Hartmann, A. F.: Subtotal resection of the pancreas for hypoglycemia. Surg. Gynecol. Obstet. 59:474, 1934.
9. Gross, R. E.: The Surgery of Infancy and Childhood. Philadelphia, W. B. Saunders Co., 1953.
10. Hamilton, J. P., Baker, L., Kaye, R., and Koop, C. E.: Subtotal pancreatectomy in the management of severe persistent idiopathic hypoglycemia in children. Pediatrics 39:49, 1967.
11. Harken, A. H., Filler, R. M., AvRuskin, T. W., and

Crigler, J. F., Jr.: The role of "total" pancreatectomy in the treatment of unremitting hypoglycemia of infancy. J. Pediatr. 6:284, 1971.

12. Hendren, W. H., Jr., Greep, J. M., and Patton, A. S.: Pancreatitis in childhood: Experience with 15 cases. Arch. Dis. Child. 40:132, 1965.

13. Hutson, D. G., Zeppa, R., and Warren, W. D.: Prevention of postoperative hemorrhage after pancreatic cystogastrostomy. Ann. Surg. 177:689, 1973.

14. Jaffe, R., Hashida, Y., Yunis, E. J.: Pancreatic pathology in hyperinsulinemic hypoglycemia of infancy. Lab. Invest. 42:356, 1980.

15. Jordan, G. L., Jr.: Complications of pancreatic and splenic surgery. *In* Artz, C. P., and Hardy, J. D. (eds.): Management of Surgical Complications, 3rd ed. Philadelphia, W. B. Saunders Co., 1975, p. 534.

16. Jordan, G. L., Jr., and Howard, J. M.: Pancreatic pseudocysts. Am. J. Gastroenterol. 45:444, 1966.

17. Ortiz, V. N., Haase, G. M., Sotos, J. F., and Clatworthy, H. W., Jr.: Reimplantation of the ampulla of Vater after total pancreatectomy for nesidioblastosis. J. Pediatr. Surg. 13:722, 1978.

18. Schumer, W., McDonald, G. O., Nichols, R. L., and Miller, B.: Transgastric cystogastrostomy. Surg. Gynecol. Obstet. 137:48, 1973.

19. Thomford, N. R., and Jesseph, J. E.: Pseudocyst of the pancreas. Am. J. Surg. 118:86, 1969.

20. Warren, W. D., Marsh, W. H., and Sandusky, W. R.: An appraisal of surgical procedures for pancreatic pseudocyst. Ann. Surg. 147:903, 1955.

21. Warshaw, A. L.: Inflammatory masses following acute pancreatitis. Surg. Clin. North Am. 54:621, 1974.

22. Welch, K. J.: The pancreas. *In* Ravitch, M. M., Welch, K. J., Benson, C. D., et al. (eds.): Pediatric Surgery, 2nd ed. Vol. 2. Chicago, Year Book Medical Publishers, 1979.

SPLEEN AND PORTAL CIRCULATION

21

Angelo J. Eraklis, M.D.

THE SPLEEN

In children, elective splenectomy is of major benefit in the management of a number of congenital and acquired diseases. The physician's decision about whether to recommend elective removal of the spleen and about the age at which that procedure should be carried out is based on the advantages and dangers of splenectomy. Since the indications for splenectomy are primarily medical, the need for and the timing of the procedure are generally decided by a medical specialist (hematologist, oncologist, or metabolic disease specialist). When splenectomy has been chosen, the role of the surgeon is to evaluate the preoperative status and requirements of the patient and to remove the spleen as safely as possible with the least morbidity and the lowest possible mortality.

Indications for Splenectomy in the Child

For the majority of children, the indication for splenectomy is a hematologic disease, primarily congenital hemolytic anemia or idiopathic thrombocytopenia.[7] Of the total number of children undergoing splenectomy, the percentage who require the procedure because of trauma varies widely. Institutions with active emergency services report a large percentage of ruptured spleens, whereas referral institutions show more elective splenectomies. Splenectomy as part of a procedure for portal vein decompression and hypersplenism is now less common. Preservation of the spleen during major surgery of the left upper quadrant, such as gastric tube formation, fundoplications, pancreatectomy, and portal vascular

264

shunts, is currently recommended. In recent years, staging of children with Hodgkin's disease has become the second most frequent indication for splenectomy. Indications for splenectomy in 1413 children are shown in Table 21–1.

The need for splenectomy in treating patients with *idiopathic thrombocytopenia* must be determined on an individual basis. Splenectomy is indicated in persons who have the acute form of this disorder if the platelet count is less than 1000/mm³ and the platelets are unresponsive to steroid therapy for more than 1 week. The absolute number of platelets may be only 5000/mm³, but their functional capacity is as good as a count of 50,000/mm³ in a normal person. These are young, highly functional platelets, as opposed to the mixed age of platelets in normal blood. For children with chronic thrombocytopenic purpura that lasts longer than 1 year and is unresponsive to steroids, removal of the spleen is indicated.

In *hereditary spherocytosis*, the red cell mass turns over at five times the normal rate and

TABLE 21–1 INDICATIONS FOR SPLENECTOMY IN 1413 CHILDREN UNDER THE AGE OF 16 YEARS

Disease	Number of Patients
Congenital hemolytic anemia	395
Trauma	348
Idiopathic thrombocytopenia	265
Portal hypertension and hypersplenism	167
Incidental to other surgery	59
Hypoplastic aplastic anemia	47
Histiocytoses and inborn errors of metabolism	32
Lymphoma, leukemia, Hodgkin's disease	20
Acquired hemolytic anemia	18
Primary splenic disease (cyst or torsion)	16
Other	46

pigment production is increased, often leading to gallstones. The role of splenectomy in this disease is also in question, and the decision to undertake it must be made on an individual basis, depending on the patient's hemoglobin level and transfusion volume requirements. The need for splenectomy in patients with *thalassemia major* is predicated on the size of the spleen and the transfusion requirements, which may be significantly decreased by removal of the organ. For an *immune hemolytic anemia* the process must be chronic, associated with a positive Coombs' test, and unresponsive to steroids. Even when these criteria are followed there is a 50 per cent chance of failure to reverse or modify the process by splenectomy. For the aforementioned hematologic conditions in which hemolysis is common, the incidence of gallstone disease is at least 10 per cent. A preoperative ultrasound study of the biliary tree is indicated in these patients, and an effort should be made to palpate the gallbladder during surgery.

In our institution, *Hodgkin's disease* has become the second most common indication for splenectomy, which is advised for all patients with the disease except those in stages IA and IV. The clinical stage of 25 per cent of all patients who are staged by laparotomy has been changed by the operative and pathologic findings. These findings include involvement of the spleen in half the patients whose stage is changed and involvement of the retroperitoneal nodes in the other half. An additional advantage of splenectomy in this disease is the avoidance of irradiation of the left upper quadrant and sparing of the lung and kidney. Partial splenectomy in patients with Hodgkin's disease is not advised, since a lesion may exist in the part not removed.

In patients with a splenic mass or trauma, the decision for or against splenectomy often rests entirely with the surgeon.[12] Patients with *nonangiomatous, nonparasitic splenic cysts* may present with chronic, intermittent abdominal or left shoulder pain and a sense of abdominal fullness. On examination, a mass in the left upper quadrant may be present. A scintiscan will show focal intrasplenic absence of isotope uptake.[10]

Torsion of the spleen with or without splenic infarction is an unusual congenital lesion. The absence of splenic uptake on scanning indicates complete vascular occlusion.[3] At operation the spleen is found to be devoid of its normal ligamentous attachments to the diaphragm and retroperitoneum.

Management of the child with an *injured spleen* is undergoing change. The majority of such children have sustained blunt trauma to the abdomen in sports or play. Associated injuries to major organs are uncommon.[6, 9] Most of these patients can be safely monitored in a surgical intensive care environment and, if necessary, given transfusions of blood.[2, 6, 7] The symptoms of almost all these young people improve during the first 24 hours, and surgical exploration or splenectomy is not required. The recent availability of scintigraphy with technetium-99m (^{99m}Tc) sulfur colloid has provided a reliable and convenient technique for diagnosing splenic injury and documenting its anatomic evolution during the healing period.[9]

At Children's Hospital Medical Center, Boston, in a 3-year period from 1976 through 1978, 91 children whose physical signs suggested splenic injury underwent ^{99m}Tc sulfur colloid scintigraphy. Thirty-four of these patients were found to have ruptured spleens. All but three were treated nonoperatively. One patient died of associated massive bodily injuries sustained in an automobile accident. One child with mononucleosis underwent splenectomy for spontaneous rupture of a large, soft spleen. The third child had a splenectomy because vital signs failed to stabilize quickly with large volume transfusions. The remaining 31 patients (87 per cent of the group with proven rupture of the spleen) were discharged without operation. More than half of these patients required blood transfusions during hospitalization. If we exclude the one child with massive injuries and the other with an underlying infection, only one child of the 32 with proven rupture of the spleen for whom a conservative program was outlined failed to respond to conservative measures and required surgery. There were no late sequelae, no delayed ruptures, and no evidence of splenosis on repeat scan. The reported high incidence of delayed rupture of the spleen (11 to 15 per cent of patients) is probably related to a delay in diagnosis of splenic rupture rather than to delayed rupture of a subcapsular hematoma. A 1 to 2 per cent incidence of delayed rupture has been reported in more recent series in which modern diagnostic methods have shown the rupture of the organ early.

As an alternative method of management, Ratner et al.[14] and Sherman and Asch[16] have recommended partial splenectomy or direct surgical repair of the ruptured spleen. The methods would not seem to apply to our three patients who ultimately required splenectomy.

The indications for nonoperative treatment are a technetium scan that shows the entire spleen to be perfused and therefore fully vascularized, no associated intra-abdominal injuries identified, and no associated systemic illness such as mononucleosis or blood clotting abnormalities. In addition, vital signs must stabilize within the first few hours after injury with modest volume transfusions.

The nonoperative management of patients sustaining blunt abdominal trauma and injury to the spleen consists of placing central lines for monitoring and transfusion, passing a nasogastric tube, and placing the child in an intensive care environment for close monitoring. Transfusions are given as indicated. The child is kept in bed with the nasogastric tube in place for 3 days. A hospital stay of 10 days has been suggested. A repeat scan is recommended within 2 weeks and a follow-up study within 3 months. No contact sports are permitted for 2 months. Of 31 patients with proven rupture of the spleen who were not operated upon, all had follow-up scans made from 6 weeks to 1 year after injury. In no patient was there evidence of regenerating ectopic splenic tissue to support the theory of splenosis after injury. Splenic cyst or pseudocyst of nonangiomatous and nonparasitic nature is said to be a late but rare complication of blunt trauma. In a series of 12 patients with splenic cysts reported by Griscom et al., only one patient had a distinct history of abdominal trauma.[10]

Splenectomy

For elective removal of the spleen, we prefer a left upper quadrant transverse incision made with the child lying in a semilat-

eral position and with a break in the table.[11] The anterior and posterior rectus fascia are incised, and the undivided rectus muscle is retracted medially. Posteriorly, the incision is continued just below the eleventh rib. This exposure allows a rapid approach to the spleen, little retraction, and ready access to the posterior aspect of the organ. With the spleen pulled downward and forward, the peritoneal and phrenic attachments are divided and the spleen is exteriorized. Once the spleen is out of the abdominal cavity, the short gastric vessels are divided. The hilus of the spleen is then clearly visualized, and the splenic artery and vein can be readily identified. Such exposure minimizes the chance of injury to the tail of the pancreas, which may need to be dissected free of the splenic vessels before division.

When the operation is done because of blunt or penetrating abdominal trauma, some surgeons prefer to use a vertical incision. In children with hemolytic disease, the gallbladder is palpated and, whenever possible, visualized. We do not carry out a cholecystectomy at the same operation, although others have done so without incident. The abdomen is closed without drains.

In children undergoing splenectomy for acquired hypersplenism and congenital hemolytic diseases, the presence and location of accessory spleens are of paramount importance. Unsatisfactory response to splenectomy may be related to the surgeon's failure to identify and remove such accessory spleens. Re-exploration may be necessary. One or more accessory spleens were found in 229 (16 per cent) of 1413 children (Table 21–2); 145 children had only one accessory spleen identified, and 10 were found to have as many as five or more accessory spleens (Fig. 21–1A). The exact

TABLE 21–2 ACCESSORY SPLEENS

Number of Accessory Spleens*	Number of Patients
1	145
2	45
3	16
4	9
5 or more	10
Unknown	4

*One or more accessory spleens were found in 229 of 1413 children (16 per cent).

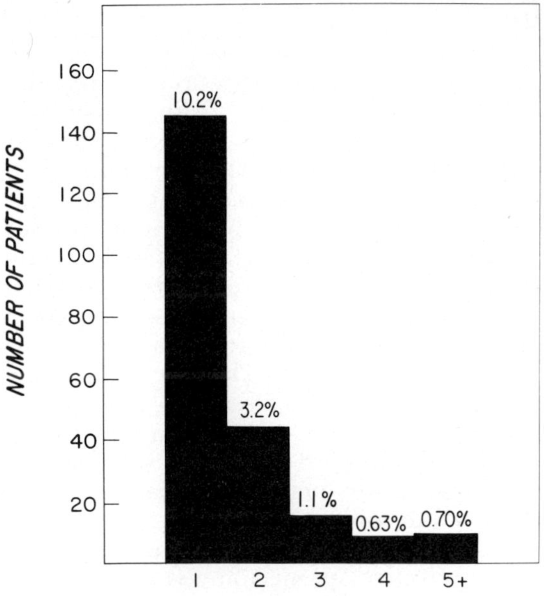

Figure 21–1 *A,* Number of accessory spleens found in 1413 children who underwent splenectomy. Sixteen per cent of all children were found to have at least one accessory spleen. *B,* Location, when noted by the surgeon, of accessory spleens in these children.

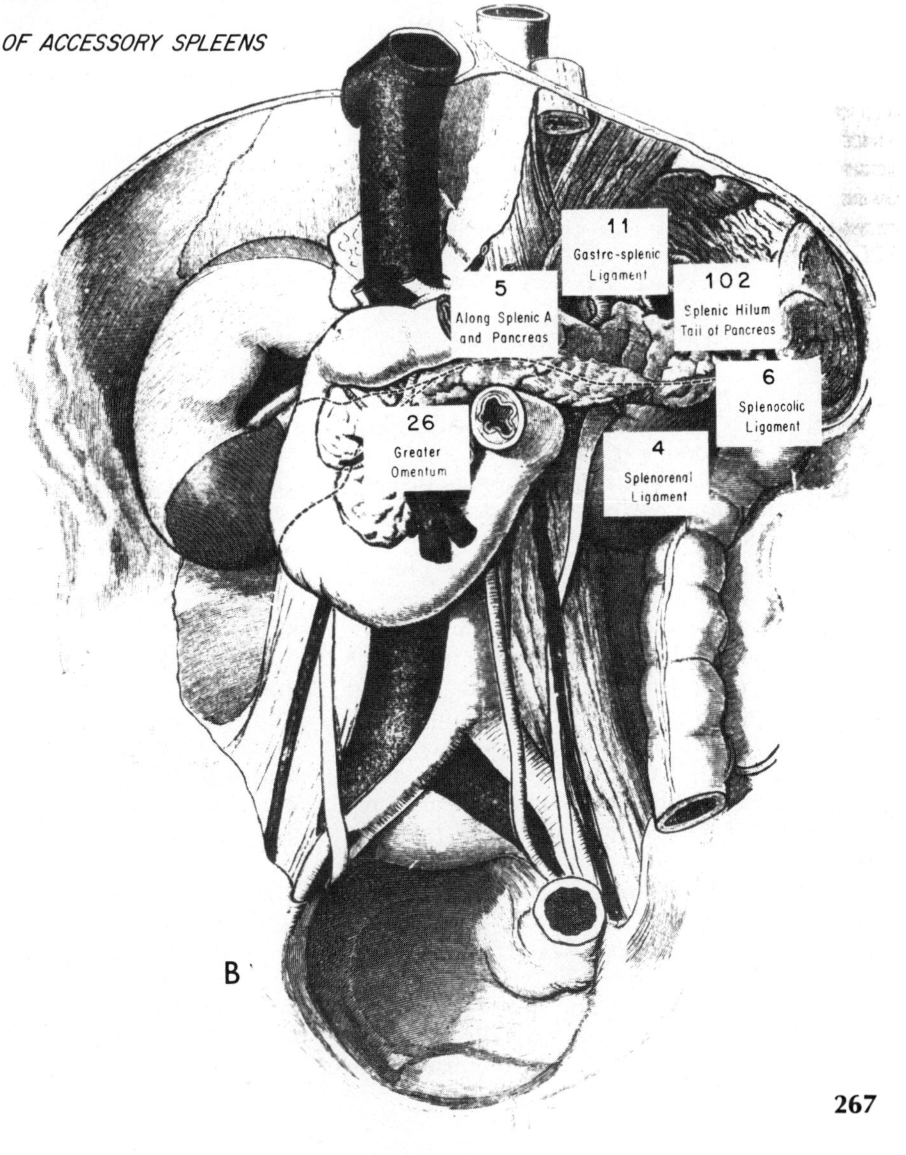

TABLE 21–3 LOCATION OF 154 ACCESSORY SPLEENS

Location of Spleens	Number of Spleens
Splenic hilum and tail of pancreas	102
Greater omentum	26
Gastrosplenic ligament	11
Along splenic artery and pancreas	5
Splenocolic ligament	6
Splenorenal ligament	4

location of 154 accessory spleens was noted; the majority were close to the hilum of the spleen or adjacent to the tail of the pancreas (Table 21–3). Twenty-six accessory spleens were found within the greater omentum, 11 within the gastrosplenic ligament, five along the splenic artery and pancreas, six within the splenocolic ligament (Fig. 21–1B), and four posteriorly within the splenorenal ligament. On the basis of these findings, a search for accessory spleens should include careful examination of the superior, inferior, and posterior supporting ligaments of the spleen as well as the omentum and upper margin of the pancreas along the splenic artery.

RESULTS OF SPLENECTOMY

In a review of 1413 children, the effect of splenectomy on the platelet count and coagulability of blood was assessed by analyzing the incidence of thromboembolic disease, the number of children treated postoperatively with heparin, and the preoperative and postoperative platelet counts.[7] The response of the peripheral platelet count to splenectomy was evaluated in 58 children with congenital hemolytic anemia and in 68 with idiopathic thrombocytopenia. For the 68 patients with idiopathic thrombocytopenia, the mean preoperative platelet count was 38,000/mm^3. On the first postoperative day, the mean platelet count for these patients was 193,000/mm^3. This rose progressively over the next 8 days to the highest level of 881,000/mm^3 (Fig. 21–2A). In children with thrombocytopenia, infusion of platelets is not indicated. Of the 265 patients in this series who had idiopathic thrombocytopenia, platelets were given preoperatively to 31 and intraoperatively to 14. In our personal experience, preoperative or intraoperative administration of platelets has not been necessary. In the 58 patients with congenital hemolytic anemia, the average preoperative platelet count was 322,000/mm^3, rising postoperatively to a high of 1,050,000/mm^3 by the ninth postoperative day (Fig. 21–2B). Only seven of the 1413 children were treated with heparin postoperatively. In our personal experience, no patient has required postsplenectomy heparinization. There was no report of thromboembolic disease in any patient. Since the platelet count continues to rise during the first 10 days after splenectomy, multiple, early peripheral platelet counts are of little value.

The hospital mortality for patients undergoing elective splenectomy is well below 1 per cent. In our experience, there have been no hospital deaths among more than 550 patients who have undergone elective splenectomy. Overall statistics are seriously modified by the mortality associated with splenectomy for trauma and compound injuries. In the review of 1413 cases, the overall mortality was 3.3 per cent (47 patients). Forty-three of the 47 patients who died had trauma and complicated medical problems. Only four of the deaths occurred in patients who were thought to have idiopathic thrombocytopenia but whose platelet counts did not respond to splenectomy.

Of the 47 patients who died, 10 died intraoperatively, all of them children with trauma or a malignancy. Of the 37 patients who died during the postoperative period, 28 died as a result of their primary disease and four of overwhelming infection. Five died of unspecified causes. Since many of the deaths occurred in children with a fatal underlying disease, it seemed useful to evaluate postoperative mortality and its relationship to the primary diagnosis. Of 395 patients with congenital hemolytic anemia, the only one who died was a 3-year-old child in whom a high fever and gastrointestinal bleeding developed. Three hospital deaths among the 265 patients with thrombocytopenia were due to intracranial bleeding in children aged 14 years, 8 years, and 6 months. In two patients the intracranial bleeding was related to thrombocytopenia persisting after splenectomy, raising serious doubts about the accuracy of the preoperative diagnosis. The 1.7 per cent mortality

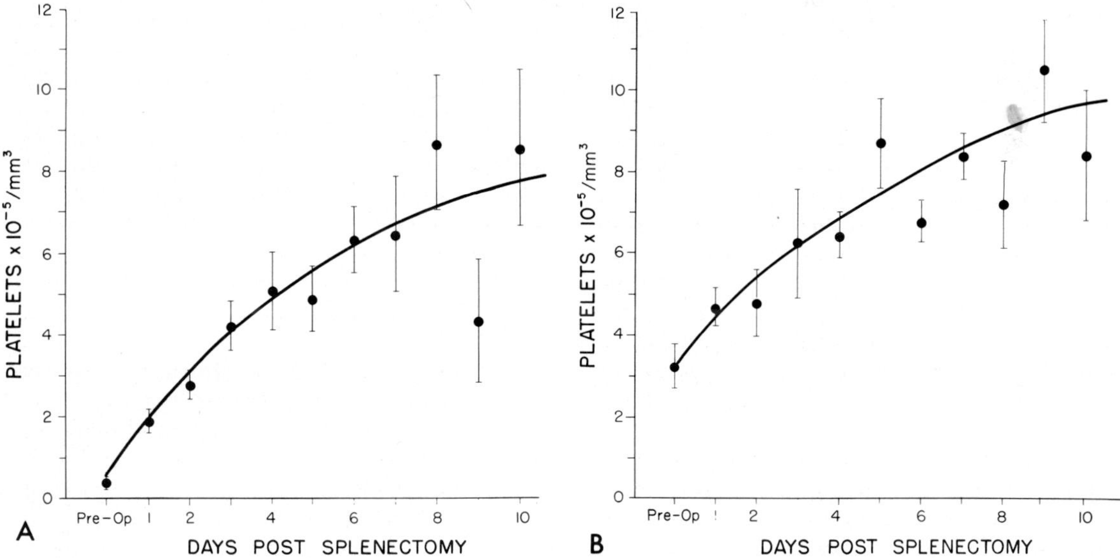

Figure 21–2 *A,* Peripheral platelet counts in 68 children following splenectomy for idiopathic thrombocytopenia. *B,* Peripheral platelet counts in 58 children after splenectomy for congenital hemolytic anemia.

noted in the 348 children with ruptured spleens was due to associated injuries, especially head trauma. The highest mortality (7.5 per cent) occurred in the group of 360 patients who underwent splenectomy for advanced malignancy, aplastic anemia, and a variety of other conditions for which splenectomy was probably of little value.

The nonfatal postoperative complication rate for the entire series was 12.6 per cent. In the 660 patients with congenital hemolytic anemia or idiopathic thrombocytopenia, the complication rate was 6.5 per cent (Table 21–4). Most of these complications were minor, leading only to slightly prolonged hospitalization. Significant pancreatitis was encountered in five children with congenital hemolytic anemia or idiopathic

TABLE 21–4 NONFATAL POSTOPERATIVE COMPLICATIONS OF SPLENECTOMY

Complications	Total Series (1413 Patients)	CHA and ITP* (660 Patients)
Incisional	47	11
Bleeding	42	6
Pancreatitis	25	5
Other	64	22
TOTAL	178 (12.6%)	44 (6.5%)

*Congenital hemolytic anemia and idiopathic thrombocytopenia.

thrombocytopenia, presumably as a result of injury to the tail of the pancreas in the process of removing the spleen.

POSTSPLENECTOMY SEPSIS

Since the initial report by King and Shumacker in 1952, a number of articles have documented the increased incidence of severe infection following splenectomy in children.[4, 7, 13, 18, 20] Subsequent authors have supported the evidence for increased susceptibility to infection after splenectomy, whereas others have presented data denying any such danger. Despite review of the histories of at least 3000 patients by more than two dozen authors, considerable confusion still exists about the degree of risk after splenectomy in infants and children. This has caused serious concern to pediatricians and surgeons confronted with conditions for which splenectomy is known to be of benefit.

Increasing evidence has shown that the risk is definite and exists when splenectomy is done for any reason and at any age. When splenectomy is done for some systemic diseases such as histiocytoses, inborn errors of metabolism, thalassemia, and portal hypertension related to hepatitis, the mortality from overwhelming postoperative sepsis ranges from 10 to 33 per cent. Even in patients with no underlying systemic illnesses, such as those who have sustained splenic trauma, a small but definite statistical incidence persists. In one series of 389 patients, a 0.25 per cent mortality from overwhelming sepsis followed splenectomy for trauma.[20] In another series of 688 patients who underwent splenectomy for trauma, the overall mortality from overwhelming sepsis in the study period was 0.56 per cent.[19] The incidence of overwhelming sepsis in the general population is 0.01 per cent.

It is estimated that there are approximately 50,000 people in this country who are functionally asplenic as a complication of sickle cell disease. An additional 35,000 patients annually undergo splenectomy for trauma, hematologic indications, and staging laparotomy for Hodgkin's disease. Therefore, the pool of patients who are potentially at risk for postsplenectomy sepsis is large.

A single experience with postsplenectomy sepsis leaves a profound impression on the physicians caring for the patient. The onset of the infection is difficult to detect, the course is extremely rapid, and the outcome is fatal in 50 to 75 per cent of those who become ill.[5] The majority of deaths follow a sudden, overwhelming bout of meningitis and septicemia. Death occurs within hours after the onset of symptoms. The terminal events include seizures, shock, and evidence of disseminated intravascular coagulation. At postmortem examination, bilateral adrenal hemorrhages (Waterhouse-Friderichsen syndrome) were commonly found.[8] The remainder of the deaths followed an acute and fulminating episode of pneumonia with septicemia not responding to antibiotics. In 50 per cent of the patients who died, *Streptococcus pneumoniae* was cultured. *Neisseria meningitidis* and *Hemophilus influenzae* organisms were found in the majority of the remaining patients.

The risk of sepsis seems to be substantially higher in very young children. In our series the mortality after splenectomy due to infection in children less than 4 years of age was 8.1 per cent; for those older than 4 years the mortality was 3.3 per cent. However, in this group the indications for splenectomy were often more urgent and, in gener-

al, the primary disease more serious and not as likely to respond to medical treatment. The interval between splenectomy and the fatal infection is significant. Eighty per cent of the deaths from infection occurred within 4 years after splenectomy, although death from overwhelming sepsis has occurred as late as 18 years after the procedure.[8]

The exact role of the spleen in preventing or suppressing bacterial infection in human beings is unknown. Removal of this organ results in a number of alterations in the defenses of the host. The spleen is an important part of the reticuloendothelial system. It acts as a filter for circulating debris, including bacteria, and is an important source of lymphoid cells and antibody production. It is known that splenectomy in animals results in decreased resistance to pneumococcal infections and depresses the serum levels of immunoglobulin M and opsonins.[19] The immunologic response to various antigens is also decreased.[15] Patients with sickle cell disease are at risk for pneumococcal infection because of deficient pneumococcal serum opsonization activity. Sophisticated immunologic studies of these patients have disclosed important differences, such as an inability to switch from immunoglobulin M to immunoglobulin G synthesis after secondary immunizations; furthermore, almost complete loss of amplified T cell function has been noted in splenectomized mice.[1] Circulating antibody levels are abnormal in splenectomized human patients following injection of heterologous erythrocytes.[15] The human spleen also produces tuftsin; absence of this material may further compromise the postsurgical patient.[4]

The onset of sepsis is so insidious and progression to death so rapid that therapy following diagnosis of postsplenectomy infection is unsatisfactory. Prophylaxis offers the best hope of dealing with the real risk of postsplenectomy sepsis. The incidence of such infection is markedly reduced when patients are given maintenance doses of prophylactic penicillin. Doses are similar to those used in the past for persons with rheumatic heart disease. Patient noncompliance and penicillin-resistant organisms are the obvious shortcomings of such a program of prophylaxis.

Recently a polyvalent pneumococcal vaccine has been developed that provides significant protection for several years. This vaccine offers insufficient prophylaxis for children less than 2 years old and does not protect against all types of pneumococcal bacteria responsible for infection in children. Patients treated for Hodgkin's disease have an impaired immune response to such vaccination.[17] Asplenic individuals also have a diminished immunologic response to such vaccination, further limiting its usefulness.

In our institution, postsplenectomy patients are started on a prophylactic regimen of penicillin G (125 mg twice daily). For patients undergoing elective splenectomy, pneumococcal immunization should be provided before surgery. Most important is an education program for patients and their families stressing the need for immediate medical attention and administration of antibiotics at the slightest evidence of an inflammatory or infectious process. Such a combined effort reduces the risk of death after splenectomy to an absolute minimum.

PORTAL CIRCULATION

In addition to cirrhosis of the liver and extrahepatic portal vein thrombosis, a number of congenital diseases such as cystic fibrosis, congenital hepatic fibrosis, and biliary atresia may lead to an elevated portal blood pressure and gastrointestinal hemorrhage. Recent knowledge of the pathophysiology of diseases such as glycogen storage disease and familial hyperlipoproteinemia has pointed out the value of shunting portal blood away from the liver in these patients.[21,27,30] Although the incidence of extrahepatic portal vein thrombosis due to omphalitis or neonatal infection has decreased, patients with cystic fibrosis and biliary atresia are now living long enough for obstructive cirrhosis to develop and are being seen with portal hypertension and its complications.[28]

The management of portal hypertension in children presents technical and diagnostic problems not encountered in adults. The small caliber of the portal venous system in children predisposes patients undergoing any of the shunt procedures to a higher rate of thrombosis. For this reason the site selected within the portal venous system should

be the largest available so that the widest possible anastomosis may be achieved. The high failure rate of peripheral splenorenal shunts led Clatworthy to recommend the more central splenorenal shunt.[23] In the very young patient, surgery should be delayed as long as possible to allow maximum growth and dilatation of these veins.

The type of shunt and its location should be determined preoperatively for each child after the anatomy has been clearly defined by angiography and ultrasonography. In children with thrombocytopenia and coagulopathies, superior mesenteric arteriography is safer than a percutaneous transsplenic puncture. Although splenectomy decreases splanchnic blood flow, preservation of the organ is most important in the young to avoid the threat of overwhelming sepsis. In children, hypersplenism is more likely to reverse spontaneously following decompression of the portal pressure and is not in itself an indication for splenectomy.

In a series of 105 patients treated at the Children's Hospital Medical Center in Boston, the site of obstruction was intrahepatic in 29 and extrahepatic in 76 (Table 21–5).[25] The age distribution at the time of splenorenal shunt is shown in Table 21–6. The method of surgical treatment of portal hypertension in these children is outlined in Table 21–7. The predominant procedure was a splenorenal shunt as the initial operation in 70 patients and as a secondary procedure in six. These children received peripheral splenorenal shunts before the central splenorenal shunt became popular.[23,24] It is of interest that in spite of their young age,

TABLE 21–5 SITE AND CAUSE OF OBSTRUCTION IN 105 CHILDREN WITH PORTAL HYPERTENSION

Site and Cause	Number of Patients
Intrahepatic	29
Hepatitis, cirrhosis	8
Cystic fibrosis	6
Wilson's disease	6
Biliary atresia	3
Anomalies of liver	2
Abdominal trauma	2
Hemophilia	1
Galactosemia	1
Extrahepatic	76
Other infection in infancy	43
Omphalitis infection in infancy	26
Anomalies of splenic or portal veins	7

TABLE 21–6　AGE DISTRIBUTION AT TIME OF SPLENORENAL SHUNT

Age	Number of Patients
2–4 yr	20
5–8 yr	24
9–12 yr	25
13–16 yr	7

their small size, and subsequent thrombosis of the shunt in many, only 14 children required subsequent surgery due to persistent or recurrent portal hypertension and bleeding.

TABLE 21–7　PORTAL HYPERTENSION IN CHILDREN — SURGICAL PROCEDURES AND RESULTS IN 105 PATIENTS

Procedure and Results	Number of Patients
Splenectomy (as sole procedure)	20
Subsequent surgery required	7
No subsequent surgery required	13
Ligation of varices	24
As initial procedure	10
As secondary procedure	14
Subsequent surgery required	12
No subsequent surgery required	12
Portocaval or mesentericocaval shunt	5
As initial procedure	5
Subsequent surgery required	1
No subsequent surgery required	4
Splenorenal shunt	76
As initial procedure	70
As secondary procedure	6
Subsequent surgery required	14
No subsequent surgery required	62
Esophagogastric resection, primary anastomosis	5
As secondary procedure	5
Subsequent surgery required	1
No subsequent surgery required	4
Esophageal resection, colonic interposition	13
As secondary procedure	13
Subsequent surgery required	0
No subsequent surgery required	13

The operation was successful in 50 per cent of children weighing less than 50 pounds at the time of surgery, whereas the success for the entire group was 70 per cent.

There were nine deaths among the 76 splenorenal shunt patients. One child died of complications of the operation. Three died of persistent or recurrent portal hypertension and bleeding. The remaining five died of their underlying disease, such as mucoviscidosis or Wilson's disease.

The major and unique complications related to shunting of portal blood to the systemic venous system are metabolic and biochemical in nature. Ammonia intoxication or portal-systemic encephalopathy, noted in 15 per cent of adults, is rarely seen in young children.[22] Postoperative hepatic failure and ascites are also seldom seen in children and are related more to poor selection of patients for surgery or to the type of shunt performed than to surgical technique. Peptic ulcer disease develops or is aggravated following portacaval shunts in approximately 15 per cent of adults.[26] Histamine is deactivated by the liver and, when bypassed, is available to stimulate gastric secretion. This problem also does not occur in children.[29]

References

Spleen

1. Amsbaugh, D. F., Prescott, B., and Baker, P. J.: Effect of splenectomy on the expression of regulatory T cell activity. J. Immunol. 121:1483, 1978.
2. Aronzon, D. Z., Scherz, A. W., Einhorn, A. H., et al.: Nonoperative management of splenic trauma in children: A report of six consecutive cases. Pediatrics 60:482, 1977.
3. Broker, F. H., Khettry, J., Filler, R. M., et al.: Splenic torsion and accessory spleen. A scintigraphic demonstration. J. Pediatr. Surg. 6:913, 1975.
4. Constantopoulos, A., Najjar, V. A., and Smith, J. W.: Tuftsin deficiency: A new syndrome with defective phagocytosis. J. Pediatr. 80:564, 1972.
5. Dickerman, J. D.: Splenectomy and sepsis: A warning. Pediatrics 6:938, 1979.
6. Douglas, G. J., and Simpson, J. S.: The conservative management of splenic trauma. J. Pediatr. Surg. 5:565, 1971.
7. Eraklis, A. J., and Filler, R. M.: Splenectomy in

childhood: A review of 1413 cases. J. Pediatr. Surg. 7:382, 1972.

8. Eraklis, A. J., Kevy, S. V., Diamond, L. K., et al.: Hazard of overwhelming infection after splenectomy in childhood. N. Engl. J. Med. 276:1225, 1967.

9. Fischer, K. C., Eraklis, A. J., Rossello, P., and Treves, S.: Scintigraphy in the followup of pediatric splenic trauma treated without surgery. J. Nucl. Med. 11:3, 1978.

10. Griscom, N. T., Hargreaves, H. K., Schwartz, M. Z., et al.: Huge splenic cyst in a newborn: Comparison with 10 cases in later childhood and adolescence. Am. J. Roentgenol. 129:889, 1977.

11. Gross, R. E.: The Surgery of Infancy and Childhood: Its Principles and Techniques. Philadelphia, W. B. Saunders Co., 1953, p. 547.

12. Kiesewetter, W. B., and Patrick, D. B.: Childhood splenectomy: Indications for and results from. Am. Surg. 37:135, 1971.

13. King, H., and Shumacker, H. B., Jr.: Splenic studies; susceptibility to infection after splenectomy performed in infancy. Ann. Surg. 136:239, 1952.

14. Ratner, M. H., Garrow, E., Valda, V., et al.: Surgical repair of the injured spleen. J. Pediatr. Surg. 12:1019, 1977.

15. Rowley, D. A.: The formation of circulating antibody in the splenectomized human being following intravenous injection of heterologous erythrocytes. J. Immunol. 65:515, 1950.

16. Sherman, N. J., and Asch, M. J.: Conservative surgery for splenic injuries. Pediatrics 61:267, 1978.

17. Siber, G. R., Weitzman, S. A., et al.: Improved antibody response to pneumococcal vaccine after treatment for Hodgkin's disease. N. Engl. J. Med. 299:442, 1978.

18. Singer, D. B.: Postsplenectomy sepsis. In Rosenberg, H. S., and Bolande, R. P. (eds.): Perspectives in Pediatric Pathology. Chicago, Year Book Medical Publishers, 1973, pp. 285–311.

19. Sullivan, J. L., Schiffman, G., Miser, J., et al.: Immune response after splenectomy. Lancet 1:178, 1978.

20. Walker, W.: Splenectomy in childhood: A review in England and Wales, 1960–1964. Br. J. Surg. 63:36, 1976.

Portal Circulation

21. Altman, R. P.: Portal hypertension. In Ravitch, M. M., Welch, K. J., Benson, C. D., et al. (eds.): Pediatric Surgery, 3rd ed. Chicago, Year Book Medical Publishers, 1979, pp. 847–856.

22. Bismuth, H., Franco, D., and Alagille, D.: Portal diversion for portal hypertension in children: The first 90 patients. Ann. Surg. 192:18, 1980.

23. Clatworthy, H. W., and Boles, E. T.: Diseases of the spleen and portal circulation. In Mustard, W. T., Ravitch, M. M., Snyder, W. H., et al. (eds.): Pediatric Surgery, 2nd ed. Chicago, Year Book Medical Publishers, 1969, pp. 777–785.

24. Gross, R. E.: The Surgery of Infancy and Childhood: Its Principles and Techniques. Philadelphia, W. B. Saunders Co., 1953.

25. Longino, L. A.: Personal communication.

26. McDermott, W. V., Jr., Pallazzi, H., Mondet, A., and Nardi, G. L.: Elective portal-systemic shunt: An analysis of 237 cases. N. Engl. J. Med. 264:419, 1961.

27. Raffensberger, J. G., Shkolnik, A. A., Bogg, J. D., et al.: Portal hypertension in children. Arch. Surg. 105:249, 1972.

28. Schuster, S. R., Shwachman, H., Toyama, W. M., et al.: The management of portal hypertension in cystic fibrosis. J. Pediatr. Surg. 12:201, 1977.

29. Silen, W., and Eiseman, B.: Evidence of histamine as agent responsible for gastric hypersecretion after portocaval shunt. Surgery 50:213, 1961.

30. Tank, E. S., Wallin, V. W., Jr., Turcotte, J. G., et al.: Surgical management of bleeding gastroesophageal varices in children. Arch. Surg. 98:451, 1969.

STOMACH AND DUODENUM

22

Clifford D. Benson, M.D., F.A.C.S.
Donald W. Hight, M.D., F.A.A.P.

Surgical correction of congenital and acquired lesions of the stomach and duodenum constitutes a significant portion of the abdominal surgery performed in infancy and early childhood. Prompt diagnosis and meticulous pre- and postoperative fluid and electrolyte administration determine ultimate success or failure of the surgical procedure, especially in the neonate. The initial correction of the disorder employing standard surgical techniques can in large part eliminate postoperative complications.

GASTRIC DISTENSION

Unrecognized gastric dilatation can have an adverse effect on intestinal motility, respiratory function, and wound healing. Use of a nipple to pacify a sick infant who is restricted from oral intake may promote air swallowing and progressive gastric distension. Postoperative ileus, occult sepsis, hypokalemia, and a painful upper abdominal incision will alter intestinal motility and delay gastric emptying.[52] A dilated stomach will elevate the left diaphragm, increase intra-abdominal pressure, cause abdominal distension, and increase the likelihood of complications in wound healing.

In infants, breathing is mostly diaphragmatic. Restriction of diaphragmatic movement will cause carbon dioxide retention, respiratory acidosis, and ventilatory insufficiency. Compensatory tachycardia and an elevated respiratory rate may be early signs of gastric dilatation, which can easily be treated by prompt nasogastric intubation and suction. By minimizing early postoperative distension, prolonged naso-gastric decompression can be avoided and early return of intestinal motility stimulated.

A nasogastric sump suction tube should be inserted whenever the risk of gastric dilatation is high. Continuous low wall suction with frequent irrigation or hourly hand aspiration by skilled nurses should be ordered to ensure tube patency. Intravenous fluids should be precisely calculated to replace fluid and electrolytes lost from gastric aspiration. Injury to gastric mucosa with consequent hemorrhage may result from uncontrolled high wall suction or occlusion of a double-lumen sump catheter. Such bleeding can be avoided by reducing the strength of wall suction to less than 40 mm of water and by re-establishing the patency of sump suction by either irrigating the tube with normal saline solution or inserting a new nasogastric catheter.

Care must be taken to fix the tube securely to the patient's nose or upper lip to prevent its from inadvertently being withdrawn and to prevent pressure necrosis of the nares. Decompression should be discontinued as soon as possible to avoid parotitis and otitis media, both complications of prolonged nasogastric suction.

GASTRIC PERFORATIONS

Isolated perforations of the gastrointestinal tract in the newborn usually occur between the third and fifth days of life. Although the cause of these lesions has been debated, regardless of their location within the intestinal tract, there are physical characteristics that suggest a localized vascular insult. Lloyd speculated that the ischemic lesions were due to circulatory redistribution of intestinal blood flow during a stressful neonatal period. A significant episode of asphyxia or hypoxia was recorded in 80 per cent of infants with gastric perforation.[33] Such perforations have been found at the site of incipient or frank necrosis and may be aggravated by an increase in gastric acid secretion.[32, 56] Whether this lesion is caused by "hypophyseal–adrenal axis stress phenomenon" has not been established.[27]

The infants at risk are usually of high birth weight and present with respiratory distress, tachycardia, and rapidly developing abdominal distension. The diagnosis is established by obtaining upright chest and abdominal roentgenograms, demonstrating free air under the diaphragms (Fig. 22–1). The distension, if massive, can cause respiratory distress, which may be dramatically relieved by needle aspiration of the peritoneal cavity. Prompt recognition, nasogastric suction, and administration of lactated Ringer's solution (120 to 150 ml/kg/24 hr) and plasma to replace third-space fluid sequestration are required to treat hypovolemic shock due to gastric acid-induced peritonitis. Prior to laparotomy, high doses of broad-spectrum antibiotics are administered intravenously. The site of gastric perforation may be along any portion of the anterior or posterior wall of the stomach, but the most common site is high on the greater curvature. The lesser sac should be entered to exclude occult or secondary gastric perforation. The defect can be easily identified by locating hemorrhage and necrosis within the gastric wall and bile staining of surrounding connective tissue. The edges of the perforation should be débrided back to fresh bleeding mucosa and muscle and then closed in two layers using nonabsorbable sutures. These sutures should be placed well beyond the margins of the perforation. A good vascular supply will ensure prompt healing and avoid reperforation. The abdomen is then copiously irrigated with warm saline solution to reduce contamination from milk curds and gastric contents. Nasogastric or gastrostomy decompression should be continued until peristaltic function returns, as evidenced by stool passage and decreasing quantities of gastric aspirate. Transperitoneal drainage is not necessary unless an established abscess cavity is found.

The mortality from this condition is related to duration of symptoms, extent of peritonitis, and reversibility of hypovolemic shock and sepsis. Although the reported mortality is high (50 per cent), prompt resuscitation and proper surgical treatment will contribute to a substantially higher salvage rate.[32, 57]

GASTROSTOMY

The use of gastrostomy in children was originally intended for feeding of infants with congenital obstructions above the level of the stomach.[23] Subsequent experience has shown gastrostomy to be an effective means of gastrointestinal decompression following major abdominal or intestinal surgery. It is also useful when dilating caustic lye strictures of the esophagus, supporting premature infants, and advancing children with short-gut syndromes to elemental diets.[6, 37] A morbidity of 2.5 to 16 per cent has been reported for this relatively simple procedure.[12, 21, 24] Before the use of hyperalimentation and elemental diets, the majority of complications were attributed to poor nutritional status and prematurity.

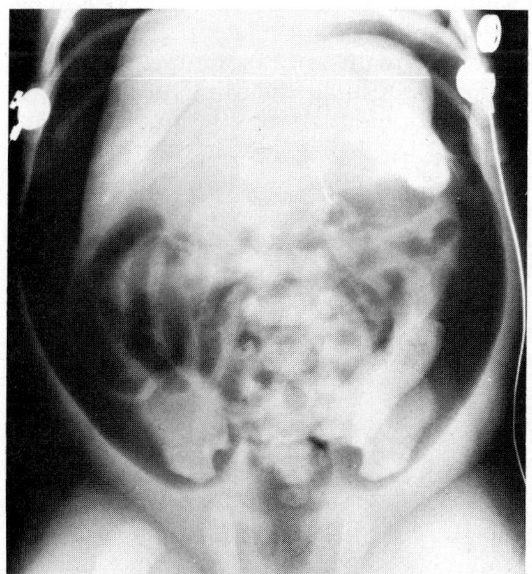

Figure 22–1 Upright abdominal roentgenogram shows massive free intraperitoneal air (pneumoperitoneum).

The gastrostomy site should lie along the anterior surface of the body of the stomach. The perimeter of the proposed site should be supported with atraumatic clamps. The central portion is grasped with a hemostat, which is then touched by an electrocautery. When this device is similarly applied to the mucosa and submucosal layers, bleeding points will be coagulated. A double purse-string suture of silk is then used to seal the gastric opening and eliminate postoperative hemorrhage from gastric mucosa. A variety of catheters have been recommended (Pezzer, Foley balloon, Malecot, Robinson) for initial use. The Malecot catheter is preferred. Forceful blind insertion can cause perforation of the posterior gastric wall, which may be avoided by carefully drawing the bulb catheter tip back against the purse-string closure. Four nonabsorbable sutures are then placed around the gastrostomy to the undersurface of the peritoneum to prevent separation.

Major complications arise from inadequate fixation of the gastrostomy tube in the stomach.[35, 51] Five to 7 days are needed for the gastrostomy and abdominal wall to establish a good seal. Inadvertent removal of the tube during the first week may lead to leakage of gastric contents with resultant peritonitis and sepsis. Reinsertion of the catheter during the early postoperative period should be performed in the operating room using a well-lubricated Foley catheter. One to 2 ml of contrast material should be injected into the catheter to verify its position in the stomach.

If the catheter is not well secured to the external abdominal wall, the balloon tip may be carried by peristaltic action into the duodenum, causing gastric outlet obstruction, gastrointestinal hemorrhage, intussusception,[21] and pyloric stenosis. Pressure necrosis of the esophagus has also been reported. Once the catheter has been inserted, a mark on its exterior can be used as a guide for proper positioning.

A progressively widening gastrocutaneous stoma will cause abdominal wall cellulitis, skin ulceration, and severe depletion of fluid and electrolytes. Supplemental parenteral nutrition, administration of trace elements, and local skin care will help to minimize irritating contact with gastric acid. Along with these measures, inserting a smaller rather than larger gastrostomy tube will allow the wound edges to close and narrow the stomal opening.

Prolapse of the gastric mucosa is frequently associated with a progressively enlarging gastrocutaneous fistula. Conservative treatment includes application of pressure binder dressings, intravenous parenteral nutrition, insertion of a small gastrostomy catheter, and meticulous local skin care.

Closure of a gastrostomy site usually occurs spontaneously within several days after the tube is removed. Once the opening has become lined with gastric and squamous epithelium, however, fistulectomy and formal closure are required. Postoperative breakdown of such a closure is common, but complete closure occurs spontaneously with good nutrition, systemic antibiotics, and local wound care.

HYPERTROPHIC PYLORIC STENOSIS

Pyloric stenosis is one of the most common lesions requiring surgical treatment in the first few weeks of life. The ratio of males to females affected is 4:1.[3] Associated major anomalies have been estimated to occur in 6 to 12 per cent of patients.[1, 48] There is a significant excess of pyloric stenosis among persons with blood group types B and O, leading some to speculate that genetically linked enzymatic and secretory functions of the gastrointestinal tract may play a role in the development of this lesion.[13] Seasonal variation in the incidence has been discredited.[10] Complacency must be avoided in managing this well-recognized pediatric problem if unnecessary complications are to be prevented.

Vomiting from pyloric stenosis begins in about 21 days, although pyloromyotomy is not performed until the patient is about 6 weeks old.[3] The diagnosis is confirmed by a history of projectile vomiting, weight loss with progressive dehydration, and constipation. With experience, palpation of a pyloric tumor ("olive") in the right upper quadrant is diagnostic. Such a tumor can be located in about 80 to 85 per cent of patients.[8] There is no intra-abdominal organ or viscus that mimics the pyloric tumor. In the Children's Hospital of Michigan series, three errors in

TABLE 22–1 INFANTILE PYLORIC STENOSIS AT CHILDREN'S HOSPITAL OF MICHIGAN, 1940–1978 (1777 PATIENTS)

Complications	Number of Patients	Per Cent
Perforation		
Duodenal	40	2.2
Gastric	2	0.1
Reoperation	10*	0.5
Wound dehiscence	2	0.1
Wound infection	4	0.2
Death	8	0.4
Unrecognized duodenal perforation	1	
Diarrhea†	4	
Malnutrition	2	
Renal failure	1	
Error in diagnosis‡	3	0.1

*Six referred from other hospitals.

†Intractable postoperative diarrhea, dehydration, 1940–1946.

‡Palpable tumor not confirmed at operation.

diagnosis (0.1 per cent) were made in which a pyloric tumor was reported to have been felt but was not confirmed at laparotomy (Table 22–1). One of these children had a horseshoe kidney with a prominent upper pole.

If the history and physical findings are inconsistent, an upper gastrointestinal tract roentgenographic series should be performed preoperatively. Chalasia and gastroesophageal reflux may mimic the symptoms of pyloric stenosis. Twenty-four hours should elapse between the barium study and surgery, during which time the stomach should be carefully lavaged of all contents. Reflux of barium or gastric acid either preoperatively or during induction of general anesthesia may lead to severe aspiration pneumonia.

Blood should be obtained to assess acid-base balance and the state of dehydration before surgery is performed. Determinations of serum potassium, chloride, and sodium; blood urea nitrogen (BUN); pH; and carbon dioxide content will substantiate the degree of dehydration. A carbon dioxide content of more than 30 mEq/l, a BUN greater than 20 mg/dl, and a potassium level of less than 3 mEq/l suggest a severely dehydrated, alkalotic infant unfit for general anesthesia. In spite of available laboratory data, the most critical factor dictating the timing of pyloromyotomy following resuscitative measures is the surgeon's clinical assessment of the baby's preoperative condition. As many as 11 per cent of infants may have an unexplained hyperbilirubinemia that resolves spontaneously following treatment.[30] Administration of 0.9 per cent normal saline solution and dextrose at a rate of 120 to 130 ml/kg/24 hr with 5 mEq/l of potassium chloride for each 250 ml of intravenous fluid will rapidly rehydrate an affected infant within 24 hours, making the patient an improved anesthetic risk. The surgical treatment of pyloric stenosis should not be considered an emergency procedure. Performing such surgery under local anesthesia should be reserved for exceptional circumstances.

Pyloromyotomy (Ramstedt procedure) is performed through a right transverse or Robertson incision above the palpable liver edge. Omentum or transverse colon is identified and used to find and deliver the stomach. The greater curvature is grasped with a wet sponge so that it is not traumatized by repeatedly slipping back into the abdomen and so that gastroepipyloric veins are not torn. The pyloric tumor is delivered into the abdominal incision and stabilized by the first assistant. The pyloromyotomy begins with a split proximal to the pyloric vein (white line) along the anterior-superior avascular portion of the tumor (Fig. 22–2). The separation is then extended proximally, exposing oblique muscle fibers of the gastric antrum.[25] Care is taken to avoid obvious venous communications along the anterior surface of the pylorus. A pyloric spreader will aid in the controlled separation of the circular muscle fibers without fragmentation until the submucosa protrudes through the muscular defect. Recurrent stenosis and outlet obstruction are more often due to an inadequate separation onto the pyloric antrum than to an inadequate split proximal to the duodenal junction. Milking the duodenum to demonstrate bile or squeezing air in the stomach across the pylorus is the best way to discover occult perforations. Mucosal defects are closed with interrupted fine silk sutures and buttressed with a pedicle of omentum. Failure either to look for or to recognize a perforation will lead to peritonitis, overwhelming sepsis, and death. One such death

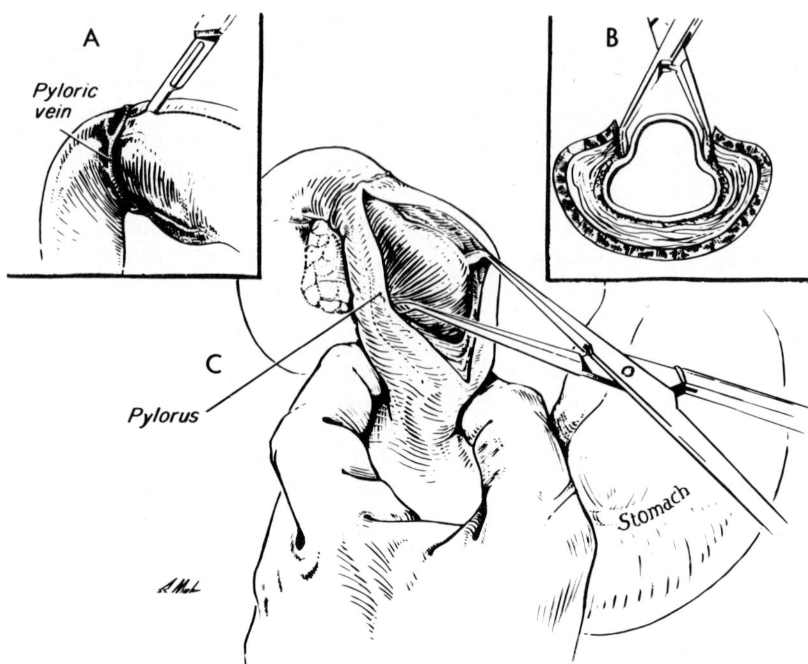

Figure 22–2   Pyloric stenosis: operative technique. *A,* Incision made on anterosuperior surface through avascular area. *B,* Cross section of hypertrophied pylorus after operation has been completed. *C,* Circular muscle has been separated, allowing submucosa to bulge into defect. (Reproduced with permission from Benson, C. D.: Infantile hypertrophic pyloric stenosis. *In* Ravitch, M. M., et al., eds.: Pediatric Surgery, 3rd edition. Vol. 2. Copyright © 1979 by Year Book Medical Publishers, Inc., Chicago.)

in our series followed an unrecognized duodenal perforation. After such a repair, the stomach should be decompressed for 48 to 72 hours before oral feeding is resumed. Bleeding from the edges of the pyloromyotomy is usually due to venous congestion caused by tension and traction of the pylorus and stomach. The ooze will stop when the viscera are replaced in the abdominal cavity. Rarely, arterial bleeding points will require suture ligature. Topical thrombin or microfibrillar collagen (Avitene) may also be applied to control venous bleeding from the cut edges.

Following pyloromyotomy, gastric peristalsis and gastric tone are greatly diminished for 18 to 24 hours.[47] Our postoperative feeding regimen begins 8 to 12 hours after surgery with 30 ml of dextrose and water and is gradually advanced to full-strength formula over a 15-hour period. Vomiting during the postoperative period is treated by gentle nasogastric lavage to evacuate residual mild curd. If vomiting persists, the baby should be given nothing by mouth for 8 to 12 hours before the feeding schedule is resumed. Upper gastrointestinal tract roentgenographic series performed during the first 3 weeks postoperatively are difficult to interpret and are seldom helpful. For the occasional infant with persistent feeding intolerance, peripheral intravenous nutrition is provided until vomiting ceases and normal gastric motility resumes. Reoperation should be postponed for 2 weeks, as nearly all vomiting will cease during this time.

Morbidity and mortality are principally related to unrecognized or inadequately treated gastric and duodenal perforations.[22] Wound infections are rare and are more apt to occur in the presence of severe malnutrition or following an inadvertent mucosal perforation. Wound disruption may be avoided by using either a muscle-retracting or a splitting incision. If the incision has been properly placed, the infant's liver edge will drop beneath the incision and buttress the closure.

From preoperative assessment to intraoperative pyloromyotomy to postoperative feeding regimen, successful treatment of pyloric stenosis depends upon close attention to every small detail of management.

NEONATAL GASTRIC HEMORRHAGE

Gastric hemorrhage in the newborn, though rare, is occasionally severe. Increased gastric acidity can be a causative factor, especially between the fourth and seventh days of life. Bleeding is usually controlled with vitamin K given intramuscularly and repeated gastric lavage using a 2 per cent sodium bicarbonate solution. Transfusion with fresh whole blood will be required in neonates who have massive bleeding, but care should be taken to avoid overtransfusion. If the prothrombin time and the partial thromboplastin time are prolonged, fresh frozen plasma should be administered once the red blood cell volume has been replaced. Conservative measures are usually successful in controlling bleeding from gastric erosions.[54] Suture ligation of the many small bleeding points is futile and should be avoided. Flexible gastroscopy should be performed to rule out a major arterial bleeding point in the stomach, pyloric canal, or proximal duodenum.

PEPTIC ULCERATION OF INFANCY AND CHILDHOOD

Peptic ulceration in children is associated with chronic illness, trauma, burns, and the ingestion of ulcerogenic medications, especially aspirin and steroids. In contrast to those in adults, acute ulcers in pediatric patients are frequently isolated lesions of the antrum or duodenal bulb.[17] Among older children with peptic ulceration, males predominate. A high incidence of peptic ulceration (35 per cent) has been found in relatives of these patients.[50] Diagnosis should be confirmed by gastroscopy and upper gastrointestinal tract roentgenographic series. Ulcerogenic medications must be discontinued and vigorous antacid therapy begun. Gastric acid studies are of no diagnostic or prognostic value in the treatment of this disease.

Duodenal ulcers in children frequently present as hematemesis in infants and as atypical abdominal pain in older children.[40] Dyspeptic symptoms may be misdiagnosed as mesenteric lymphadenitis or gastroenteritis. Perforation is an uncommon but serious complication associated with a high mortality, particularly in young patients. Follow-up studies suggest there is a 50 per cent chance that a duodenal ulcer beginning in childhood will cause symptoms when the patient reaches adolescence or adulthood.[39]

Emergency operative treatment should be reserved for patients with uncontrolled gastric or duodenal hemorrhage or free perforation. Symptoms of duodenal obstruction and chronic epigastric pain may improve with medical management alone. Before operative intervention, adequate replacement of circulating blood volume using lactated Ringer's solution and whole blood is required. Antibiotics are administered. Endoscopy is used to locate the site of hemorrhage. Diagnostic angiography is recommended if the rate of bleeding is life-threatening in a poor risk patient in whom the use of intra-arterial vasopressin is considered.

The surgical procedure of choice is vagotomy and pyloroplasty.[17] Intraoperative suture ligation of specific bleeding sites may be necessary to establish hemostasis, but simple plication, ligation of bleeding points alone, and gastroenterostomy are associated with a high rate of recurrent ulceration and bleeding and should be avoided.[17, 43, 45, 50] There have been conflicting follow-up data regarding growth and development after 75 to 90 per cent gastrectomy.[16, 41] Bilateral vagotomy and antrectomy is the procedure of choice for older children in whom symptoms recur after pyloroplasty and vagotomy.

MALROTATION

Anomalies of intestinal rotation and mesenteric fixation are associated with a variety of surgical problems ranging from midgut volvulus and intestinal infarction to abnormal displacement of the right colon and appendix. They are thought to be an asymptomatic finding in 0.2 per cent of patients undergoing barium studies at any age. The threat of sudden torsion around the superior mesenteric artery and infarction of the dependent intestinal viscera dictates the need for careful work-up of any child with bilious vomiting or chronic abdominal symptoms.[55] Mortality of 10 to 15 per cent in patients with midgut volvulus is due to infarcted small and large bowel with perforation, peritonitis, and associated congenital anomalies.[29, 46, 49]

Most frequently, patients with anomalies of intestinal rotation present with symptoms of partial or complete duodenal obstruction due to extrinsic compression from duodenal bands. The diagnosis is made by demonstrating an abnormally positioned cecum outside the right lower quadrant. Abnormal fixation of the duodenum and small bowel has been demonstrated on upper gastrointestinal tract roentgenographic series despite a normally located cecum.[31, 53] Once the diagnosis of incomplete intestinal rotation has been made in the symptomatic child, surgical correction is indicated.

When laparotomy is performed for malrotation, several steps in the surgical treatment must be followed. Through a right supraumbilical transverse incision, the abdominal cavity must be completely eviscerated and the base of the mesentery visualized. Torsion of the mesentery must be reduced by two or three counterclockwise rotations of the small bowel. Adequate reduction is ensured when the mesentery lies flat against the retroperitoneum. The vascular supply to ischemic viscera may improve substantially once the volvulus has been reduced, circulation re-established, and the obstructive intestine decompressed. Intestinal resection should be conservative as long as the viability of the ischemic intestine is questionable. Judgment is important in estimating the extent of infarcted viscera. Delay of resection for 24 to 36 hours with re-exploration has been advocated.[29] Areas of infarcted gut will be obvious, thereby establishing the extent of resection and the possibility of a primary anastomosis. The postoperative management of massive small and large bowel resections will require the use of intravenous parenteral nutrition until the intestinal absorptive surface area has regenerated. The use of a gastrostomy feeding tube inserted during the initial operation will simplify the subsequent graduated transition to elemental feeding.

Duodenal bands extending from the lateral peritoneal reflection of the right upper quadrant across the anterior surface of the second and third portion of the duodenum must be completely divided. The fibers should be carefully dissected free of the lateral and anterior duodenal surface. Pancreatic and biliary ducts, as well as the blood supply to the duodenum, enter along the medial surface. The distal duodenum runs into the base of the small bowel mesentery and must also be completely mobilized. The duodenum, once freed of all peritoneal attachments including segments of the ligament of Treitz, lies in a cephalad-to-caudad plane along the right side of the midline and appears to have redundant convoluted folds.

Intrinsic obstructions, i.e., webs and stenosis, must be excluded after all superficial attachments lying on the surface of the duodenum have been divided.[20] Through a small antral gastrotomy, a #10 or 12 Foley balloon catheter should be inserted through the duodenum, inflated, and then withdrawn without resistance. If the balloon becomes caught in the duodenum, suggesting an intrinsic duodenal narrowing, a vertical duodenotomy over the anterior surface must be performed. Webs and windsock anomalies may be simply divided or resected circumferentially, leaving submucosa and muscular layers intact. The duodenum is then closed transversely to prevent cicatrizing stenosis.

Bill and Grauman have advocated suture fixation of small and large bowel to minimize the risk of recurrent volvulus.[7] This controversial procedure may lead to postoperative intestinal obstruction. In reviewing the surgical procedure performed on 441 patients, Welch noted only four recurrences (0.9 per cent) and advocated only appendectomy and placement of the duodenum and small bowel to the right of the midline, with the cecum and large bowel positioned in the left flank.[57]

CONGENITAL ANTRAL WEB AND PREPYLORIC DIAPHRAGM

Obstructing prepyloric diaphragms or webs of the gastric antrum are a rare cause of gastrointestinal symptoms in children. In infants these defects must be differentiated from hypertrophic pyloric stenosis. The symptoms of pyloric atresia or complete antral membrane in the neonate should lead to prompt recognition and surgical treatment of the condition.[9] In contrast, partially obstructing lesions of the gastric outlet may produce intermittent symptoms of vomiting, weight loss, and abdominal pain, leading to an erroneous diagnosis and delay in definitive therapy until later childhood. The condition is recognized in most patients in the first, sixth, or seventh decade of life.[59]

Prepyloric webs are best diagnosed by barium contrast studies, which demonstrate the linear defect in the gastric antrum. The radiographic findings may be mistaken for a deformity of duodenal ulcer disease. Frequently, several radiologic examinations will be required to identify this thin diaphragm.[11] Excessive instillation of barium sulfate into the stomach can obscure a web, which may be diagnosed only after using multiple spot views and air-contrast techniques.[2] When the radiographic diagnosis is in doubt, gastroscopy is helpful in clarifying the cause of outlet obstruction.

Correction of the diaphragm or web is accomplished after the stomach and duodenum are fully exposed through an upper abdominal right transverse incision. The stomach and duodenum, once fully mobilized, may be palpated for evidence of intraluminal narrowing or formation of septa. There is seldom external evidence to aid in identifying the location of the diaphragm. Intraluminal inspection of the lesion is accomplished through a longitudinal gastrotomy in the distal body of the stomach. Correction of pyloric atresia will require segmental resection and gastroduodenostomy. A web is most accurately located by inserting a #10 or 12 Foley catheter into the duodenum, inflating the balloon, and withdrawing the catheter until the obstructing diaphragm is encountered and prolapsed through the gastric opening. Once the web is located, the gastrotomy is extended to a point just proximal to the lesion. Excision of the web involves complete resection of the mucosa and redundant submucosa. The muscular layers are rarely involved and need not be removed with the specimen. Careful approximation of the mucosal edges at the margins of the resection will ensure hemostasis, prompt healing, and

minimal circumferential narrowing. The gastrotomy is closed transversely using a two-layer hemostatic closure technique. Wedge excision, antrectomy, and gastrojejunostomy are not recommended forms of surgical treatment. Proximal gastric ulcer formation is a secondary phenomenon due to chronic gastric stasis and distension. This inflammatory process will heal rapidly once normal gastric emptying has been re-established. Vagotomy and pyloroplasty are not indicated as part of the treatment of antral web.[19]

Coexistent congenital anomalies have been reported in as many as 50 per cent of patients.[2, 26] After correction of either pyloric atresia or complete antral membrane in the newborn, careful inspection must exclude secondary atresias in the distal intestinal tract.[44]

ATRESIA AND STENOSIS OF THE DUODENUM

Congenital intrinsic duodenal obstruction occurs with such regularity as to be high on the list of possible diagnoses for every newborn with persistent bilious vomiting. Delay in diagnosis of 3 to 10 days is attributed to the degree of intraluminal obstruction, ranging from complete atresia to partial stenosis of the annular pancreas, windsock, and incomplete diaphragm. The site of obstruction is most frequently postampullary (65 per cent).[14] Polyhydramnios in the maternal history is an important diagnostic sign and can be elicited in more than 50 per cent of cases.[14] There is a higher incidence of coexistent congenital anomalies than with any other form of intestinal atresia. Down's syndrome, tracheoesophageal fistula, imperforate anus, urinary tract anomalies, and congenital heart disease are seen either singly or in combination with duodenal atresia. Secondary distal intestinal obstruction occurs less often than with primary atresias of the small and large bowel. Hyperbilirubinemia may be severe enough to necessitate exchange transfusion, although bilirubin levels rapidly return to normal once intestinal continuity and bowel motility are re-established.

Plain roentgenograms of the abdomen are diagnostic in about 50 per cent of patients.[14] A "double bubble" sign in the upright abdominal x-ray film is pathognomonic of duodenal atresia. An emergency barium enema study should be done in patients with partial duodenal obstruction to rule out malrotation and midgut volvulus. An upper gastrointestinal tract roentgenographic series may be necessary if vomiting is intermittent and plain roentgenograms suggest gastric and duodenal dilatation.

Operative exposure of the duodenum is accomplished through a right transverse supraumbilical incision. Duodenal atresia is easily recognizable by the large, distended proximal portion and the small distal segment entering the jejunum. Obstruction may be caused by an anterior portal vein,[36] annular pancreas,[38] or atretic segment of the duodenum. The corrective surgical procedure is a bypass duodenoduodenostomy rather than an attempted segmental resection.[14, 15, 58] When the duodenal segments are widely separated and a duodenoduodenostomy is not possible, a retrocolic duodenojejunostomy should be done. No attempt should be made to resect the anterior aspect of an annular pancreas or prepyloric portal vein. A diamond-shaped anastomosis (described by Kimura et al.) takes advantage of the large redundant portion of obstructed duodenum and eliminates the need for dissection along the posterior wall near the ampulla of Vater.[28] Localized areas of stenosis and partial membranes or windsocks (Fig. 22–3) should be excised through a ventral duodenostomy with precise mucosal approximation and transverse closure to avoid luminal narrowing.

The dilated proximal duodenum, once reanastomosed in continuity with the distal duodenum, may exhibit ineffective peristaltic activity for a prolonged period. Peripheral parenteral nutrition will provide adequate postoperative calories. Gastrostomy tubes are necessary only in premature, low-birth-weight infants or in those with multiple anomalies such as imperforate anus or esophageal atresia.[15] There has been no significant benefit from transanastomotic feeding tubes, which are often difficult to insert and stabilize and do not reduce postoperative convalescence.

A survival of 65 to 75 per cent should be expected following correction of a duodenal

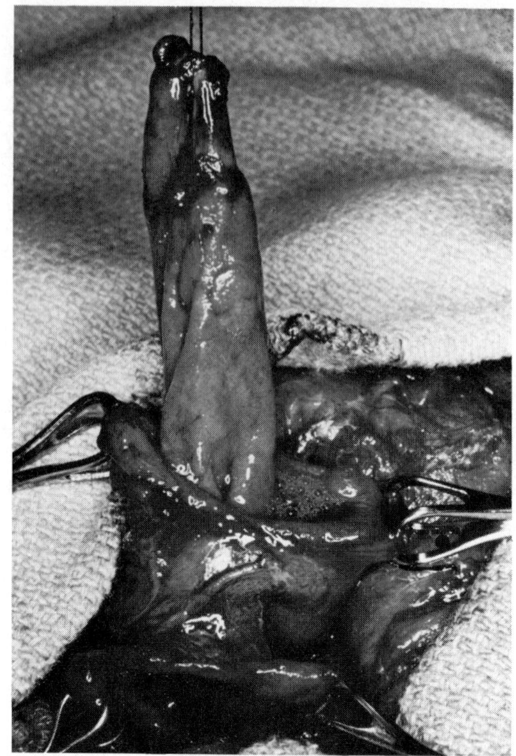

Figure 22–3 Windsock anomaly prolapsed through transverse duodenotomy. The lesion is excised by dividing its attachment to inner wall of duodenum. (Reproduced with permission from Lynn, H. B.: Duodenal obstruction: atresia, stenosis and annular pancreas. *In* Ravitch, M. M., et al., eds.: Pediatric Surgery, 3rd edition. Vol. 2. Copyright © 1979 by Year Book Medical Publishers, Inc., Chicago.)

obstruction. The majority of perioperative deaths are attributed to respiratory complications (28 per cent), associated malformations (30 per cent), prematurity (20 per cent), and anastomotic complications (16 per cent).[14, 20] Late deaths are often due to lethal congenital anomalies.

FOREIGN BODIES IN STOMACH AND DUODENUM

The management of ingested foreign bodies lying in the intestinal tract is often a cause of debate regarding attempted endoscopic extraction or removal by laparotomy. Once the object has passed the esophageal inlet and inferior pharyngeal constrictors, however, even the most angulated foreign body will traverse the gastrointestinal tract with little risk of causing intestinal perforation or obstruction. In a series of 766 infants and children, Gross found only 43 in whom the foreign body had to be removed by laparotomy.[18]

Conservative management is recommended, and hospitalization is usually not necessary for the majority of patients. A special diet is of little value, but the child's parents should be alert for symptoms of abdominal pain, and the stool should be inspected for 5 days following ingestion. If the object has not been recovered by 7 days, a repeat radiograph should be taken to verify the location of the foreign body. If the object has passed the duodenum without causing abdominal pain, vomiting, or melena, continued observation is recommended. Once signs of vomiting, gastric dilatation, or ileus occur, hospitalization and laparotomy are indicated. Sharp objects may perforate the duodenum, causing urinary complications, or may lodge in a congenital duodenal diverticulum.[5, 42]

Surgical judgment will dictate the timing of laparotomy for foreign bodies that remain lodged in the duodenum for an extended period. After being located by palpation, the object can be removed through a vertical duodenotomy, which is closed transversely to avoid subsequent stenosis. Transperitoneal drainage is not indicated unless established abscess formation from a localized perforation is encountered.

Trichobezoar of the stomach must be surgically removed. Such large collections of foreign matter and undigested food are best extracted through a small longitudinal incision in the body of the stomach. Attempts should be made to isolate the site of gastrotomy from the peritoneal cavity to reduce the risk of peritoneal contamination. Closure of the stomach using a two-layer technique minimizes the risk of postoperative bleeding or intraperitoneal leakage of gastric contents.

References

1. Ahmed, S.: Infantile pyloric stenosis associated with major anomalies of the alimentary tract. J. Pediatr. Surg. 5:660, 1970.
2. Bell, M. J., Ternberg, J. L., McAlister, W., et al.: Antral diaphragm — a cause of gastric outlet obstruction in infants and children. J. Pediatr. 90:196, 1977.
3. Benson, C. D.: Infantile pyloric stenosis. Progr. Pediatr. Surg. 1:63, 1970.
4. Benson, C. D.: Infantile hypertrophic pyloric stenosis. *In* Ravitch, M. M., et al. (eds.): Pediatric Surgery, 3rd Ed. Chicago, Year Book Medical Publishers, 1979.
5. Benson, C. D., Lloyd, J., Jr.: Stomach and Duodenum. *In* Ravitch, M. M., et al. (eds.): Pediatric Surgery, 3rd Ed. Chicago, Year Book Medical Publishers, 1979, pp. 897–902.
6. Berg, R. B., Schuster, S. R., and Colodny, A. L.: The use of gastrotomy in feeding premature infants. Pediatrics 33:287, 1964.
7. Bill, A. H., and Grauman, D.: Rationale and technique for stabilization of the mesentery in cases of nonrotation of the midgut. J. Pediatr. Surg. 1:127, 1966.
8. Bishop, H. C.: Diagnosis of pyloric stenosis by palpation. Clin. Pediatr. 12:226, 1973.
9. Brown, R. P., and Hertzler, J. H.: Congenital prepyloric gastric atresia. J. Dis. Child. 97:857, 1959.
10. Campbell, D. P., Vanhoutte, J. J., and Smith, E. I.: Partially obstructing antral web — a distinct clinical entity. J. Pediatr. Surg. 8:723, 1973.
11. Campbell, M. A.: A question of seasonal variation of pyloric stenosis. J. Pediatr. 74:1006, 1969.
12. Connar, R. G., and Sealy, W. C.: Gastrostomy and its complications. Ann. Surg. 143:245, 1956.
13. Dodge, J. A.: Abnormal distribution of ABO blood groups in infantile pyloric stenosis. J. Med. Genet. 8:468, 1971.
14. Fonkalsrud, E. W., deLorimier, A. A., Hays, D. M.: Congenital atresia and stenosis of the duodenum. Pediatrics 93:79, 1969.
15. Girvan, D. P., and Stephens, G. A.: Congenital intrinsic duodenal obstruction: A 25 year review of its surgical management and consequences. J. Pediatr. Surg. 9:833, 1974.
16. Green, T. H., and Hendren, W. H.: Subtotal gastrectomy for bleeding duodenal ulcer in childhood. Report of 3 cases with 6 year followup study in one. N. Engl. J. Med., 262:118, 1960.
17. Grosfeld, J. L., Shipley, F., Fitzgerald, J. F., and Ballantine, T V: Acute peptic ulcer in infancy and childhood. Am. Surg. 44:13, 1978.
18. Gross, R. E.: The Surgery of Infancy and Childhood, Philadelphia, W. B. Saunders Co., 1953, pp. 250–252.
19. Hait, G., Esselstyn, C. B., and Rankin, G. B.: Prepyloric mucosal diaphragm (antral web). Arch. Surg. 105:486, 1972.
20. Haller, J. A., and Cahill, J. L.: Combined congenital gastric and duodenal obstruction: Pitfalls in diagnosis and treatment. Surgery 63:503, 1968.
21. Haws, E. B., Sieber, W. K., and Kiesewetter, W. B.: Complications of tube gastrostomy in infants and children; 15 year review of 240 cases. Ann. Surg. 164:284, 1964.
22. Hayes, M. A., and Goldenberg, I. S.: The problems of infantile pyloric stenosis. Int. Abstr. Surg. 104:105, 1957.
23. Holder, T. M., and Gross, R. E.: Temporary

gastrostomy in pediatric surgery experience with 187 cases. Pediatrics 26:36, 1960.

24. Holder, T. M., Leape, L. L., and Ashcraft, K. W.: Gastrostomy: Its use and dangers in pediatric patients. N. Engl. J. Med. 286:1345, 1972.

25. Javett, S. L., Jackson, H., and Utian, H. L.: Torgensen's muscle and infantile hypertrophic pyloric stenosis. J. Pediatr. Surg. 8:383, 1973.

26. Kekomaki, M., and Kuitunen, P.: Simultaneous occurrence of congenital pyloric web and hiatal insufficiency in an infant. Helv. Paediatr. Acta 29:595, 1974.

27. Kiesewetter, W. B.: Spontaneous rupture of the stomach in the newborn. J. Dis. Child. 91:162, 1956.

28. Kimura, K., Tsugawa, C., Ogawa, K., et al.: Diamond-shaped anastomosis for congenital duodenal obstruction. Arch. Surg. 112:1262, 1977.

29. Krasna, I. H., Becker, J. M., Schwartz, D., and Schneider, K.: Low molecular weight dextran and reexploration in the management of ischemic midgut-volvulus. J. Pediatr. Surg. 13:480, 1978.

30. Levine, G., Favara, B. E., Mierau, G., et al.: Jaundice, liver ultrastructure, and congenital pyloric stenosis. A study in infants. Arch. Pathol. 95:267, 1973.

31. Lewis, J. E.: Partial duodenal obstruction with incomplete duodenal rotation. J. Pediatr. Surg. 1:47, 1966.

32. Linkner, L., and Benson, C. D.: Spontaneous perforation of the stomach in the newborn. Ann. Surg. 149:525, 1959.

33. Lloyd, J. R.: The etiology of gastrointestinal perforation in the newborn. J. Pediatr. Surg. 4:77, 1969.

34. Lynn, H. B.: Duodenal obstruction. *In* Ravitch, M. M., et al. (eds.): Pediatric Surgery, 3rd edition. Chicago, Year Book Medical Publishers, 1979.

35. Martin, L. W., and Fultz, C. T.: Use of gastrostomy in pediatric surgery. Arch. Surg. 78:904, 1959.

36. McCarten, K. M., and Littlewood Teele, R.: Preduodenal portal vein: Venography, ultrasonography, and review of the literature. Ann. Radiol. 21:155, 1978.

37. Meeker, I. A., and Snyder, W. H.: Gastrostomy for the newborn surgical patient: A report of 140 cases. Arch. Dis. Child. 37:159, 1962.

38. Merrill, J. R., and Raffensperger, J. G.: Pediatric annular pancreas: twenty years' experience. J. Pediatr. Surg. 11:921, 1976.

39. Michener, W. M., Kennedy, R. L. J., and DuShane, J. W.: Duodenal ulcer in childhood. Am. J. Dis. Child. 100:814, 1960.

40. Milliken, J. C.: Duodenal ulceration in children. Gut 6:25, 1965.

41. Moore, T. C.: Gastrectomy in infancy and childhood. Ann. Surg. 162:91, 1965.

42. Pellerin, D., Fortier-Beaulieu, M., and Gueguen, J.: The fate of swallowed foreign bodies. Experience of 1250 instances of subdiaphragmatic foreign bodies in children. Progr. Pediatr. Radiol. 2:286, 1969.

43. Ravitch, M. M., and Duremdes, G. D.: Operative treatment of chronic duodenal ulcer in childhood. Ann. Surg. 171:641, 1970.

44. Richardson, W. R., and Martin, L. W.: Pitfalls in the surgical management of incomplete duodenal diaphragm. J. Pediatr. Surg. 4:303, 1969.

45. Rosenlund, M. L., and Koop, C. E.: Duodenal ulcer in childhood. Pediatrics 45:283, 1970.

46. Saltz, N. J., and Luttwak, E.: Volvulus of the midbowel and its resulting intestinal obstruction. Arch. Surg. 76:633, 1958.

47. Scharli, A. F., and Leditschke, J. F.: Gastric motility after pyloromyotomy in infants: A reappraisal of postoperative feeding. Surgery 64:1133, 1968.

48. Scharli, A., Sieber, W., and Kiesewetter, W. B.: Hypertrophic pyloric stenosis at Children's Hospital of Pittsburgh from 1912 to 1967. J. Pediatr. Surg. 4:108, 1969.

49. Schneider, A. J.: Volvulus and massive gangrene with survival. Arch. Surg. 76:1004, 1958.

50. Seagram, C. G. F., Stephens, G. A., and Cumming, W. A.: Peptic ulceration at the Hospital for Sick Children, Toronto, during the 20 year period 1949–1969. J. Pediatr. Surg. 8:407, 1973.

51. Senter, K. L.: Complications of temporary tube gastrostomy. Arch. Surg. 81:103, 1960.

52. Signer, E., and Fridrich, R.: Gastric emptying in newborns and young infants. Acta Paediatr. Scand. 64:525, 1975.

53. Slovis, T. L., Klein, M. D., and Watts, F. B., Jr.: Incomplete rotation of intestines with normal cecal position. Surgery 87:325, 1980.

54. Stanley-Brown, E. G., and Stevenson, S. S.: Massive gastrointestinal hemorrhage in the newborn infant. Pediatrics 35:482, 1965.

55. Stewart, D. R., Colodny, A. L., and Daggett, N. C.: Malrotation of the bowel in infants and children: A 15 year review. Surgery 79:716, 1976.

56. Touloukian, R. J.: Gastric ischemia: The primary factor in neonatal perforation. Clin. Pediatr. 12:219, 1973.

57. Welch, K. J.: Stomach and duodenum. *In* Ravitch, M. M., et al. (eds.): Pediatric Surgery, 3rd edition. Chicago, Year Book Medical Publishers, 1979, p. 923.

58. Wesley, J. R., and Mahour, G. N.: Congenital intrinsic duodenal obstruction: A 25 year review. Surgery 82:716, 1977.

59. Woolley, M. M., Gwinn, J. L., and Mares, A.: Congenital partial gastric antral obstruction, an elusive cause of abdominal pain and vomiting. Ann. Surg. 180:265, 1974.

23

SMALL INTESTINE

Arvin I. Philippart, M.D.
Reuben S. Dubois, M.B., B.S.

Complications of small bowel surgery in children arise from errors in preoperative diagnosis and intraoperative assessment as well as from errors in the execution of the surgical procedure. Delay in diagnosis may increase the frequency of surgical intervention, as in necrotizing enterocolitis or intussusception, or increase the magnitude and extent of the procedure, as in intussusception or midgut volvulus. Such delays may also result from the limitations of radiologic evaluation of the small bowel, which necessitate greater reliance on clinical judgment. Early recognition of complications in the neonate will minimize morbidity from depletion of fluid and electrolytes, aspiration, and ischemic perforations. A correct preoperative and intraoperative diagnosis expedites the procedure and results in less postoperative morbidity and mortality.

Supportive management throughout the perioperative period is particularly critical in the neonate. Recent advances in neonatal survival have resulted as much from improved supportive care as from improved surgical techniques.

ATRESIAS AND ANASTOMOSES

Successful resection and anastomosis of small intestine require correct assessment of the abnormality, adequate blood supply and neuromuscular function at the margins of resection, absence of distal obstruction, and meticulous surgical anastomotic technique. Failure to fulfill these requirements results in postoperative obstruction, perforation, or fistula formation.

These principles are best exemplified in the management of the neonate with jejun-oileal atresia. Small bowel atresias and stenoses are attributed to mesenteric vascular accidents that occur in utero.[17] These accidents may or may not be associated with a pre-existing disease, such as cystic fibrosis, or anomaly, such as volvulus. Most occur early in fetal life. The severity of the insult and the chronicity of the obstruction determine the extent of secondary changes. The proximal gut is markedly dilated. Wall thickness is greatly increased. Muscular elements are disorganized and neural plexuses absent or diminished in the end of the proximal segment. The distal segment is small and its wall is thin, but again there is neuromuscular disorganization.

Simple anastomosis of the atretic segments will produce anatomic patency but functional obstruction. The proximal segment must be resected[2] or tapered[29] or both to provide adequate function. Poor survival before the advent of total parenteral nutrition resulted largely from anastomotic dysfunction and from insufficient absorptive surface subsequent to in utero losses of long intestinal segments.

Associated distal obstructions occur in approximately 10 per cent of patients with atresia. This may result from additional atresias, intraluminal obstruction as in meconium ileus, or dyskinetic gut as seen with ruptured cord hernias. Preoperative contrast enemas followed by intraoperative instillation of saline solution into the small bowel distal to the atresia will detect these obstructions. The fluid column should reach the residual barium in the cecum to rule out associated intraluminal obstruction. Such maneuvers are not used in the patient with ruptured cord hernia when the gut is reduced into the abdomen and the atretic

285

ends are exteriorized through the abdominal defect as dual enterostomies until motility returns.

Jejunal atresia with a helical or "apple-peel" ileum requires specific comment. This anomaly results from loss of superior mesenteric artery circulation distal to the right branch of the middle colic artery. Much gut is frequently lost, and the proximal end of the distal segment functions poorly, necessitating more extensive distal resection.[34] It is critical that the ileum not be untwisted, as this will cause torsion of the blood supply to the residual small bowel.

Before primary anastomosis became popular, the Mikulicz dual enterostomy with application of a spur-crushing clamp was used.[21] After a period of obturation of the stoma with vented overflow and proven distal patency, the stoma was closed extraperitoneally. The advantages were the lack of an intraperitoneal anastomosis and proof of distal function before closure. The disadvantages were the need for multiple procedures, an unacceptable incidence of anastomotic leaks at final closure, and late blind loop syndromes. Alternatives are the Bishop-Koop and Santulli enterostomies.[7] The former has been more widely used. The advantage of the Bishop-Koop procedure is a less frequent need for secondary anastomosis. The disadvantages are the presence of an intraperitoneal anastomosis, delayed closure of the mucus fistula, and late blind loop syndromes. Despite the current widespread application of primary anastomosis, each of these staged techniques is still useful when there is the possibility of distal obstruction (ileal atresia, ruptured cord hernia, or complicated meconium ileus).

Primary anastomosis is now the preferred technique in most circumstances when distal patency has been established. Because of the secondary changes in residual gut after ischemia, side-to-side and end-to-side anastomoses are not used. Such anastomoses produce anastomotic dysfunction, ineffective proximal peristalsis, and blind loop syndromes. Resection followed by end-to-end/oblique anastomosis is now preferred, with or without proximal jejunal tapering for jejunal atresias. A single layer of interrupted, inverting, fine (5-0 or 6-0) suture is used with knots within the lumen. An in-

complete second seromuscular layer may be used in questionable areas. No running hemostatic suture is used. Minimal wall is inverted. Such techniques produce the least anastomotic obstruction and little risk of leak.

MECONIUM ILEUS

This disease presents as distal small bowel obstruction in two forms, both associated most commonly with cystic fibrosis. In simple meconium ileus, terminal ileal obstruction results from obturation of the lumen by viscid meconium resulting from in utero deficiency of pancreatic enzymes and abnormal intestinal mucus. The gut wall is intact. In complicated meconium ileus, a superimposed in utero vascular accident produced perforation or atresia with or without meconium peritonitis. For this reason, all patients with distal atresia should eventually be evaluated for cystic fibrosis.

Surgical complications have been many through the years. Early approaches utilized resection of the maximally dilated gut with creation of stomas. Since cystic fibrosis produces primary malabsorption, gut resection should be avoided whenever possible. More recently, meglumine diatrizoate (Gastrografin) enemas have been used to avoid operation in patients with simple meconium ileus.[18] Hyperosmolar dehydration may occur when such enemas are given without intravenous fluid replacement. An alternative is enema evacuation of the colon with Gastrografin relieving distal obstruction, followed by operative irrigation and evacuation through an ileotomy, which can then be closed without resection, stomas, or danger of disruption because the colon is patent.

Meconium ileus should not be confused with Hirschsprung's disease with an ileal transition zone. The appearance of the ileum on barium enema studies and the nature of the meconium should allow differentiation. However, a biopsy for ganglion cells can be helpful in the unusual situation.

In complicated meconium ileus the associated atresia or perforation can be managed by primary anastomosis, if distal patency is certain, or by stomal diversion, if patency is uncertain or if there is meconium peritonitis with pseudocyst formation.

NECROTIZING ENTEROCOLITIS

Necrotizing enterocolitis results in hemorrhagic intestinal infarction and occurs most commonly in stressed premature infants. The etiology is multifactorial, but mesenteric ischemia is common to all.[19] Most patients are managed successfully without operation. Indications for operation include those complications of the disease producing peritonitis, perforation, or obstruction.

The entire gut demonstrates some pathologic changes. Necrosis necessitating resection usually involves the ileum and right colon. Conservative resections should be done and dual unmatured stomas created. With infrequent exception, primary anastomosis should be avoided because residual gut also demonstrates histologic ischemic changes. Although unreported, perforations occurred frequently in the past when resection and primary anastomosis was performed. If diverted, marginal gut may be left distally. Contrast evaluation of the defunctionalized colon is necessary before continuity is re-established. Late cicatricial stenosis is not infrequent.

Postoperative care is complex, and venous alimentation is generally necessary. Injudicious early feeding may produce severe fluid losses or reactivate the disease. Surprisingly few late mechanical or metabolic complications have emerged in this group of patients.

INTUSSUSCEPTION

Intussusception is the invagination of proximal intestine into distal intestine. Its clinical features are well discussed elsewhere.[22] Alternative forms of management include hydrostatic reduction, operative reduction, and resection.

Most complications of this disease begin with delay in diagnosis. Such delay increases the derangements consequent to intestinal obstruction, the ischemia due to mesenteric vascular compression, and the likelihood of operative management. The most frequent cause of delay is failure to consider the diagnosis if the child is older than 1 year or has had antecedent gastroenteritis. Other atypical presentations causing diagnostic delay occur when intussusception is secondary to a disease, such as anaphylactoid purpura or cystic fibrosis, or to a recent operation. Delay results from the similarity of symptoms of the primary disease and the intussusception. Atypical intussusceptions seldom have a colonic component visible on barium enema studies.

Complications of hydrostatic reduction should be rare if the reservoir is kept no more than 30 to 36 inches above the x-ray table and there is no manipulation. Failure to demonstrate reflux into the terminal ileum mandates exploration unless there is marked clinical improvement. Intussusception recurs in 3 to 5 per cent of all patients, with no difference in incidence between operative and nonoperative reduction. A decision must be made about the management of a patient with recurrence. If the initial intussusception was recently reduced hydrostatically, a second attempt at hydrostatic reduction is appropriate. A second recurrence is reduced operatively so that the surgeon can look for an underlying lesion or "lead point." If intussusception recurs soon after operative reduction and appendectomy, reoperation is preferred. A later recurrence may be managed by hydrostatic reduction. In the rare circumstance of multiple recurrences without a recognized lead point, a "blind" segmental ileocolectomy has been recommended.[28] Such occurrences are fortunately rare, and resection is not a panacea.

Complications of operative reduction should also be few. Proper operative reduction is accomplished by gentle retrograde compression without traction. The major difficulties for the less experienced surgeon occur in recognizing lead points that require resection. Most intussusceptions reduced operatively reveal intramural thickening secondary to venous congestion, edema, and hypertrophied Peyer's patches. These do not require resection. Specific lesions such as Meckel's diverticulum, duplications, or polyps can be differentiated. Patients with these conditions require resection.

Resection of an intussusception should be necessary only infrequently. True irreducibility is an indication, but has been unusual in our experience. If reduced, the involved ileum may be markedly discolored. Rather than immediate resection, observation for 10 to 15 minutes will ordinarily indicate adequate return of perfusion to preclude resection. If required, resection should include the intussusceptum. The intussuscipiens is adequately perfused. Failure to recognize that difference can lead to anastomotic disruption.

Intussusception following an unrelated operation requires special comment. Even experienced physicians may not diagnose the condition immediately.[6] It follows major extraperitoneal as well as intraperitoneal and occasionally thoracic procedures. The condition is recognized late because it is superimposed on an expected ileus, the mass is rarely palpable, and the colon is uninvolved. Operation is required when there is persistent clinical and radiologic evidence of small bowel obstruction. A high index of suspicion is necessary.

Fever is a frequent complication after reduction of an intussusception. It is usually low grade but may be high and associated with hypotension. It is thought to be due to reperfusion of previously ischemic gut with mobilization of lysosomal enzymes or endotoxin. Appropriate management includes administration of antibiotics and volume expansion. Such fevers occur within the first postoperative hours. Perforation rarely occurs this early.

CROHN'S DISEASE

The indications for surgical intervention in patients with Crohn's disease are the complications of the disease, including obstruction, perforation, hemorrhage, and growth failure. Complications of surgical management are largely determined by the mode of presentation and the adequacy of preparation. Elective resections after thorough metabolic and intestinal preparation are rarely associated with complications. The complication rate is high when emergency intervention is required in the catabolic patient with sepsis who has been treated with steroids and immunosuppressive agents. Whenever possible, operation should be delayed to permit treatment with antibiotics, intestinal decompression, and total parenteral nutrition. This is usually possible in children with acute exacerbations, partial obstruction, or fistulae. Such temporizing will ordinarily allow primary resection, obviating bypass and secondary operations with their attendant complications. Delay is not possible in the presence of free perforation or acute and massive blood loss.

Complications of elective resections include wound infection, obstruction, perforation, and fistula formation — the complications that follow small bowel resections for any disease. Earlier reports record a higher incidence of complications of Crohn's disease than has been our recent experience in performing elective resections in well-prepared patients.[10]

In the chronically ill patient with acute complications a lesser operation may be justified. A major disadvantage in this group is the frequent lack of adequate assessment of the extent of their disease prior to their emergency presentation to the surgeon because of acute illness. Bypasses or exclusion procedures have been widely used. Complications of these procedures include retention of diseased bowel with toxicity, fistulae, and blind loop syndromes. For very sick patients we have preferred excision of the acutely perforated bowel, creation of temporary dual stomas, and performance of interval enteroenterostomy after adequate evaluation and metabolic preparation. This alternative approach is used when primary resection and enteroenterostomy is inadvisable.

Although total parenteral nutrition now plays a major role in treatment of this disease and has diminished surgical complications, it has also been associated with an increased frequency of seizures and coma. In our experience this has been associated with low serum levels of magnesium and zinc. Others have suggested that water intoxication, steroids, and hypertension are causative.[16] Catabolic patients have diminished host-defense mechanisms, if not secondary to immunosuppressive therapy, then secondary to malnutrition. As a result of diminished defenses and the primary disease, systemic sepsis is frequent and must be anticipated.

The major complication of resections for Crohn's disease in children is recurrent disease. Although the presence of grossly visible disease at resection margins appears to increase recurrence rates and postoperative complications, there is no definitive evidence that the extent of resection of bowel or mesentery or the presence of nonspecific microscopic submucosal inflammation alters the incidence of complications or recurrences.[24]

MECKEL'S DIVERTICULUM

Meckel's diverticulum is a remnant of the omphalomesenteric duct located on the antimesenteric border of the distal ileum. It is found in 2 per cent of the population. Acute complications necessitating surgical intervention include hemorrhage, perforation, and obstruction due to intussusception or vitelline duct remnants.[1] The frequency of these complications is widely reported as 25 per cent, but it is more likely closer to 4 per cent, as calculated by Soltero and Bill.[27]

Complications in management of the acute disorders of Meckel's diverticulum begin with delay in diagnosis. Hemorrhage is the most common complication in children, who present with painless bleeding sufficient to necessitate replacement of blood. Radiographic evaluation is rarely helpful except to rule out other lesions. Isotopic imaging is useful only if it provides positive evidence of ectopic gastric mucosa in a child with lower gastrointestinal tract bleeding. Reliance on a negative study will miss as many as 50 per cent of cases. Operative identification is rarely difficult when laparotomy is done for hemorrhage. When a Meckel's diverticulum is not found, more careful inspection is necessary. The vitelline artery may be recognized by its course over the surface of the ileum to the antimesenteric border or to a retracted, fixed diverticulum attached to the mesentery. Resection of the diverticulum for hemorrhage may be done with or without an ileal resection. If adjacent ileum is not excised, careful inspection of the specimen is required to establish

that both the ectopic mucosa and the ulcer are contained in the resected diverticulum. The bleeding site may be in the ileum and not in the diverticulum. A diverticulum that has been the lead point of an intussusception may require ileal resection because of marginal viability of adjacent ileum at the head of the intussusception.

Technical complications following resection of an incidentally recognized diverticulum are those that follow any enterotomy with anastomosis no matter what technique is used. A more important question is, When should an incidentally discovered Meckel's diverticulum be removed? Those with scarring, palpable ectopic mucosa, or narrow bases and those attached to the parietes should be removed. Restraint should be exercised when the primary procedure is extensive, when there is a more distal anastomosis, and when the abdomen is uncontaminated. Although no statistics are available for complications of removal of the incidental Meckel's diverticulum, the complications of enterotomy are known.

ENTERIC FISTULAE

Fistulae result from the external drainage of enteric perforations. Such perforations

TABLE 23–1 CAUSES OF FISTULAE

Iatrogenic
  Anastomotic failure
    Ischemia
    Suture technique
  Wound closure
  Retained foreign body

Residual Pathology
  Ischemia
    Necrotizing enterocolitis
    Midgut volvulus
  Distal obstruction
    Intraluminal
      Meconium ileus
      Unrecognized atresia
    Intramural
      Hirschsprung's disease
      Dyskinesia
    Adhesive

Other
  Crohn's disease
  Radiation enteritis

may be iatrogenic or the result of a pathologic process (Table 23–1). They present as a wound infection with drainage of enteric contents after wound drainage, the appearance of enteric contents at a previously placed drain site, or as free perforation and peritonitis necessitating drainage at a secondary procedure.

Iatrogenic causes of anastomotic failures include excessive mesenteric devascularization and inadequate suture placement. Erosion or fixation of bowel by the sutures in a laparotomy closure occur more frequently in older patients than in neonates in whom closure is rarely difficult. An exception is the infant with an abdominal wall defect such as an omphalocoele or ruptured cord hernia. A retained intra-abdominal foreign body should always be considered in any patient with a fistula.

Residual enteric pathology is the more frequent cause of fistulae. Ischemic lesions resulting in extensive small bowel necrosis and the consequent need to salvage all possible gut include necrotizing enterocolitis and malrotation with midgut volvulus. The attempt to salvage gut of marginal variability with concurrent anastomosis will frequently lead to anastomotic leak and fistula formation. In our view, more gut of marginal viability can be salvaged, and the complications of anastomosis avoided, by initial dual stomas followed by later enteroenterostomy.[19]

A second major cause of anastomotic failure and fistula formation is unrecognized distal obstruction. Intraluminal obstructions, already discussed, include meconium ileus and unrecognized secondary atresia. Intramural obstructions include the dysmotility states in aganglionosis (Fig. 23–1) and the dyskinetic state associated with ruptured cord hernias.

Fistulization may occur at a distance from a suture line with radiation enteritis or Crohn's disease. The former is infrequent in children owing to current radiotherapeutic techniques. Ileal fistula formation after appendectomy is a classically recurring presentation of Crohn's disease.

The management of small bowel fistulae has been greatly simplified by the widespread use of total parenteral nutrition.

Nevertheless, initial principles of management are unchanged. Adequate drainage of the recent fistula is important to minimize intra-abdominal accumulations and sepsis. Administration of antibiotics is required for the patient with systemic sepsis. Such measures are less critical in the nonseptic patient with a well-organized fistulous tract.

Subsequent evaluation of the patient should include review of all pathologic material for evidence of Crohn's disease or other inflammatory processes. Plain films of the abdomen are reviewed for evidence of retained foreign bodies, abscess cavities, or intestinal obstruction. Contrast radiographs through the mature fistula will help locate the level of perforation (Fig. 23–1). Enteric

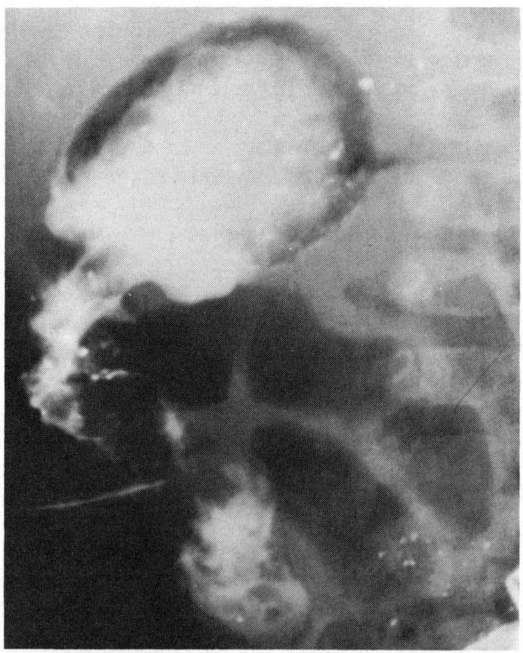

Figure 23–1 Fistulogram in 10-month-old child who weighed 9 pounds at the time of transfer for persistent ileal and colonic fistulae, malnutrition, and persistent intestinal obstruction after multiple previous laparotomies. Fistulogram of ileum demonstrates right colon transition zone of Hirschsprung's disease confirmed by rectal biopsy. After a period of decompression and total parenteral nutrition, the fistulae at sites of prior anastomoses in the ileum and cecum were surgically closed, and a transition zone colostomy was performed. The child thrived and has undergone subsequent successful reconstruction.

contrast studies assess associated proximal or distal disease, particularly distal obstruction. Rectal biopsy is appropriate if Hirschsprung's or inflammatory bowel disease is suspected.

Central to management are treatment of sepsis and provision of adequate calories to produce anabolism. Although "feed me, drain me" catheter techniques and oral elemental diets have been recommended, the simplest and most rapidly effective technique is total parenteral nutrition. In the absence of distal obstruction, most fistulae will close without operation. If reoperation is required because of distal obstruction or a residual pathologic process, nutritional preparation will allow an appropriate definitive surgical procedure without the need for staged bypasses and exclusions described in older surgical texts.

ILEOSTOMY

The complications of ileostomy are largely determined by the indications for which they are done and the planned duration of the stoma. Temporary stomas, particularly the Mikulicz type, were widely used in neonates with intestinal obstruction before primary anastomosis became popular in the 1960's. Their complications are discussed in the section on meconium ileus. Successful surgical management of necrotizing enterocolitis and the frequency of that disease have again led to common use of temporary, separate enterostomies in small, sick, premature infants. In this situation, two technical points are germane. All stomas must be sutured to each fascial layer of the abdominal wall to avoid dehiscence, evisceration, and prolapse. Primary maturation is unnecessary. Dysfunction is rarely an issue in patients with extensive resections for ischemia because few are fed significant amounts orally prior to closure.

Permanent ileostomies have been created after total colectomy for inflammatory bowel disease and polypoid syndromes. In recent years, many pediatric surgeons have adapted the endorectal pull-through procedure following colectomy for ulcerative colitis and polypoid disease, markedly diminishing the number of permanent ileostomies. Granulomatous disease is now the primary indication for permanent ileostomy. Stenosis, retraction, prolapse, and parastomal hernias are the result of errors in technique.[9] The Brooks stoma with primary maturation should avoid dysfunction. Stomal stenosis and dislocations ordinarily require operative revision for optimal function, appliance fit, and hygiene. Fistulae may result from transmural suture fixation or from active Crohn's disease. The acute single fistula frequently clears with superficial drainage, antibiotics, and an elemental diet. Reactivation or chronicity necessitates local revision with excision of the tract. Multiple fistulae or extensive undermining of the subcutaneous tissue often necessitates excision of the stoma and relocation elsewhere. We have not been impressed by results produced by total parenteral nutrition or 6-mercaptopurine in the patient with chronic fistula.

The continent ileostomy has been used less extensively in children than in adults because of growth considerations and the availability of the alternative endorectal pull-through. Neither the reservoir ileostomy nor the pull-through has been done long enough for late results to be evaluated. Partial obstruction is a critical and common complication of the continent ileostomy. Concern that growth of the ileum may increase obstruction has limited popularity of the Kock procedure for growing children.[15] Application of the technique to the adolescent without a rectum and a prior end ileostomy is appropriate when one is certain that the patient does not have Crohn's disease and when one is aware of the complications.[15, 30]

POSTOPERATIVE OBSTRUCTION

Failure of normal progressive peristalsis to return after operation has classically been separated into early and late, mechanical and adynamic causes. In the child, the usual period of adynamic ileus is shorter and associated with fewer secondary wound and pulmonary sequelae than in the adult. However, in specific instances this period may be

TABLE 23–2 INDICATIONS FOR INITIAL LAPAROTOMY IN PATIENTS WITH LATE POSTOPERATIVE INTESTINAL OBSTRUCTION*

Indication	Number of Patients
Abdominal wall defects	16
Hirschsprung's disease	13
Intestinal atresia	9
Malrotation	6
Diaphragmatic hernia	5
Appendicitis	14
Tumor	7
Other	21
Total	91

*Experience at Children's Hospital of Michigan, 1970–1978.

markedly prolonged. Intestinal atresias and ischemic diseases have already been discussed. The classic lesion leading to prolonged ileus is the ruptured cord hernia. In the patient with this condition, sufficient progressive peristalsis to permit survival on oral intake alone may not occur for 3 to 4 weeks and occasionally not for 6 to 9 months. Total parenteral nutrition is required for survival. Other poorly understood dysmotility states may present as pseudo-obstructions with normal ganglion cell distribution.[25, 26]

A review of our own recent experience (Table 23–2) reveals that mechanical obstructions occur most often after extensive intestinal procedures in the neonate and young infant. The initial procedure preceding obstruction was performed during the first 3 months of life in 34 per cent of patients, during the first year in 49 per cent, and during the first 2 years in 65 per cent. Obstructive episodes occurred soon after operation. Sixty-three per cent of obstructions occurred within 3 months after operation and 78 per cent within the first year.

Operation was required in 75 of 91 patients (82 per cent). Nonoperative management with tube decompression was used successfully in 16 of 91 (18 per cent). Nonoperative management was successful most often in older children with complicated illnesses following perforative appendicitis, repair of abdominal wall defects, or multiple previous obstructive episodes.

Postoperative obstructions were largely adhesive. However, four patients had small bowel intussusceptions (discussed earlier). All occurred during the initial hospitalization and were recognized only because a high index of suspicion led to exploration.

SHORT BOWEL SYNDROME

Extensive bowel resection produces alterations in intestinal motility, secretion, digestion, and absorption.[13, 23, 31] The availability of total parenteral nutrition in recent years has increased the number of survivors and, therefore, the need for greater understanding of enteric feeding. The difficulties encountered are proportional to the amount and locations of gut resected and the functional status of the remaining intestine.

Pathologic processes most commonly associated with functional short bowel syndromes are necrotizing enterocolitis and extensive intestinal atresias in the neonate, malrotation with midgut volvulus in patients of all ages, and Crohn's disease in older children. When ischemic lesions are present, residual gut is abnormal but has potential for recovery and compensatory growth. In Crohn's disease, residual gut may become increasingly abnormal, superimposing additional malabsorption on deficiencies in gut length.

Normal Digestion and Absorption

The normal sites of digestion and absorption of nutrients are schematically represented in Figures 23–2 and 23–3. The duodenum and jejunum absorb all substrates except vitamin B_{12} and bile acids, which are absorbed in the ileum. Dietary carbohydrate must be digested by pancreatic and brush border enzymes. The disaccharidases are highly susceptible to depletion in a number of enteropathic states. The most widely appreciated of these enzymes is lactase. Proteins are enzymatically converted to peptides and subsequently to amino acids for transport. Di- and tripeptides containing glycine, proline, and/or hydroxyproline are absorbed as the intact peptide. A fact of interest and possible therapeutic importance is that these peptides are transported more readily than the component amino acids. Long-chain triglyceride (LCT) is the

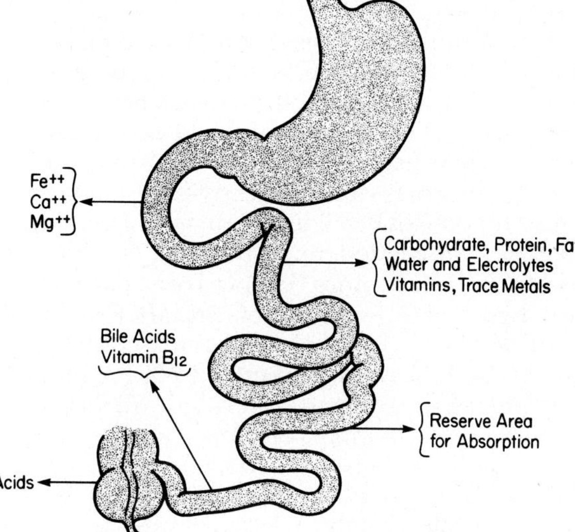

Figure 23-2 Sites of absorption of dietary nutrients and bile acids.

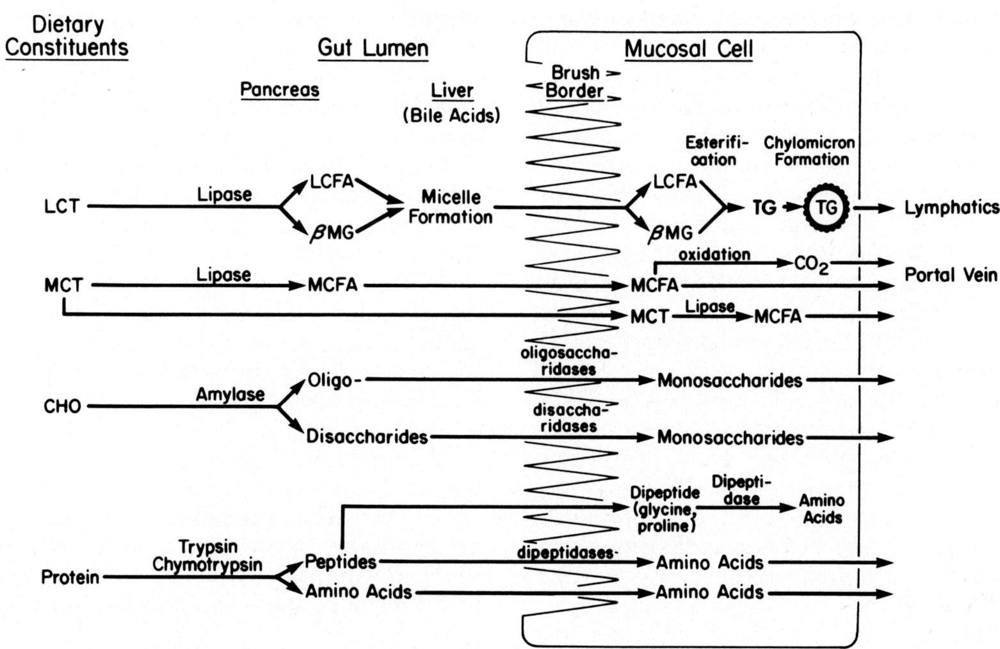

Figure 23-3 Normal digestion and absorption of dietary fat, protein, and carbohydrate. (LCT = long-chain triglyceride; MCT = medium-chain triglyceride; LCFA = long-chain fatty acid; MCFA = medium-chain fatty acid; βMG = beta monoglyceride; CHO = carbohydrate; TG = triglyceride.

predominant dietary fat and requires intraluminal lipolysis and micellar solubilization for absorption. For this reason, medium-chain triglycerides (MCT) are used extensively in the short bowel syndrome.

Intraluminal lipolysis of MCT by pancreatic and gastric lipase is more rapid than that of LCT. Both medium-chain fatty acids (MCFA) and MCT are absorbed in the absence of bile salts. MCT, however, are more slowly absorbed than the fatty acids. MCT enter the mucosal cell in the intact form and may be hydrolyzed by a mucosal lipolytic system, which is quite distinct from pancreatic lipase. The majority of the MCFA are transported as fatty acids in the portal venous blood. Certain amounts of MCFA may be elongated, oxidized, esterified, or incorporated into chylomicrons and transported in the lacteals. It is important to stress that luminal disappearance of MCT and MCFA may not necessarily correlate with active absorption of lipid or its availability as an effective source of calories.[11]

Metabolic Consequences of Small Bowel Resection

Various factors determine the severity of the complications and metabolic sequelae following small bowel resection. Lesser resections are usually well tolerated because the intestine has significant functional reserve and capacity for adaptation. Large extents of the mid small bowel, a reserve area for absorption, can be resected without causing serious complications (see Fig. 23–2), and extensive resection of the distal small intestine may be well tolerated provided the ileocecal valve remains intact. Preservation of the ileocecal sphincter seems important, since its absence predisposes the remaining small intestine to bacterial contamination and appears to increase transit time. The exact mode of action of the ileocecal valve remains obscure.

Following extensive intestinal resection, most nutrients, including fat, protein, carbohydrate, vitamins, trace metals, and water and electrolytes, are absorbed subnormally. The amount of small bowel remaining after resection and its functional condition, as well as that of the colon and other digestive organs, are of prime importance in determining the severity of the complications.

Initially, water and electrolyte malabsorption is of major concern. As time progresses, the consequences of malabsorption of other nutrients, especially fat and lactose, become evident.

In addition to these generalized sequelae, certain specific pathophysiologic abnormalities may occur. Hypergastrinemia and gastric hypersecretion are common.[4] The length of small bowel resected correlates with the degree of hypersecretion. This occurs within 24 hours after resection and decreases with time. The precise cause is unknown but may be decreased gastrin catabolism or removal of inhibitory peptides that are produced in the resected bowel. Gastric hypersecretion may lead to decreased luminal pH and interference with pancreatic enzyme function. In addition, the large volumes secreted may contribute to the diarrhea observed initially in the postoperative period. Gastric hypersecretion may lead to peptic ulceration, although this is not common in children. Possible beneficial aspects of gastric hypersecretion and hypergastrinemia include a role in the adaptive process and prevention of secondary bacterial overgrowth in the remaining small intestine.

Malabsorption of bile acids and their excessive entry into the colon will lead to diarrhea.[13] Free bile acids impair water absorption in the large bowel and in sufficiently high concentrations will result in cyclic AMP–mediated active secretion of water and electrolytes into the lumen of the residual colon. Similarly, unabsorbed fatty acids that enter the colon are β-hydroxylated by the action of bacteria and lead to impaired colonic water absorption or secretion.

Although not commonly reported in the pediatric age group, gallstones increase in incidence after intestinal resection. They are probably secondary to interruption of the enterohepatic circulation of bile salts or to bacterial contamination and altered composition of bile.

Resection of the distal ileum leads to vitamin B_{12} malabsorption, as the specific transport mechanism for intrinsic factor–bound vitamin B_{12} absorption is localized in the ileal mucosa. Thus, patients with sufficiently extensive ileal resection will, in due course, become vitamin B_{12} deficient. Megaloblastic anemia, peripheral neuropathy, and subacute combined degeneration of the spinal cord appear to be uncommon complications in children with the short bowel syndrome. Vitamin B_{12} malabsorption may be compounded by pancreatic exocrine insufficiency and also by bacterial metabolism in those patients with small bowel contamination, even in the presence of an adequate amount of ileum.

Hyperoxaluria and calcium oxalate nephrolithiasis are not uncommon in patients with the short bowel syndrome, especially in those who have an intact colon. Enteric hyperoxaluria results from increased absorption of oxalate in patients with fat maldigestion. Dietary oxalate is usually rendered insoluble, and therefore is poorly absorbed, by intraluminal calcium. In patients with steatorrhea, the concentration of ionized calcium is decreased because of precipitation with fatty acids, so binding to oxalate may be reduced and oxalate absorption increased.[8]

An increasing number of elements, in trace quantities, are known to be of nutritional importance. Deficiency of these elements, particularly copper and zinc, is common in children with the short bowel syndrome. Copper deficiency appears to be secondary to intestinal malabsorption. This may be compounded by normally low levels of copper in premature infants and the interruption of the recently postulated enterohepatic circulation of this trace metal. Copper deficiency may lead to anemia, neutropenia, and bone changes. The latter may be associated or confused with scorbutic or rachitic changes. Zinc deficiency is probably secondary to malabsorption, although the exact mechanism is unknown. Recent evidence, however, suggests a deficiency of a zinc-binding ligand found in pancreatic secretions. The main clinical features of zinc deficiency are poor growth and impaired wound healing.

Intestinal Adaptation Following Small Bowel Resection

Both structural and functional adaptation occur in the bowel remaining after intestinal resection.[32, 33] Adaptation is a slow process that takes several weeks. Of prognostic significance is the fact that the ileum has a greater capacity to adapt than does the jejunum.

Structural or morphologic adaptive changes after massive intestinal resection include increased diameter of the intestine and mucosal cell hyperplasia, leading to an increased total number of absorptive cells per unit length of villus.

Functional adaptation after small bowel resection includes both increased nutrient absorption and increased specific activity of certain mucosal enzymes. Functional adaptation appears to be related to increased numbers of absorptive cells rather than to increased transport capacity. In fact, some metabolic functions are decreased, suggesting functional immaturity of these cells, which resemble crypt cells rather than mature villus tip cells.

Various mechanisms have been postulated as a cause of small bowel mucosal hyperplasia following intestinal resection. These include the trophic effects of enteric hormones and increased concentrations of intraluminal nutrients in the remaining bowel. The effect of intraluminal substrate appears to be dependent upon nutrient absorption. However, the effect of secondarily stimulated biliary and pancreatic secretions or even enteric hormones cannot be excluded. Intraluminal factors play a major role in adaptive hyperplasia and stress the importance of early oral alimentation in the management of patients with the short bowel syndrome. There is very suggestive evidence, however, that the trophic effects of enteric hormones, altered innervation, proportional blood flow, and bacterial flora of the bowel may also influence epithelial cell proliferation. Of the enteric hormones, gastrin has received most attention. However, experimental data do not suggest that this hormone has an important role in adaptive hyperplasia of the residual intestine after resection. Although they have not been well studied, other enteric hormones such as cholecystokinin, secretin, and enteroglucagon may play a role in the adaptive process.[14]

Management of Short Bowel Syndrome

Management of the infant who has had massive small bowel resection requires an understanding of the pathophysiologic and adaptive processes so that optimal and logical nutritional and drug therapy may be provided. In general, these patients require a combination of parenteral nutrition and careful enteral alimentation with either elemental or predigested formula. Although the techniques of total parenteral nutrition have improved to the point that infants can be completely nourished by intravenous infusions, even in the home, the goal should be to establish the patient on a program of oral feedings that meet all nutritional needs. Most infants will require total parenteral nutrition in the immediate postoperative period. It should be planned initially to give all needed calories and essential nutrients, including vitamins and trace metals, by venous infusion. Parenteral alimentation alone, however, leads to mucosal hypoplasia. It is therefore important to commence enteral feedings with elemental or predigested formula as soon as practical.[12] In general, these formulas contain amino acids or casein hydrolysate, monosaccharides or glucose polymers, and MCT. Initially, feedings should be given frequently in small volume and low concentration, but they may be progressively increased as tolerated. Some infants cannot tolerate bolus feeding, and continuous enteral alimentation will be required.[5]

The most common problem associated with feeding is the development of osmotic diarrhea. Electrolytes and osmolarity of stool supernatant should be checked frequently to detect this complication. The major advantage of elemental and predigested formulas lies in the fact that they are lactose-free, are nonantigenic, and contain MCT. Their major drawback is their high osmotic load, due largely to amino acids and monosaccharides. Polycose and other glucose polymers require enzymatic digestion by brush border oligosaccharidases (see Fig. 23–3). The major advantage of these substances is that oligosaccharidases are less susceptible to depletion than are the disaccharidases. Furthermore, carbohydrate in this form makes only a minor contribution to the total osmolar concentration of the dietary load.

Most infants need at least 120 calories/kg/24 hr, in combined intravenous infusions and enteral feedings, to gain weight, to grow satisfactorily, and to compensate for continuing malabsorption. Once the parenteral alimentation is discontinued, trace metals and vitamin supplements, especially fat-soluble A, D, E, and K, are essential. Both calcium and magnesium supplements will also be required, especially if severe malabsorption is present. Infants who have undergone extensive ileal resection may need regular injections of vitamin B_{12}.

Before discussing the treatment of specific problems, a comment regarding the use of antidiarrheal agents is necessary. In general, these are of little or no beneficial effect and may increase abdominal distention. Adequate doses, however, may effectively reduce transit time and cramps and may be of value when attempting to wean an infant from parenteral alimentation.

If there is evidence of gastric hypersecretion, cimetidine or antacids may be useful to improve absorption.

Bacterial overgrowth is common in those infants without an ileocecal valve or those who have significant dysmotility and stasis. The risk of this complication is increased in infants with iatrogenic achlorhydria induced by cimetidine. Courses of antibiotics such as ampicillin or trimethoprim and sulfamethoxazole may be of benefit in improving absorption and controlling diarrhea.

Bile acid–induced diarrhea may be controlled by cholestyramine; however, this therapy is of value only in patients who have had a limited ileal resection. In general, children who have had resection of more than 100 cm respond as adults do, benefiting more from MCT than from cholestyramine because the diarrhea is secondary to the presence of long-chain β-hydroxy fatty acids in the residual colon. Cholestyramine therapy may lead to significant complications. Of these, metabolic acidosis, intestinal obstruction, and hypernatremia are the most common. The precise mechanism of the metabolic acidosis is controversial. Improvement occurs, however, with dose reduction and sodium bicarbonate supplementation. In addition, cholestyramine may interfere with the absorption of many drugs and nutrients.

Hyperoxaluria can also be treated with

cholestyramine. It is more effectively controlled, however, by decreasing dietary intake of oxalate and improving fat absorption or providing a low-fat diet.

Secondary pancreatic exocrine insufficiency is not uncommon in patients with the short bowel syndrome, especially if the infant has significant malnutrition. As MCT are more slowly absorbed than MCFA, and as many predigested and elemental formulas contain significant amounts of LCT, due consideration should be given to pancreatic enzyme replacement in infants whose weight gain is poor despite adequate caloric intake.

References

1. Benson, C. D.: Surgical implications of Meckel's diverticulum. *In* Ravitch, M. M., et al. (eds.): Pediatric Surgery, 3rd edition. Chicago, Year Book Medical Publishers, 1979, p. 955.
2. Benson, C. D., Lloyd, D. R., and Smith, J. D.: Resection and primary anastomosis in the management of stenosis and atresia of the jejunum and ileum. Pediatrics 26:265, 1960.
3. Bohane, T. D., Hara-Ikse, K., Bigger, W. D., et al.: A clinical study of young infants after small intestinal resection. J. Pediatr. 94:552, 1979.
4. Buxton, B.: Progress report. Small bowel resection and gastric hypersecretion. Gut 15:229, 1974.
5. Christie, D. L., and Ament, M. E.: Dilute elemental diet and continuous infusion technique for management of short bowel syndrome. J. Pediatr. 87:705, 1975.
6. Cox, J. A., and Martin, L. W.: Postoperative intussusception. Arch. Surg. 106:263, 1973.
7. DeLorimier, A. A., Fonkalsrud, E. W., and Hays, D. M.: Congenital atresia and stenosis of the jejunum and ileum. Surgery 65:819, 1969.
8. Dobbins, J. W., and Binder, H. J.: Effect of bile salts and fatty acids on the colonic absorption of oxalate. Gastroenterology 70:1096, 1976.
9. Goldblatt, M. S., Corman, M. L., Haggitt, R. C., et al.: Ileostomy complications requiring revision: Lahey Clinic experience, 1964–1973. Dis. Colon Rectum 20:209, 1977.
10. Goligher, J. C.: Surgery of the Anus, Rectum, and Colon, 3rd edition. London, Bailliere, Tindall & Cox, 1975, p. 843.
11. Greenberger, N. J., and Skillman, T. G.: Medical Progress. Medium chain triglycerides. Physiological considerations and clinical implications. N. Engl. J. Med. 280:1045, 1969.
12. Greene, H. C., McCabe, D. R., and Merenstein, G. B.: Protracted diarrhea and malnutrition in infancy: Changes in intestinal morphology and disaccharidase activities during treatment with total intravenous nutrition or oral elemental diets. J. Pediatr. 87:695, 1975.
13. Hofmann, A. F., and Poley, J. R.: Role of bile acid malabsorption in pathogenesis of diarrhea and steatorrhea in patients with ileal resection. I. Response to cholestyramine or replacement of dietary long chain triglyceride by medium chain triglyceride. Gastroenterology 62:918, 1972.
14. Hughes, C. A., Bates, T., and Dowling, R. H.: Cholecystokinin and secretin prevent the intestinal mucosal hypoplasia of total parenteral nutrition in the dog. Gastroenterology 75:34, 1978.
15. Kock, N. G., Darle, N., Hulten, L., et al.: Ileostomy. Curr. Probl. Surg. 14(8):1, 1977.
16. Levine, A. M., Pickett, L. K., and Touloukian, R. J.: Steroids, hypertension and fluid retention in the genesis of postoperative seizures with inflammatory bowel disease in childhood. J. Pediatr. Surg. 9:715, 1974.
17. Louw, J. H., and Barnard, C. N.: Congenital intestinal atresia: Observations on its origin. Lancet 2:1065, 1955.
18. Noblett, H.: Meconium ileus. *In* Ravitch, M. M., et al. (eds.): Pediatric Surgery, 3rd edition. Chicago, Year Book Medical Publishers, 1979, p. 943.
19. Philippart, A. I., and Rector, F. E.: Necrotizing enterocolitis. *In* Ravitch, M. M., et al. (eds.): Pediatric Surgery, 3rd edition. Chicago, Year Book Medical Publishers, 1979, p. 970.
20. Pitchumoni, C. S.: Pancreas in primary malnutrition disorders. Am. J. Clin. Nutr. 26:374, 1973.
21. Randolph, J. G., Zollinger, R. M., and Gross, R. E.: Mikulicz resection in infants and children: A 20-year survey of 196 patients. Ann. Surg. 158:481, 1963.
22. Ravitch, M. M.: Intussusception. *In* Ravitch, M. M., et al. (eds.): Pediatric Surgery, 3rd edition. Chicago, Year Book Medical Publishers, 1979, p. 989.
23. Roy, C. C., Silverman, A., and Cozzetto, F. J.: Malabsorption syndrome. *In* Silverman, A., et al. (eds.): Pediatric Clinical Gastroenterology, 2nd edition. St. Louis, C. V. Mosby Co., 1975.
24. Schneider, K. M., and Becker, J. M.: Inflammatory bowel disease. *In* Ravitch, M. M., et al. (eds.): Pediatric Surgery, 3rd edition. Chicago, Year Book Medical Publishers, 1979, p. 1010.
25. Shaw, A., Shaffer, H., Teja, K., et al.: A perspective for pediatric surgeons: Chronic idiopathic intestinal pseudoobstruction. J. Pediatr. Surg. 14:719, 1979.
26. Sieber, W. K., and Girdany, B. R.: Functional intestinal obstruction in newborn infants with morphologically normal gastrointestinal tracts. Surgery 53:357, 1963.
27. Soltero, M. J., and Bill, A. H.: The natural history of Meckel's diverticulum and its relation to incidental removal. Am. J. Surg. 132:168, 1976.
28. Soper, R. T., and Brown, M. J.: Recurrent acute intussusception in children. Arch. Surg. 89:188, 1964.
29. Thomas, C. G., and Carter, J. M.: Small intestinal atresia: The critical role of a functioning anastomosis. Ann. Surg. 179:663, 1974.

30. Thow, G. B.: Symposium: Present status of the continent ileostomy. Dis. Colon Rectum 19: 189, 1976.
31. Wesser, E., Fletcher, J. T., and Urban, E.: Clinical conference short bowel syndrome. Gastroenterology 77:572, 1979.
32. Williamson, R. C. N.: Medical Progress. Intestinal adaptation. Part 1. Structural, functional and cytokinetic changes. N. Engl. J. Med. 298:1393, 1978.
33. Williamson, R. C. N.: Medical Progress. Intestinal adaptation. Part 2. Mechanisms of control. N. Engl. J. Med. 298:1444, 1978.
34. Zerella, J. T., and Martin, L. W.: Jejunal atresia with absent mesentery and a helical ileum. Surgery 80:550, 1976.

24

COLON AND RECTUM

Lester W. Martin, M.D.
Richard E. Black, M.D.

Certain anatomic considerations influence the complications that may arise from surgery of the colon and rectum. The colon traverses all quadrants of the abdominal cavity and lies both intraperitoneally and extraperitoneally. The rectum is adjacent to the genitourinary tract and pelvic nerves and vessels. The perineal structures are not as readily accessible to operative exploration as other areas of the body. The principles of prevention and management of specific complications that follow operations related to colonic and anorectal disease will be discussed, with minimal attention given to systemic complications that may follow any type of operation.

APPENDICITIS

There are few complications of acute appendicitis as long as the infection is contained within the appendix, but once the infecting bacteria have penetrated the serosa or have entered the regional circulation, a series of complications may result[4] (Table 24–1). Emphasis is placed on early removal of the inflamed appendix to prevent complications. The diagnosis of appendicitis cannot be made with complete accuracy prior to operation. To prevent perforation, therefore, it is generally accepted that in 15 to 20 per cent of patients operated upon for acute appendicitis, the appendix will be normal. Conversely, even with the most sophisticated diagnostic facilities, the early signs and symptoms of appendicitis may be so subtle and varied that on rare occasions, perforation may occur even while the child is under hospital observation by an experienced clinician. Most complications of acute appendicitis are a result of infection and may

present clinically as wound infection, peritonitis, sepsis, intra-abdominal abscess, and formation of fistulae to surrounding organs.[5, 15]

Peritonitis develops following perforation of the appendix. It may be localized initially and then become generalized with the spread of contamination in the peritoneal cavity. Clinical symptoms include diffuse abdominal tenderness, fever, recurrent vomiting, rigidity of abdominal wall musculature, tachycardia, and leukocytosis. Progression leads to paralytic ileus and abdominal distension. Treatment includes nasogastric suction to decompress the stomach and bowel, intravenous fluids, and appropriate antibiotics and operative intervention after adequate fluid resuscitation. Intra-abdominal abscesses are frequent complications in the pediatric population. Periappendicular abscesses occur 3 to 7 days

TABLE 24–1 POSTOPERATIVE COMPLICATIONS OF 1987 APPENDECTOMIES*

Complication	Number
Wound infection	22
Pelvic abscess	20
Intra-abdominal abscess	5
Subphrenic abscess	4
Fecal fistula	4
Empyema	1
Evisceration	1
Intestinal obstruction (requiring surgery)	12
Hematoma of wound	3
Incisional hernia	1
Leukemia	3
Measles	4
Chickenpox	1
Total	81

*From Martin, L. W.: Appendicitis. *In* Benson, C. D., et al. (eds.): Textbook of Pediatric Surgery, 1st ed. Chicago, Year Book Medical Publishers, 1962.

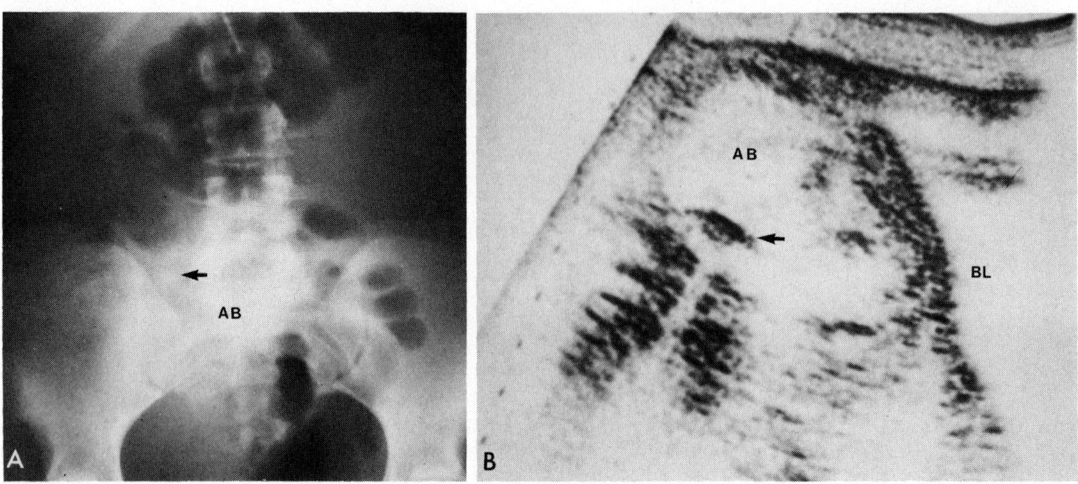

Figure 24–1 *A,* Upright anteroposterior roentgenogram of abdomen showing appendiceal abscess (AB) with fecalith *(arrow)* lying superior and lateral to the deformed bladder. There is moderate increased gas and dilation of the terminal ileum. *B,* B scale sonogram showing abscess cavity (AB) and the fecalith *(arrow),* which is echogenic. The bladder (BL) is to the right and adjacent to the abscess. (Courtesy of R. Teele).

following onset of symptoms as the result of a perforation that has been walled off locally by loops of bowel, omentum, and abdominal wall to prevent generalized contamination (Fig. 24–1*A, B*). A tender, palpable mass in the right lower quadrant, fever, and leukocytosis coupled with an extended history suggest the diagnosis. This complication may be handled in one of two ways: either by exploration and drainage of the localized abscess, or by intravenous fluids, antibiotics, and nasogastric suction until resolution of the acute symptoms and mass, with interval appendectomy in 6 to 8 weeks.

The pelvis is the most frequent site of postappendectomy abscess. Abscess usually becomes manifest 4 to 5 days after operation by persistent fever, localized tenderness, a palpable abdominal or rectal mass, and leukocytosis. Many pelvic infections subside with antibiotic therapy and probably represent a phlegmon or cellulitis with agglutinated loops of bowel rather than a true abscess. Rectal examination or abdominal palpation or both will usually identify the pelvic abscess. Abdominal radiographs, ultrasound studies, barium contrast studies, and radionuclide-labeled leukocyte studies are useful diagnostic aids. The majority of pelvic inflammatory masses that develop following appendectomy will resolve with the aid of broad-spectrum antibiotics. Some will progress to frank suppuration, character-

ized by continued systemic signs of infection and localized fluctuation of the mass upon examination, which constitute indications for surgical drainage. This may be accomplished by the abdominal, rectal, or vaginal route, depending on the location of the abscess and where the abscess most closely approaches the surface (Fig. 24–2).

Subphrenic and subhepatic abscesses result from a contamination extending along the paracolic gutters. Spiking fevers, anorexia, occasionally diarrhea, and leukocytosis are clinical manifestations. Abdominal radiographs may show pleural effusion and gas bubbles or air fluid levels in an abscess cavity. Ultrasonography and radionuclide-labeled leukocyte scanning are also helpful diagnostic aids. The preferred method of drainage is extraperitoneal through the flank or the bed of the twelfth rib.

Interloop abscesses may occur anywhere in the abdominal cavity. These are difficult to detect and localize. They often resolve with antibiotic therapy but may require open drainage.

Wound infections are the most common complications of appendicitis. Between the fourth and eighth postoperative days, erythema, swelling, and tenderness along with fever and leukocytosis herald the onset of a wound infection. Removal of skin sutures, evacuation of purulent material, and open packing of the wound lead to resolution of

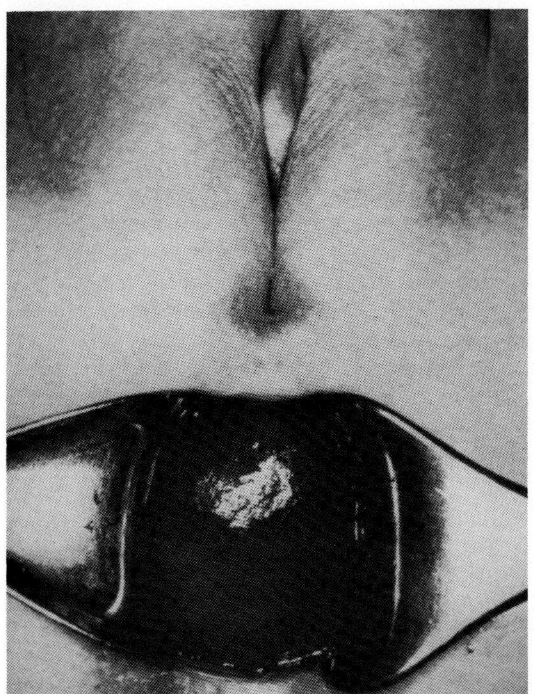

Figure 24–2 After dilation of the anus and insertion of McBurney retractors, a large pelvic abscess is seen bulging forward and continuing upward to the cul-de-sac. The abscess was drained at the point of maximal fluctuation in the midline with a Kelly clamp after incision of the mucosa and submucosa. (From Martin, L. W.: Appendicitis. *In* Benson, C. D., et al., eds.: Textbook of Pediatric Surgery, 1st edition. Chicago, Year Book Medical Publishers, 1962.)

the symptoms. Local care produces a satisfactory scar even with secondary wound healing. The incidence of wound infection can be minimized if certain precautions are observed. Care should be taken not to contaminate the wound edges when a nonperforated appendix is removed. Hemostasis is mandatory, since hematomas beneath the surface provide ideal culture media in an anaerobic environment. If the appendix is found to be perforated, the operative wound immediately becomes contaminated. Consequently, to suture it closed is to invite infection. Any sutures placed in such a wound, except to close the peritoneum, create an environment ideal for proliferation of anaerobic organisms. Their necrotizing capabilities with destruction of normal tissue may lead to fistula formation if adjacent to the bladder or ureter, or may result

in exsanguinating hemorrhage if adjacent to the ileac vessels.[10]

Pylephlebitis, or suppurative phlebitis of the portal vein, may develop as a complication of appendicitis and peritonitis. The suppurative process extends into the liver parenchyma, producing multiple liver abscesses. The causative organism is generally a gram-negative rod. The symptoms are chills, intermittent fever, tachycardia, septic shock, and sometimes mild jaundice. The diagnosis can generally be confirmed by ultrasound studies. Treatment includes general supportive measures as well as large doses of intravenous antibiotics directed at gram-negative organisms as well as anaerobes. Surgical drainage is indicated for any complicating liver abscesses that can be demonstrated and localized by ultrasound. Mortality, even with modern antibiotics and supportive measures, approaches 25 per cent. Liver abscesses following appendicitis are usually multiple, may or may not communicate with each other, and are deceptively inapparent to the surgeon at the time of operation. With preoperative ultrasound studies as a guide, repeated needle aspirations of the areas of nonechogenicity will yield pus, which can then be drained.. Extraperitoneal drainage is preferred, if it is possible, and is accomplished by inserting a large rubber catheter or multiple Penrose drains into the abscess cavity. Further needling of the liver parenchyma frequently identifies additional abscesses, all of which must be drained. Continuation of spiking fever postoperatively indicates additional undrained collections, necessitating reoperation. Ultrasound studies have proved most helpful in demonstrating such additional undrained abscesses. Of our last four patients with suppurative liver abscesses, three have required a second operation. All four survived, but a significant mortality must be anticipated.

Small bowel obstruction will develop after perforated appendix and peritonitis in approximately 15 per cent of patients. They may be divided into three groups. Obstruction during the septic phase of peritonitis is generally a result of "obstructive ileus" caused by infection adjacent to a loop of bowel. The treatment consists of nasogastric suction, surgical drainage of any purulent collection, and administration of appropriate antibiotics. The second variety occurs following recovery from the septic phase, generally 10 to 14 days postoperatively. Filmy adhesions tend to obstruct and kink the bowel. This noninflammatory type of obstruction responds well to treatment with a "long tube." When it occurs within 6 weeks after operation, a long tube should be passed as soon as the diagnosis is evident. Fluoroscopy is often of value in placing the tip of the tube into the duodenum. Suction decompression of the small bowel will generally result in relief of the obstruction within 2 to 3 days. Daily re-evaluation is mandatory until the obstruction is relieved. In the event of lack of improvement, laparotomy is indicated. The third type is small bowel obstruction occurring later than 6 weeks following operation. In this group of patients, the adhesions are characteristically firm and fibrous. Prompt laparotomy with

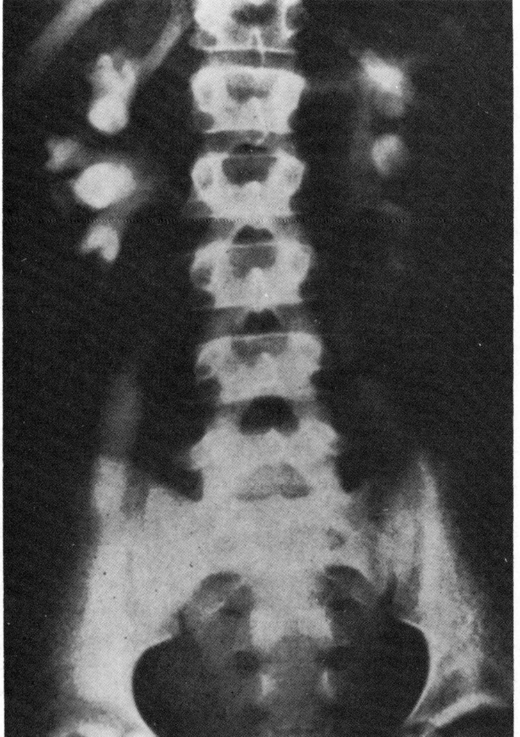

Figure 24–3 Bilateral hydroureteronephrosis demonstrated by intravenous pyelogram (IVP) and resulting from a pelvic abscess of 12 days' duration. The IVP returned to normal 6 weeks later. (From Martin, L. W.: Appendicitis. *In* Benson, C. D., et al., eds.: Textbook of Pediatric Surgery, 1st edition. Chicago, Year Book Medical Publishers, 1962.)

operative release of the obstruction is obligatory for this type of obstruction.

Persistent wound drainage with sinus formation generally indicates a retained foreign body. This is most frequently a fecalith, which may eventually be spontaneously extruded, following which the sinus will heal. At the time of operation for a perforated appendix, a search for and recovery of a fecalith from the local area will avoid several weeks of morbidity associated with a draining sinus. Occasionally the foreign body is not extruded spontaneously and may act as a nidus for persistent infection. It then requires surgical removal along with drainage of the associated recalcitrant abscess.

Sterility in the female patient is a not uncommon late complication of pelvic inflammation associated with perforation of the appendix. Fibrous adhesions about the fallopian tubes can result in an occlusion of the tubes similar to that which follows gonococcal salpingitis. The incidence of this complication is uncertain because of lack of long-term follow-up. Temporary bilateral hydroureteronephrosis is common and can be documented by intravenous pyelogram but requires no surgical intervention (Fig. 24–3).

INFLAMMATORY BOWEL DISEASE

Ulcerative colitis is an inflammatory disease of the rectal and colonic mucosa. Limited extension into the ileum in the form of "backwash ileitis" is probably of little clinical significance. In contrast to ulcerative colitis, granulomatous colitis (or Crohn's colitis) may involve the small bowel as well. Unlike ulcerative colitis, granulomatous colitis initially and predominantly involves the submucosa and then progresses transmurally. The complications seen in persons with these two inflammatory bowel diseases reflect this basic pathology.

Complications of chronic inflammatory bowel disease are numerous and varied and are of sufficient gravity of themselves to demand early, definitive surgical therapy of the primary colonic disease. Systemic complications include electrolyte deficiencies, anemia, hypoproteinemia, avitaminosis, amyloidosis, osteoporosis, amenorrhea, re-

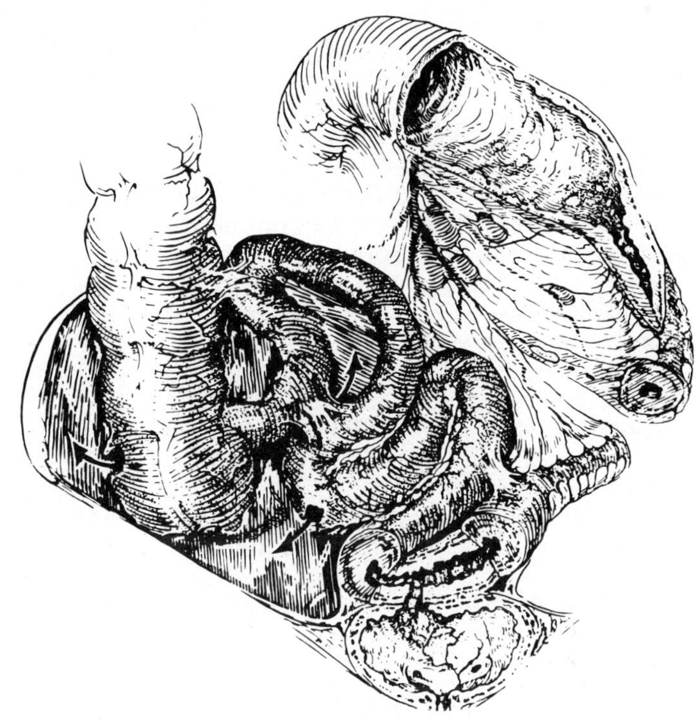

Figure 24–4 Various features of advanced granulomatous ileocolitis with maximal involvement of the distal ileum and ascending colon. These include multiple abscesses within the mesentery and between bowel segments, fistulae between large and small bowel segments, fistulae to the bladder and to the perineum, and free lateral colonic perforation. Cicatricial narrowing leads to chronic intermittent proximal small bowel obstruction. (From Welch, K. J.: Regional enteritis. *In* Benson, C. D. et al., eds.: Textbook of Pediatric Surgery, 1st edition. Chicago, Year Book Medical Publishers, 1962.)

tarded sexual development, and retarded growth. Serious complications in other organ systems include arthritis, arthralgias, spondylitis, uveitis, iritis, fatty liver, hepatitis, cirrhosis, pyroderma gangrenosum, erythema nodosum, renal glomerular changes, nephrolithiasis, interstitial pancreatitis, peripheral neuritis, vascular thrombosis, and stomatitis. Colonic complications of ulcerative colitis include gross hemorrhage; stricture formation with partial obstruction; perforation, either free, producing peritonitis, or confined, with abscesses and fistulae; malabsorption; carcinoma of the colon; and toxic megacolon (Fig. 24–4). Perianal ulcers and fistulae occur in association with granulomatous colitis. The more significant acute and chronic complications leading to surgical intervention will be discussed in detail.

Growth retardation and delay in development of secondary sex characteristics have been reported in 30 to 50 per cent of children with inflammatory bowel disease. The mechanism of such retardation is obscure, but poor nutrition, corticosteroid therapy, and secondary hypopituitarism are probably contributory. Persistence of this process through puberty frequently prevents the child from achieving full growth potential. Patients operated upon before epiphyseal closure have resumed a normal or near-normal growth pattern when all the diseased bowel has been excised or bypassed. Unremitting major hemorrhage may occur in patients with ulcerative colitis as well as in those with granulomatous colitis. Sigmoidoscopy can be useful in revealing the area of bleeding. Occasionally the bleeding point can be coagulated, but in extreme situations, resection or proctectomy may be the only means of preventing exsanguination.

Strictures are more common in patients with granulomatous disease than in those with ulcerative colitis and occur much earlier in the course of the disease. They are usually benign and may be so treated until signs of obstruction supervene. In contrast, strictures in persons with ulcerative colitis that cannot be differentiated from carcinoma necessitate colectomy. Free perforation is more common in ulcerative colitis than in granulomatous colitis. It occurs more frequently in the splenic flexure of the sigmoid loop during the course of fulminant disease and need not be preceded by toxic dilatation. Perforation occurs occasionally with the first attack and, whether early or late in the course of the disease, has a significant mortality. Free perforation in persons with granulomatous colitis is almost always associated with distal obstruction. Immediate exploration and resection of the diseased bowel with proximal diversion is indicated.

Perianal disease complicating granulomatous colitis is an indication of continued activity of the inflammatory bowel process. Conservative measures such as meticulous local hygiene and early incision and drainage of abscesses will maintain a reasonable state of well-being, but persistent and recalcitrant infection is an indication for total bowel rest with nutritional support by total parenteral nutrition.[3]

The risk of malignancy is of particular importance in the child with ulcerative colitis. The incidence of carcinoma is directly proportional to the duration of disease and increases markedly after 10 years. Carcinoma is an indication for colectomy. The risk of malignancy exists with granulomatous disease, particularly when it begins in childhood, but it is much less than the risk with ulcerative colitis.

Toxic megacolon, a dreaded complication of ulcerative colitis, occurs in a small percentage of patients. It usually is a manifestation of fulminant disease and may occur with the initial acute episode, less frequently during a relapse, and rarely in the chronic forms. The diagnosis should be suspected in any patient with active colitis who has a decreased number of daily stools, abdominal distension, fever, lethargy, and signs of toxicity.

Toxic megacolon warrants only a brief trial of intense nonoperative therapy, including intestinal decompression, administration of antibiotics, correction of electrolyte deficits, discontinuance of opiates and anticholinergic medications, and administration of blood and albumin transfusions and corticosteroids. Deterioration or failure to improve within 24 to 36 hours following institution of therapy mandates surgical intervention.[1] The procedure of choice is total or subtotal colectomy with ileostomy.

In Crohn's colitis, the full-thickness involvement of the bowel wall leads to penetration of adjacent viscera with the development of fistulae to various other organs, i.e., small bowel, bladder, adjacent colon, or

through the abdominal wall to the skin. Extension of the infection posteriorly may result in a psoas abscess or retroperitoneal abscess requiring surgical drainage.

Hydronephrosis may result from ureteral compression by an abscess, inflammation, or, later, fibrosis. The process can generally be reversed by drainage of the abscess and resection of the diseased bowel. Occasionally, periureteral lysis may be required.

Complications Following Total Colectomy and Endorectal Ileoanal Anastomosis

In recent years, there has been a trend toward treating ulcerative colitis in children and young adults with total colectomy, mucosal proctectomy, and ileoanal anastomosis, thus preserving anal continence.[14] Early in our experience with this operation, complications were both frequent and serious. Lessons learned from experience with earlier patients have resulted in only rare and minor complications in our most recent 15 patients.[13]

Postoperative diarrhea was troublesome for the first year following closure of the ileostomy. This has been largely overcome by construction of a reservoir with terminal ileum just inside the anus. This "storage area" has changed the intolerable diarrhea to a tolerable situation in which six to eight stools are passed daily, immediately following closure of the ileostomy.

Pelvic sepsis and cuff abscess can be largely avoided by drainage of the cuff and establishment of a temporary diverting ileostomy to divert the fecal stream until complete healing of the rectal anastomosis occurs. It is also important that the rectum be mechanically cleansed by saline irrigation just prior to beginning dissection of the rectal cuff. A period of 4 to 6 weeks of preoperative total parenteral alimentation and vigorous medical therapy will, in most instances, permit healing of the rectal mucosa, which is a necessity if it is to be dissected free without perforation.

Stenosis at the ileoanal anastomosis is generally mild and responds to digital dilatation. Occasionally, a significant stricture will require dilatation with the patient under general anesthesia. We have encountered one patient with severe stricture secondary to pelvic sepsis. The original operation, performed elsewhere, was attempted without a proximal ileostomy. Abdominoperineal resection of the strictured area was required 3 years after the original operation. Results were excellent, with the patient regaining total continence.

HIRSCHSPRUNG'S DISEASE

Following operation for Hirschsprung's disease, a number of complications have been encountered. Small bowel obstruction, adhesions, small bowel intussusception, wound dehiscence, and infections are common to any laparotomy.[2] Those more specifically related to the operation for Hirschsprung's disease, including enterocolitis, anastomotic leak with pelvic abscess, stenosis of the suture line, and incontinence, will be considered in more detail.

Enterocolitis is a dreaded and life-threatening complication characterized by sudden onset of abdominal distension, explosive gas and liquid stools, fever, vomiting, dehydration, and shock (Fig. 24–5). The condition may progress rapidly to death, or it may present in a chronic form with malabsorption and, in extreme examples, a protein-losing type of colitis with hypoproteinemia, edema, and failure to thrive. The cause is a distal functional obstruction. Enterocolitis may be seen either prior to or following the definitive operation. The basic objective of treatment is relief of the distal obstruction. When enterocolitis is encountered before the definitive operation, initial treatment consists of colonic decompression with a rectal tube, nasogastric suction, intravenous replacement of fluid and electrolyte losses, correction of anemia, administration of antibiotics, and, in severe cases, parenteral alimentation. When the patient's general condition has stabilized, a diverting colostomy is established. It is important that the colostomy be placed proximal to the area of inflammation and that it be completely diverting.

Any child in whom enterocolitis develops preoperatively is likely to experience enterocolitis after the definitive operation. The complication can be avoided if certain precautions are observed: (1) The definitive operation should be delayed at least 6 months to allow adequate healing of the colonic ulcerations in the involved colon; (2) it is imperative that all of the ulcerated area be completely defunctionalized by proximal diversion of the fecal stream; (3) little or no

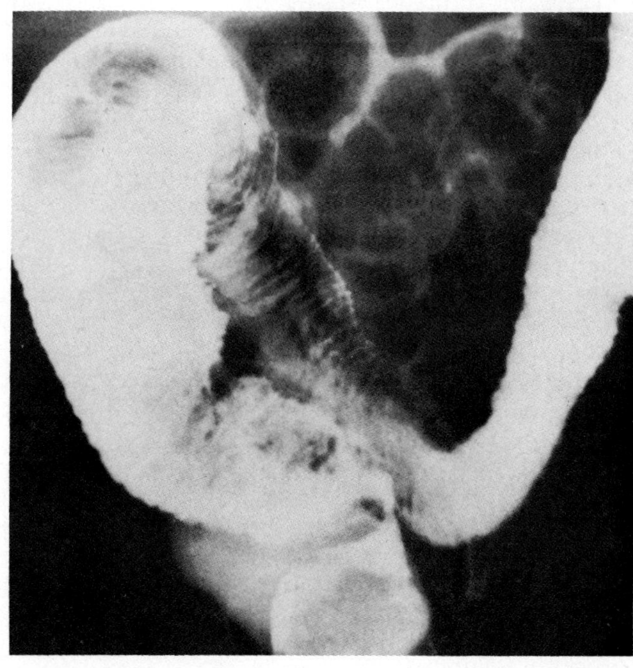

Figure 24–5 Fulminating and at times fatal colitis may occur with undiagnosed Hirschsprung's disease in infancy. In this barium enema study there is dilation and mucosal feathering of the rectosigmoid above the aganglionic segment due to multiple mucosal and submucosal ulcers. (From Martin, L. W.: Hirschsprung's disease. *In* Holder, T. M., and Ashcraft, K. W., eds.: Pediatric Surgery. Philadelphia, W. B. Saunders Co., 1980.)

aganglionic internal sphincter should be permitted to remain after the definitive operation; and (4) the rectal suture line should be protected by the proximal colostomy until complete rectal healing has occurred. By observing these precautions, we have been successful in avoiding the complication of postoperative enterocolitis in virtually all of our patients for the past several years. If enterocolitis should develop in a patient after the definitive operation, the colon should be carefully studied by proctoscopy or colonoscopy and by barium contrast radiography. If no cause is found, consideration should be given to transanal resection of additional aganglionic internal sphincter. If significant ulceration of the colon or an anastomotic leak is encountered, proximal diversion of the fecal stream may be required until complete healing has occurred.[8]

Anastomotic leak with pelvic abscess is an avoidable complication that may develop when the definitive pull-through anastomosis is performed without adequate bowel preparation or without protection of the suture line by proximal diversion of the fecal stream. This complication can lead to significant morbidity and even mortality. If the child recovers, pelvic sinuses and anastomotic strictures may permanently preclude normal bowel function.

Fecal incontinence results if too much aganglionic internal sphincter is left behind or if too much is removed. If the length of residual rectal cuff is too long, partial obstruction may result in spillover and soilage. This condition can be corrected by removal of a transverse ellipse of rectal wall routinely to include the old suture line and additional internal sphincter. If too much rectal wall has been removed, incontinence will result because of lack of sensation within the anal canal. It is important that the anal columns be preserved at the time of the original operation. Occasionally, mild fecal soilage will be encountered for several months following closure of the colostomy and will spontaneously improve with the passage of time, growth, healing, and psychologic maturation of the patient.

Disorders of sexual function following abdominoperineal procedures for Hirschsprung's disease have received little attention but are a distinct consideration in any abdominoperineal procedure. In adults, both impotence and failure of ejaculation are thought to be related to disruption of the parasympathetic and sympathetic nerve supply in the immediate area about the rectum. Some problems with sexual function have been reported in as many as 40 per cent of male adults less than 60 years of age at the time of proctectomy. This possible complication has influenced some surgeons to prefer either the Duhamel[12] or the Soave-type procedure to the Swenson resection, even though a search of the literature has failed to reveal reports of sexual dysfunction following the Swenson operation.

Skip areas in Hirschsprung's disease are rare but have been reported.[11] They must be considered when symptoms of constipation and abdominal distension persist after the definitive operation.

TOTAL COLONIC AGANGLIONOSIS

Total colonic aganglionosis presents a special problem of surgical management. The operation that we have performed preserves a major portion of the aganglionic colon with a side-to-side anastomosis between it and the terminal small intestine. Certain complications have been encountered.[6]

Regrowth of the septum between the rectum and colon has occurred in the rectal area when anastomosis is performed with the mechanical stapler. Since encountering this in one patient and learning of its occurrence elsewhere, we have elected to continue using the stapler but, in addition, to oversew the suture line from the inside with a running chromic catgut suture. There has been no regrowth of the septum since we adopted this technique. The method, incidentally, also provides additional hemostasis, which is sometimes not completely assured with the stapler.[7]

In one patient we found perforation of a retained segment of defunctionalized colon. The defunctioned aganglionic segment of transverse colon proximal to the long side-to-side anastomosis had been retained in our first patient. A fecaloma in this defunctionalized aperistaltic segment of colon had eroded through the bowel wall and resulted in perforation and an abscess requiring operation. Since this experience, any defunctionalized bowel in subsequent patients has been resected.

We have not encountered postoperative peritonitis in any of our patients, although this is a constant threat. It is difficult to mechanically cleanse the aganglionic, aperistaltic colon prior to operation. It has been our policy to insert a rectal tube preoperatively. After the abdomen is opened at the time of the definitive procedure, the rectal tube is used to irrigate the colon. The surgeon then massages the colon to milk out retained stool and debris and mechanically cleanse the colon prior to opening into its lumen for anastomosis. The rectal tube is then removed and the lumen of the colon may be opened, diminishing concern about peritoneal contamination.

For the first year following operation, bowel movements are frequent, unformed, and associated with a certain amount of perineal excoriation. Medications may be used to decrease intestinal peristalsis, but the most effective means of managing this condition is periodic forceful dilatation of the anal sphincter to relieve any spasm of retained internal sphincter.

In one child, fecal incontinence resulted from inadvertent placement of the anastomosis too low on the posterior wall of the anorectal canal. This was corrected 2 years later by a posterior approach, plicating the posterior rectal wall as far proximal as the puborectalis muscle.

MALFORMATIONS OF THE RECTUM AND ANUS

Great variations in anorectal malformations necessitate that the operation be tailored to fit the particular malformation. An improperly chosen operation may result in a lifetime of incontinence, whereas a simpler procedure properly performed could provide completely normal bowel control. A thorough understanding of the particular malformation is therefore vital to a successful outcome.

Supralevator atresias are best managed with a diverting colostomy and a definitive operation when the child is 6 to 12 months of age. The exact approach used by the surgeon is a matter of choice. The important consideration is placement of the rectum through the puborectalis sling and placement of the external opening within the external sphincter muscle without undue tension and without prolapse.

Infralevator malformations may be corrected surgically during the first week of life when the bowel still contains meconium and before there is formed stool to contaminate and disrupt the suture line. After this time, a proximal diverting colostomy is mandatory until the anorectal suture line has completely healed. Incontinence may result from misplacement of the rectum outside the puborectalis sling, damage to the delicate nerves of the area, stenosis, prolapse, or sometimes the basic malformation. In some instances, a high atresia associated with sacral malformations will have defective nerve supply to the pelvic area, and subsequent control is not possible regardless of the type of operation performed. This is particularly true in patients with vertebral malformations of the lower spine. The associated congenital neurologic deficit may affect both the rectum and the urinary tract.

Anal stenosis results from contraction of a circular scar of the anastomosis. If the epithelial surfaces are accurately approximated and primary healing is achieved, stenosis does not occur. If the epithelial surfaces are not accurately approximated, or if disruption occurs because of excessive suture-line tension, poor blood supply to the area, or passage of large stool through the new anastomosis, the distance between the epithelial surfaces is replaced by granulation tissue, including fibroblasts, which contract in all directions as part of the healing process. Stricture is the result. Most mild strictures may be treated by simple dilatations. Severe strictures may require surgical release. Since scar tissue contracts for at least 6 months following complete healing, it is preferable that the surgical release of a stricture be deferred for at least 6 months, if possible. Release can generally be accomplished by means of a simple Y-V advancement of anal skin across the strictured segment. This, if necessary, may be performed on opposite sides of the anal canal and will provide adequate relief of stricture.

Prolapse of anorectal mucosa will result in a "wet bottom" with persistent seepage and incontinence. It can be corrected by simple excision of the mucosal prolapse.

Hyperchloremic acidosis may sometimes occur before the definitive operation because of reabsorption of urine, which may flow retrograde through the rectovesical fistula and into the colon. A suprapubic cystostomy may be required to divert the urinary stream and obviate this complication before the definitive abdominoperineal operation.

Constipation following operation for imperforate anus is common because prenatal obstruction has resulted in significant rectosigmoid dilatation that persists after anoplasty. It is important that the child be followed up carefully by the surgeon until several years of age and until bowel habits are well established. Constipation that develops in the interim may be treated by any one of several methods, as long as secondary megacolon, with its various associated problems, is not permitted to develop.

Recurrent rectourinary fistulae may result from incomplete initial repair or may develop secondary to local infection, with the necrotizing effect of anaerobic organisms forming a new communication between the rectum and urethra. Repair of recurrent fistulae is difficult and generally requires an abdominoperineal procedure protected by a proximal diverting colostomy.

COLOSTOMY

A colostomy in a child is significantly more likely to result in complications than is a colostomy in an adult because of the patient's poor cooperation and prolonged straining when crying. Special care and meticulous technique are required for construction of a colostomy in an infant or small child. Most complications result from technical error during initial construction of the colostomy. A functioning colostomy should never be brought through a working incision unless the incision is small enough that its entire circumference is utilized for the colostomy. The colostomy should be sutured to all layers of the abdominal wall and should be constructed with care whether it is to be temporary or permanent.

Necrosis of the colostomy is due to inadequate blood supply because of either misjudgment of the circulation or excessive tension. Necrosis may be mucosal only, or it may involve only that portion of the bowel which lies exterior to the peritoneum. In these instances, the colostomy itself need not be disturbed, although it must be observed for the possible development of subsequent stricture. If the bowel is necrotic through the abdominal wall and into the abdominal cavity, reoperation is necessary for reconstruction of the colostomy.

Retraction of the stoma may occur as a result of necrosis of the stoma or because of inadequate mobilization of the bowel with placement of the stoma under tension. A retracted stoma may function adequately, but consideration should be given to reoperation and reconstruction with further mobilization of the colon to gain additional length.

Stricture formation is seen more commonly when colostomies are constructed by the technique of natural sloughing with a clamp. Modern techniques of primary suture maturation have largely eliminated this problem. Strictures at the skin level may be treated adequately by simple excision of the mucocutaneous junction including the stricture, or by simple release with a Heineke-Mikulicz procedure to the narrowed area. Deeper strictures may occur as a result of hematoma with subsequent fibrosis in the subcutaneous tissues. A significant deep stricture may require circumferential excision and further mobilization of the bowel in order that a satisfactory colostomy may be reconstructed.

Prolapse of an end colostomy is unusual. Most instances of colostomy prolapse involve the distal segment of a double-barreled colostomy that prolapses in retrograde fashion. This complication generally requires division of the loop and either closure of the distal segment or construction of a new distal stoma in a separate stab wound.

Herniation about a colostomy generally results from inadequate suturing of the peritoneum around the circumference of the colostomy. If herniation occurs about a permanent colostomy, repair will be necessary because, with time, the herniation will interfere with colostomy function and with application of the colostomy appliance.

Bleeding from the stoma generally results from trauma to the exposed bowel by gauze bandages, appliances, clothing, or irrigating catheters. Care must be taken to prevent such trauma, and consideration should be given to the possibility that bleeding may be coming from a lesion higher in the gastrointestinal tract.

A patient with small bowel obstruction due to internal herniation about a colostomy or to adhesions adjacent to the colostomy may require operation to relieve the obstruction.

Infection at the site of a colostomy is unusual unless the colostomy has been performed through a working incision or unless the mucosa has not been accurately sutured to the skin.

Perforation of the colon during colostomy irrigations may cause peritonitis, necessitating immediate operation. Generally, the simplest and most effective method of management is to establish an additional new colostomy at a higher level of the colon to divert the fecal stream from the perforation and leave the old colostomy undisturbed.

COLONOSCOPY

Complications following colonoscopy performed for diagnostic or therapeutic reasons include perforation, hemorrhage, intracolonic explosion, electrical burns, respiratory problems, and transient bacteremia.

Perforation occurs in less than 0.2 per cent of procedures performed by experienced surgeons. It is more likely to occur during polypectomy than during a diagnostic procedure and is more common when an attempt is made to remove a sessile polyp. If the perforation is recognized, immediate operation to close it is mandatory. If perforation with signs of peritonitis becomes evident only during the postoperative period, laparotomy with exteriorization of the perforation may be the treatment of choice.

Bleeding following polypectomy may result immediately but can develop within 24 hours or even as long as 1 week following the procedure when the coagulated area sloughs. Such bleeding is usually self-limited and rarely is of such a degree as to require laparotomy, except in patients with some form of coagulopathy. Screening for coagulation disorders, including aspirin ingestion, is recommended before colonoscopy, as it is before any operative procedure.

Intracolonic explosions due to ignition of methane gas in the lumen of the bowel have been reported. These generally can be avoided by adequate preoperative evacuation of the colon and aspiration of all air from the lumen of the bowel prior to reinflation and use of the coagulation current.

Respiratory problems related to excessive sedation have been reported and are probably best obviated by use of a general anesthetic for the small or uncooperative child when performing colonoscopy.

Transient bacteremia associated with colonoscopy is of significance for patients with associated valvular heart disease. For these patients, administration of systemic antibiotics prior to endoscopy is recommended. Care should be taken to thoroughly cleanse and disinfect the colonoscope between patients. A 2 per cent glutaraldehyde soak for 10 minutes, followed by rinsing with tap water, is advised as a precaution to prevent contamination of patients with microorganisms from previous patients.

ANORECTAL TRAUMA

Anorectal trauma with extraperitoneal perforation of the rectum caused by automobile accidents, inserted foreign bodies, rectal thermometers, improperly administered enemas, or traumatic endoscopic examinations can result in pelvic sepsis, abscess, sinus tracts, or other serious problems. Treatment depends on the extent of the injury. Minor lacerations require no specific treatment if the bleeding stops spontaneously. More serious injury to the pelvic and sphincter muscles may require surgical reconstruction with the protection of a proximal diverting colostomy. Penetration into the extraperitoneal structures with abscess formation will generally necessitate surgical drainage.

Injury from rectal thermometers warrants special consideration, since retention of mercury outside the bowel lumen in the tissues of the pelvis can be followed by absorption and subsequent mercury poisoning. Mercury within the lumen of the bowel is not absorbed and can generally be evacuated with the aid of a suppository. Radiographic demonstration of retained mercury in the soft tissues necessitates surgical removal.

References

1. Adams, J. T.: Toxic dilatation of the colon. A surgical disease. Arch. Surg. 106:678, 1973.
2. Cox, J. A., and Martin, L. W.: Postoperative intussusception. Arch. Surg. 106:263, 1973.
3. Fischer, J. E., Foster, G. S., Abel, R. M.; et al.: Hyperalimentation as primary therapy for inflammatory bowel disease. Am. J. Surg. 125:165, 1973.
4. Fitz, R. H.: Perforating inflammation of the vermiform appendix; with special reference to its early diagnosis and treatment. Am. J. Med. Sci. 1:277, 1886.
5. Martin, L. W.: Appendicitis. *In* Benson, C. D., et al. (eds.): Textbook of Pediatric Surgery, 1st ed. Chicago, Year Book Medical Publishers, 1962.
6. Martin, L. W.: Surgical management of Hirschsprung's disease involving the small intestine. Arch. Surg. 97:183, 1968.
7. Martin, L. W.: Surgical management of total colonic aganglionosis. Ann. Surg. 176:343, 1972.
8. Martin, L. W.: Hirschsprung's disease. *In* Hardy, J. D. (ed.): Rhoads Textbook of Surgery, 5th Edition. Philadelphia, J. B. Lippincott Co., 1977.
9. Martin, L. W.: Hirschsprung's disease. *In* Holder, T. M., and Ashcraft, K. W. (eds.): Pediatric Surgery. Philadelphia, W. B. Saunders Co., 1980, pp. 389–400.
10. Martin, L. W., Altemeier, W. A., and Reyers, P. M., Jr.: Infections in pediatric surgery. Pediatr. Clin. North Am. 16:735, 1969.
11. Martin, L. W., Buchino, J. J., LeCoultre, C., et al.: Hirschsprung's disease with skip area (segmental aganglionosis). J. Pediatr. Surg. 14:686, 1979.
12. Martin, L. W., and Caudill, D. R.: A method for elimination of the blind rectal pouch in the Duhamel operation for Hirschsprung's disease. Surgery 62:951, 1967.
13. Martin, L. W., and LeCoultre, C.: Technical considerations in performing total colectomy and Soave endorectal anastomosis for ulcerative colitis. J. Pediatr. Surg. 13:762, 1978.
14. Martin, L. W., LeCoultre, C., and Schubert, W. K.: Total colectomy with mucosal proctectomy and preservation of continence in ulcerative colitis. Ann. Surg. *186*:477, 1977.
15. Martin, L. W., and Perrin, E. V.: Neonatal perforation of the appendix in association with Hirschsprung's disease. Ann. Surg. 166:799, 1967.
16. Welch, K. J.: Regional enteritis. *In* Benson, C. D., et al. (eds.): Textbook of Pediatric Surgery, 1st ed. Chicago, Year Book Medical Publishers, 1962.

GENITOURINARY SYSTEM | 5

25

KIDNEYS AND URETERS

W. Hardy Hendren, M.D.

PHILOSOPHIC CONSIDERATIONS

Major complications of pediatric surgery do not occur unpredictably. Most result from something the surgeon has done or has not done. They can be avoided by using precise surgical technique and paying strict attention to preserving blood supply, avoiding tension in anastomoses, handling tissues gently, and all the other surgical principles that deserve more than lip service. More complications result from the surgeon's cutting corners in an effort to "avoid doing too much" than result from dealing with a problem in a thorough manner. Often there are alternative ways of handling a particular problem. The surgeon whose armamentarium includes a variety of techniques will have patients with fewer complications than the surgeon whose repertoire is limited to one way of dealing with an entity.

The speed with which an operation is done deserves special mention. Many years ago, prolonged surgery was not possible, because anesthesia was inadequate. Success depended on speed. This is seldom true today with modern techniques of anesthetic management, intraoperative monitoring, and postoperative intensive care. This should not encourage procrastination, but it does allow spending enough time to do a first-class job. Many complications I have seen resulted from trying to "beat the clock." A surgeon can usually predict how long an operation will take if it is one he performs frequently. But sometimes an operation will take longer than expected. If temperament, or ego, prevents taking the extra time required, catastrophe can result. Surgeons with great experience have fallen into this trap, which could have been avoided by slowing the pace.

Finally it is a sound principle never to conclude an operation until completely satisfied that the task has been done well. That which looks questionable at the operating table nearly always has an outcome as bad as was feared, or worse.

SURGERY OF THE KIDNEY

The most common renal operations in children are pyeloplasty, nephrectomy, partial nephrectomy, nephrostomy, and pyelolithotomy.

Pyeloplasty

Repair of ureteropelvic junction obstruction is the most frequently performed renal operation in childhood. It is followed by an unnecessarily high number of serious complications, most of which are avoidable. As a first consideration, many kidneys are removed needlessly. A review of series from various centers shows that the rate of nephrectomy ranges from 5 to 36 per cent.[29, 33, 34, 46, 48] About 19 of 20 kidneys with pyeloureteral obstruction have enough cortex to merit a salvage operation. Indeed, there are examples of patients with giant hydronephrosis in whom renal function can be surprisingly good after obstruction is relieved.[10] In evaluating function by intravenous pyelography, it is important to obtain delayed films 4 to 8 hours after injection of contrast medium. Sometimes early films will show "nonfunction," but later films can demonstrate considerable excreted contrast medium. A radionuclide scan can be helpful in deciding whether a kidney should be removed or repaired. Percutaneous nephrostomy (see later) can be a helpful short-term measure in an occasional patient. It can provide temporary drainage to assess function and can facilitate treatment of infection if present before surgical repair.

For operative exposure of the kidney for

pyeloplasty, I prefer a subcostal extraperitoneal flank incision. Rib resection is seldom needed in children. If both sides are involved, each is done through its own incision. Some surgeons have advocated a transverse upper abdominal incision for simultaneous exposure of both kidneys. This does not provide any advantage, in my opinion, and it gives the added complication of possible intestinal obstruction from adhesions. In some cases an anterior approach to the ureteropelvic junction is easiest, retracting the lower pole of the kidney down and back. In others, however, a posterior exposure is easier, retracting the lower pole of the kidney forward and up. The practice of completely mobilizing the kidney and ureter from the renal fossa and delivering it onto the surface of the wound for repair should be discouraged. It is unnecessary and is more likely to result in an angulated anastomosis when the kidney is replaced in its position. Another practice to be discouraged is that of passing a tape around the ureteropelvic junction and delivering it up for easy access. This is not necessary, and

such mobilization is likely to injure the blood supply to the ureter.

A variety of techniques of pyeloplasty have been described, including the Foley Y-V principle,[16] spiral flap pyeloplasty,[11] and intubated ureterotomy.[12] I am convinced that dismembering pyeloplasty is applicable in nearly all cases (Fig. 25–1).[2] After appropriate retraction of the kidney, the fascia overlying the ureteropelvic junction is incised. The stenotic segment is divided, leaving the ureter in situ. The dilated renal pelvis is grasped with blunt forceps (never tooth forceps!), and the dependent part of the renal pelvis is dissected free. This will allow tension-free anastomosis in most cases. If more slack is needed, such as when there is a long, narrow segment, the kidney can be mobilized and pexed downward. With a fine traction suture in the tip of the divided ureter, the ureter is spatulated for 2 to 3 cm along its lateral wall, opposite the main longitudinal blood supply, until the lumen is clearly of ample width. The renal pelvis is cut across obliquely so that it may be joined to the spatulated opening in the

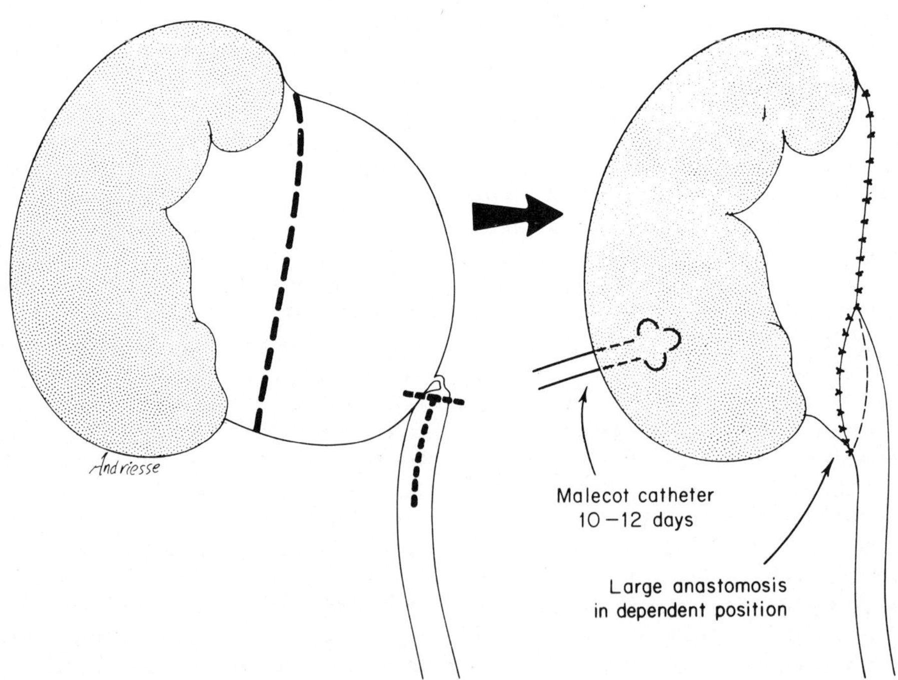

Figure 25–1   Dismembering pyeloplasty. Renal pelvis is reduced in size in about half of patients, when it is excessively dilated.

ureter. The anastomosis is made using interrupted sutures of fine chromic catgut, with the knots on the outside. Usually the anastomosis begins inferiorly and works upward. Running suture technique is possible, but interrupted technique provides greater accuracy. It is easy to lose orientation when matching the spatulated ureter to the renal pelvis. I have seen three instances of the upper end of the ureter being sewn to the lower edge of the renal pelvis, 180 degrees askew.

The controversy over stents and nephrostomy drainage will never be resolved. A good anastomosis of adequate size is not made better, in my opinion, by placing a stent within it. Therefore, we seldom use stents. Pyeloplasty anastomoses should be made watertight. Postoperative perinephric extravasation of urine is an invitation to periureteral scarring and obstruction. In most cases, therefore, we use nephrostomy drainage of the kidney for about 1 week postoperatively, especially when the kidney is very hydronephrotic. The tube is a small Malecot catheter, which is placed in a dilated calyx and brought out the flank. Seven to 10 days later, contrast medium is introduced through the nephrostomy tube. If the substance goes easily through the anastomosis and there are no leaks, the tube is withdrawn. Nephrostomy drainage is not used if the ureter and renal pelvis are of ideal quality and the kidney is minimally dilated. It may, indeed, be undesirable to leave a nephrostomy in these circumstances, since placing the tube through parenchyma of almost normal thickness can injure a segment of the kidney. Although stents are usually unnecessary and nephrostomy drainage is optional, a gutter drain should be placed during every pyeloplasty so that any urine that leaks will be evacuated. Healing is poor when the repair is bathed in urine. When the kidney is very hydronephrotic, its lower pole can compress the ureter. This can be averted by pexing the lower pole of the kidney laterally.

COMPLICATIONS

Anastomotic Leak. If a postoperative nephrostogram shows leakage of contrast medium, nephrostomy drainage is contin-ued until subsequent study 1 or more weeks later shows that the leak has sealed, which it will have done in nearly every case.

Temporary Anastomotic Obstruction. Postoperative edema can temporarily obstruct the anastomosis. If contrast medium does not pass easily at satisfactory pressure (15 cm of water or less), the tube remains until a subsequent examination shows good drainage. If the anastomosis fails to "open up" after 4 to 5 weeks of observation, we pass a small panendoscope through the nephrostomy tract with the patient under anesthesia. In two such patients we found edematous mucosa at the lower edge of the anastomosis that was causing functional obstruction. Light figuration of the edematous mucosa with a coagulating Bugbee electrode solved the problem.

Persistent Anastomotic Obstruction. Failure of a ureteropelvic junction repair is nearly always the result of a technical error, e.g., angulation, loss of blood supply, tension, or inadequate caliber of the anastomotic site. Reoperation should not be performed until several months have elapsed to allow subsidence of postoperative induration and edema. Early reoperation is an invitation to another failure. A patient with an obstructed kidney should be maintained on temporary nephrostomy drainage until sufficient time has passed to ensure optimal conditions for reoperation. Of the 130 children in whom we performed pyeloplasty, 15 had been referred for reoperation after prior operative failure.[29] In each, reoperation using previously cited principles corrected the obstruction. Figures 25–2 and 25–3 show one of these cases and its repair. Occasionally the renal pelvis is scarred or too small to be anastomosed to the ureters. Calicoureterostomy, a possible alternative, is shown in Figures 25–4 through 25–6. A wedge of adjacent parenchyma must be removed to avert compression of the anastomosis.

Miscellaneous Complications. Although no patient in our own series had anastomotic obstruction, one required reoperation for talc granulomas encasing and compressing the upper third of the ureter. The ureter was decorticated and wrapped with omentum, with successful results. About one in five of these patients has an aberrant

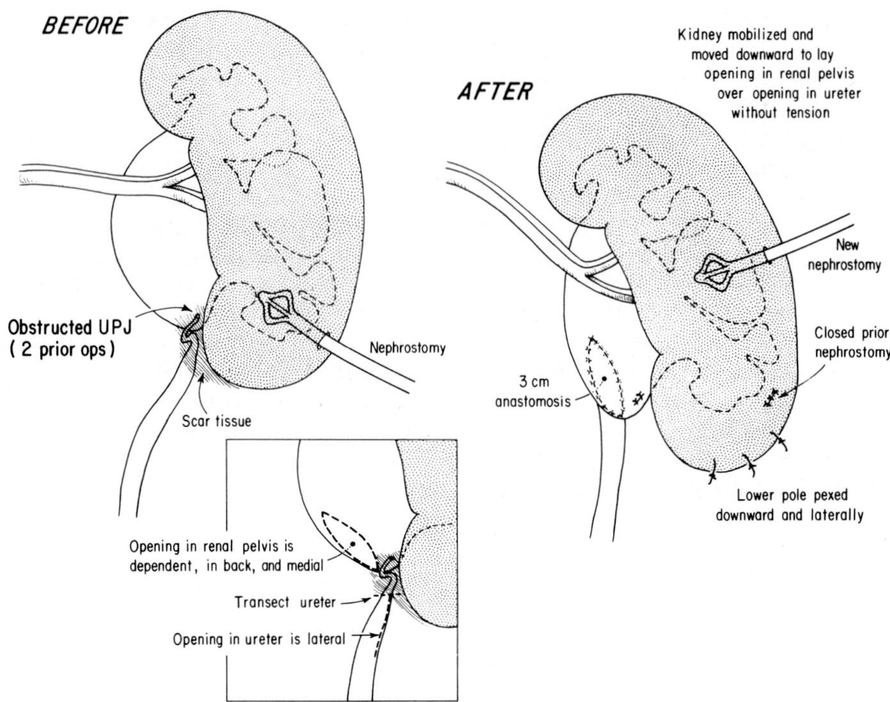

Figure 25–2   A typical case of twice-failed pyeloplasty and its surgical correction by wide spatulation of ureter and downward displacement of kidney to obtain tension-free anastomosis.

vessel crossing the ureteropelvic junction. It should *never* be cut as described in the older literature. That can produce segmental renal ischemia with secondary hypertension. The ureteropelvic junction should be dismembered and reanastomosed, usually anterior to the vessel. Vesicoureteral reflux is seen in some patients with pyeloureteral obstruction. Sometimes the pyeloureteral obstruction is more apparent than real and is caused by tortuosity of the upper ureter secondary to reflux. If that appears to be the case, an antireflux operation is done first, following which the ureteropelvic junction will often straighten and become normal. On the other hand, if the pyeloureteral obstruction is real, which can be shown by antegrade pressure-perfusion study, the pyeloplasty is done first, followed later by correction of reflux.

HORSESHOE KIDNEY

This is a common malformation. Sometimes there is hydronephrosis of one or both halves of the horseshoe kidney. Traditional teaching had held that the ureter becomes partially obstructed as it crosses the isthmus of the kidney. This has led to cutting the isthmus and rotating the halves of the kidney laterally to "unobstruct the ureter." I have never seen a bona fide example of this problem, nor have several surgeons of considerable experience whom I have questioned on this subject. Hydronephrosis is usually caused by insertion of the ureter high on the renal pelvis, with or without stenosis of the actual ureteropelvic junction. Obstruction can be relieved by performing a side-to-side pyeloplasty to provide dependent drainage of the renal pelvis.

Nephrectomy

Complete nephrectomy is an easier operation than pyeloplasty or partial nephrectomy. The most common indication in childhood is congenital multicystic kidney, which usually presents as a unilateral flank mass in the newborn. Intravenous pyelography usually fails to visualize the multicystic kidney. Other indications in-

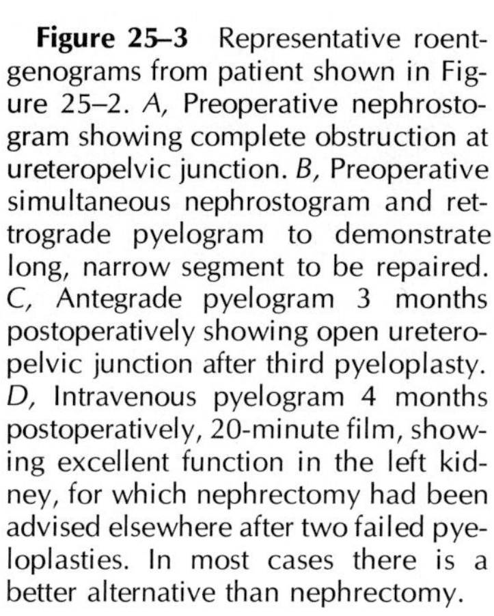

Figure 25–3 Representative roentgenograms from patient shown in Figure 25–2. *A,* Preoperative nephrostogram showing complete obstruction at ureteropelvic junction. *B,* Preoperative simultaneous nephrostogram and retrograde pyelogram to demonstrate long, narrow segment to be repaired. *C,* Antegrade pyelogram 3 months postoperatively showing open ureteropelvic junction after third pyeloplasty. *D,* Intravenous pyelogram 4 months postoperatively, 20-minute film, showing excellent function in the left kidney, for which nephrectomy had been advised elsewhere after two failed pyeloplasties. In most cases there is a better alternative than nephrectomy.

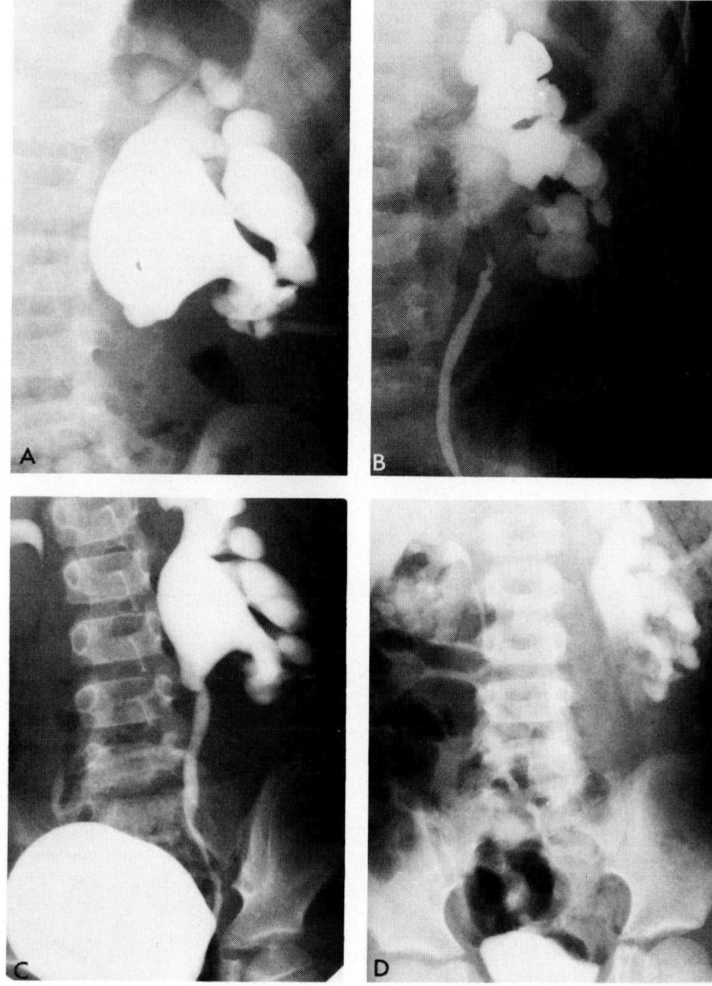

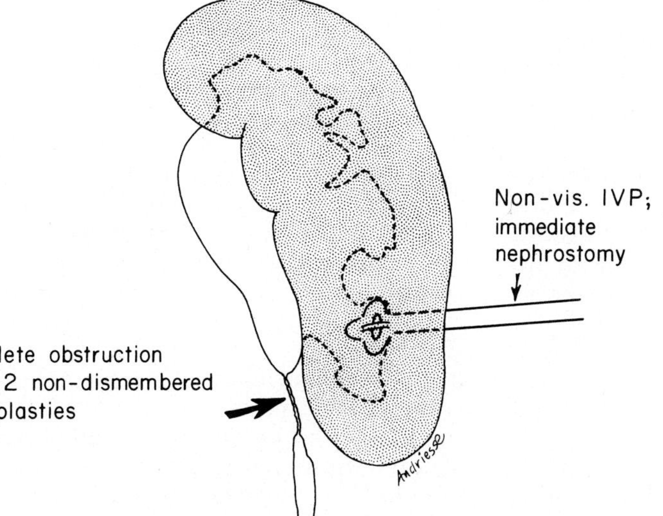

Figure 25–4 Anatomy in an 11-year-old boy referred after two failed pyeloplasties. Nonvisualization on intravenous pyelogram prompted immediate reinsertion of a nephrostomy tube. One week later reoperation was performed.

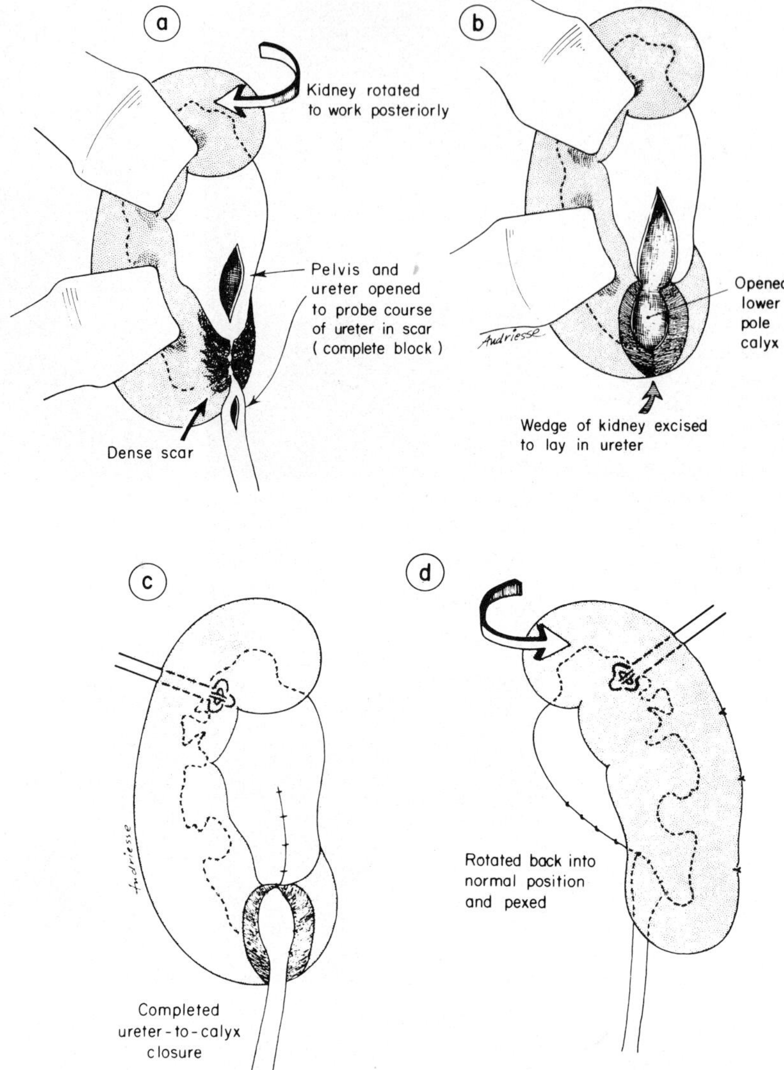

Figure 25–5   Technique for caliciureterostomy in the patient shown in Figure 25–4, for whom a third ureteropelvic junction repair proved unfeasible. It is important to resect a wedge of kidney adjacent to the anastomotic site.

clude end-stage pyelonephritis, usually resulting from massive reflux; dysplastic kidney, sometimes causing hypertension; ureteropelvic junction obstruction with no functional parenchyma; and a number of infrequent causes such as various infections, including tuberculosis. Nephrectomy is a technically simple procedure, yet certain precautions are in order. The renal vessels should be identified and ligated individually. In ligating the renal vein, care must be taken not to put excessive traction on it as the ligature is tied, thereby tenting up the vena cava and partially occluding it with the tie. A torn vein can hemorrhage, which is frightening to the inexperienced surgeon and which can prove fatal to the patient if it is mishandled. A frantic attempt to control hemorrhage with sutures or clamps with inadequate exposure can be disastrous. As in any vascular injury, bleeding should be controlled by an assistant's finger placed on the hole or by an atraumatic side-occluding clamp. Additional exposure should then be obtained to control the cava above and below the point of injury. Only after such

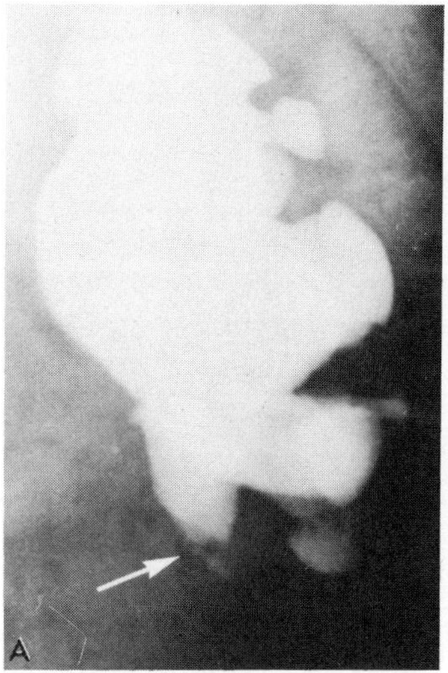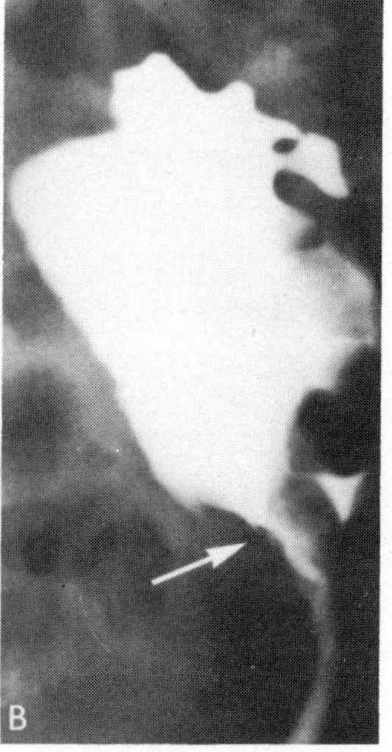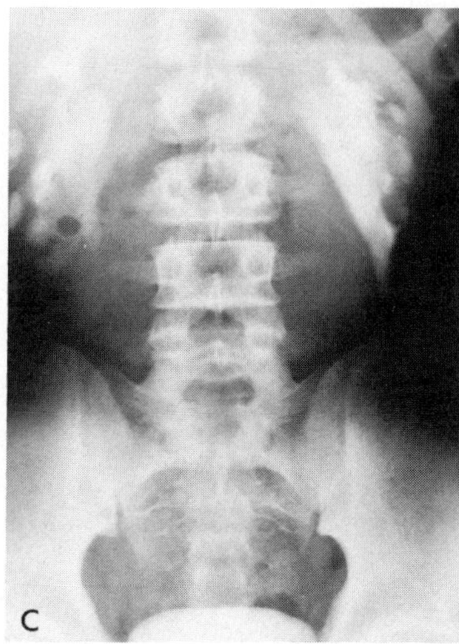

Figure 25–6   Representative roentgenograms of patient shown in Figures 25–4 and 25–5. *A,* Preoperative nephrostogram showing complete obstruction (*arrow*). *B,* Retrograde pyelogram 6 months postoperatively showing open anastomosis (*arrow*). *C,* Intravenous pyelogram three years postoperatively showing excellent function of left kidney and open anastomosis. The patient also had successful pyeloplasty on the opposite side.

control is obtained should the site of injury be inspected and closed appropriately under direct vision.

Injury to adjacent structures during nephrectomy is avoided by being aware of their presence and not inflicting trauma by direct dissection or rough retraction (on the right, the liver, duodenum, right colon, and vena cava; on the left, the spleen, tail of pancreas, aorta, and left colon). Rough retraction is usually avoided by working through incisions of adequate size! Inadvertent entry into the pleural space is possible during nephrectomy, especially if a rib is resected. This presents no problem if recognized. It is best to make certain that the hole is *large enough* to allow free escape of air from the pleural space when the lung is expanded by the anesthesiologist. Too small an opening can cause ball-valve trapping of air and tension pneumothorax. No attempt should be made to close the leak when it is first noted. It is safer to do so at the end of the operation when the wound is closed, while the anesthesiologist inflates the lung appropriately.

Whether the ureter should be removed during nephrectomy depends on its condition. If the ureter is normal, it can be ligated in the gutter below the kidney and left in place. An abnormal ureter is best removed. Examples include ureters with vesicoure-

teric reflux, which may trap urine and perpetuate infection, and ureters that enter ectopically outside the bladder, which may harbor chronic infection if not removed. If the lower ureter cannot be reached through the flank incision, it can be approached through a second small lower abdominal incision. If dissection is carried close onto the ureter, removal should not injure adjacent structures that it crosses. If there is a second ipsilateral ureter to be saved, it can be helpful to place a ureteral catheter into the better ureter to facilitate its recognition during removal of the diseased ureter.

Partial Nephrectomy

Some of the conditions for which partial nephrectomy may be needed in children are shown in Figure 25–7. Most common is a duplex collecting system with severe damage of one renal moiety, usually the upper pole. Often the upper pole ureter ends in an ectopic location. It may terminate as a ureterocele, either normotopically in the bladder or ectopically in the urethra. Sometimes the upper pole is a tiny, multicystic, dysplastic segment, scarcely more than a nubbin, and it may be joined to a ureter that empties distal to the external urethral sphincter, causing the female patient to be "wet all the

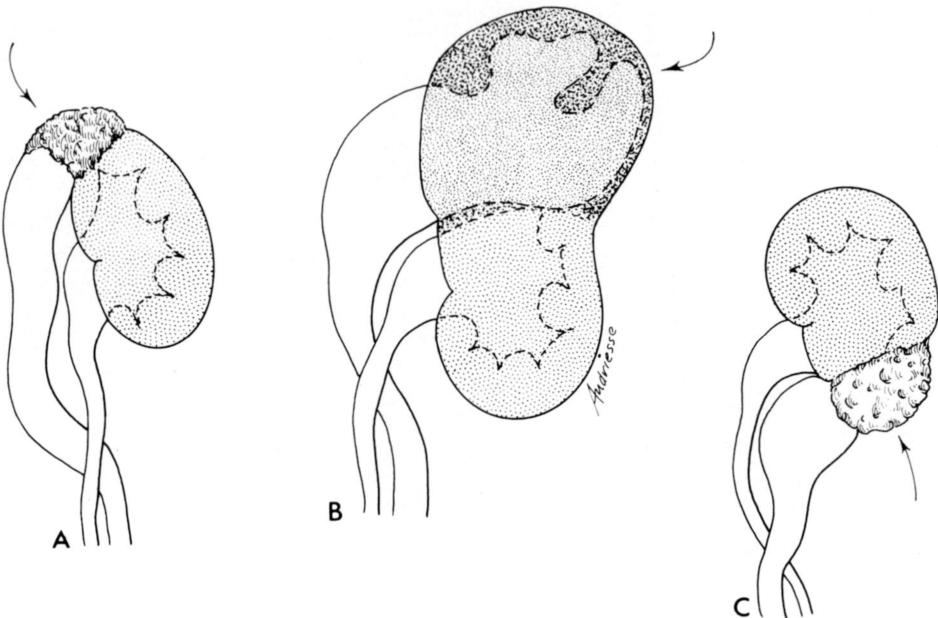

Figure 25–7 Some anatomic indications for heminephrectomy. *A,* Dysplastic upper pole (*arrow*), which may accompany ectopic ureter or ureterocele. Often not visualized by intravenous pyelogram. *B,* Severe hydronephrosis of upper pole (*arrow*), most often associated with ureterocele. *C,* Selective atrophy of lower pole (*arrow*), which can be shrunken or hydronephrotic. Usually associated with massive reflux to lower pole.

time." In other patients usually the female infant with a ureterocele, the upper pole shows extreme hydronephrosis. Upper pole nephrectomy is very simple when there is a cleft-like demarcation between the two renal moieties. In other patients, however, the segment to be removed is enveloped by the adjacent better pole to be spared. In any event, several precautions can prevent complications during partial nephrectomy (Fig. 25–8). Methylene blue can be instilled into the ureter of the segment to be removed, staining the tissues to be resected. There are separate vessels to the upper pole. They should be ligated close to the specimen to be removed, to minimize inadvertent damage to the lower pole vessels to be saved. It is sometimes helpful to have placed a ureteral catheter from below into the ureter of the better renal segment, attaching it to an extension tubing through which saline solution is instilled by a circulating nurse to distend the renal collecting system to be preserved. This can also help demonstrate any leaks in the retained kidney after partial

nephrectomy. In theory, it is useful to preserve some capsule of the specimen being removed to cover the raw surface of the remaining kidney. In practice, this is usually not possible. Sometimes the raw surface can be closed with a few mattress sutures, all of which are placed before any are tied. Large sutures should be avoided to prevent compromising the remaining renal parenchyma. Gerota's fascia can be used to cover the raw surface of kidney after partial nephrectomy. Most important in avoiding postoperative complications, however, is accurate suture control of blood vessels or openings in the collecting system to be spared. A drain should be placed in the renal fossa and remain until absence of drainage is assured. When removal of one renal moiety and its ureter is performed, one must pay careful attention to which ureter is removed, especially if two incisions are used. In Figures 25–9 and 25–10 is shown a patient referred for reconstruction after inadvertent interruption of the lower ureter during upper pole nephrectomy.

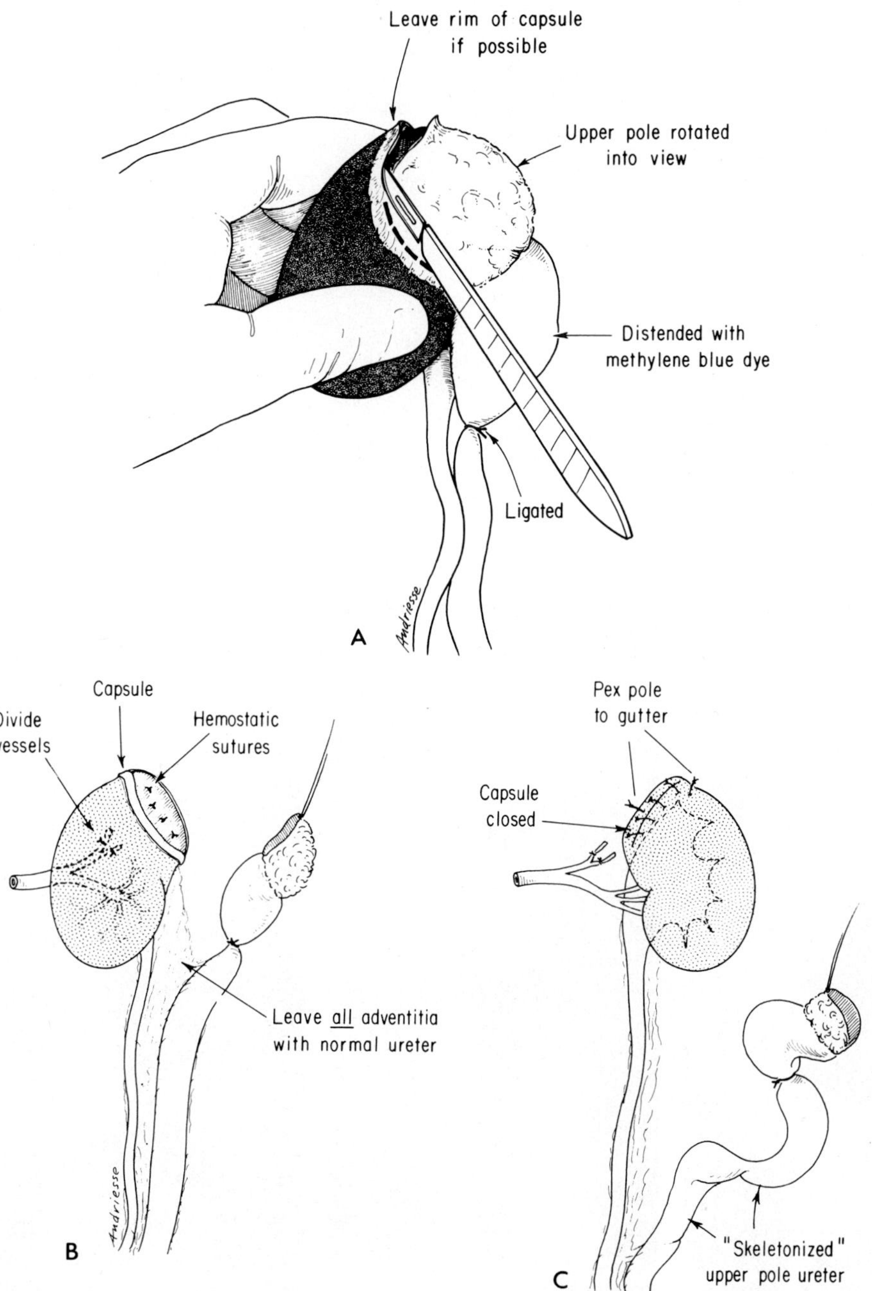

Figure 25–8 Technique of heminephrectomy. *A,* Collecting system of segment to be removed is distended with methylene blue, a useful aid in demarcating the segment to be resected. *B* and *C,* Further steps in removing diseased moiety and its ureter.

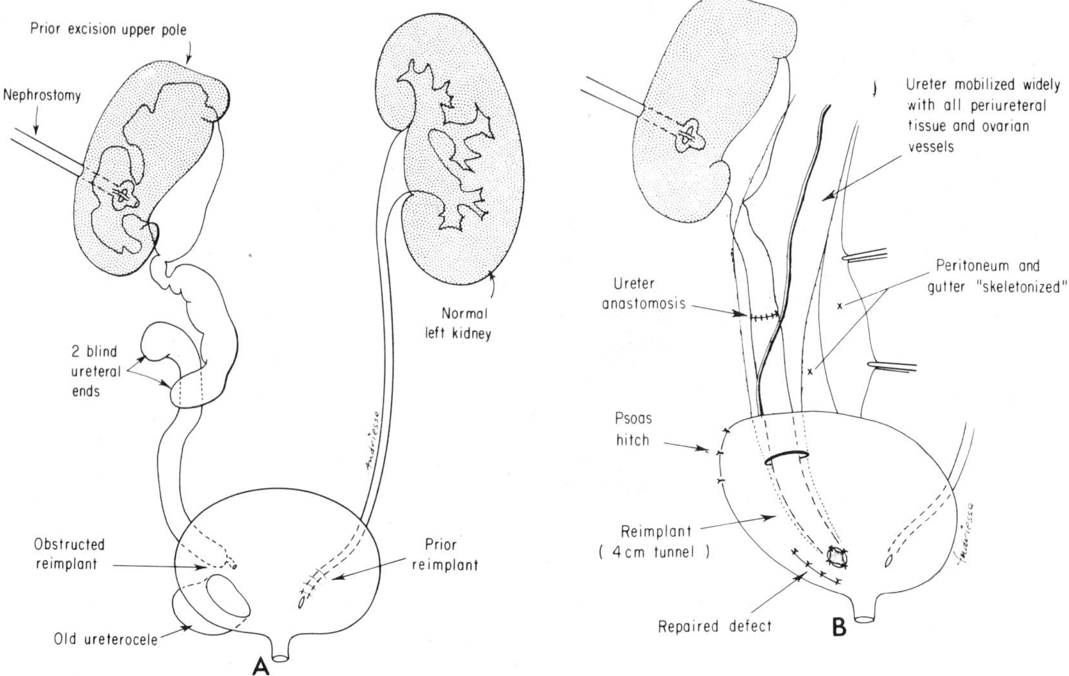

Figure 25–9 Anatomy before (A) and after (B) repair in child referred with discontinuity of remaining ureter, an operative mishap during excision of upper pole.

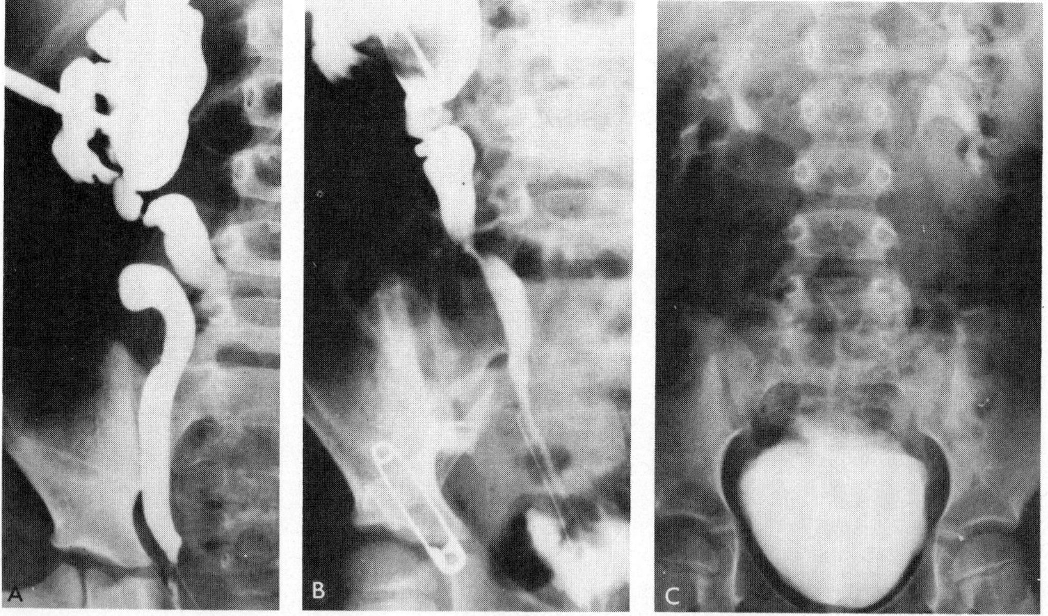

Figure 25–10 Representative roentgenograms of patient shown in Figure 25–9. A, Simultaneous preoperative nephrostogram and retrograde pyelogram, showing discontinuity of remaining ureter. B, Nephrostogram 10 days following repair. There is a stent in the lower ureter following its repeat reimplantation. C, Intravenous pyelogram 1 year later. Excellent function of right kidney, for which nephrectomy had once been advised.

Nephrectomy for Tumor

Nephroureterectomy for Wilms' tumor presents entirely different considerations than nephrectomy for benign disease. Blood loss can be great. An intravenous cutdown catheter should be placed in the upper extremity, where it is easily available to the anesthesiologist. I have seen two deaths occur when the cutdown was placed in an ankle. In one patient it became disconnected, and the infused blood drained beneath the drapes, not into the patient. In another, hemorrhage necessitated cross-clamping of the vena cava. This impeded central return of blood being infused into the leg. We use not only a central infusion line in the upper extremity but also an arterial monitoring catheter for constant direct blood-pressure recording.

Ideal operative exposure of a large Wilms' tumor, or neuroblastoma adjacent to the kidney, can be obtained through a generous transabdominal incision. Some surgeons prefer a transverse abdominal incision to permit routine inspection of the other kidney, which in 5 per cent of patients will also be involved with tumor. The thoracoabdominal incision gives optimal exposure from all sides. It avoids the need for excessive handling and retraction of the tumor during dissection posterolaterally from the gutter and diaphragm. Retracting these tumors can cause intraoperative embolization or iatrogenic rupture. Despite the large size of the thoracoabdominal wound, it is followed by few complications. Since it violates only the lower thorax, pulmonary and pleural complications are rare. Since it approaches the tumor from behind and laterally, and the small bowel lies forward, requiring little if any handling, intra-abdominal complications are unusual. A chest tube should always be used. I recall a child who died of postoperative intrathoracic hemorrhage from an intercostal vessel. The hemorrhage was not detected early because no chest tube had been placed.

In removing Wilms' tumors, it is theoretically desirable to first approach the renal hilum to ligate the vessels. In practice, this is often impossible. A large tumor can distort the vessels, making their early identification difficult. This is especially true when a tumor crosses the midline or surrounds the great vessels. Constant thought about the vessels to be spared is the best safeguard against their inadvertent transection. Vessels I have seen inadvertently divided include the aorta, the vena cava, the superior mesenteric artery, and the opposite renal artery. These tumors may extend along the renal vein into the vena cava. It is useful to obtain the preoperative intravenous pyelogram by injecting contrast medium into the saphenous vein, thereby visualizing the vena cava. If tumor is seen in the vena cava, preparations can be made for its removal, using cardiopulmonary bypass if necessary. In one of our patients, intracaval tumor blocked not only the inferior vena cava but also the hepatic veins, producing the Budd-Chiari syndrome. Removal of the tumor and its extension, plus chemotherapy and radiation therapy for pulmonary metastases, has resulted in 10-year survival of this child. If tumor in renal veins is not suspected, ligation of the vein can cause intraoperative embolization of tumor. We reported such a case involving a right adrenal tumor.[9] The surgeon who approaches a large Wilms' tumor must be prepared to deal with surgery of the aorta and vena cava, colonic resection if the adjacent mesocolon is involved, or partial hepatectomy if the tumor cannot be separated from the liver. To be ill prepared invites the complication of local recurrence from inadequate resection.

Nephrostomy

Long-term tube nephrostomy should be avoided because it will inevitably be accompanied by chronic urinary traction infection with secondary loss of renal function. Long-term tube drainage also commonly results in stone formation. Today there is virtually no indication for its use in a young patient with benign disease. Short-term nephrostomy, on the other hand, can be of great value. As shown in Figure 25–11, the renal collecting system is identified by passing into it a #22 spinal needle, injecting a small amount of contrast medium, and visualizing its position in the collecting system roentgenographically. A small trocar is then inserted parallel to the spinal needle. Through the

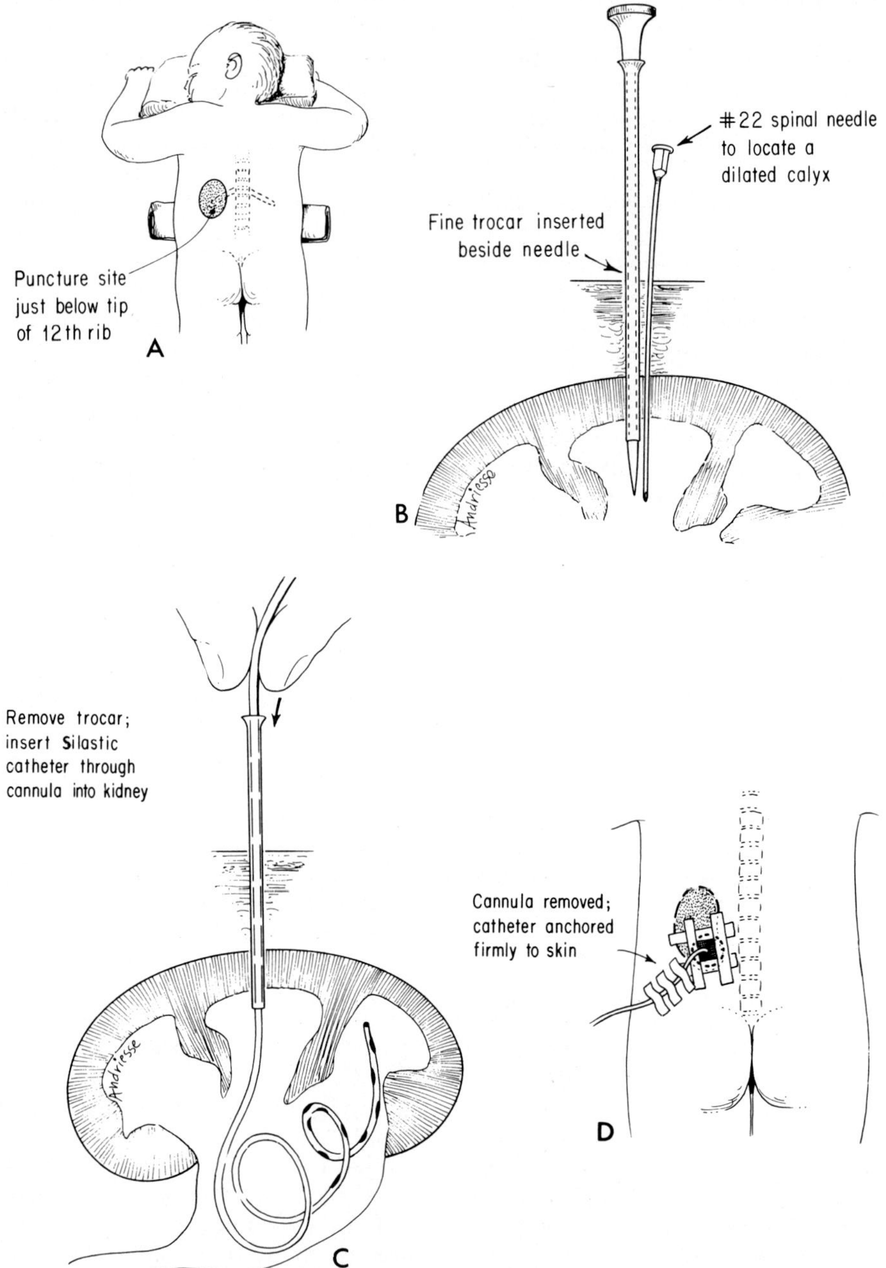

Figure 25–11   Technique of percutaneous temporary nephrostomy using nonreactive Silastic tubing.

trocar a length of soft, nonreactive Silastic catheter tubing is passed into the renal pelvis. This can provide temporary drainage for an obstructed kidney while definitive correction is prepared for. If percutaneous drainage is not feasible, open nephrostomy can be performed. When the renal cortex is thick, a probe is passed through a small opening in the renal pelvis into the lower pole calyx and out the renal cortex. Through that tract, a small Malecot catheter is led into the kidney. If the kidney is hydronephrotic, opening the renal pelvis is not necessary. The tube can be inserted directly through the cortex at a thin spot. Circle nephrostomy has been advocated for easy replacement of a long-standing nephrostomy tube. Although this technique is applicable in adult patients, I believe it should be discouraged in children. We have treated one patient in whom the renal pelvis was destroyed in this manner. In another, the circle tube was brought through the ureteropelvic junction and out the upper ureter, creating obstruction at a previously normal ureteropelvic junction. This necessitated a difficult secondary pyeloplasty. The most commom complication of nephrostomy in children is inadvertent pulling out of the tube. This can be avoided by anchoring the tube securely with adhesive. When a tube is pulled out, it should be replaced immediately, for the tract can close in just a few hours. The tract should be explored gently with sound to check the direction and depth of the tube. If a tube of the same size will not pass readily, especially in a relatively new tract, a well-lubricated tube of smaller size should be passed immediately and its position checked by injection of contrast medium. Pushing hard on a tube that does not pass easily nearly always results in its placement somewhere outside the kidney.

Pyelolithotomy

Renal stones are more common in some parts of the world than in others. Principles of their surgical management in children do not differ from those in adults. The surgeon should not only remove the stones but also correct the problem that caused them to form, if possible. Stones can result from stasis caused by obstruction or from infection due to reflux. A metabolic disorder such as cystinuria may be the underlying problem, controllable by appropriate medical management. Routine analysis of stones can often shed light on their cause and serve to direct therapy aimed at preventing recurrence.

Many complications can result from surgery for stones, especially in a patient undergoing reoperation whose kidney may be encased in chronic inflammatory tissue, which makes difficult accurate identification of hilar structures. Careful dissection of the renal hilum is mandatory to prevent injury to its vessels. It is important to compress the ureter gently to prevent downward passage of stones during manipulation of the kidney. Stones should be removed in the manner least likely to injure renal parenchyma. This will depend on the size of the stone, whether it has staghorn branches, its location, and the thickness of the cortex. An isolated stone in a dilated calyx is often best removed by incising thin cortex and retrieving the stone through the nephrotomy. In some patients, however, it is best done by opening the renal pelvis and grasping the stone from below. Pelvotomy should be well away from the ureteropelvic junction lest iatrogenic stenosis result. Occasionally, ureteropelvic junction obstruction is the primary cause of stone formation. In that case, pyeloplasty should be done.

A common complication of renal stone surgery is incomplete removal. Several precautions will reduce the likelihood of that complication. One is routine nephroscopy to search the interior of the kidney. This is easier in patients with hydronephrosis. Unfortunately, there are limitations to this technique, because today's instruments are not ideal. Rigid nephroscopes have excellent optics, but their rigidity limits their utility. The flexible instruments lack clarity and have not yet been miniaturized enough for practical use in smaller patients. Operative radiography is a useful adjunct in locating radiopaque stones. Recently, coagulum pyelolithotomy has proved very helpful in patients with multiple stones.[45] Solutions of cryoprecipitate, thrombin, and calcium chloride are introduced into the kidney, forming a jelly-like coagulum that traps small stone particles. A cast of the collecting system is pulled from the kidney with blunt forceps, removing entrapped stones. Generous irrigation of the collecting system is important to wash out small retained fragments. All these techniques require less time and patience, but they are well worth the effort if they can avoid the need for a repeat operation. If the kidney is hydronephrotic, we place a Malecot nephrostomy tube to allow postoperative irrigation. In some patients, Renacidin solution* can be used to dissolve retained stone fragments post-

---

*Guardian Chemical Corp., Hauppauge, New York.

operatively.[14] Indeed, some stones can be dissolved without open operation by inserting two irrigating catheters percutaneously. Complications of this therapy include septicemia, hypermagnesemia, and inflammation of the collecting system. Every patient in whom stones have formed should be taught that intake of large quantities of water is essential to prevent recurrence.

SURGERY OF THE URETER

A large share of urologic surgery centers on the ureter. We will consider the most common operations involving the ureter in children, including repair of megaureter, transureteroureterostomy, excision of ureterocele, cutaneous ureterostomy, ileal loop urinary diversion, colon conduit urinary diversion, ureterosigmoidostomy, and construction of a ureter from small bowel. Ureteral reimplantation is discussed in Chapter 26.

Repair of Megaureter

Until recently, the dilated and often tortuous ureter was considered an uncorrectable problem.[5, 45] In the past 20 years or more, its repair has become commonplace.[6, 7, 18, 23, 32] In Figure 25–12 are shown the principle types of megaureter, those with obstruction and those with massive reflux. They can be subdivided into various classifications according to their etiology.[43] However, in those for which repair is indicated, the task is basically the same. It requires tapering and reimplanting the lower ureter so that it will drain normally and not reflux. The tip of the ureter is resected if it is obstructed.

The most common complications after surgery for megaureter are shown in Figure 25–13. Reflux usually results from a tunnel that is too short relative to the diameter of the ureter. The ratio of tunnel length to ureter diameter should be about 5:1. In some patients, reflux will persist despite a

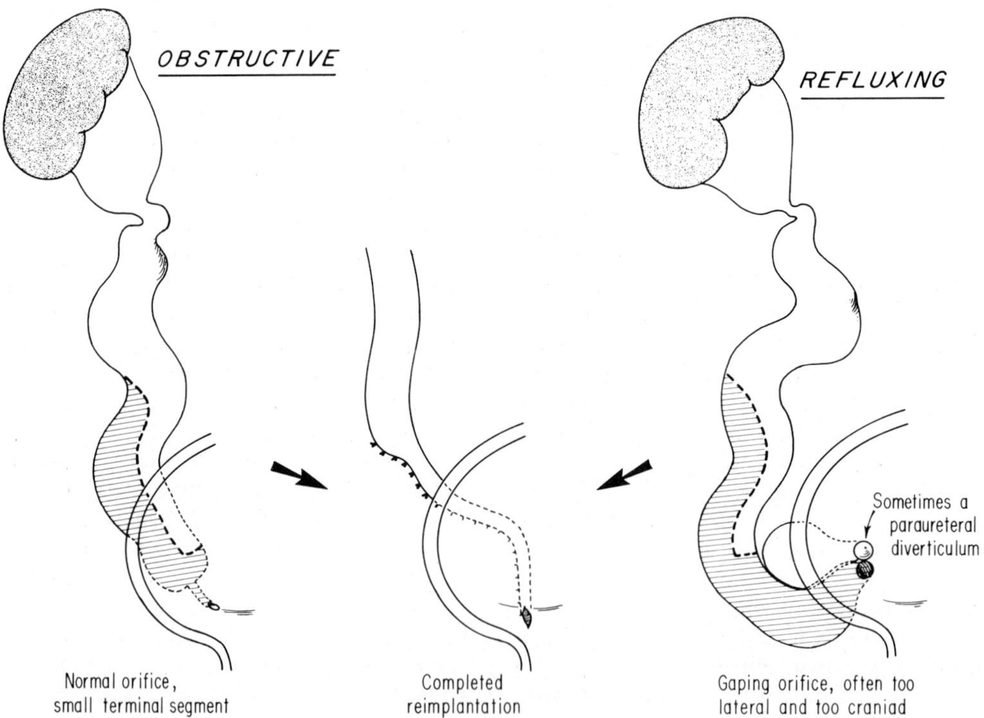

Figure 25–12   The principal anatomic types of megaureter and scheme of operative repair.

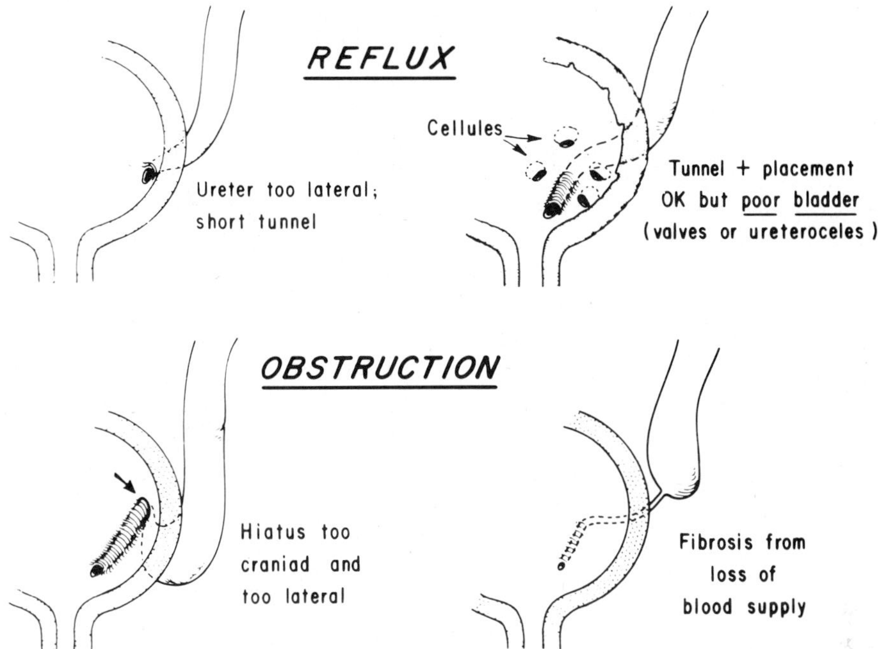

Figure 25–13 The most common complications after megaureter repair.

long tunnel. These are usually persons whose bladder and ureter are scarred and less pliable than normal. Obstruction after tapering and implantation usually results from placing the ureteral hiatus too far craniad or too far laterally, causing angulation when the bladder fills. Fibrosis of the distal ureter results from loss of its blood supply.

Certain precautions will minimize the incidence of complications. Initially, mobilization is best done intravesically. This avoids injury to bladder innervation, which can occur after paravesical dissection of the ureter. During further mobilization extravesically, the dissection should preserve ureteral adventitia for collateral blood supply. Surrounding structures should be skeletonized, not the ureter. In tapering, the ureter should be narrowed enough to obtain a satisfactory ratio of tunnel length to ureter diameter, but not so much as to cause obstruction. Accurate placement of the hiatus in the back wall of the bladder, not the side, is important to avoid angulation. Watertight closure of the longitudinal ureteral resection is important to prevent postoperative leakage. Tapering is not extended above the

level of the iliac artery to avoid devascularization of the lower ureter. Postoperative drainage is maintained with a soft plastic catheter threaded up to the kidney. In patients who have had a prior high diversion, a stent should be placed in the lower ureter during healing, because a "dry reimplant" can seal completely. Stiff catheters should never be used as drainage stents. They can erode the ureteral wall, causing ureterovesical fistulae.

Complications will occur more often in reimplanting tapered megaureters than in reimplanting nondilated ureters. There is nearly always an option for correction of a complication. To consider diversion is an unnecessarily pessimistic view.[13] A representative case is shown in Figures 25–14 and 25–15. This child's problem of massive reflux was not solved until a third operation was done. In some cases the best solution consists of long tunnel reimplantation of the better ureter, combined with psoas hitch, and transureteroureterostomy or transureteropyelostomy for drainage of the other kidney. We have done this in 53 patients, all of whom needed difficult reoperations, with success in most.[26]

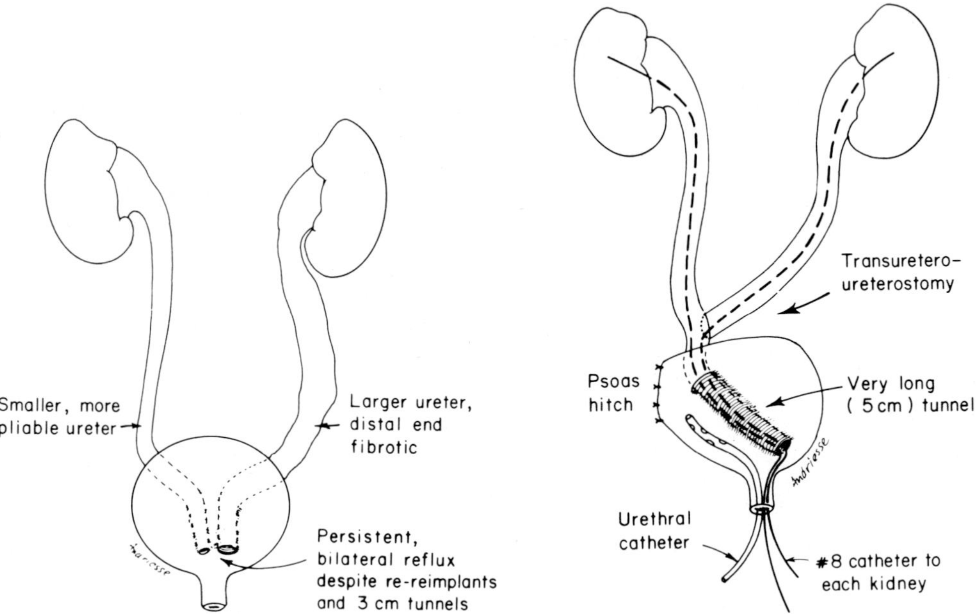

Figure 25–14 Failure to correct reflux in megaureters, managed by unilateral repeat reimplantation of right ureter for a third time and left-to-right transureteroureterostomy.

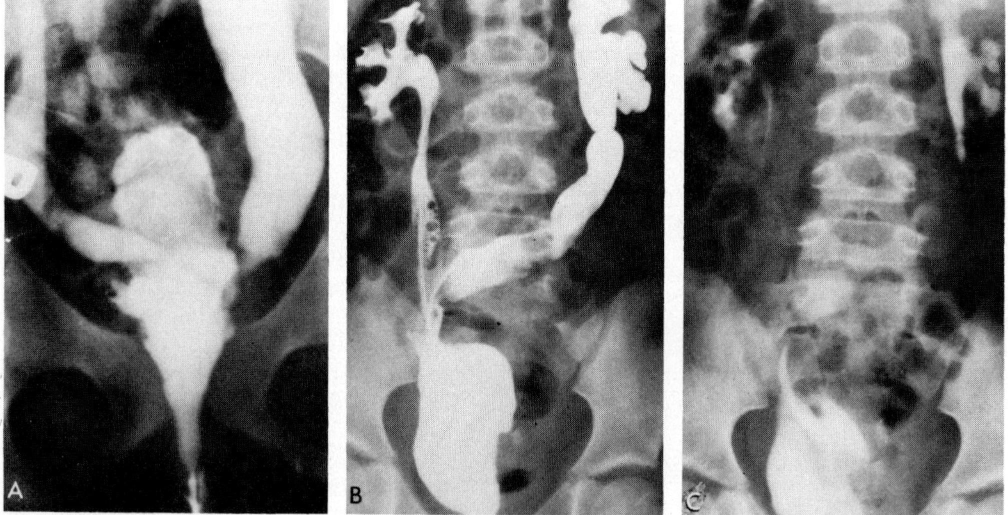

Figure 25–15 Representative roentgenograms from patient shown in Figure 25–14. *A,* Preoperative voiding cystourethrogram showing massive reflux, despite long tunnels, which is not rare when ureters and trigone are very abnormal, such as in boys with urethral valves or girls with ureteroceles. *B,* Injection of catheter stents 10 days after reconstruction. Note psoas hitch of bladder on right and transureteroureterostomy. *C,* Intravenous pyelogram 4 weeks after reconstruction. Note diagonal course of ureter across the trigone, and its long tunnel. Cystogram showed absence of reflux. The patient is clinically well, with stable upper tracts and no urinary infection 4½ years later.

Transsureteroureterostomy

Transureteroureterostomy has gained popularity in recent years since the demonstration by Hodges et al. that it is a safe procedure with a wide variety of uses.[27, 30] Essentials of the technique are shown in Figure 25–16. It can be used when one ureter is not long enough to be implanted into the bladder but can be joined to the opposite ureter. The ureter to be drained must be mobilized enough to allow it to be brought to the other side without tension. Its periureteral adventitia must be spared to preserve collateral blood supply coming from above. It must not be angulated be-

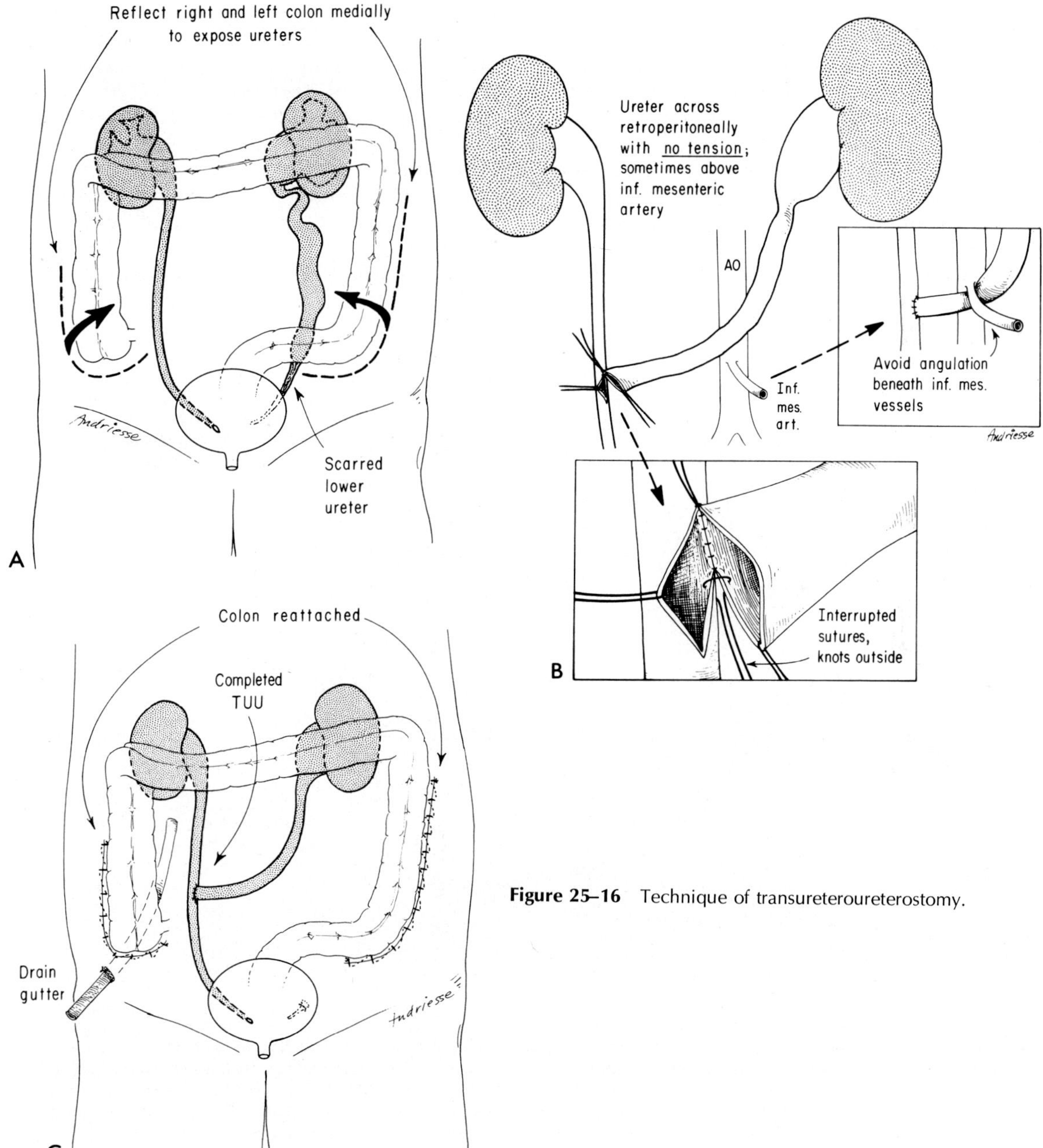

Figure 25–16 Technique of transureteroureterostomy.

neath the inferior mesenteric artery. Anastomosis to the contralateral ureter must be watertight and should be in the side wall of the recipient ureter not anteriorly, lest angulation cause obstruction. The recipient ureter should not be mobilized and displaced toward the ureter to be drained. Complications of transureteroureterostomy include obstruction, angulation, leakage, and loss of blood supply. They are preventable by taking the precautions outlined above. Depending on whether transureteroureterostomy is an isolated procedure or one done with other maneuvers in complicated reconstructions, drainage stents may or may not be used. In any case, a retroperitoneal drain should be used in the event that there is temporary leakage.

Wide mobilization of the ureter with preservation of its blood supply is necessary not only in transureteroureterostomy but also in other types of reconstructive operations.

Retaining the gonadal vessels with the ureter for added collateral circulation is a useful measure that can help prevent loss of blood supply. This is shown in Figure 25–17.

Ureterocele

There are many complications after surgery for ureteroceles in infants and children. In patients with a single ureter, optimal treatment is excision of the ureterocele and reimplantation of the ureter. When the ureter is widely dilated, it should be tapered. Unroofing was formerly popular, but it substituted reflux for obstruction. Unroofing should be condemned today except in most unusual circumstances.

More difficult is the management of patients with duplex collecting systems. Op-

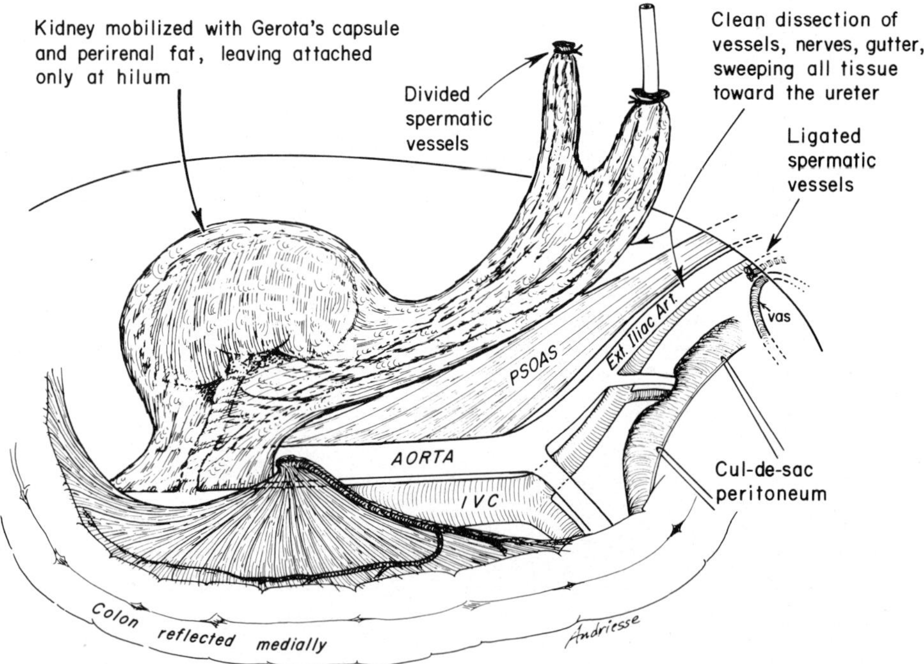

Figure 25–17 Technique for wide mobilization of ureter often needed in repeat reimplantation of ureter, transureteroureterostomy, and other reconstructive operations. The ureter is dissected free from adjacent structures, sweeping all periureteral tissue toward it, as in radical retroperitoneal lymphadenectomy. The gonadal vessels are maintained with the ureter for additional collateral blood supply. A little additional length can be obtained by mobilizing the kidney from its bed and pexing its lower pole inferiorly. Autotransplantation of the kidney is another option to consider but is seldom indicated in children, in whom the vessels are small and the kidneys often already badly damaged. Wide mobilization of the ureter, together with upward fixation of the bladder by psoas hitch, will often allow reimplantation that would be impossible by ordinary means.

timal treatment depends on the age and condition of the child and on whether one or both sides are involved.[28] Figure 25–18 shows a scheme of various approaches that might be used. In an older child with one side involved, one-stage complete repair may be feasible. However, in a sick infant with bilateral involvement, removal of dysplastic upper poles and the associated ureters may be wisest, leaving the lower reconstruction until later. Indeed, if there is no reflux up the lower pole ureter, some surgeons postpone the lower reconstruction indefinitely.[4]

Many complications are possible in these patients. In most, the upper pole is best removed. If the upper pole appears salvageable, it can be anastomosed to the adjacent lower pole. In some of our patients, however, later follow-up showed that the retained upper pole needed to be removed. In managing duplex ureters with reflux into one,

reimplantation of both ureters in a common sheath is a satisfactory procedure. When one of the two ureters is greatly dilated, however, as it usually is in patients with ureterocele, complications can occur after double reimplantation, even if the larger one is tapered. An alternative — removing the dilated ureter and sparing the blood supply of the better ureter — is shown in Figure 25–19. Figures 25–20 and 25–21 show a patient in whom complications resulted from ureteral reimplantation of two ureters, one of which was grossly dilated.

When removing ureteroceles, it is important not to leave a distal lip that can act as an obstructing urethral valve. Failure to repair the bladder neck and trigone at the site of a ureterocele can cause two complications. One is stress incontinence, resulting from an inadequate bladder neck. The second is formation of a diverticulum proximal to the bladder neck.[3] This causes the bladder neck

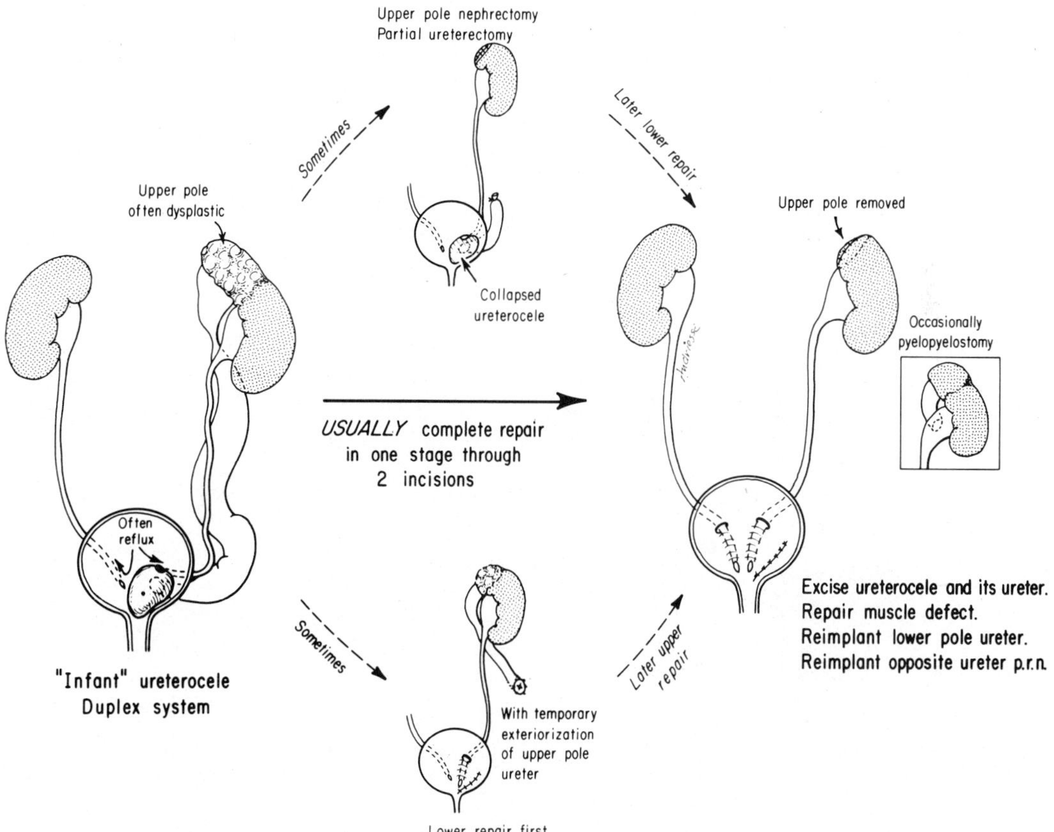

Figure 25–18 Methods of managing ureterocele with duplex collecting system, which is about twice as common as ureterocele with single collecting system.

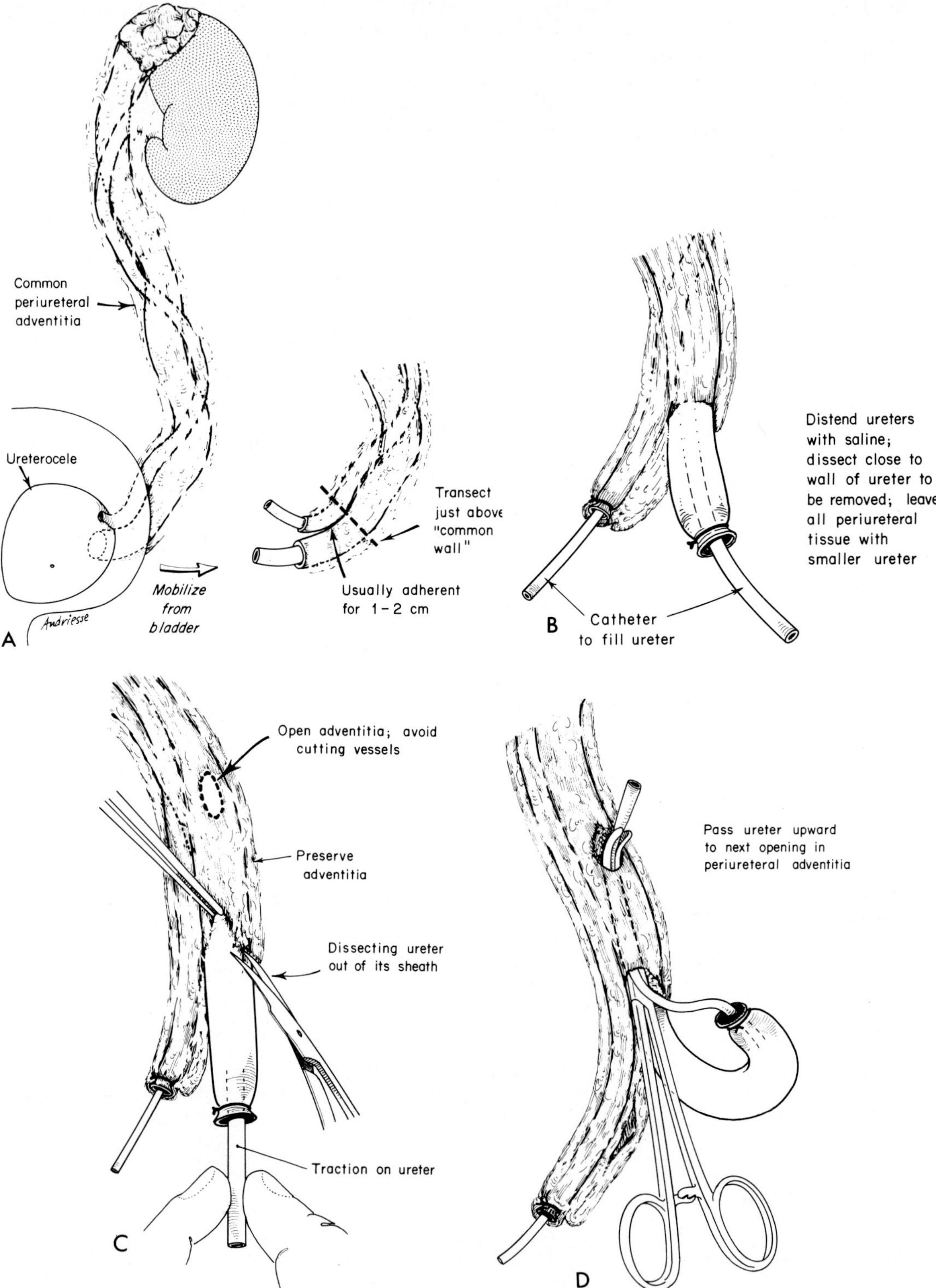

Figure 25–19　Technique for separating two ureters while preserving blood supply of the lower pole ureter to be spared and reimplanted. By making ''stair step'' incisions in periureteral adventitia instead of opening it widely, more collateral blood supply is spared, reducing the likelihood of ischemia to the better ureter.

Illustration continued on opposite page

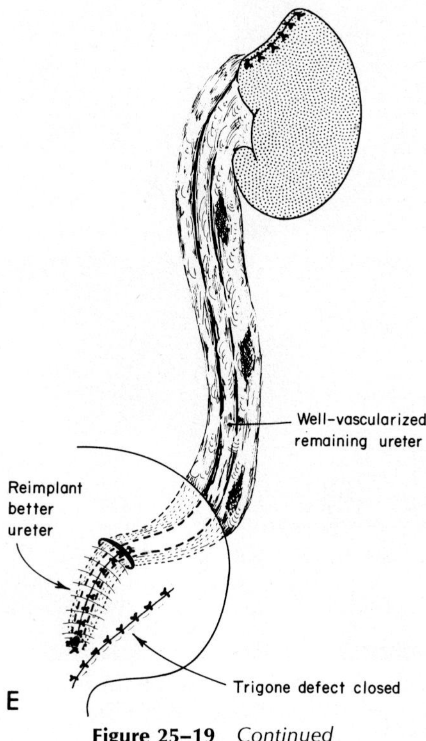

Figure 25–19 *Continued*

Figure 25–20 Anatomy before and after reoperation in an 8-year-old girl with lower ureteral obstruction. The original problem had been left ureterocele with a duplex collecting system. Double tapered reimplants had been performed, resulting in obstruction of both ureters. The condition was managed by reimplanting a better ureter (lower pole) and by pyelopyelostomy.

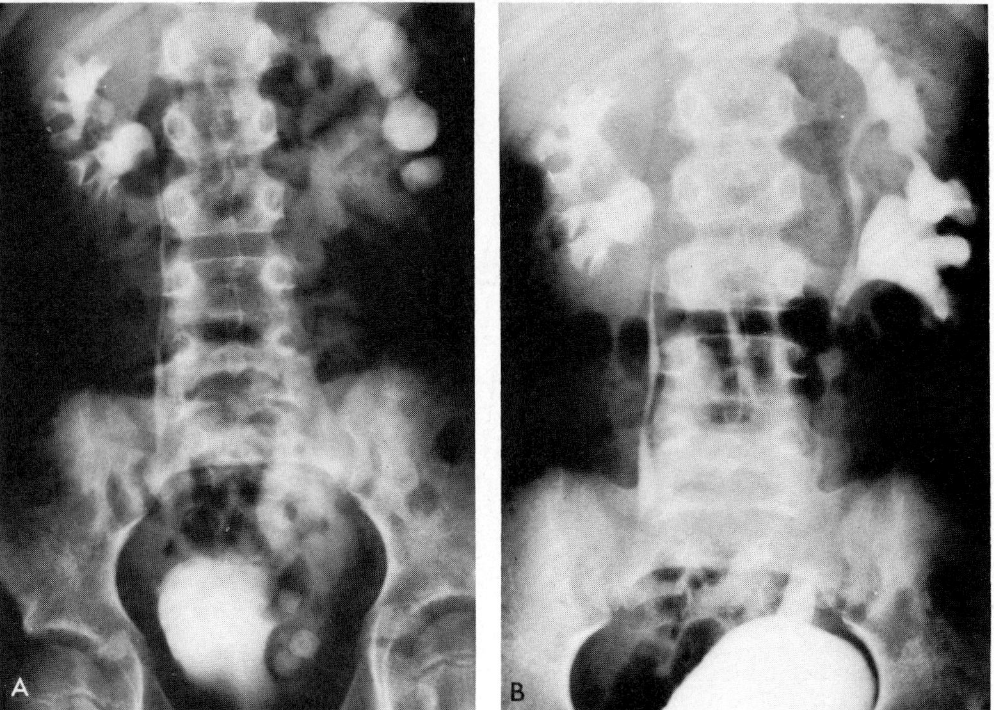

Figure 25–21 Roentgenograms from patient shown in Figure 25–20. *A,* Original intravenous pyelogram before first operation elsewhere, showing multiple stones in ureterocele and its ureter. Hydronephrosis of both renal segments. *B,* Intravenous pyelogram 2 months following reoperation. In most duplex collecting systems where there is marked enlargement of one or both ureters, it is best to remove the larger, reimplanting the better one and draining the other renal moiety by transureteropyelostomy.

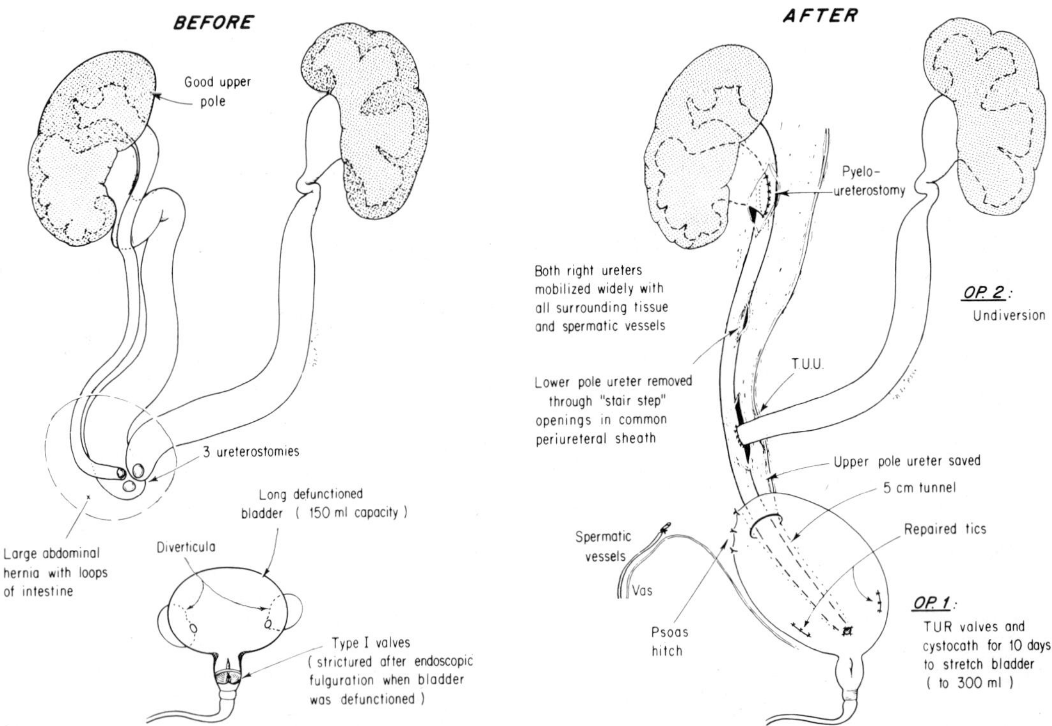

Figure 25–22 A 15-year-old boy was referred for undiversion 8 years after end ureterostomies had been performed. Case demonstrates that extensive surgery can be done on a ureter if its periureteral adventitia and gonadal vessels are maintained for blood supply. Note that the right upper pole ureter was operated on at three levels — high (pyeloureterostomy), middle (transureteroureterostomy), and low (reimplantation into bladder) — and that, in addition, the adjacent lower pole ureter was dissected away from it.

to act as an obstructing valve during micturition. Incomplete removal of a ureterocele and its ureter can also produce the complication of stasis and infection in the retained stump. Figures 25–22 and 25–23 show what extensive manipulation can be done in repair of a ureter if its blood supply is carefully preserved.

Ureterostomy

Loop cutaneous ureterostomy has been used widely during the past 20 years for temporary drainage of the upper tract in infants with severe obstructive uropathy who are too young to undergo definitive repair.[31, 38] It is a procedure that, in my opinion, has been greatly overused. It can be followed by numerous complications.[24] Other techniques of ureterostomy include Roux-en-Y ureterostomy,[44] ring ureteros-

tomy,[47] and end ureterostomy.[15] Many of the patients we have seen for subsequent reconstruction were much more difficult to treat because of prior ureterostomies. Reconstruction in these patients is usually best done in a single stage, closing the ureterostomy and repairing other problems simultaneously. In Figures 25–24 and 25–25 is shown a patient in whom the ureterostomies tethered the ureters upward, making satisfactory reimplantation of the ureters impossible. The child was referred for repeat operation.

If ureterostomy is elected, the opening should be high in the ureter, not in the midureter where it can complicate subsequent reconstruction by interfering with blood supply. End ureterostomy has been advocated for both temporary and permanent drainage in children. Complications include stenosis of the cutaneous opening, especially if the ureter is not dilated; failure

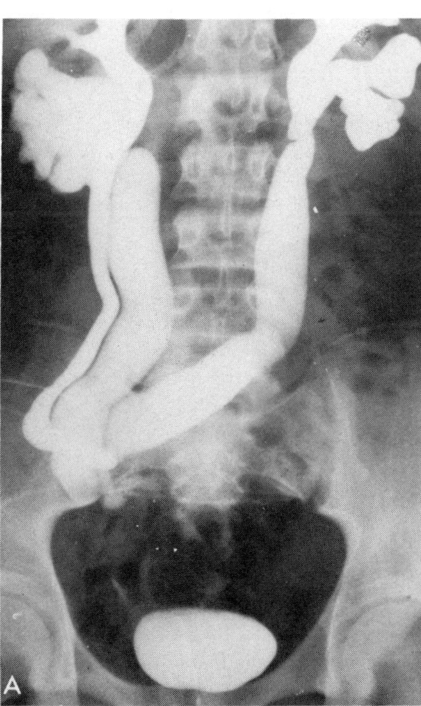

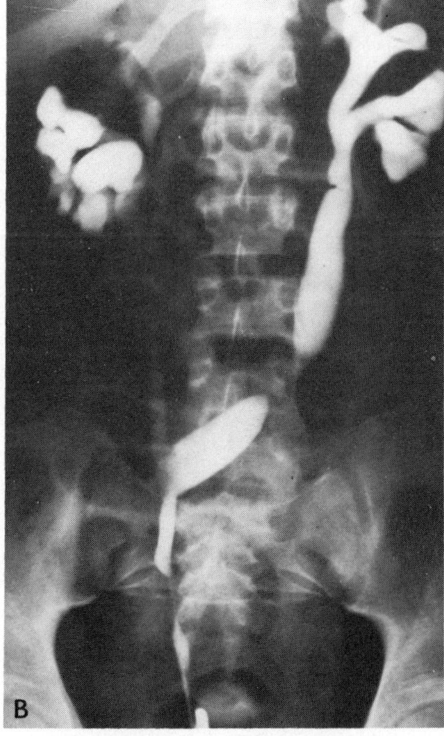

Figure 25–23 Roentgenograms from patient shown in Figure 25–22. *A,* Simultaneous preoperative cystogram and ureterogram to demonstrate anatomy to be reconstructed. Small bladder was first stretched up by filling through the cystocath inserted during cystoscopy. *B,* Retrograde pyelogram made 4 months postoperatively to outline the reimplanted right ureter, pyeloureterostomy, and transureteroureterostomy. Cystogram showed no reflux. The patient is well and free of infection 2 years postoperatively.

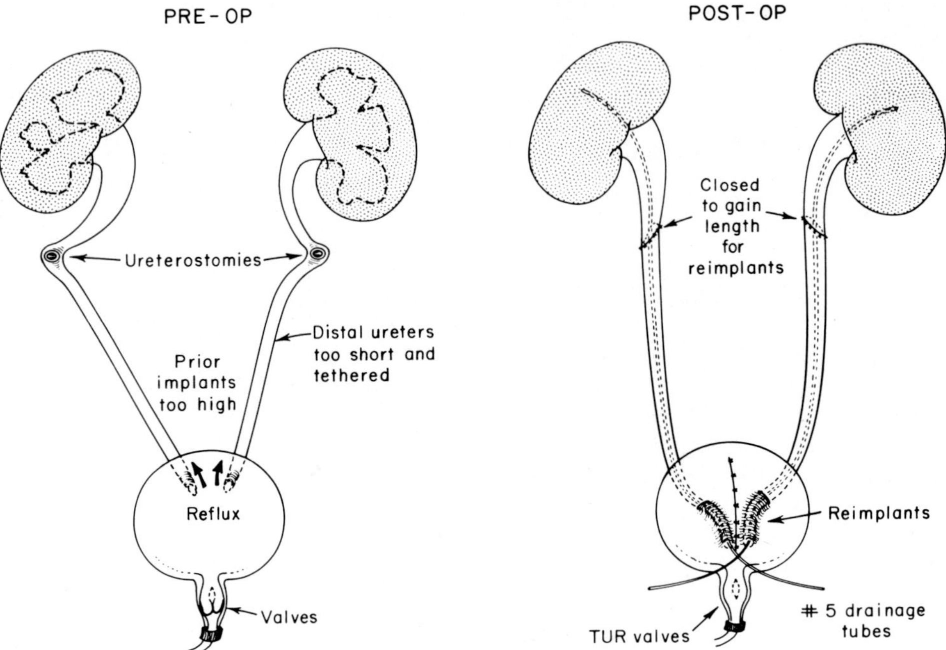

Figure 25–24   One of the complications of loop ureterostomies. The patient had reflux, but lower ureters were too short to be reimplanted, because they were tethered up by ureterostomies. The patient was referred for a second attempt. In a single operative session, the ureterostomies were taken down for closure, which allowed satisfactory repeat reimplantation.

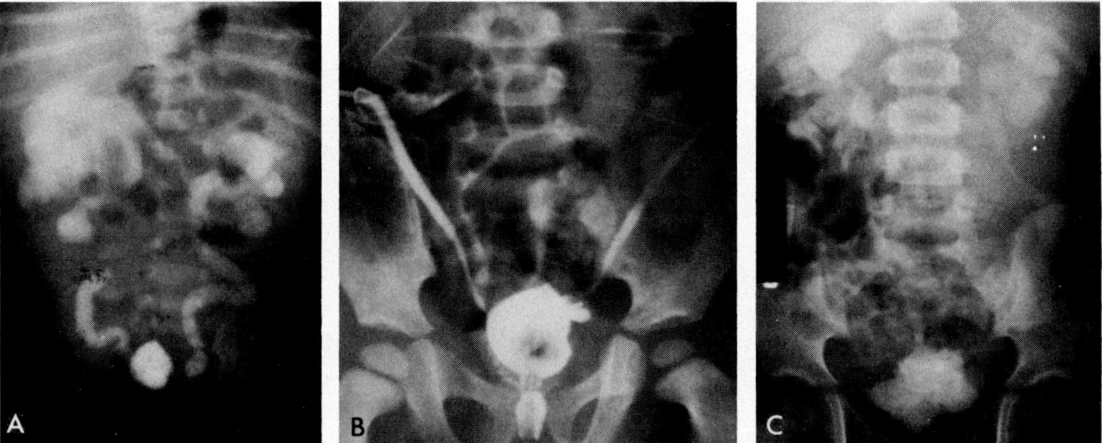

Figure 25–25   Representative roentgenograms from patient shown in Figure 25–24. *A,* Intravenous pyelogram at age 2 months. Note bilateral hydronephrosis and spontaneous extravasation of contrast medium around right kidney. *B,* Cystogram at age 2½ years, showing reflux up both ureters. Note their straight course upward, tethered at the site of ureterostomies. *C,* Intravenous pyelogram made 3½ years after undiversion. Patient is now 9 years old. Despite badly damaged upper tracts, he has reasonable renal function (blood urea nitrogen, 14 mg/dl; serum creatinine, 0.4 mg/dl; and creatinine clearance, 86 l/M² body surface area).

to drain adequately if the ureter is atonic; and chronic urosepsis from contamination by contents of the collecting bag. I believe that the best way to avoid ureterostomy complications is to avoid doing the operation! Many of the so-called temporary ureterostomies are unnecessary and could be avoided by doing a definitive operation.[17] It is my opinion that those children who require permanent cutaneous diversion are better served if it is done by means of a colon conduit. The colon conduit should include nonrefluxing technique to prevent ascent of bacteria to the upper tract.

Ileal Loop Urinary Diversion

Ileal loop urinary diversion was introduced 30 years ago by Bricker for use in patients undergoing exenteration for cancer.[8] Soon it was applied to many youngsters with myelodysplasia or obstructive uropathy thought too severe to permit reconstruction. Long-term follow-up of children after ileal loop urinary diversion has shown an unacceptable rate of upper tract deterioration.[36, 42] Many patients with ileal loops have chronic bacilluria, probably entering from the appliance. There is free reflux from the loop to the upper tract, which causes infection, stones, and deterioration. Stenosis of the stoma is common and aggravates this. It is my firm belief that ileal loops should not be used in young patients who have a long life expectancy. We have not performed the operation in more than 10 years. Instead, during the past decade our efforts have centered on undiversion of the urinary tract in young patients with ileal loops and other diversions.[20, 21] Of 113 patients undiverted as of September 1981, 44 had ileal loops. Some of the options used in these reconstructions are shown in Figure 25–26.

ILEAL LOOP UNDIVERSION

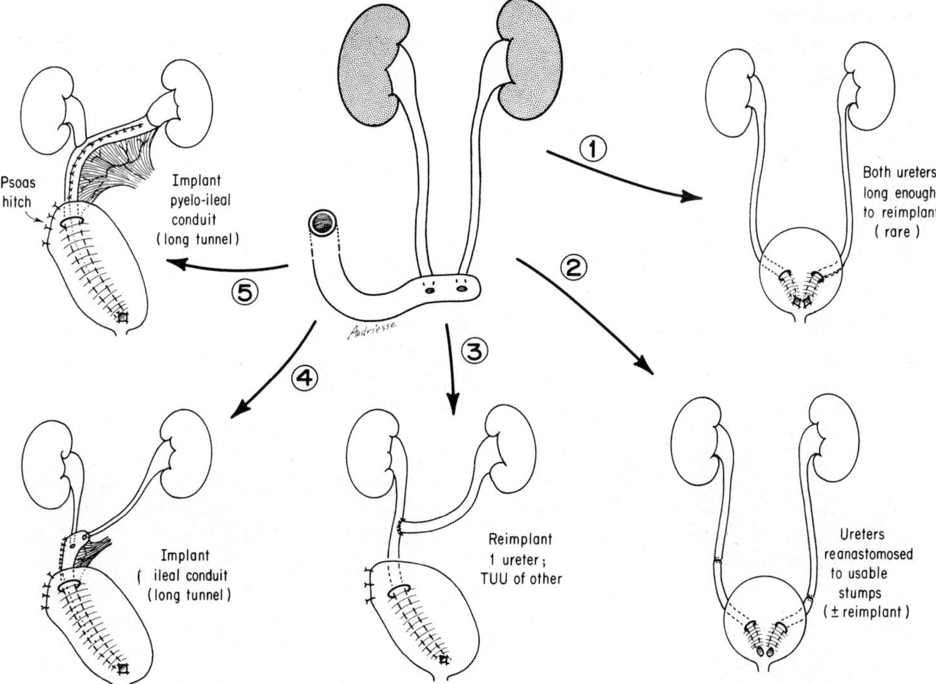

Figure 25–26   The most common options in undiverting urinary tract of patient with prior ileal loop urinary diversion. Every effort should be made to use ureters if possible, but in the majority of our patients it was necessary to use bowel segment implanted into bladder. This should not be done in small, fibrotic bladders where a very long tunnel cannot be made.

Colon Conduit Urinary Diversion

Experimental study of dogs subjected to an ileal loop urinary diversion of one ureter and a nonrefluxing colon conduit urinary diversion of the other ureter showed a marked difference in the incidence of pyelonephritis.[39] On the ileal loop side it was 83 per cent, whereas on the colon conduit side, where reflux was prevented, it was only 7 per cent. Although nonrefluxing colon conduits have not yet been studied for as long as ileal loops, their component parts have been used for many years. Mogg used the colon with satisfactory long-term experience.[37] Leadbetter described the tunneling and anastomosis technique three decades ago.[35] Stomal stenosis is much less common in colon conduits than in ileal conduits. The blood supply must be carefully chosen and maintained during creation of a colon conduit. An ample length of colon should be used, because there is a tendency for the colon to shorten during preparation of the conduit. Ureter tunnels should be long enough to prevent low-pressure reflux. Angulation and compression can be avoided by meticulous preparation of the tunnel. Small traps beneath the mesentery of the loop should be closed lest a loop of bowel become caught. It is not so important to close the gutter lateral to the conduit itself. A completed colon conduit diversion is shown in Figure 25–27. Some patients with colon conduits have the option of later anastomosis of the conduit to the rectosigmoid,[1, 22] as shown in Figure 25–28, thereby accomplishing staged ureterosigmoidostomy. This should not be considered if there is low-pressure reflux on loopogram or if the upper tracts are very dilated and damaged.

Diversion of urine to the colon carries the risk of hyperchloremic acidosis. Although good kidneys can handle the additional work of re-excreting solute reabsorbed from the colon, that is not possible in patients with marginal renal function. Liberal intake of water is needed even for patients with good upper-tract functional reserve to re-excrete the excess solute load. Serum electrolytes should be monitored periodically. If the serum bicarbonate level falls below 20 mEq/l, supplementary sodium bicarbonate (2 to 4 mEq/kg body weight) is administered by mouth. Supplementary potassium should be given if there is hypokalemia, another complication of diverting the urine into the colon. One of our patients became very weak as a result of hypokalemia and was thought at first to have an acute neurologic disorder. Potassium cured the problem immediately.

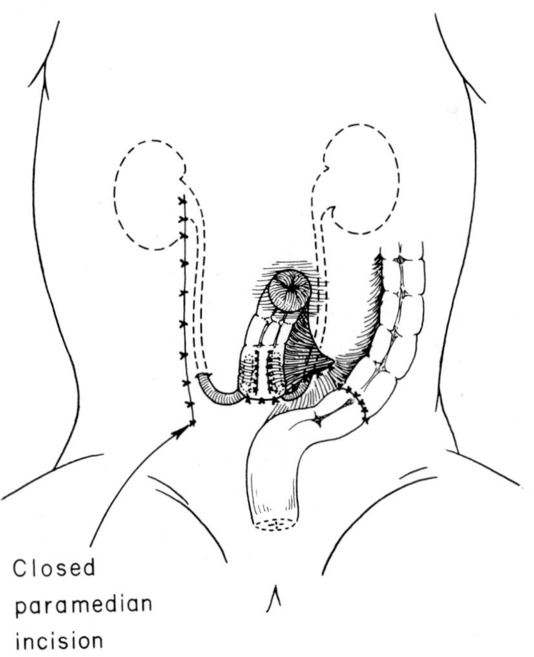

Figure 25–27   Anatomy of a colon conduit urinary diversion. Stoma can be placed in left, center, or right of abdomen, depending on the previous incisions.

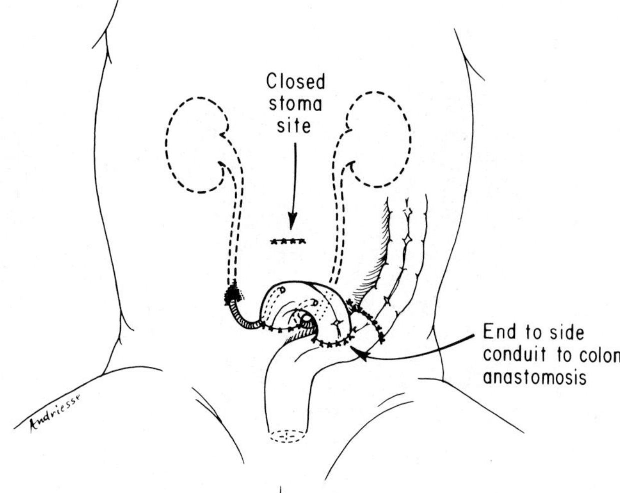

Figure 25–28 Subsequent reimplantation of colon conduit into colon by end-to-side technique, using two layers of chromic catgut (running technique for inner layer to ensure a watertight anastomosis, and interrupted technique for seromuscular layer). Nonabsorbable sutures should not be used, for they can result in stones.

The colon conduit has proved an excellent alternative in patients with long-standing ileal loops who are showing progressive upper-tract deterioration. In these patients, the ureters are often too short for two good, nonrefluxing ureteral anastomoses to be constructed. In this circumstance, the better ureter should be anastomosed to the conduit and the other drained by transureteropyelostomy, as shown in Figure 25–29. One good anastomosis to the bowel conduit is better than two poor ones.

Ureterosigmoidostomy

Direct ureterosigmoidostomy has been used widely in children, mainly those with exstrophy of the bladder. When the ureteral anastomoses are performed with good tunnels that prevent reflux and are not obstructed, long-term results can be excellent. Anastomotic complications, however, produce rapid deterioration of the upper tract. Local revision can be accomplished in some. In others, an extensive reoperation is better. One of the approaches we have used is shown in Figure 25–30. This technique facilitated making very long tunnels for ureters that were slightly dilated, one of the contraindications for performing primary ureterosigmoidostomy. There is an increased incidence of carcinoma of the colon at the site of ureterosigmoidostomy. These patients should be instructed to watch for blood in their stool, the presence of which should mandate endoscopic visualization. Barium enema should *not* be performed lest barium pass up the ureter into the kidney. Some patients in whom carcinoma developed had the old-fashioned type of ureterosigmoidostomy in which the tip of the ureter was simply dunked into the bowel lumen instead of being anastomosed to the mucosa. In some of them an inflammatory polyp formed at the tip of the ureter. This may be a factor in the development of carcinoma. Whether this complication will occur in patients after the currently used method of operation remains to be seen.

Small Bowel Ureter

For patients in whom neither ureter is long enough for satisfactory anastomosis to the bladder, there is the option of making a substitute ureter from intestine. This technique has been used in adults with recurrent renal stones.[17, 41] In such patients, prevention of reflux has not been so important. Most will do well with the full caliber of the bowel joined to the bladder without antireflux technique. In young patients, however, we have found it important to taper the bowel to prevent reflux.[25] A patient for whom this was done is shown in Figures 25–31 and 25–32. When tapered small bowel is implanted in the bladder, it must

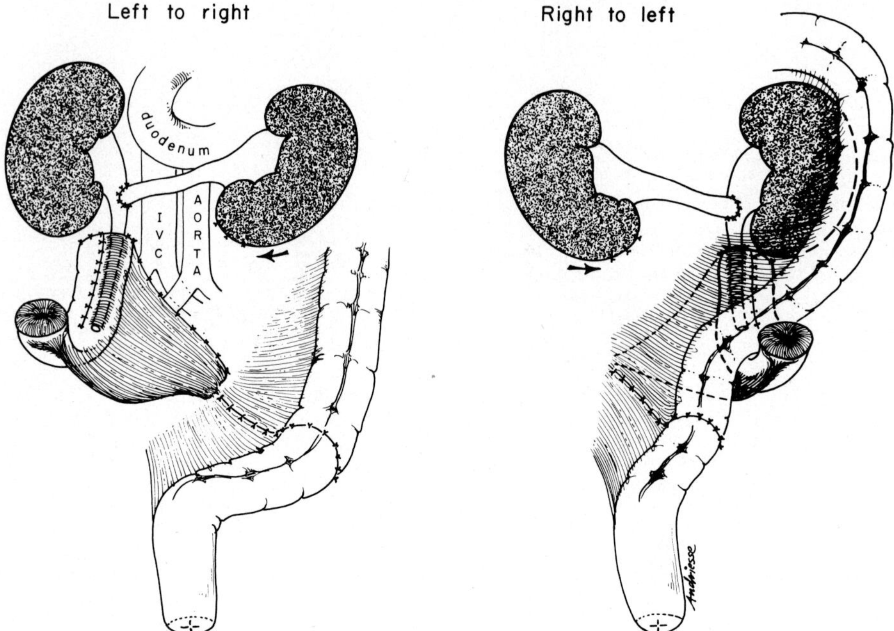

Figure 25–29 A method for colon conduit diversion in patient whose ureters are not suited for two tunneled, nonrefluxing anastomoses.

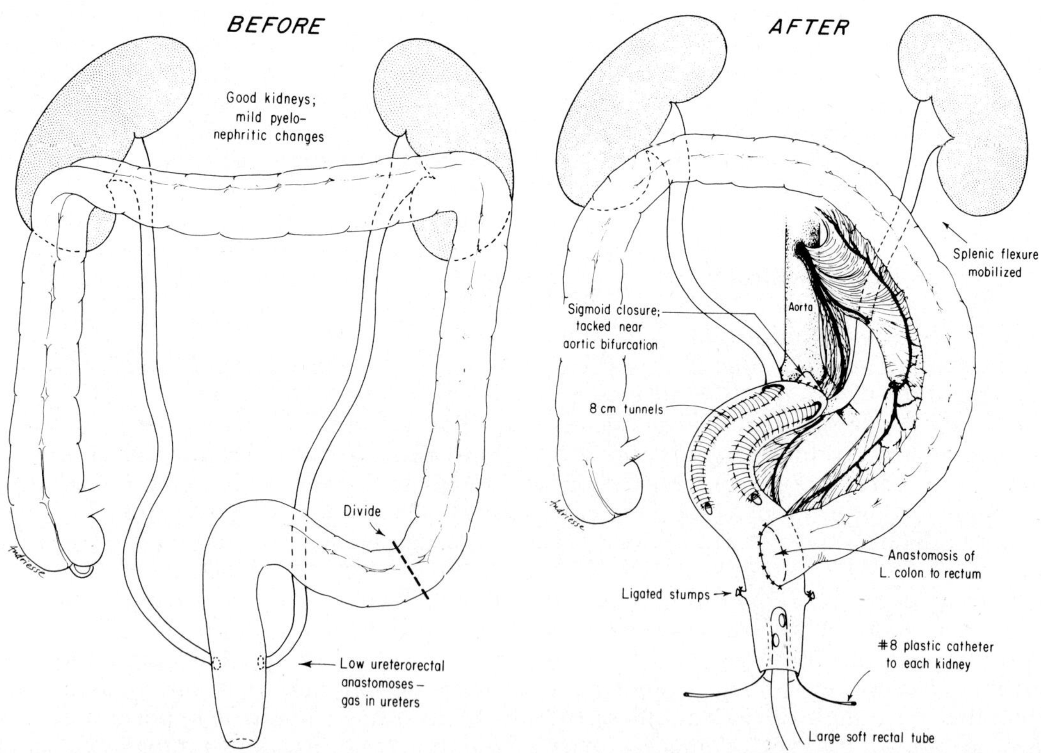

Figure 25–30 Anatomy before and after revision of ureterosigmoidostomies in 25-year-old man with chronic pyelonephritis. Original indication for operation had been exstrophy of the bladder. Because ureters were somewhat dilated and slightly inflamed, it was necessary to construct very long tunnels to stop coloureteral reflux. This was accomplished by the technique shown. In some patients with shorter ureters, a Roux-en-Y limb of colon has been brought to an even higher point in the abdomen to achieve this end.

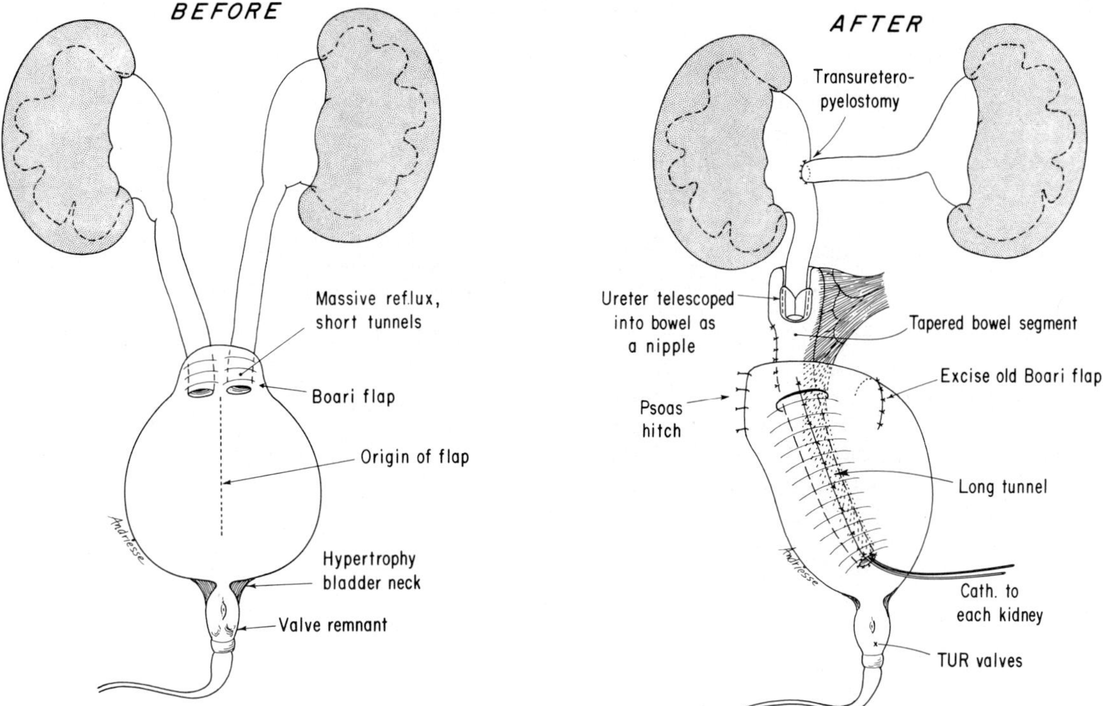

Figure 25–31   Anatomy before and after reconstruction in 24-year-old medical student with recurrent pyelonephritis from massive reflux. Neither ureter was satisfactory for tunneled reimplantation. A tapered segment of small bowel was used as a substitute ureter with long tunneled reimplantation to avert reflux. It is easier to join one ureter to bowel conduit and drain the other as transureteropyelostomy or transureteroureterostomy.

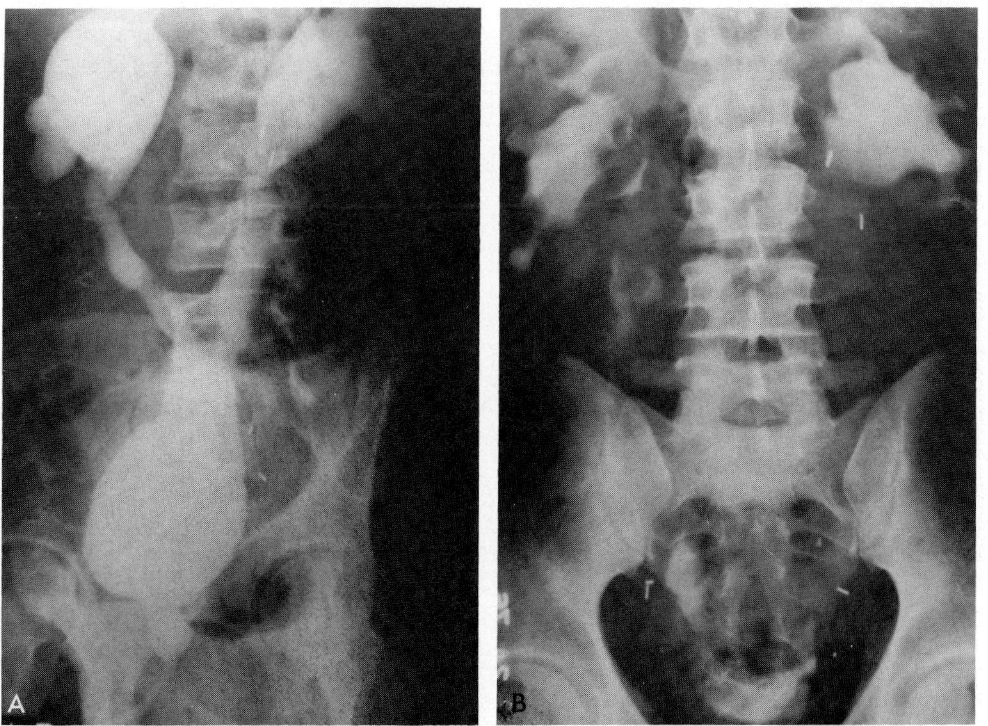

Figure 25–32   Roentgenograms from patient shown in Figure 25–31. *A,* Preoperative cystogram showing massive reflux up the ureters previously implanted into Boari flap. *B,* Intravenous pyelogram after reconstruction. Note less dilated upper tract and tapered bowel conduit visible in the right gutter. Five years postoperatively, the patient is free of infection and actively working full time as a physician.

341

have a very long tunnel (6 to 10 cm) to prevent reflux. Psoas hitch is necessary to accomplish this. A nipple anastomosis of the ureter to the upper conduit will prevent slight reflux from reaching the kidney, but massive reflux will overcome the nipple and reach the kidney. Tapering the caliber of the conduit improves its peristaltic emptying and also facilitates obtaining a satisfactory ratio of tunnel length to "ureter" diameter. The conduit should not be trimmed too narrow lest it become obstructed. Late stenosis is a recognized complication of ileal loop urinary diversion. We have also observed this complication in three patients who had tapered bowel substituting for ureter. There was a diaphragm of mucosa in each. In two, open resection was performed. In one, the diaphragm was incised endoscopically after a telescope was passed up the conduit at cytoscopy. It is futile to attempt tunneling small bowel into a small, fibrotic bladder when a long tunnel implantation is impossible. In such patients, the bladder should be augmented with cecum. The terminal ileum should be intussuscepted for several centimeters to form an antireflux nipple.[26] This is facilitated by removing the mesentery from the segment to be intussuscepted and crosshatching the bowel wall so it will remain intussuscepted. Other techniques we have used have failed to prevent reflux.

CONCLUSION

Most major complications of surgery of the kidneys and ureters are preventable. When complications occur, they can usually be corrected without resorting to nephrectomy or permanent urinary diversion.

References

1. Althausen, A. F., Hagen-Cook, K., and Hendren, W. H.: Non-refluxing colon conduit: Experience with 70 cases. J. Urol. 120:35, 1978.
   Follow-up of complications in colon conduits in children and adults at the Massachusetts General Hospital.
2. Anderson, J. C.: Hydronephrosis: A fourteen years' survey of results. Proc. Roy. Soc. Med. 55:93, 1962.
   Technique and results of dismembering pyeloplasty.
3. Ashcraft, K. W., and Hendren, W. H.: Bladder outlet obstruction after operation for ureterocele. J. Pediatr. Surg. 14:819, 1979.
   Complications resulting from failure to repair the muscle defect in bladder during ureterocele surgery.
4. Belman, A. B., Filmer, R. B., and King, L. R.: Surgical management of duplication of the collecting system. J. Urol. 112:316, 1974.
   Management of duplex systems, including upper pole excision only to defunction ureteroceles when reflux is not present.
5. Bergman, H.: The Ureter. New York, Harper & Row, 1967.
   A book describing diseases of the ureter in which megaureter is not considered a surgical entity. (The second edition, published recently, contains a chapter on repair of megaureter. Bergman, H.: The Ureter. New York, Springer-Verlag, 1981.)
6. Bischoff, P.: Megaureter. Br. J. Urol. 29:416, 1957.
   One of the late Dr. Bischoff's pioneering articles on ureteral modellage to improve emptying. The ureter was not reimplanted with present tunneling technique.
7. Bjordal, R., Eek, S., and Knutrud, O.: Early reconstruction of wide ureter in children. Urology 11:326, 1978.
   An extensive experience from Norway with megaureter repair in young children, with excellent results.
8. Bricker, E. M.: Bladder substitution after pelvic evisceration. Surg. Clin. North Am. 30:1511, 1950.
   Introducing the ileal conduit for urinary diversion.
9. Case Records of the Massachusetts General Hospital. Adrenal carcinoma with sexual precocity. N. Engl. J. Med. 287:1033, 1972.
   Embolization of adrenal tumor that had extended into the vena cava.
10. Crooks, K. K., Hendren, W. H., and Pfister, R. C.: Giant hydronephrosis in children. J. Pediatr. Surg. 14:844, 1979.
    A series of 20 patients with giant hydronephrosis (kidney occupied hemiabdomen, met or crossed midline, and was at least five vertebrae in length), of whom 16 had ureteropelvic obstruction. A reconstructive operation was accomplished in 14 of 20 patients.
11. Culp, O. S., and DeWeerd, J. H.: A pelvic flap operation for certain types of ureteropelvic obstruction: Observations after two years' experience. J. Urol. 71:523, 1954.
    Spiral flap pyeloplasty technique from the Mayo Clinic.
12. Davis, D. M.: Inbubated ureterotomy. Surg. Obstet. Gynecol. 76:513, 1943.
    A technique for managing long, narrow ureteral stenosis (prior to development of current, more reliable methods).
13. Derrick, F. C., Jr.: Management of the large, tortuous, adynamic ureter with reflux. J. Urol. 108:153, 1972.
    Presents a discouraging outlook in megaureter repair, advocating diversion instead.
14. Dretler, S. P., Pfister, R. C., and Newhouse, J. H.:

Renal stone dissolution via percutaneous nephrostomy. N. Engl. J. Med. 300:341, 1979.
Describes the solution hemiacidrin and its dangers, and cites six cases in which it was used successfully.

15. Eckstein, H. B., and Kapila, L.: Cutaneous ureterostomy. Br. J. Urol. 42:306, 1970.
The use of end ureterostomy in children.

16. Foley, F. B.: A new plastic operation for stricture at the ureteropelvic junction. J. Urol. 38:643, 1937.
The Y-V repair of ureteropelvic junction obstruction.

17. Goodwin, W. E., Winter, C. C., and Turner, R. D.: Replacement of the ureter by small intestine: Clinical application and results of the "ileal ureter." J. Urol. 81:406, 1959.
An early paper from UCLA on small bowel "ureter."

18. Hendren, W. H.: Operative repair of megaureter in children. J. Urol. 101:491, 1969.
A series of 45 megaureters in 29 infants and children, operated on from 1960 to 1968, describing technical aspects of tapering and reimplantation.

19. Hendren, W. H.: A new approach to infants with severe obstructive uropathy: Early complete reconstruction. J. Pediatr. Surg. 5:184, 1970.
Early definitive repair in infants as an alternative to "temporary diversion."

20. Hendren, W. H.: Urinary tract refunctionalization after prior diversion in children. Ann. Surg. 180:494, 1974.
Urinary tract undiversion. An experience with 32 children from 1969 to 1974.

21. Hendren, W. H.: Refunctionalizing the urinary tract after prior diversion. Contemp. Surg. Nov. 1975.
Experience in reconstructing 49 prior urinary diversions, in a 6-year period from 1969 to 1975.

22. Hendren, W. H.: Nonrefluxing colon conduit for temporary or permanent urinary diversion in children. J. Pediatr. Surg. 10:381, 1975.
A technique for constructing colon conduit with nonrefluxing ureterocolonic tunnels.

23. Hendren, W. H.: Complications of megaureter repair in children. J. Urol. 113:238, 1975.
A series of 160 megaureters in 14 years, emphasizing complications encountered and their management.

24. Hendren, W. H.: Complications of ureterostomy. J. Urol. 120:269, 1978.
Problems seen in 36 patients referred for reconstructive operations after ureterostomy.

25. Hendren, W. H.: Tapered bowel segment for ureteral replacement. Urol. Clin. North Am. 5:607, 1978.
Tapered small bowel was reimplanted with a tunnel to prevent reflux in 28 patients, with success in 21. Seven had reoperation for reflux. In four, making a longer tunnel solved the problem. In three, ileocecal bladder augmentation was done because the bladders were small and fibrotic.

26. Hendren, W. H.: Reoperative ureteral reimplantation: Management of the difficult case. J. Pediatr. Surg. 15:770, 1980.

A description of various techniques useful in secondary problem cases.

27. Hendren, W. H., and Hensle, T. W.: Transureteroureterostomy: Experience with 75 cases. J. Urol. 123:826, 1980.
A series illustrating the many uses of this procedure and its low rate of complications.

28. Hendren, W. H., and Mitchell, M. E.: Surgical correction of ureteroceles. J. Urol. 121:590, 1979.
Describes the spectrum of ureteroceles and their management based on 73 cases.

29. Hendren, W. H., Radhakrishnan, J., and Middleton, A. W.: Pediatric pyeloplasty. J. Pediatr. Surg. 15:133, 1980.
A series of 153 pyeloplasties in 130 children, stressing technical details of operative correction. In the 17 years of this series, eight other children underwent nephrectomy instead of repair of ureteropelvic obstruction, a rate of 5 per cent.

30. Hodges, C. V., Moore, R. J., Lehman, T. H., and Behnam, A. M.: Clinical experiences with transureteroureterostomy. J. Urol. 90:552, 1963.
One of a series of papers from the University of Oregon that established transureteroureterostomy as an important part of the urologic surgeon's armamentarium.

31. Johnston, J. H.: Temporary cutaneous ureterostomy in the management of advanced congenital urinary obstruction. Arch. Dis. Child. 38:161, 1963.
A paper describing the use of temporary upper-tract diversion in infants with severe hydronephrosis (a technique Mr. Johnston rarely uses today).

32. Johnston, J. H.: Reconstructive surgery of megaureter in childhood. Br. J. Urol. 39:17, 1967.
Mr. Johnston's experience with obstructive megaureter, using terminal resection, tapering, and tunneled reimplantation.

33. Johnston, J. H., Evans, J. P., Glassberg, K. I., et al.: Pelvic hydronephrosis in children: A review of 219 personal cases. J. Urol. 117:97, 1977.
A series of 219 pyeloplasties from the Alder Hey Children's Hospital in Liverpool with 10 per cent nephrectomy rate in children with pyeloureteral obstruction.

34. Kelalis, P. P., Culp, O. S., Stricker, G. B., et al.: Ureteropelvic obstruction in children: Experience with 109 cases. J. Urol. 106:418, 1971.
A series of 109 cases of ureteropelvic junction obstruction in children at the Mayo Clinic, with nephrectomy rate of 24 per cent.

35. Leadbetter, W. F.: Consideration of problems incident to performance of ureteroenterostomy: Report of a technique. J. Urol. 65:818, 1951.
A description of tunneling and direct primary anastomosis of the ureter to colon mucosa as a better method than the Coffey technique, wherein the tip of the ureter was simply dunked into the bowel, where it healed secondarily (or failed to heal and formed an inflammatory pseudopolyp).

36. Middleton, A. W., Jr., and Hendren, W. H.: Ileal conduits in children at the Massachusetts General Hospital from 1955 to 1970. J. Urol. 115:591, 1976.
One of many papers in the literature pointing out the

less than favorable long-term results of ileal loops in children.

37. Mogg, R. A.: The treatment of neurogenic incontinence using the colonic conduit. Br. J. Urol. 37:681, 1965.
    A large and early experience using colon instead of small bowel as a urinary conduit.

38. Perlmutter, A. D., and Patil, J.: Loop cutaneous ureterostomy in infants and young children: Late results in 32 cases. J. Urol. 107:655, 1972.
    Use of loop ureterostomy and subsequent reconstruction in children with severe uropathy.

39. Richie, J. P., Skinner, D. G., and Waisman, J.: The effect of reflux on the development of pyelonephritis in urinary diversion: An experimental study. J. Surg. Res. 16:256, 1974.
    An experimental study in dogs showing a much greater rate of pyelonephritis in renal units diverted by ileal loop (83 per cent) than in those diverted by nonrefluxing colon conduit (7 per cent).

40. Scherer, J. F.: Cryoprecipitate coagulum pyelolithotomy. J. Urol. 123:621, 1980.
    Reviews history of this technique and describes illustrative cases.

41. Skinner, D. G., and Goodwin, W. E.: Indications for the use of intestinal segments in management of nephrocalcinosis. J. Urol. 113:436, 1975.
    An update of the large experience at UCLA in use of small bowel as a substitute "ureter."

42. Smith, E. D.: Follow-up studies on 150 ileal conduits in children. J. Pediatr. Surg. 7:1, 1972.
    An important paper from the Royal Children's Hospital in Melbourne, Australia, emphasizing that deterioration is noted even in once-normal renal units after ileal loop diversion.

43. Smith, E. D., et al.: Report of working party to establish an international nomenclature for the large ureter. Birth Defects: Original Article Series, Vol. 13, No. 5, pp. 3–8. The National Foundation, 1977.
    Classification of various types of megaureter.

44. Sober, I.: Pelvioureterostomy-en-Y. J. Urol. 107:473, 1972.
    A Roux-en-Y technique for ureteral exteriorization.

45. Stephens, F. D.: Treatment of megaureters by multiple micturition. Aust. N. Z. J. Surg. 27:130, 1957.
    A palliative method of managing refluxing megaureters prior to era of reconstructive surgery.

46. Uson, A. C., Cox, L. A., and Lattimer, J. K.: Hydronephrosis in infants and children. II. Surgical management and results. JAMA 205:75, 1968.
    A series of 126 children with hydronephrosis at Babies Hospital in New York. There were 91 pyeloplasties and 45 nephrectomies (36 per cent).

47. Williams, D. I., and Cromie, W. J.: Ring ureterostomy. Br. J. Urol. 47:789, 1975.
    A ring technique for temporary exteriorization of the ureter in children with uropathy.

48. Williams, D. I., and Kenawi, M. M.: The prognosis of pelviureteric obstruction in childhood. A review of 190 cases. Eur. Urol. 2:57, 1976.
    A series of 190 children with ureteropelvic junction obstruction from the Hospital for Sick Children, Great Ormond Street, London, with 4.8 per cent nephrectomy rate.

26

BLADDER AND URETHRA

Lowell R. King, M.D.

Some complications of surgery of the bladder and urethra in children can be avoided by selecting only suitable candidates for each specific procedure. Such selection may mandate a little or a lot of preoperative evaluation. Surgical technique is also of prime importance. Postoperative problems often may be avoided by careful attention to minute details and meticulous postoperative care. Some complications are specific to a particular procedure. This chapter will discuss briefly the indications for operation, alternatives when they exist, important points in the performance of the procedure, how best to check the operation at its completion, and special or specific care needed in the postoperative period.

CYSTOURETHROGRAPHY AND CYSTOSCOPY

Cystourethrography and cystoscopy are diagnostic tools of the utmost importance and usefulness in evaluation of the bladder and urethra. Cystography is usually performed in the awake child. A small polyethylene feeding tube, usually 5 French in infants and 8 French in older children, is lubricated and inserted into the bladder. Small latex Foley catheters are avoided in boys, as they may curl up in the urethra. Subsequent inflation of the balloon may then result in rupture of the urethra. The bladder is filled with contrast material by gravity drip. Spot films are usually made of the full bladder, and the renal fossae are screened fluoroscopically for reflux. When voiding begins, the catheter is quickly removed and oblique views of the urethra are exposed.[39] The upper tracts are checked again for reflux just after voiding. Using this technique, much important information

is obtained.[19] Voiding films are particularly important, since the appearance of various obstructions in the male urethra is often diagnostic, and less specific dilatation of the posterior urethra may give a clue to sphincter dyssynergia in either sex.[3] Residual urine is estimated, although only an empty appearance of the bladder on the postvoiding film is completely reliable. Dysuria resulting from catheterization, or incomplete bladder filling, may be the cause of apparent residual urine that is misleading and inconsistent.

In children, cystoscopy is almost always performed after evaluation of the urinary tract by voiding cystourethrogram and intravenous pyelogram. Because cystoscopy requires that the patient be under general anesthesia, its use is limited. The procedure may be used to evaluate the ureterovesical junction in reflux, to get split cultures to localize infection and check for cystitis cystica or cystitis glandularis in children with otherwise unexplained frequent and recurrent infection, and to prepare the patient for some types of urodynamic studies and for retrograde pyelography. Cystoscopy is sometimes necessary but usually unrewarding in the evaluation of microscopic hematuria when a bladder lesion is not suspected on physical examination or intravenous pyelography, and in the routine evaluation of children with occasional urinary tract infections in whom the aforementioned x-ray studies show no abnormality.

When cystoscopy is elected, it is desirable to obtain as much information from the test as possible. After the child is anesthetized, the urethra and meatus are calibrated with bougies à boule of progressively larger size. The narrowest part of the urethra, usually the meatus or distal urethra in girls[45, 46] and the meatus or urethra near the penoscrotal junction in boys,[2, 54] is noted. Girls are over-dilated to 28 to 32 French to rupture the distal urethral ring in order to obviate this structure as a possible cause of obstruction or "irritation," even though it now seems certain that the distal urethral ring is a normal structure and is unlikely to play a role in the onset or persistence of infection.[23, 35] Overdilatation of the urethra in girls does not add to the morbidity of simple cystoscopy.

If a stricture is encountered in boys, filiforms are employed, and the screw-on Le-Fort following sounds are preferred for dilatation to prevent any risk of urinary extravasation. The male urethra should not be overdilated, as tearing of the tissue results in more scar deposition and worsening of the stricture.

The cystoscope selected should be smaller than the largest bougie and capable of being inserted and withdrawn with ease. The urethra may be inspected as the cystoscope is inserted — a useful technique to visualize a stricture or suspected valve — or, more often, the cystoscope is inserted into the bladder with the obturator in place. Urine is obtained for culture prior to washing the bladder and inserting the lens. The interior of the bladder can then be studied, the ureteral orifices identified, and further tests performed.[9] If split renal cultures are desired to localize infection, the bladder is washed with 2 to 3 liters of sterile water before insertion of catheters to collect urine from the upper tracts. We prefer to evaluate the refluxing orifice by gauging its morphology (stadium, horseshoe, golf-hole configuration), degree of laterality, and width, and by estimating the length of the intravesical ureter by passing a ureteral catheter and comparing the length of elevated intravesical ureter with the centimeter markings on the catheter.[29, 37]

URETHRAL VALVES

Urethral valves in male infants are most simply treated by resection or fulguration endoscopically.[13] This is most safely done by inserting the miniature resectoscope through a perineal urethrostomy, entering the urethra where it is of relatively wide caliber. This prevents stricture formation, which may occur when the delicate urethra of the male infant is traumatized by over-dilatation.

Urethral valves occur in the membranous urethra (posterior urethral valves), the pendulous urethra, and the bulbous urethra. There are several varieties. Posterior urethral valves are most common, and their direct treatment is described in the preceding paragraph. A Young's Type III valve (congenital stricture) is often adequately treated by a single dilatation, rupturing this obstructive membrane.[16] Anterior valves may be resected endoscopically. On occasion the valve may be the anterior lip of a urethral diverticulum that requires open excision, at which time the leaflet is also removed[17] (Fig. 26–1).

The management of urethral valves deserves more than passing comment. The younger the boy at the time of presentation, the more severe the degree of obstruction is apt to be, the more likely is renal dysgenesis, and the more life-threatening is the disease.[33] Valves may be treated directly, as described above, or by temporary urinary diversion to preserve renal potential (especially to permit eradication of infection that persists despite treatment[57]), or by "total reconstruction" of the urinary tract, that is, by valve resection and reimplantation of refluxing or obstructed ureters at the same operation.[26, 27] Deciding which approach to employ in each baby presenting with retention, urinary ascites, or palpable bladder and kidneys is truly the art of pediatric urology.[81]

In general, a direct attack on the valve by transurethral resection is warranted when the urine is uninfected and renal function is adequate, as reflected in a serum creatinine level below 4 mg/dl. If the resection goes smoothly and bleeding is minimal, do not use a catheter postoperatively, thus minimizing the risk of infection. The bladder is often so obstructed that decompensation has occurred. Overflow incontinence may continue for several months before the return of bladder tone eliminates residual urine. If infection intervenes, some form of temporary diversion such as cutaneous vesicostomy may be necessary until the bladder improves.[8]

Reflux is common in conjunction with obstruction due to valves. This is the reason

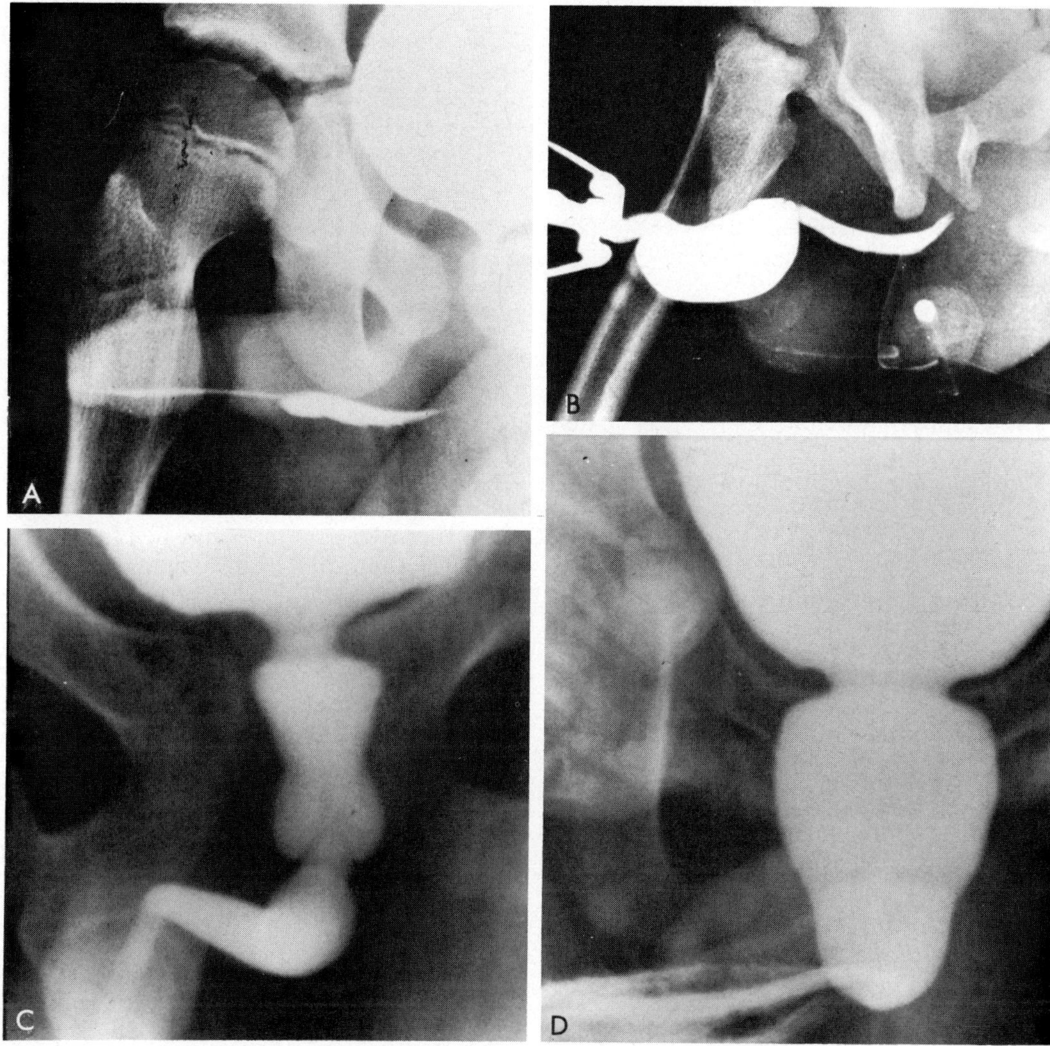

Figure 26–1 Urethral configurations seen with various types of valves. *A,* An anterior urethral valve in the penile urethra seen on a voiding film. Note the poor stream distal to the obstruction. The valve was resected endoscopically. *B,* A retrograde urethrogram demonstrating a large urethral diverticulum. In this instance the anterior lip of the diverticulum moved upward and forward, obstructing the urethra, as urination occurred. This obstructive "valve" was resected when the diverticulum was excised. *C* and *D,* Type I valves, as seen on voiding films. Note the dilatation and elongation of the posterior urethra and, in *D,* the poor stream distal to the valve. Both were resected endoscopically. At cystoscopy, elevation of the bladder neck, with detrusor hypertrophy, is a striking finding. The bladder neck is not the site of obstruction, however.

"total correction" was introduced. The procedure can work exceptionally well, solving all associated problems with a single operation. The drawbacks are that "total correction" is a lengthy operation for a sick infant. If obstruction occurs at the site of ureteral implantation, kidney function may be further impaired. Reflux stops in 50 to 60 per cent of ureters with reflux after the valve is resected. Johnston and Kulatilake[33] have

shown that when reflux continues with reimplantation after obstruction has been relieved, the associated kidney is often dysgenetic or dysplastic and has little potential for function. They believe that the refluxing ureter need be treated only if the residual refluxed urine is the likely cause of persistent infection, and that nephroureterostomy is usually preferable to reimplantation because of the poor kidney function. In this view, total reconstruction is seldom the most reasonable approach. Reflux can be treated specifically if it persists after obstruction is relieved.

Young infants with valves may present with urinary ascites. The bladder is trabeculated and the kidneys hydronephrotic, but renal function is often surprisingly good. Diagnosis of urinary ascites is established by detection of coexisting urinary tract abnormalities and is confirmed by determining the urea nitrogen and creatinine content of the ascitic fluid, which will be greater than similar values in the serum.[70]

It is usually impossible to identify a discrete source of the urinary extravasation radiographically. Intraperitoneal rupture of a bladder diverticulum is an occasional cause, but usually the urine appears to be a transudate, passing out of the collecting system through the thin calyceal musculature near the renal sinus and into the adjacent peritoneum. The perirenal tissues are usually edematous.

The most secure form of treatment is usually bilateral retroperitoneal flank drainage, renal biopsies, and temporary urinary diversion. In these instances, nephrostomy has a definite role when overall renal function is good. The nephrostomy tube introduces infection, but if the valve can be resected within a few days, the tubes may be needed for only a few weeks. Their removal is so much simpler than reversing even a planned temporary upper tract diversion that their interim use should be considered in suitable patients.

Temporary upper tract diversion, such as loop ureterostomy,[57] Roux-en-Y (Sober),[67] or ring ureterostomy,[79] is best employed in children with marked hydronephrosis when infection is present before the valve is discovered and the infection cannot be eradicated, presumably because of the large amount of residual urine. In such patients, valve resection alone will not solve the problem fast enough, as bladder function takes time to recover. Total correction is chancy because of the presence of active infection and the risk that even transient obstruction of the reimplanted ureters, due to postoperative edema, could worsen kidney function. In addition, infection often must be eradicated before upper tract tone will improve. The most reliable way of salvaging this situation is with high, temporary diversion. The high ureteral stoma site minimizes the risk of postoperative residual urine and continuing infection. The externalized segment of the ureter is excised, and ureteral continuity is restored by end-to-end ureteroureterostomy after infection has resolved and renal function has stabilized.

URETHRAL STRICTURE

Stricture of the urethra results in a thin urinary stream and eventually in bladder decompensation and dribbling incontinence. Congenital strictures are often called Type III valves, particularly when they are found in the posterior urethra. These circumferential strictures may be filmy and can often be ruptured by dilatation.[61] When they are thicker, transurethral excision using a miniature resectoscope is required.

Acquired strictures in children are caused by rupture of the urethra due to a fall astride, iatrogenic trauma, or crushing injury. Those seen in conjunction with fracture of the bony pelvis are usually the most severe. Fragments of the pubis sever the urethra at the apex of the prostate. The resulting hematoma elevates the bladder and prostate and widely separates the prostatic apex and urethral stump. The diagnosis is suspected because of the pelvic fracture, blood at the meatus, and mass found on rectal examination. Initial treatment consists of transfusion while the child is being checked for other injuries. After the patient becomes stable, treatment should consist of cytostomy with or without evacuation of the hematoma and realignment of the urethra.[18, 48, 53, 73, 74] In either instance, a stricture will result. However, if the ends can be brought together, the stricture will be shorter, making eventual repair simpler. I favor this approach. A longitudinal extraperitoneal lower midline incision is employed. Clot is evacuated anterior and lateral to the bladder, and the cystostomy tube is inserted. A Foley catheter is then inserted through the urethra, facilitating identification of the transected stump, which will have retracted beneath pubic fragments. After two or three heavy (2-0) chromic sutures are placed in the lateral margins of the urethra and in the ventral midline, the catheter is threaded through the prostate and into the bladder, and the balloon is inflated. The sutures are then continued through the prostatic apex. Gentle pressure on the catheter leads the prostate and bladder to the urethral stump, at which point the sutures are tied. Drains are placed and the wound is closed. The cystostomy is maintained for 4 to 6 months. At that time, simultaneous antegrade and retrograde urethrography delineates the length of the stricture, usually 1 or 2 cm. Several methods of urethroplasty can be employed. I think the most versatile and reliable approach is the technique of Waterhouse and coworkers — transpubic excision of the stricture with mobilization of the distal corpus spongiosum to allow anastomosis of the mobilized urethra to the prostatic apex without tension. Since adequate blood supply for the urethra comes from the glans, the entire urethra can be dissected free of attachments to the corpora cavernosa. Even long strictures (5 to 7 cm in older children) can be bridged in this manner.[76]

A drawback to this operation is that the procedure is carried out in an area in which the anatomy is very distorted owing to the pelvic fracture. Sequestrum may be present. Removal of bone leaves spaces that are not immediately filled by the rigid, inflamed soft tissues. To prevent hematoma, seroma, and resulting infection, Hemovac drains are placed adjacent to the anastomosis. A better method is to fill the "dead space" with omentum to prevent infection. Omentum is quite pliable and vascular, and when detached from the greater curvature of the stomach, as described by Turner-Warwick and Ashken, it will easily reach the operative area.[75]

Short or more distal strictures are easier to treat. First, the extent of the stricture must be accurately defined. This is usually best done by retrograde urethrography performed several weeks or months after dilatation. Short strictures may be incised endoscopically with a miniature scalpel that mounts on the resectoscope and can be moved back and forth with the ratchet arm.[38] Cuts are made through the stricture and across its full length into the corpus spongiosum at three or four points, usually 2, 6, and 10 o'clock in the cytoscopic view (Fig. 26–2). Incisions at the 12 o'clock position, carried into the corpora cavernosa, have been reported to result in chordee, probably because of associated urinary extravasation.

Longer or more dense strictures require open urethroplasty. One- or two-stage techniques may be employed. In the Johansen procedure the stricture is opened longitudinally in the ventral midline.[30] The urethral incision extends at least 1 cm into healthy urethra proximally and distally. The urethra is then marsupialized by sewing the edges of open urethra to adjacent skin edges. This procedure is versatile in that posterior strictures can be marsupialized by turning a flap of perineal skin up to the prostatic apex, approximating healthy

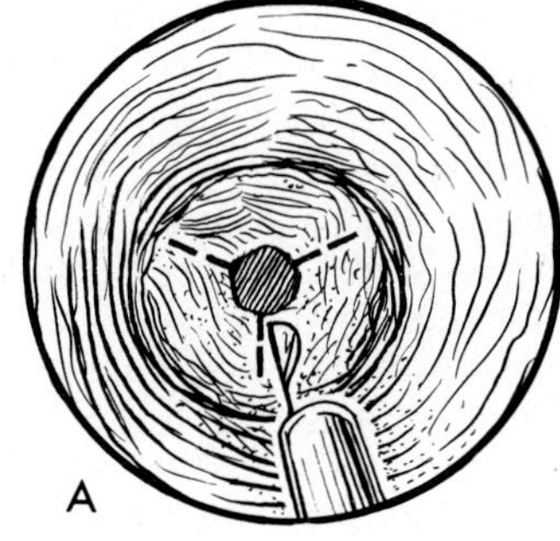
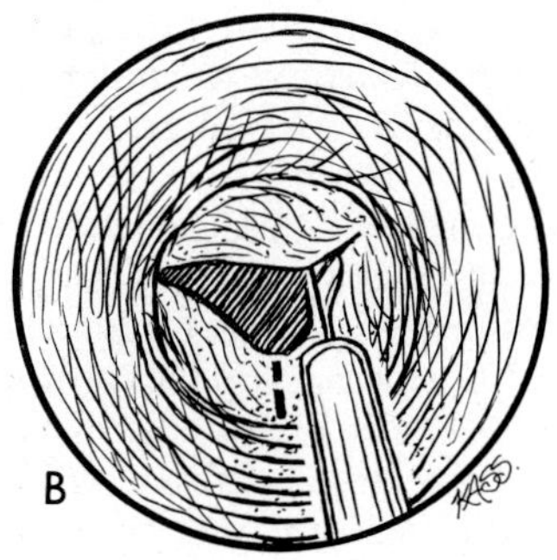

Figure 26–2 *A,* Endoscopic appearance of a urethral stricture, showing incisions to be made under direct vision. *B,* The stricture is being incised at the 2 o'clock position. Incision at the 10 o'clock position has already been performed, followed by incision at the 6 o'clock position.

skin to the opened, strictured posterior urethra.[10, 52, 72] Catheter drainage is employed for a few days postoperatively. Strips of skin parallel to the externalized urethra will be turned in to increase the diameter of the urethra during the second stage. This is done 4 to 6 months after the first operation so that the skin left attached to the urethral strip in the second stage will have developed a good blood supply from the urethra. The interval is used to depilate the skin that will be turned in to form the neourethra and to calibrate the urethral stoma at either end of the open urethral segment. If the stoma is narrow, meatotomy should be done before closure so that the result of the meatotomy can be ascertained before the second stage. In this way, the risk of recurrent stricture is minimized.

At times, when plenty of local skin is available on the penile shaft, a full-thickness island flap graft can be employed to repair a stricture in a single operation. The longitudinal incision used to expose the strictured urethra is 1 cm lateral to the midline, as the midline skin will be turned in to form the ventral portion of the new urethra. The stricture is delineated and opened longitudinally into urethra of normal caliber. A strip of skin in the ventral midline, usually 1.5 cm in uniform width, is outlined and detached at the skin edges, keeping the blood supply intact. The skin surface is rotated 180 degrees as the island graft and is sewn to the edges of the opened urethra. As in all urethral reconstructions, as many layers as possible are approximated over the neourethra, using absorbable suture material or pull-out wires. Closure should be carried out without tension. One simple way to get an extra layer to close, with offset suture lines, is to use Smith's maneuver. A strip of epithelium only is resected along one of the skin edges to be closed to a depth of 4 to 6 mm, leaving the underlying dermis in place. This denuded dermis is sutured to the subcuticular tissue about ½ cm lateral to and below the opposite skin edge. The knots are buried. The epidermis is then closed, resulting in a two-layer closure that helps to minimize fistula formation.[65]

A potent topical antibiotic is applied to the wound beneath the dressing. The urine is diverted by catheter through a perineal urethrostomy or by a suprapubic cystos-tomy, depending on the age and size of the boy.

In infants, indwelling catheters through the urethra, a perineal urethrostomy, or a cystostomy tube almost always induce bladder spasms. When it is important that the child not void across the urethra until healing has occurred, belladonna and opium suppositories, one half given every 4 hours when the child is awake, are a good preventative. Perineal urethrostomy is a comfortable form of urinary drainage and is employed in older boys in whom a Foley catheter of adequate caliber (I like a 14 French or larger) can be inserted.

Cystostomy is a more versatile form of temporary urinary diversion. Intubated cystostomy is employed for 5 to 10 days in most small boys undergoing hypospadias repair as well as after surgical correction of stricture while healing occurs. The procedure is also indicated after rupture of the bladder or urethra, most antireflux surgery, excision of bladder diverticula, and bladder surgery in general.[6] Cystostomy tubes (Pezzer or Malecot catheters) are usually inserted through a relatively small transverse suprapubic incision. The main complications to be avoided are placing the catheter into the peritoneal cavity and kinking the tube within the bladder so that it will not drain properly. Both can be avoided if the catheter is irrigated before the wound is closed. A problem in identifying the bladder is best resolved by filling the bladder through the urethra before it is opened to elevate the peritoneum, which can then be swept off the anterior bladder wall. The filled bladder can also be identified by aspiration. Irrigation before closure, which should yield quantitative fluid return, remains the best way of preventing malfunction of the cytostomy in the postoperative period.

Tubeless or cutaneous vesicostomy is a means of establishing bladder-level drainage without the catheter, which may introduce infection. Since surgical closure of the vesicostomy is necessary, this procedure is occasionally used for extended or medium- to long-term drainage in many different situations in which, for one reason or another, it is deemed desirable to defer definitive surgery. If cutaneous vesicostomy is elected, the dome of the bladder should be brought out on the skin between the pubis and umbilicus. If the anterior wall of the bladder is sutured to the skin, the bladder may prolapse as the child strains. In extreme instances the ureters herniate and upper tract obstruction may result. In performing this operation, the bladder is filled by urethral catheter. The skin incision, a rectangle 3 cm broad and 2 cm high, is centered just below the dome. In children, this skin window is excised. The peritoneum is dissected off the bladder, and the dome is externalized to form a stoma at least 2 cm in diameter. Eventual closure is quite simple, as the bladder need only be detached and returned to the pelvis after the stoma is closed.[8, 14]

URETERAL REIMPLANTATION

Ureteral reimplantation is required in many situations to correct obstruction or reflux. Intrinsic obstruction of the ureter, usually just above the ureterovesical junction, causes ureterectasis and hydronephrosis. Typically the affected ureter is quite dilated but not very tortuous, and it funnels to a bulbous end just above the bladder. Reflux may coexist. When the ureterectasis is segmental and calycectasis is slight or absent, the lesion may be congenital ureterectasis without obstruction, which requires no treatment except surveillance.[20, 68] Generally speaking, the differential diagnosis is made on the basis of presence or absence of a hydronephrotic drip at the time of cystoscopy, drainage time of the dilated segment after retrograde pyelography or on renal scan after furosemide (Lasix) administration,[55] or results of the Whitaker test.[77, 78] During this procedure, the pressure in the dilated upper tract is monitored as fluid passes down the ureter at a high rate (10 ml/min). False negative tests are sometimes

TABLE 26–1 CHARACTERISTICS OF PRIMARY REFLUX DUE TO PARTIAL ABSENCE OF THE INTRAVESICAL URETER

Orifice is open (stadium configuration) or appears as an inverted horseshoe
Short intravesical ureter
Lateral orifice position (large trigone)

encountered after surgery, possibly because progressive maturation of scar tissue worsens obstruction with time. The test is valuable in children who have not been operated on, typically those with the prune-belly syndrome in whom the degree of ureterectasis is often dramatic, even in the absence of obstruction.[20]

VESICOURETERAL REFLUX

Vesicoureteral reflux is much more common than primary obstructive megaureter and until recently was the cause of much debate about which children required surgical correction. First, there are several causes of reflux.[37] Primary reflux, which is congenital, sometimes hereditary, and characterized by absence of part or all of the intravesical ureter, is the most common cause of persistent reflux (Table 26–1). Inflammation due to cystitis can produce reflux in the marginal ureterovesical junction, which is competent in the healthy person and becomes so again after infection is eradicated. Ureters in which the orifice is located in a bladder diverticulum reflux, and paraureteral diverticula may also displace the muscle buttressing the intravesical ureter, resulting in reflux.[4] Loss of the detrusor buttress may also result from iatrogenic causes, neurogenic bladder, thin bladders with deficient musculature as encountered in exstrophy and epispadias, and ectopic ureter.

Different criteria have evolved for the optimal management of reflux. They vary depending on the cause. Cytoscopy is usually needed to ascertain the appearance of the refluxing orifice[44] and its degree of laterality, and to rule out small associated diverticula. The length of intravesical ureter is then estimated by passing a urethral catheter, and the width of the ureter is noted.[29] This is important, since a 4:1 or 5:1 ratio of length to width of the intravesical ureter is necessary to prevent reflux.[56]

When the orifice appears normal, the intravesical ureter is nearly 1 cm long (shorter in infants); gross anatomic changes are absent; and reflux is likely to be mild (no hydronephrosis on intravenous pyelogram) or due to cystitis, causing reduced compliance in the roof of the intravesical ureter, which in the healthy person functions as a flap valve to prevent reflux. Often only surveillance is necessary, as such reflux usually stops soon after the infection is eradicated. Ureters entering diverticula or associated with large paraureteral diverticula require reimplantation, as do ectopic ureters and those continuing to reflux 6 to 12 months after previous surgery, as such reflux will be lifelong. There is little suggestion and no convincing evidence that sterile reflux, in the absence of obstruction, adversely affects renal growth or damages renal function. However, continuing reflux does predispose to infection and requires surveillance and follow-up, which becomes tedious and impractical.

One can, however, make a strong case for nonoperative management of some children with primary reflux characterized by absence of part, but not all, of the intravesical ureter and infection that can be eradicated, or prevented, while one waits to see whether growth of the intravesical ureter will correct the reflux. This happens in at least 60 per cent of such patients. Relative indications for early antireflux surgery or a trial of nonoperative surveillance to see whether reflux will stop are listed in Table 26–2. The results, judged in terms of progressive renal scarring, are now statistically similar. One can therefore make a stronger case for early antireflux surgery than one could in the recent past, when the complication rate was clearly lower in those patients who were given antibacterial prophylaxis

when there seemed some chance on cystoscopic evaluation that reflux would stop before full growth was achieved. Series vary, but further renal scars are now seen in only 1 to 5 per cent of children managed in either fashion.

The principles of antireflux surgery are applicable when the ureteral reimplantation is performed for obstruction, for reflux, or for ureteral ectopia. Whenever possible, urinary tract infection should be eradicated well before such surgery, as results are better when there is no active inflammation at the time of the operation. A transverse incision, which is eventually concealed by pubic hair, can usually be employed. The incision should be generous to permit easy exploration of the lateral perivesical spaces. When dealing with a very dilated or tortuous ureter, a midline incision is preferable because it can be extended as needed to permit dissection of the lower ureter with careful preservation of its blood supply.[28]

Several techniques of ureteral implantation are in general use. These include an extravesical procedure (Lich-Grégoir), which has the advantage that the bladder is not opened.[5] Hematuria or urine leakage from the incision is therefore unlikely, and the patient often may be discharged 2 to 4 days after surgery. This procedure is not applicable when ureterectasis is extreme or when the ureter is obstructed.

Transvesical advancements of the ureter (Glenn)[21, 22] are simple in concept and execution and may be combined with incision

TABLE 26–2 MANAGEMENT OF PRIMARY REFLUX

Indications for Early Operative Correction	Indications for Trial of Nonoperative Management
Relatively wide ureter with short submucosal segment or golf-hole orifice	Relatively long intravesical ureter
Older child (not much growth potential remaining)	Infant or younger child
Noncompliant patient Fails to return for follow-up visits Won't take medications	Returns readily for urine checks
Recurrent urinary tract infections, especially if these are not symptomatic	No recurrent infections when receiving prophylactic chemotherapeutic antibacterial agent (antibiotics not required)

of the detrusor cephalad to the ureteral hiatus (the opening in the detrusor through which the ureter passes) to move the new hiatus rostrally and thereby increase the intravesical length that can be achieved (Stephens, Anderson and Glenn)[69] (Fig. 26–3). Nonetheless, length-to-width measurements of the new intravesical ureter are marginal when these procedures are employed with widely dilated ureters. When the ureter is 1 cm or more wide in its collapsed state (20 French), other procedures are more reliable in preventing reflux. The Politano-Leadbetter procedure, modified so that the ureter is detached, identified, and dissected extravesically, permits construction of a longer intravesical tunnel because the ureter is drawn through an entirely new hiatus above and medial to the original site. Problems with this approach are avoided by placing the new hiatus properly. It should not be on the lateral bladder wall, and the

course through the detrusor should be straight.[27, 58, 59] To prevent partial obstruction by angulation, the umbilical and hypogastric arteries overlying the mobilized urether should be divided between ligatures.[24]

Another approach to implantation is that of Cohen and Ahmed.[1] In this operation the ureter is mobilized intravesically or extravesically. Often, the original hiatus can be preserved. The ureter is implanted transversely across the bladder base, so the length of the intravesical ureter is not limited to the distance between the hiatus and the bladder neck. When the original hiatus can be preserved, the risk of postoperative obstruction due to compression or angulation of the ureter is minimized (Fig. 26–4).

When the ureter is grossly dilated, some tapering of the portion that is to become the new intravesical segment is necessary. The dilated ureter is more subject to ischemic

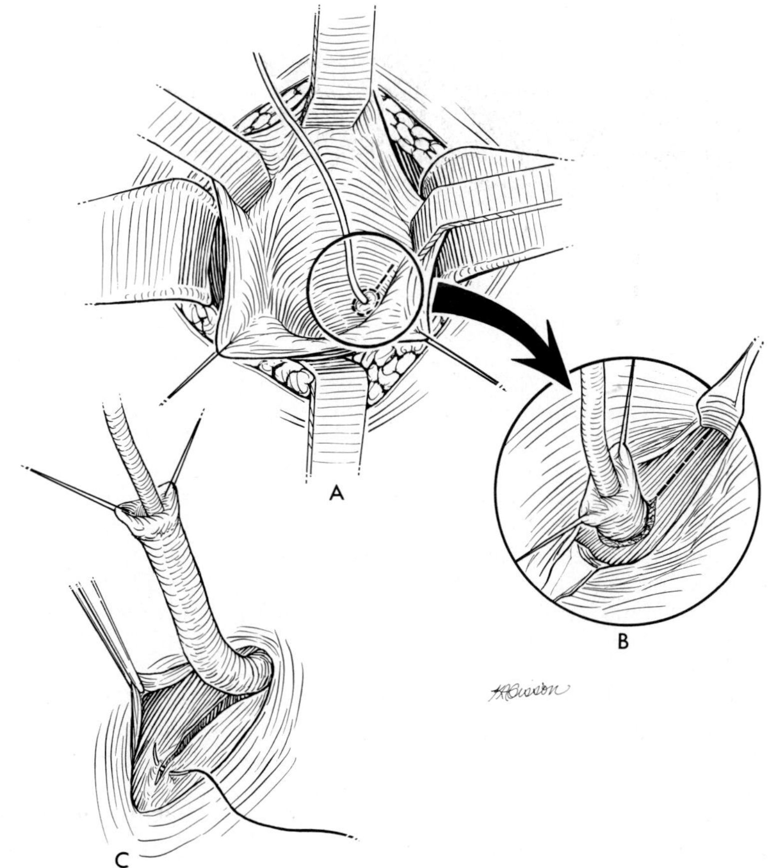

Figure 26–3 The Stephens recession-advancement technique of ureteral reimplantation. The bladder has been exposed through a transverse suprapubic incision and opened in the anterior midline. *A,* The orifice of the ureter to be reimplanted is circumscribed, and the mucosal incision is extended rostrally in the axis of the ureter *(B).* *C,* The detached ureter slides freely into the bladder within Waldeyer's fascia. The original hiatus is closed, moving the ureter's point of entry cephalad to gain greater intravesical length.

Illustration continued on following page

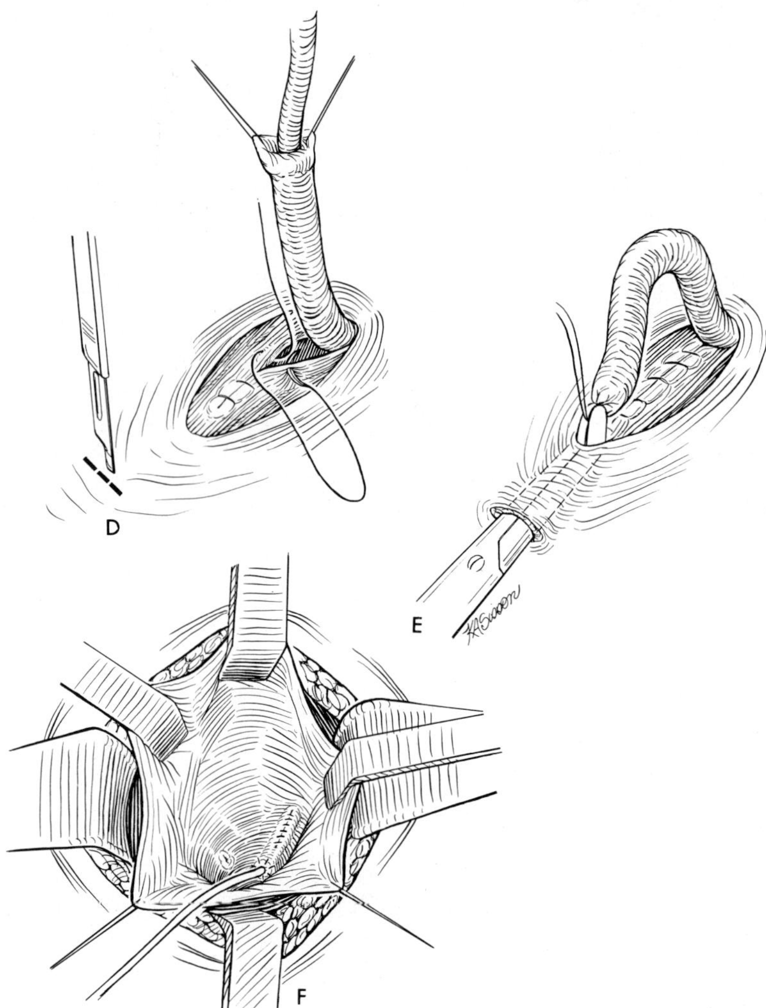

Figure 26–3 *Continued.* *D,* A new orifice site, near the bladder neck, is chosen. *E,* The ureter is placed in the new submucosal tunnel, and mucosal edges are reapproximated. *F,* The reimplantation is completed. This technique is not suited to implantation of the grossly dilated ureter in which tapering is needed to achieve an adequate intravesical ratio of length to width.

stenosis than is a ureter of near-normal caliber. Transvesical or extravesical mobilization may be employed, but special care must be exercised to preserve the adventitia and blood supply.[71] Only the portion to be transposed into the bladder need be straightened or tapered. If obstruction and reflux are prevented, the ureter of the growing child will narrow and align with time.[62] Upper tapering is seldom required.

Tapering may be done around a catheter — usually 12 French — by trimming away the excess ureter and closing the edges with a running 5-0 chromic stitch. The adventitia is loosely approximated over the closure line with another suture. The tapered segment is then implanted into the bladder using the Politano or Cohen technique, orienting the suture line in the urether against the underlying detrusor.[25, 27] A ureteral stent, generally a 10 French polyethylene feeding tube, is usually left in place for 6 to 10 days when the ureter has been tapered. Other types of reimplantation, in which the ureter is not tapered, may also be stented, but this is seldom required. A stent probably does no harm, but it will not correct a surgical misadventure such as a problem with ureteral angulation. Passage of a catheter into the newly reimplanted ureter, however, is a useful test at the conclusion of surgery. With retractors out of the bladder, the stent should pass easily. Difficulty in negotiating the new hiatus suggests J-hooking, which should be investigated and corrected before the

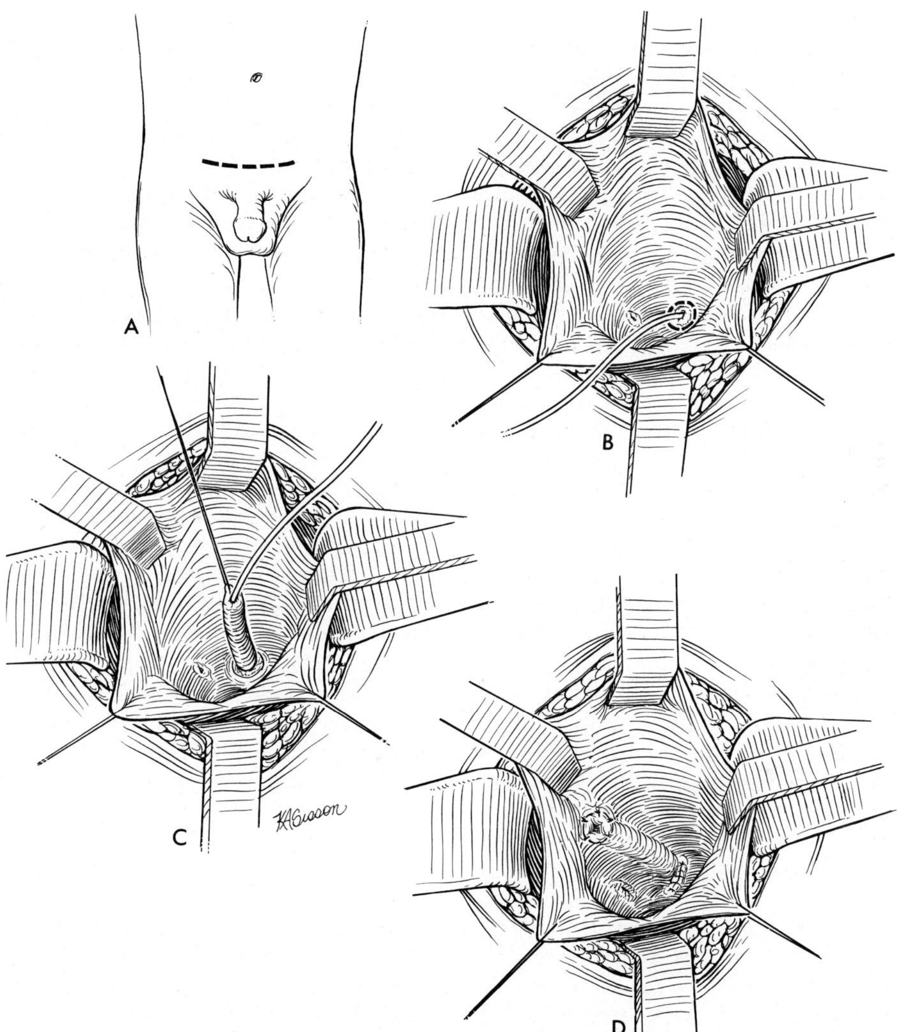

Figure 26–4   The Cohen-Ahmed technique of ureteral reimplantation. *A,* The bladder is exposed through a transverse suprapubic incision, and the anterior bladder wall is opened longitudinally. *B,* The refluxing orifice is circumscribed, and the ureter is mobilized intravesically, retaining the original vesical hiatus *(C)*. *D,* A submucosal tunnel is developed in transverse fashion, and the ureter is transposed across the bladder base to gain needed length. The contralateral ureter is avoided or, if both ureters are to be reimplanted, one is placed above the other. Since the original hiatus is preserved, the chance of extravesical obstruction due to angulation is minimized. Dilated ureters may be tapered and reimplanted in this manner.

wound is closed. Catheter drainage of the bladder is needed until the urine becomes grossly clear.

EXSTROPHY OF THE BLADDER

Exstrophy of the bladder has been termed the ultimate challenge in pediatric urology. The bladder is open on the lower abdominal wall, the pubis is separated, and the penis is short and stubby.[50] In the early days of exstrophy surgery, the immediate challenge was to close the bladder in a way that incorporated enough relief of tension on the abdominal wall reconstruction for healing to occur without bladder dehiscence.[42, 66] This was solved in various ways. For example, large flaps of external oblique fascia based on the edge of the defect through which the open bladder protruded could be turned back upon themselves to permit tension-free closure of the abdominal defect.[51] Later, posterior iliac osteotomies at the time of the bladder closure were used to facilitate abdominal wall repair while also correcting, to some extent, the tendency to a waddling gait seen in children with exstrophy.

Other major problems of children with exstrophy are urinary control and, in boys, penile length. These are solved, in many patients, by a two-stage reconstruction technique employed with success by Jeffs in a large series.[34] In brief, the bladder is closed when the child is first seen. This often means that posterior iliac osteotomies and bladder closure are performed within a few days or a week after birth. Such early surgery probably has no effect on the eventual outcome so far as continence is concerned, but the osteotomy is certainly easier, and early closure simplifies the baby's care. No attempt is made to form a urinary sphincter or produce continence at this stage. The bladder neck is left open and the epispadias is left unrepaired. In male patients, the penis is lengthened using Duckett's maneuver, in which the dorsal urethral plate is divided and the corpora cavernosa are dissected free toward their base, detaching them from the separated pubic bones.[15, 36] The length thus achieved is preserved by suturing the corpora together in the midline. Mucosa-like skin from the inferior mar-

gins of the exstrophy is then used to cover the dorsal proximal portion of the newly lengthened penis. Ureteral catheters and cytostomy drainage are employed in the postoperative period to keep the wound as dry as possible during healing.

The second procedure is usually performed when the child is about 4 years of age. If the bladder is very small, urinary diversion or some type of cytoplasty is required. Most children, however, are candidates for the usual second-stage bladder reconstruction, which involves formation of a tube of bladder muscle from the posterior trigone to serve as a sphincter, antireflux reimplantation of the ureters above the trigonal tube, epispadias repair, and revision of the abdominal wall closure. The bladder is opened through a midline incision that is extended inferiorly into the open urethra. Any sizable bladder diverticula are removed and the ureters are detached. The trigone is measured, and a strip 35 mm long and 18 mm wide, beginning above the urethra, is outlined by sutures or a marking pencil. The mucosa of the strip is rolled into a tube after the lateral mucosa of the trigone has been removed. The denuded muscle is then incised laterally at right angles at the proximal end of the tubularized mucosa, which becomes the bladder neck, and the muscle flaps so formed are then imbricated over the mucosal tube so that the newly formed sphincter is snug around a 12 French catheter.[32, 43, 80]

The ureters are then implanted into the posterior bladder wall using the Cohen technique so that an adequate length-to-width ratio is achieved to prevent reflux. Ureteral stents are usually employed again, and the bladder is closed around a cystostomy tube. Urethral length is maintained by urethral suspension, sewing the adventitia near the bladder neck to the rectus muscle and adjacent fascia as the bladder is closed.[51]

Attention is turned next to the epispadias. In girls, the labia are approximated over the urethra after removal of the triangle of skin in the midline that separates them. A good cosmetic result is easily achieved. In boys, an artificial erection should be effected to ascertain that reverse (dorsal) chordee has been corrected by lengthening of the penis. If chordee persists, it should be corrected by removal of ellipses of corpora cavernosa from the ventral aspect of the penis or by Z-plasty before the urethroplasty is performed. If the penis is straight, a strip of dorsal midline penile skin is outlined and rolled into a tube, carrying the meatus to the tip of the glans. Glandular tissue and the corpora cavernosa are approximated over the newly formed urethra, giving the penis its normal cylindrical appearance and covering the urethra with a thick layer of healthy tissue that will help to prevent fistula formation. The foreskin, represented by a ventral hood, is detached at the corona, unrolled, and transposed to the dorsum of the penis to cover the distal penile shaft, helping to provide needed coverage to preserve penile length.[31] Proximally, the lateral skin edges are approximated in the midline. Cytostomy drainage is usually maintained for about 21 days to give the urethra and sphincter a chance to heal solidly. The cystostomy catheter is clamped before removal to ascertain that the child can void. If passage of urine is difficult, the new urethra can be gently dilated using filiforms and following sounds under cystoscopic control.

When this technique is used, about 40 per cent of children with exstrophy achieve near-normal urinary control, about 20 per cent have very good control for a limited period, and 20 per cent have some usable control. In 20 per cent of patients the procedure is an outright failure owing to incontinence or urinary obstruction.[34] When renal function is normal, or nearly normal, patients in the last group are often best treated by ureterosigmoidostomy. The pitfalls of this procedure are discussed in Chapter 25. Suffice it to say that since most children with exstrophy have normal function of the anal sphincter (although the anus is often somewhat anterior), urinary control can be achieved in this manner.

Ureterosigmoidostomy is also the primary mode of therapy in babies in whom the exstrophic bladder is too small to close with expectation of adequate reservoir capacity — less than 25 mm wide at birth, in my opinion. Other approaches to the management of such small bladders deserve mention. One attractive idea is to divert the urine by antirefluxing sigmoid conduit while elongating the bladder and rolling it into a tube 18 to 20 mm in diameter

(French). During the second stage, after the sigmoid conduit has been tested to be certain no reflux is present, the distal end of the conduit is detached from the skin and anastomosed to the proximal end of the tubularized bladder.[5] Control is often achieved, perhaps partly because the sigmoid conduit is a relatively low pressure system. Abdominal muscle contraction and Valsalva maneuver are needed to initiate voiding. Thus, the sphincter mechanism required may need not to exert as strong and exact an amount of tone as when the bladder is used as a reservoir.

The principles of the Young-Dees-Leadbetter incontinence procedure were outlined earlier in conjunction with exstrophy reconstruction.[12, 40, 43] The procedure is also applicable in children with incontinence due to epispadias without exstrophy and in girls with absence of the urethra in whom bladder innervation is normal. In the Young-Dees operation the ureters are not reimplanted, as the tube of trigonal muscle rolled to form the sphincter consists of the distal trigone only. Many children with epispadias reflux. Ureteral reimplantation is often required even when the trigone is of adequate length. I prefer to make the new sphincter from a strip of mucosa 4 cm long and 18 to 20 mm wide, with the muscle flaps fabricated to make the closure tight around a 12 French catheter. The urethra is suspended as described earlier to maintain urethral length.

Implantable artificial urinary sphincters can be employed with good expectation of success in older children who are incontinent. Such devices are usually used in children whose incontinence is due to neurogenic bladder (typically a result of myelomeningocele or sacral agenesis), but they may also be used as an alternative to the incontinence procedures discussed previously in patients with potentially normal bladder function. The Scott prosthesis has been in use the longest.[64, 65] It consists of an inflatable cuff that is placed around the bladder neck. This is connected to inflation and deflation pumps and a fluid reservoir by a series of valves. The pumps are placed in the labia or scrotum, while the reservoir lies above the bladder in the subcutaneous fat. As the inflation bulb is compressed, fluid is pumped from the reservoir into the cuff at the mouth of the bladder, obstructing the urethra and producing continence. The reverse pump deflates the cuff and permits voiding. When employed in suitable candidates — those with total incontinence who leak urine from an empty bladder — a 70 per cent continence rate has been achieved at several different centers.[11] Thus, the artificial sphincter complements intermittent catheterization in the management of children with neurogenic bladder. When urinary retention is present, intermittent catheterization works very well and produces continence. In those who are totally incontinent, artificial sphincters are becoming attractive alternatives to urinary diversion.[41, 47] Mechanical sphincters are being simplified and made more durable, so improved results can be expected shortly.

CLOACAL ANOMALIES

A word should be said about cloacal anomalies and persistence of the urogenital sinus, which often results in infravesical urinary obstruction in female infants.

In simple hydrocolpos the urethra and distal vagina may share a common channel, the urogenital sinus, as the upper vagina is blocked by a transverse septum. The bladder is displaced anteriorly and inferiorly by the distended vagina, and hydronephrosis is often present. Early treatment consists of decompression of the distended vagina by vaginostomy and perforation or excision of the obstructing vaginal septum or by posterior vaginal pull-through, preserving the urogenital sinus as the urethra. The short urethra may result in urinary incontinence, which then must be treated when the child is 3 or 4 years old. Ectopic ureters and associated ureteroceles may necessitate ureteral implantation into the bladder or, if renal function is very limited, urinary diversion. Double collecting systems are often present. Nonfunction of one or more renal segments may mandate heminephroureterectomy.

Cloacal anomalies are diverse. The urethra, vagina, and rectum may enter the common cloaca at various levels; the vagina and rectum may join proximal to the point of entry of the urethra; or either the vagina or the rectum may be blind.[7] Treatment must be individualized. Injection of contrast material into the cloaca often reveals the point of entry of vagina and rectum. Pyelography is helpful in delineating the degree of hydronephrosis, the number of ureters, and the probable site of the ureteral orifices.

Raffensperger has shown that early total correction of these anomalies minimizes morbidity and mortality.[60] Combined vaginal and rectal pull-throughs are performed, and the urinary tract is reconstructed if compromised in some way other than simple compression by the dilated vagina. Residual urinary incontinence is not corrected surgically until the child is 3 or 4 years old.

References

1. Ahmed, S.: Ureteral reimplantation by the transverse advancement technique. J. Urol. 119:547, 1978.
2. Allen, J. S.: Meatal calibration of newborn boys. J. Urol. 107:498, 1972.
3. Allen, T. D.: Non-neurogenic neurogenic bladder. J. Urol. 117:232, 1977.
4. Amar, A. D.: Vesicoureteral reflux associated with congenital bladder diverticulum in boys and young men. J. Urol. 107:966, 1972.
5. Arap, S., Cabral, A. D., and DeCamposFreire, J. G.: The extra-vesical anti-reflux plasty: Statistical analysis. Urol. Int. 26:241, 1971.
6. Bauer, S. B., and Retik, A. B.: Bladder diverticula in infants and children. Urology 3:712, 1975.
7. Belman, A. B., and King, L. R.: Urinary tract abnormalities associated with imperforate anus. J. Urol. 108:823, 1972.
8. Belman, A. B., and King, L. R.: Vesicostomy: A useful means of reversable urinary diversion in selected infants. Urology 1:208, 1973.
9. Berci, G., Getzoff, P. L., and Kont, L. A.: An improved concept in optics applied to cystoscopy. J. Urol. 104:542, 1970.
10. Blandy, J. P., Singh, M., and Tresidder, G. C.: Urethroplasty by scrotal flaps for long urethral strictures. Br. J. Urol. 40:261, 1968.
11. Cook, W. A., Babcock, J. R., Swenson, O. S., and King, L. R.: Incontinence in children. Urol. Clin. North Am. 5:353, 1978.
12. Dees, J. E.: Congenital epispadias with incontinence. J. Urol. 62:513, 1979.
13. Duckett, J. W.: Current management of posterior urethral valves. Urol. Clin. North Am. 1:471, 1974.
14. Duckett, J. W., Jr.: Cutaneous vesicostomy in childhood: The Blocksom technique. Urol. Clin. North Am. 1:485, 1974.
15. Duckett, J. W., Jr.: Epispadias. Urol. Clin. North Am. 5:107, 1978.
16. Field, P. L., and Stephens, F. D.: Congenital urethral membranes causing urethral obstruction. J. Urol. 111:250, 1974.

17. Firlit, C. F., and King, L. R.: Anterior urethral valves in children. J. Urol. 108:972, 1972.
18. Gibson, G. R.: Urological management and complications of fractured pelvis and ruptured urethra. J. Urol. 111:353, 1974.
19. Gildersleeve, S., and Poznanski, A. K.: A simple technique for obtaining voiding urethrograms in children. Radiology 131:538, 1979.
20. Glassberg, K. I.: Dilated ureter — classification and approach. Urology 9:1, 1977.
21. Glenn, J. F., and Anderson, E. E.: Distal tunnel ureteral reimplantation. J. Urol. 97:623, 1967.
22. Gonzales, E. T., Glenn, J. F., and Anderson, E. E.: Results of distal tunnel ureteral reimplantation. J. Urol. 107:572, 1972.
23. Graham, J. B., King, L. R., and Kropp, K. A.: The significance of distal urethral narrowing in young girls. J. Urol. 97:1045, 1967.
24. Hendren, W. H.: Reoperation for the failed ureteral reimplantation. J. Urol. 111:403, 1974.
25. Hendren, W. H.: Complications of ureteral reimplantation and megaureter repair. *In* Smith, R. B., and Skinner, D. G. (eds.): Complications of Urologic Surgery. Philadelphia, W. B. Saunders Co., 1976, pp. 151–208.
26. Hendren, W. H.: Complications of urethral valve surgery. *In* Smith, R. B., and Skinner, D. G. (eds.): Complications of Urologic Surgery. Philadelphia, W. B. Saunders Co., 1976, pp. 303–335.
27. Hendren, W. H.: Reconstructive surgery of the urinary tract in children. Curr. Probl. Surg., May 1977.
28. Hodgson, N. B., and Thompson, L. W.: Technique of reductive ureteroplasty in the management of megaureter. J. Urol. 113:118, 1975.
29. Ireland, G. W., and Cass, A. S.: The clinical measurement of the ureteral submucosal tunnel. J. Urol. 107:564, 1972.
30. Johansen, B.: Reconstruction of the male urethra in strictures. *In* E. W. Riches (ed.): Modern Trends in Urology. London, Butterworth & Co., 1953, pp. 344–357.
31. Johnston, J. H.: The genital aspects of exstrophy. J. Urol. 113:701, 1975.
32. Johnston, J. H., and Kogan, S. J.: The exstrophic anomalies and their surgical correction. Curr. Probl. Surg., August 1974.
33. Johnston, J. H., and Kulatilake, A. E.: The sequelae of posterior urethral valves. Br. J. Urol. 43:743, 1971.
34. Jeffs, R. D.: Exstrophy and cloacal exstrophy. Urol. Clin. North Am. 5:127, 1978.
35. Kelalis, P. P.: Distal urethral stenosis. Mayo Clin. Proc. 54:690, 1979.
36. Kelley, J. H., and Eraklis, A. J.: A procedure for lengthening of the phallus in boys with exstrophy of the bladder. J. Pediatr. Surg. 6:645, 1971.
37. King, L. R., Kazmi, S. O., and Belman, A. B.: Natural history of vesicoureteral reflux. Urol. Clin. North Am. 1:441, 1974.
38. Kirchheim, D., Tremann, J. A., and Ansell, J. S.: Transurethral urethrotomy under vision. J. Urol. 119:496, 1978.
39. Kjellberg, S. R., Ericsson, N. O., and Rudhe, V.: The Lower Urinary Tract in Childhood: Some Correlated Clinical and Roentgenographic Observations. Chicago, Year Book Medical Publishers, 1957.
40. Klauber, G. T., and Williams, D. I.: Epispadias and incontinence. J. Urol. 111:110, 1974.
41. Lapides, J., Diokno, A. C., Gould, F., et al.: Further observations on self-catheterization. J. Urol. 116:169, 1976.
42. Lattimer, J. K., and Smith, M. J. V.: Exstrophy closure: A followup on 70 cases. J. Urol. 95:356, 1966.
43. Leadbetter, G. W., Jr.: Urethral reconstruction for incontinence in children. *In* Johnston, J. H., and Goodwin, W. E. (eds.): Reviews in Pediatric Urology. Princeton, Excerpta Medica, 1974, pp. 117–130.
44. Lyon, R. P., Marshall, S., and Tanaglo, E. E.: The ureteral orifice: Its configuration competency. J. Urol. 102:504, 1969.
45. Lyon, R. P., and Marshall, S.: Urinary tract infections and difficult urination in girls: Long-term followup. J. Urol. 105:314, 1971.
46. Lyon, R. P., and Smith, D. R.: Distal urethral stenosis. J. Urol. 89:414, 1963.
47. Lyon, R. P., Scott, M. P., and Marshall, S.: Intermittent catheterization rather than urinary diversion in children with myelomeningocele. J. Urol. 113:409, 1975.
48. Malek, R. S., O'Dea, M. J., and Kelalis, P. O.: Management of ruptured posterior urethra in childhood. J. Urol. 117:105, 1977.
49. Marshall, V. F., Marchetti, A. A., and Krantz, K. E.: The correction of stress incontinence by simple vesicourethral suspension. Surg. Gynecol. Obstet. 88:509, 1949.
50. Marshall, V. F., and Muecke, E. C.: Variations of exstrophy of the bladder. J. Urol. 88:766, 1962.
51. Marshall, V. F., and Muecke, E. C.: Functional closure of typical exstrophy of the bladder. J. Urol. 104:205,1970.
52. McGuire, E. J., and Weiss, R. M.: Serotal flap urethroplasty for strictures of the deep urethra in infants and children. J. Urol. 110:599, 1973.
53. Morehouse, A. D., Belitsky, P., and MacKinnon, K. J.: Rupture of the posterior urethra. J. Urol. 107:255, 1974.
54. Morton, H. G.: Meatus size in 1,000 circumcised boys from two weeks to sixteen years of age. J. Fla. Med. Assoc. 50:137, 1963.
55. O'Reilly, P. H., Testa, H. J., Lawson, R. S., et al.: Diuresis renography in equivocal urinary tract obstruction. Br. J. Urol. 50:76, 1978.
56. Paquin, A. J., Jr.: Ureterovesical anastomosis: The description and evaluation of a technique. J. Urol. 82:573, 1959.
57. Perlmutter, A. D., and Tank, E. S.: Loop cutaneous ureterostomy in infancy. J. Urol. 99:559, 1968.
58. Politano, V. A., and Leadbetter, W. F.: An operative technique for the correction of vesicoureteral reflux. J. Urol. 79:931, 1958.
59. Politano, V. A.: One hundred reimplantations and five years. J. Urol. 90:696, 1963.

60. Raffensperger, J. G.: Anomalies of the female genitalia. *In* Kelalis, P. P., and King, L. R. (eds.): Clinical Pediatric Urology. Philadelphia, W. B. Saunders Co., 1976, pp. 669–679.

61. Robertson, W. B., and Hayes, J. A.: Congenital diaphragmatic obstruction of the male posterior urethra. Br. J. Urol. 41:592, 1969.

62. Robinowitz, R., Bartin, M., Schillinger, J. F., et al.: The influence of etiology on the surgical management and prognosis of the massively dilated ureter in children. J. Urol. 119:808, 1978.

63. Scott, F. B.: The artificial sphincter in the management of incontinence in the male. Urol. Clin. North Am. 5:375, 1978.

64. Scott, F. B., Bradley, W. E., and Timms, G. W.: Treatment of urinary incontinence by an implantable prosthetic urinary sphincter. J. Urol. 112:75, 1974.

65. Smith, D.: A de-epithelialized overlap, flap technique in the repair of hypospadias. Br. J. Plast. Surg. 26:106, 1973.

66. Smith, M. J. V., and Lattimer, J. K.: The management of bladder exstrophy. Surg. Gynecol. Obstet. 123:1015, 1966.

67. Sober, I.: Pelvioureterostomy-en-Y. J. Urol. 107:473, 1972.

68. Stephens, F. D.: The ABC of megaureters. Birth Defects Original Article Series 5:1–8, 1977.

69. Stephens, F. D.: The vesicoureteral hiatus and paraureteral diverticula. Trans. Am. Assoc. Genitourin. Surg. 70:47, 1978.

70. Sullivan, M. J., Lackner, L. H., and Banowsky, L. H. W.: Intraperitoneal extravasation of urine BUN/serum creatinine disproportion. JAMA 221:491, 1972.

71. Tanagho, E. A.: Ureteral tailoring. J. Urol. 106:194, 1971.

72. Turner-Warwick, R. T.: The repair of urethral strictures in the region of the membranous urethra. J. Urol. 100:303, 1968.

73. Turner-Warwick, R. T.: Three approaches to the management of acute disruption of the membranous urethra. *In* R. Scott, Jr. (ed.): Current Controversies in Urologic Management. Philadelphia, W. B. Saunders Co., 1972, pp. 144–150.

74. Turner-Warwick, R.: A personal view of the immediate management of pelvic fracture urethral injuries. Urol. Clin. North Am. 4:81, 1977.

75. Turner-Warwick, R., and Ashken, M. H.: The use of the omental pedicle graft in the repair and reconstruction of the lower urinary tract. Br. J. Surg. 54:849, 1967.

76. Waterhouse, K., Abrahams, J. I., Gruber, H., et al.: The transpubic approach to the lower urinary tract. J. Urol. 109:486, 1972.

77. Whitaker, R. H.: Equivocal pelviureteric junction obstruction. Br. J. Urol. 47:377, 1976.

78. Whitaker, R. H.: Investigating wide ureters with ureteral pressure flow studies. J. Urol. 116:81, 1976.

79. Williams, D. I., and Cromie, W. J.: Ring ureterostomy. Br. J. Urol. 47:789, 1975.

80. Williams, D. I., and Keeton, J. E.: Further progress with reconstruction of the exstrophied bladder. Br. J. Surg. 60:203, 1973.

81. Williams, D. I., Whitaker, R. H., Barrett, T. M., and Keeton, J. E.: Urethral valves. Br. J. Urol. 45:200, 1973.

27

THE MALE EXTERNAL GENITALIA

William E. Kaplan, M.D.
A. Barry Belman, M.D., M.S.

THE PENIS

Circumcision

Circumcision is the most frequently performed surgical procedure. Gee and Ansell reviewed 5882 newborn circumcisions and found that the complication rate was 0.2 per cent.[5] These were primarily due to *infection*. Complications were more frequent when the Plastibell device was used than when the Gomco clamp was chosen.

The most common complication of circumcision is *hemorrhage*. Everyone who has performed circumcision has encountered skin-edge bleeding or a subcutaneous hematoma. Prevention requires control of all bleeding sites prior to skin closure. Nevertheless, occasional delayed bleeding may occur whether vessels are tied or electrocoagulated. Treatment may require return-

ing the child to the operating room, although a compression dressing sometimes suffices. Insertion of an indwelling urethral catheter and application of an elastic compression dressing for 12 hours has occasionally proved effective.

Another complication is *fibrous adherence of the foreskin to the glans*. In the newborn and young child, the foreskin and glans have not separated. In the process of forcibly separating these layers in preparation for circumcision, the skin of the glans is superficially de-epithelialized. Incomplete removal of foreskin may cause the cut skin edge to override the corona and adhere to the glans. Permanent scarring may then result (Fig.

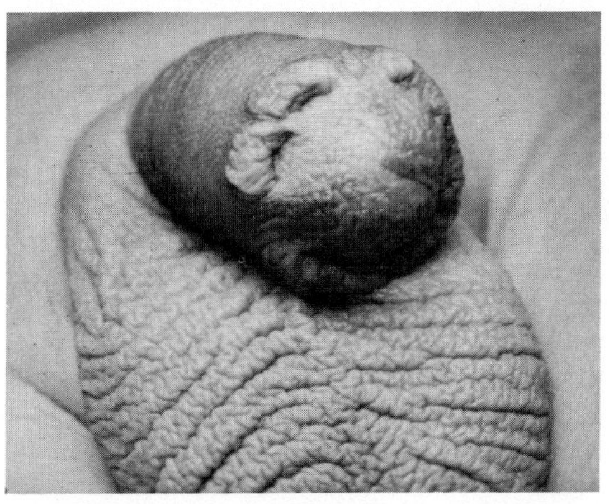

Figure 27–1 Adhesions between residual foreskin and glans.

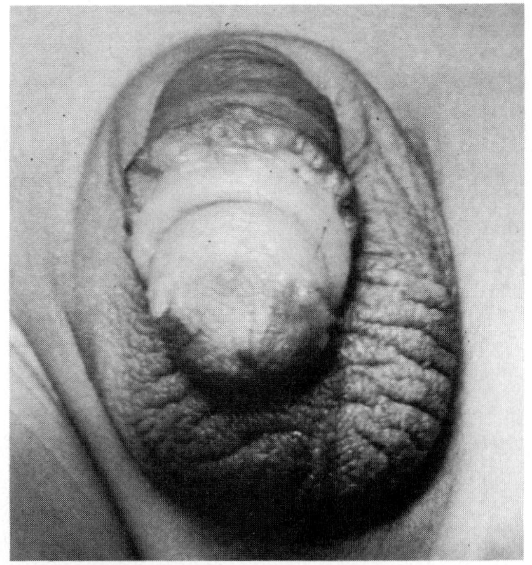

Figure 27–2 Result following revision of circumcision that required sharp dissection to release glanular adhesions.

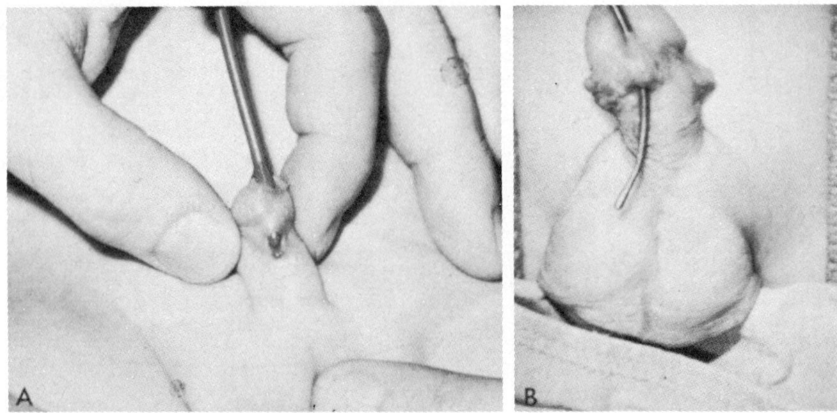

Figure 27–3   Two examples of circumcision injuries with secondary coronal fistulae. (From Belman, A. B.: The penis. Urol. Clin. North Am. 5:17, 1978.)

27–1). Sharp dissection becomes necessary to free these adhesions (Fig. 27–2). This problem can be avoided by seeing the child within 7 to 10 days post-circumcision to ensure that residual skin is not overriding the corona.

Rarely, *urethral fistulae* can result from circumcision (Fig. 27–3). We assume that there are the result of excessive ventral skin being pulled through the clamp during any of the "blind" clamp-type procedures. This is a serious problem.

We have seen one serious complication caused by a circumferential dressing. Failure to remove the dressing resulted in a gradual tourniquet effect over several days. The right corpus was completely transected, as were the urethra and part of the left corpus (Fig. 27–4). Fortunately, complete tourniquet amputation did not result. The postoperative dressing, if used at all, must be removed either before the baby is sent home after circumcision or within 24 hours.

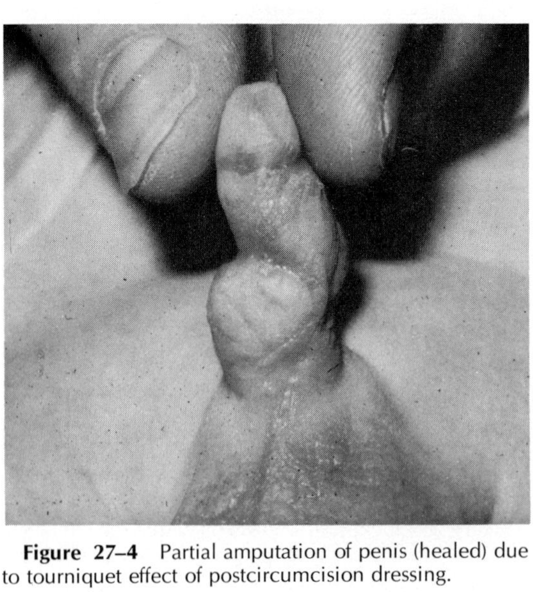

Penile necrosis may result from use of electrocautery as an adjunct to metal clamp circumcision. Electrocautery should *not* be used in conjunction with any clamp device that completely surrounds a portion of the penis.

Sharp *penile amputation* is an unlikely iatrogenic injury, but it has occurred during orchiopexy. Complete or incomplete amputation of the penis should be repaired immediately.[13, 16] Reapproximation of the corpora and the dorsal bundles with a microscope and without delay provides the best opportunity for salvage of the penis in this situation.

Hypospadias and Epispadias

The goal in both hypospadias and epispadias reconstruction is the creation of a straight phallus with the urethral meatus as far distal on the glans as possible. One of the avoidable complications is *failure to correct chordee.* Artificial erection, accomplished by injecting sterile saline solution into the corpora with a tourniquet applied to the base of the penis, allows intraoperative evaluation

Figure 27–4   Partial amputation of penis (healed) due to tourniquet effect of postcircumcision dressing.

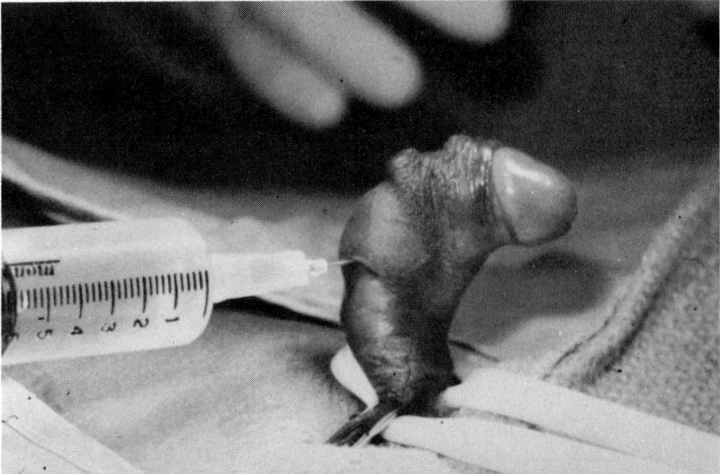

Figure 27–5 The artificial erection. The corpora are filled with sterile saline solution after application of a tourniquet to the base of the penis. This child has chordee without hypospadias.

of chordee (Fig. 27–5). Formation of the neourethra should never be initiated until adequate correction of chordee has been achieved.

Urethral fistulae are so common a problem in repair of hypospadias and epispadias that their occurrence must be anticipated in a certain percentage of patients (Fig. 27–6). The incidence of this complication can be reduced by carefully following basic surgical rules. Tissue edges should not be traumatized, fine suture should be used to invert the skin edges when closing the urethra, and the neourethra must be of adequate caliber and must not be closed under tension. Suture lines should not cross, and

multiple layers of tissue should be interposed between the urethra and skin.

Failure of the repair can be guaranteed if necrosis of skin flaps occurs. Infection can also destroy a beautiful repair. In children with a history of urinary tract infection and in those who have had multiple previous attempts at repair, a urine culture should be obtained a few days before surgery to ensure sterility of urine before surgical reconstruction.

Repair of urethral fistulae should be delayed for 6 months. This allows for resolution of induration and provides more mobile tissue to achieve a satisfactory result. The urethra distal to the fistula must not be

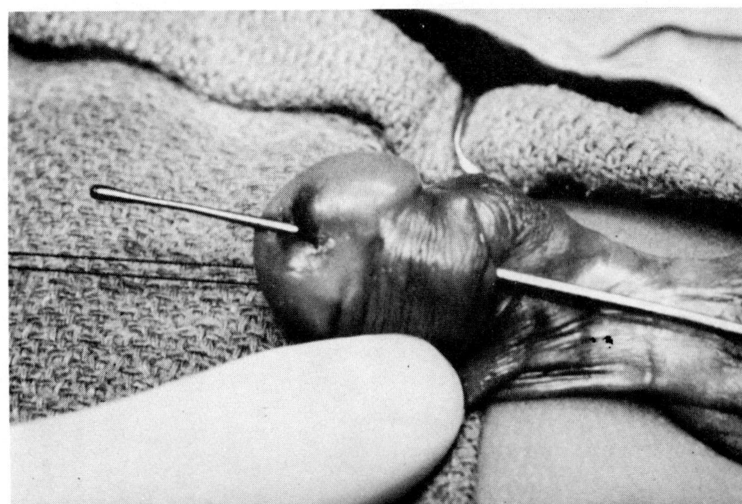

Figure 27–6 Posthypospadias urethrocutaneous fistula.

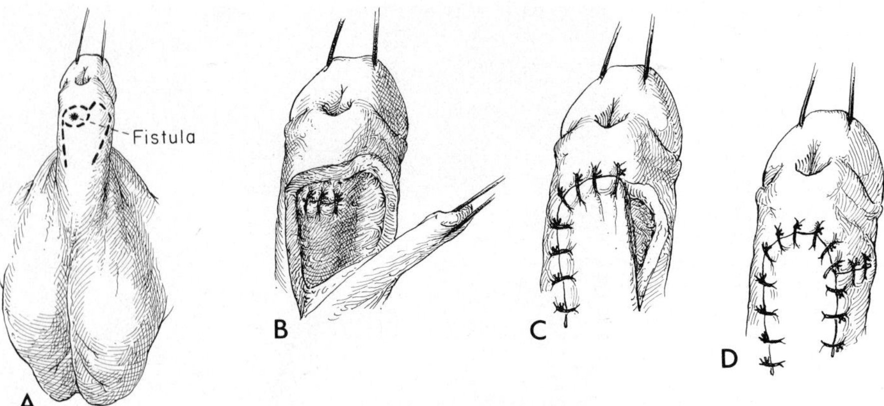

Figure 27–7 A method of closing a urethral fistula. Following closure of the fistula, a pedicle graft of penile skin completely covers the suture lines. This greatly lessens the chance of recurrence. (From Belman, A. B., and King, L. R.: Anomalies of the urinary tract — Urethra. *In* Kelalis, P. P., King, L. R., and Belman, A. B., eds.: Clinical Pediatric Urology. Volume One. Philadelphia, W. B. Saunders Company, 1976, p. 593.)

stenotic. Distal obstruction is one of the underlying causes of urethral fistula.

Correction of most fistulae can be accomplished without urinary diversion. Using fine 6-0 Dexon or chromic catgut, the circumscribed fistula is closed with an inverting subcuticular suture and reinforced with a closure of subcutaneous tissue. A pedicle flap of tissue can then be developed and rotated to avoid crossing suture lines (Fig. 27–7). The wound is covered with collodion. Double-layer closure using the vest-over-pants technique of Smith is also satisfactory.[15]

There is an increased risk of *urethral stenosis or stricture* when an end-to-end anastomosis is used to form the neourethra, as with the free graft technique of Devine and Horton[2] or the foreskin tube of Hodgson.[7] Incorporating the hypospadiac meatus in a tube rolled distal to that meatus decreases but does not eliminate this risk (Fig. 27–8). Creation of a wide-caliber spatulated junction between the original and the new urethra may prevent narrowing in all types of repairs.

Visual internal urethrotomy has become the procedure of choice for managing urethral stricture after hypospadias repair. In some patients, reoperation may be necessary. Repeated, periodic, and prolonged urethral dilatation is no longer acceptable in the managment of urethral strictures in children.

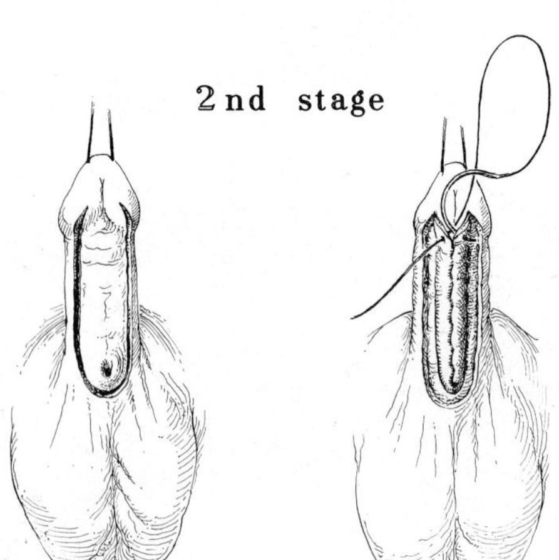

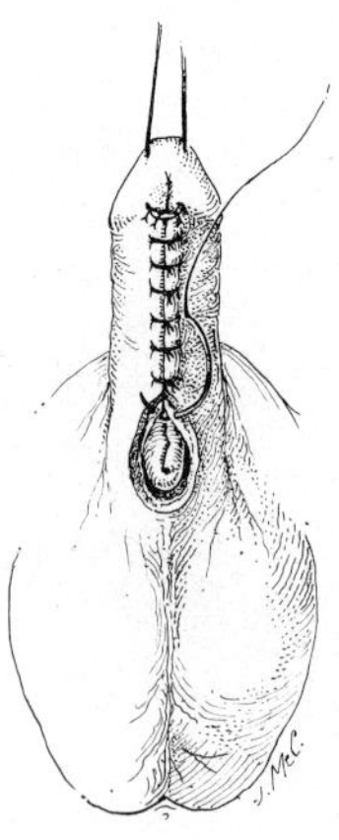

Figure 27–8 Second stage of planned two-stage repair of hypospadias (Byars modification) in which a tube is rolled distal to the hypospadiac meatus. (From Belman, A. B, and King, L. R.: Anomalies of the urinary tract — Urethra. *In* Kelalis, P. P., King, L. R., and Belman, A. B., eds.: Clinical Pediatric Urology. Volume One. Philadelphia, W. B. Saunders Company, 1976, p. 590.)

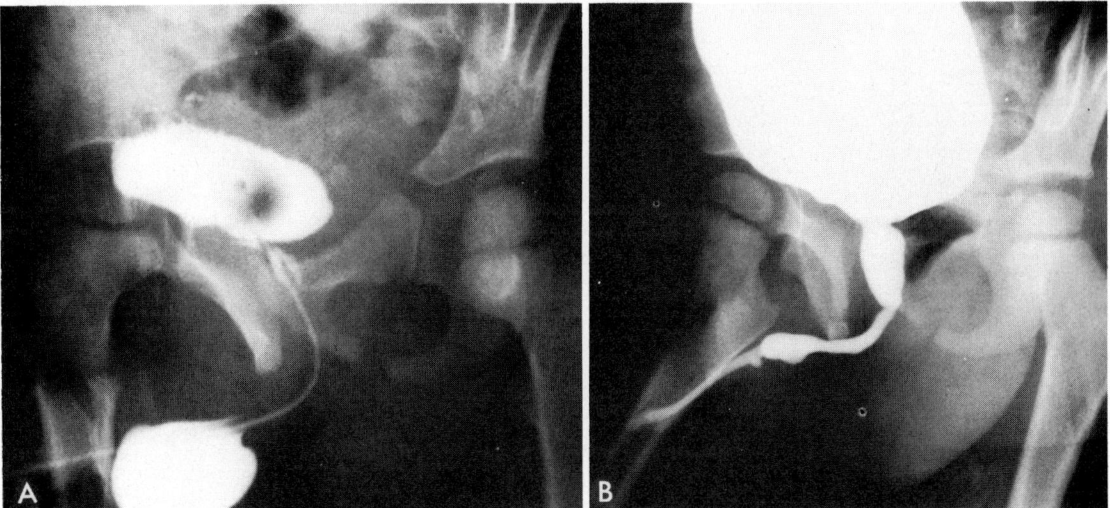

Figure 27–9 *A,* Large diverticulum at site of junction of hypospadiac meatus and new urethra. *B,* Postoperative urethrogram after repair of diverticulum. (From Belman, A. B., and King, L. R.: Anomalies of the urinary tract — Urethra. *In* Kelalis, P. P., King, L. R., and Belman, A. B., eds.: Clinical Pediatric Urology. Volume One. Philadelphia, W. B. Saunders Company, 1976, p. 594.)

Urethral diverticula are generally the result of distal obstruction, postoperative infection, or both. The result may be a huge pocket (Fig. 27–9) that requires excision and urethral closure for correction.

Meatal stenosis is a frequent complication but can generally be avoided by creating a well-vascularized distal urethra of adequate caliber. Placing the meatus at the tip of the glans, currently a popular technique, creates a higher risk of stenosis. However, the result, a cosmetically and functionally normal penis, justifies this risk.

Hematoma formation and voiding through the healing urethra can cause skin flap disruption with exposure and breakdown of the neourethra. Postoperative care of the child with hypospadias is as important for a satisfactory result as the surgical procedure itself. The manner of urinary diver-

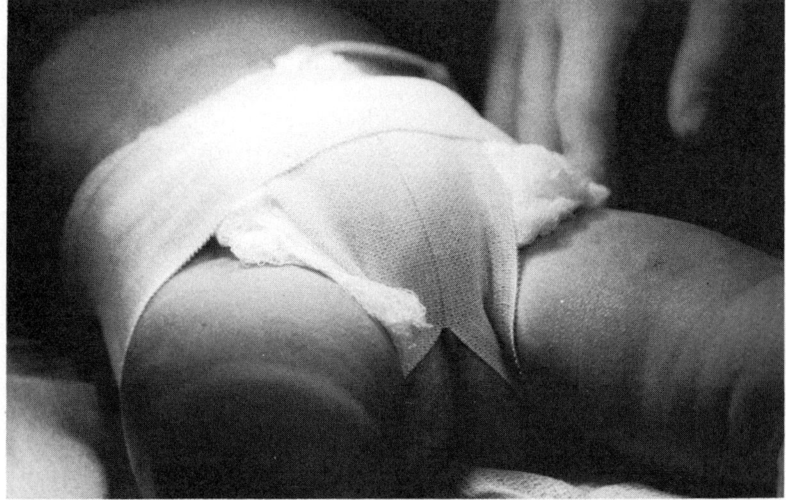

Figure 27–10 Elastoplast compression dressing for hypospadias. (From Falkowski, W. S., and Firlit, C. F.: The X-shaped hypospadias dressing. J. Urol., 123:904–906, 1981. © 1981, The William & Wilkins Co., Baltimore.)

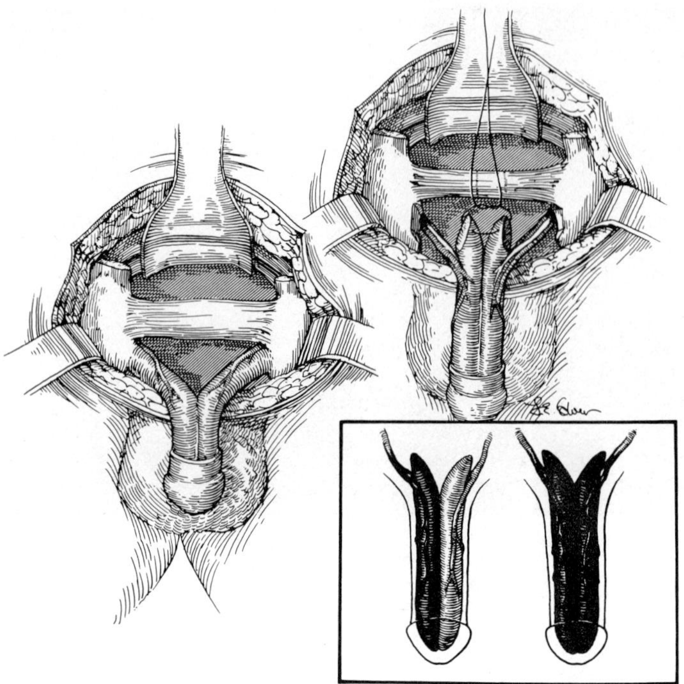

Figure 27–11 Dissection of the neurovascular bundle for penile lengthening in epispadias associated with exstrophy of the bladder. *Inset,* Thrombosis of one or both corpora due to vascular trauma. (From Peters, P. C.: Complications of penile surgery. *In* Smith, R. B., and Skinner, D. G., eds.: Complications of Urologic Surgery: Prevention and Management. Philadelphia, W. B. Saunders Company, 1976, p. 416.)

sion is individualized. One of us (W.E.K.) uses a Silastic indwelling urethral catheter for 10 to 14 days, whereas the other (A.B.B.) favors a Silastic suprapubic Cystocath and urethral stent for 7 days. Both agree that an elastic compression dressing for the first 72 hours is essential to avoid hematoma formation. The penis is wrapped initially with nylon (Owen's gauze), and then one or two layers of Elastoplast are applied (Fig. 27–10) over a fluff compression dressing. Sedation with diazepam (Valium) during the first postoperative days and use of an anticholinergic (Pro-Banthine or Ditropan) help to ensure an intact, dry dressing.

One problem for which there is no answer at present is the management of penile erections in the male adolescent after hypospadias surgery. Tension on the suture line secondary to these erections, as well as increased risk of wound infection related to the presence of hair follicles, reduces the likelihood of a successful result. Prevention of the problem by being aware of the necessity of completing surgical correction before the child starts school appears self-evident. Yet we continue to see an occasional child in whom repair has been inexplicably postponed until puberty.

A complication unique to the problem of epispadias in the child with bladder exstrophy relates to the desirability of penile lengthening. Separation of the corpora cavernosa as a result of the bony pelvic abnormality in patients with bladder exstrophy causes a stubby penis that points upward. Freeing the proximal corpora by dissecting the corpora off the ischia to produce a straighter and longer penis can result in penile necrosis if the neurovascular bundles are interrupted (Fig. 27–11).[10] Less aggressive mobilization of the corpora reduces the risk of devascularization, yet substantially lengthens the penis that points forward or downward.[8]

Priapism

Priapism occurs infrequently in children and is rarely idiopathic or secondary to excessive sexual stimulation.[1] In most patients an underlying cause can be determined and treated. Surgical treatment has generally been unsuccessful. Sickle cell disease is the most common predisposing factor. Transfusion with non-hemoglobin S packed cells is the treatment of choice. Children with acute leukemia may experience priapism secondary to sludging of cells in the corpora. Chemotherapy or irradiation rather than surgery appears to be the proper therapeutic approach.

An addition to the surgical treatment of priapism has recently been introduced by Winter.[17] The glans penis is an extension of and part of the spongiosum system and is therefore separate from the engorged corpora. Creation of a fistula between the glans and corpora can reduce the erection. With the patient under local or general anesthesia, a large-bore biopsy needle is introduced through a small dorsal glanular incision into each lateral corpus. The fibrous septum between the corpora and glans is partially disrupted, creating a means of bloody egress from each corpus. The skin defect in the glans is then closed with a few interrupted sutures.

Corporosaphenous and corporospongiosum shunts appear to have little applicability in children. Embolization or impotence secondary to a corporosaphenous shunt that persists after resolution of the priapism may necessitate ligation of that shunt.

A satisfactory postoperative result, i.e., a flaccid penis with the potential for future erection, is seldom achieved. Impotence may necessitate insertion of an artificial erectile device in adult life.

THE TESTES

Cryptorchism

Complications of untreated cryptorchism include inguinal hernia, testicular torsion, infertility, and neoplasia. A patent processus vaginalis is virtually always present, and its repair is an important part of the orchiopexy. Failure to recognize its presence may result in the need for herniorrhaphy in the future as well as reduced ability to adequately mobilize the cord.

Torsion of the undescended testis may occur. The diagnosis must be considered when a boy with an undescended or nonpalpable testis presents with abdominal pain.

Nine to 12 per cent of *testis tumors* arise in cryptorchid testes. Therefore, the undescended testis is at 35 to 40 times greater risk of malignant degeneration than is the normal testis. It is unknown whether early orchiopexy reduces the risk of malignancy in testes that were at one time undescended.

Infertility is another recognized problem related to cryptorchism. As with testis tumors, it is unknown whether early orchiopexy will influence fertility rates in this population.

Surgical complications of orchiopexy include disruption of the vas or vessels and bleeding as a consequence of overly vigorous retroperitoneal dissection. Inadequate dissection, on the other hand, results in a testis that cannot be properly placed in the scrotum. Testicular atrophy can occur when either the internal or the external inguinal ring is closed too tightly, compressing the cord and its vessels.

It should be possible to achieve cord length adequate to place in the scrotum any testis that *can be palpated preoperatively.* Rarely, a two-stage procedure may be necessary.[18] For those testes that are *not palpable preoperatively*, our preference is to attempt more adequate mobilization by approaching the testis through a midline extraperitoneal approach.[4] The Fowler-Stephens technique may then be employed if it becomes apparent that vascular length is not adequate.[6] Care must be taken with the Fowler-Stephens procedure to recognize in advance of dissection the need to divide the spermatic vessels. Perfusion of the testis after division of the spermatic vessels is dependent upon an intact distal arcade derived from the superior vesical artery (Fig. 27–12). Dissection of the vas or distal cord prior to division of the spermatic vessels negates the success of this approach. Ligation of the spermatic vessels too close to the testis also lessens the chance of success.

We advise the dartos pouch technique for fixation of the testis in all forms of orchiopexy. A separate, superficial scrotal incision with creation of the pouch may be accompanied by either internal suture fixation of the testis to the lower portion of the scrotum or cautious tightening of the scrotal fascia through which the cord passes to hold the testis in place. Rubber-band fixation of the testis to the thigh is archaic.

Inadequate mobilization of the cord with placement of the testis in the scrotum under

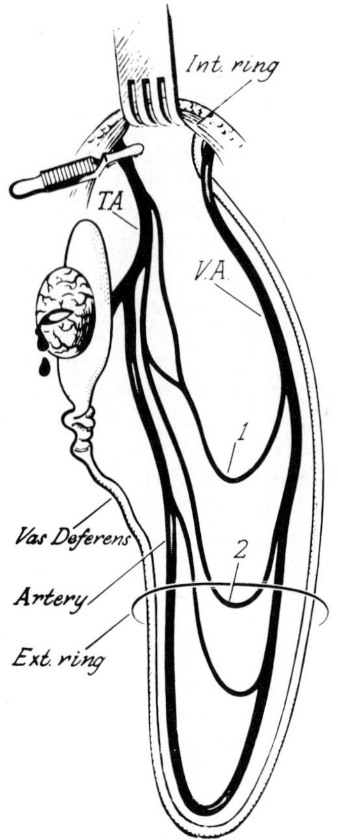

Figure 27–12 Technique of Fowler and Stephens for determining adequacy of collateral circulation to the testis. The testicular artery is occluded by a noncrushing arterial clamp, and a nick is made in the tunica albuginea of the testis to observe for arterial backflow. If arterial bleeding is demonstrated, the collateral circulation from the artery of the vas is adequate and the testicular artery may be sacrificed. (From Fowler, R., Jr., and Stephens, F. D.: The role of testicular vascular anatomy in the salvage of high undescended testes. Aust. N. Z. J. Surg. 29:92, 1959. By permission.)

tension predictably results in testicular retraction and a testis that is ultimately fixed at the pubic tubercle. Secondary operation, which carries a high risk of testicular devascularization, becomes necessary.

Torsion

Testicular torsion is a common scrotal emergency of childhood. Two forms exist: extravaginal torsion, in which the entire intrascrotal contents, includng testis, epididymis, and tunica vaginalis, rotate on the cord; and intravaginal torsion, in which the testis and epididymis rotate within the tunica vaginalis.

Extravaginal torsion is a disorder of the newborn and may well be a prenatal event (Fig. 27–13). Surgical exploration is probably not justifiable unless it is likely that the torsion occurred after birth and is an acute event. To our knowledge, testicular salvage has not been reported with extravaginal torsion. Unfortunately, the condition may be bilateral.

Intravaginal torsion occurs most commonly in the postpubertal boy.[14] Complications following simple orchiopexy after reduction of torsion of the cord (Fig. 27–14) are rare. We have seen recurrence of torsion due, most likely, to inadequate fixation. The underlying anatomic abnormality, inadequate attachment of the tunica vaginalis to the epididymis and testis, can be bilateral. Therefore, bilateral fixation must be performed at the time of exploration.

The most significant error in the care of the patient with testicular torsion is failure to recognize the possibility of torsion. Too often, sexually mature boys are treated for epididymitis when they present with scrotal pain and swelling. The result is loss of the testis.

Preoperative diagnostic evaluation using the Doppler ultrasonic stethoscope has had disappointing results in ascertaining testicular perfusion.[11] Radioisotope scanning of the scrotum using technetium has proved effective in making an accurate preoperative diagnosis of torsion (Fig. 27–15). Interpretation of the scan requires considerable experience. Unless isotope scanning can be carried out immediately and is done at a center whose staff is accustomed to the use of this modality, the delay in exploration is not justifiable when testicular torsion is suspected. Most errors results from failure to perform early surgical exploration.

Torsion of a testicular appendage appears to occur more commonly in prepubertal boys.[12] Exploration is not required if the diagnosis can be made with a high degree of certainty. Pinpoint local tenderness at the head of the epididymis and visibility of the necrotic appendage through the scrotal skin (blue dot sign) are reliable evidence of torsion.[3]

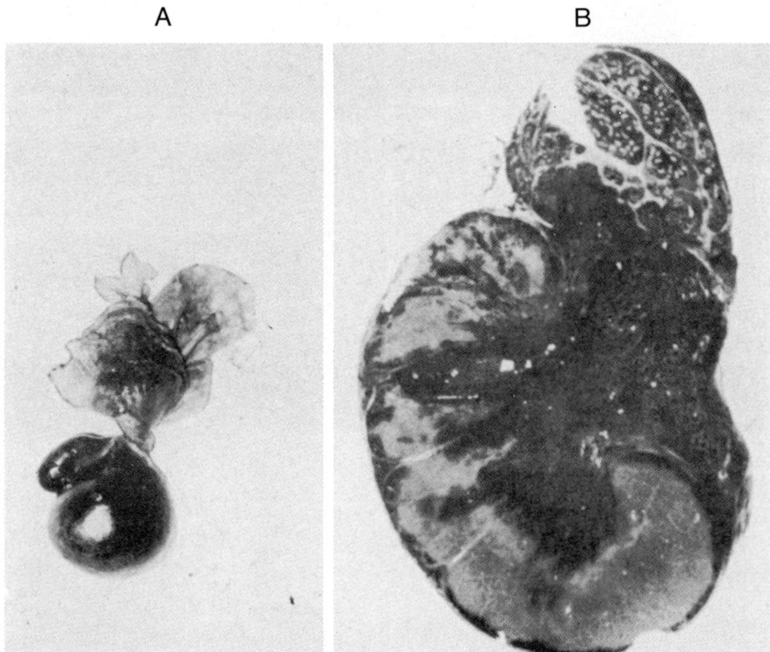

Figure 27–13 Intravaginal torsion of the testis. *A,* External appearance of a torted testis removed because of infarction and gangrene. *B,* Section of an infarcted testis showing hemorrhage. (From Allen, T. D.: Disorders of the male external genitalia. *In* Kelalis, P. P., King, L. R., and Belman, A. B., eds.: Clinical Pediatric Urology. Volume Two. Philadelphia, W. B. Saunders Company, 1976, p. 651.)

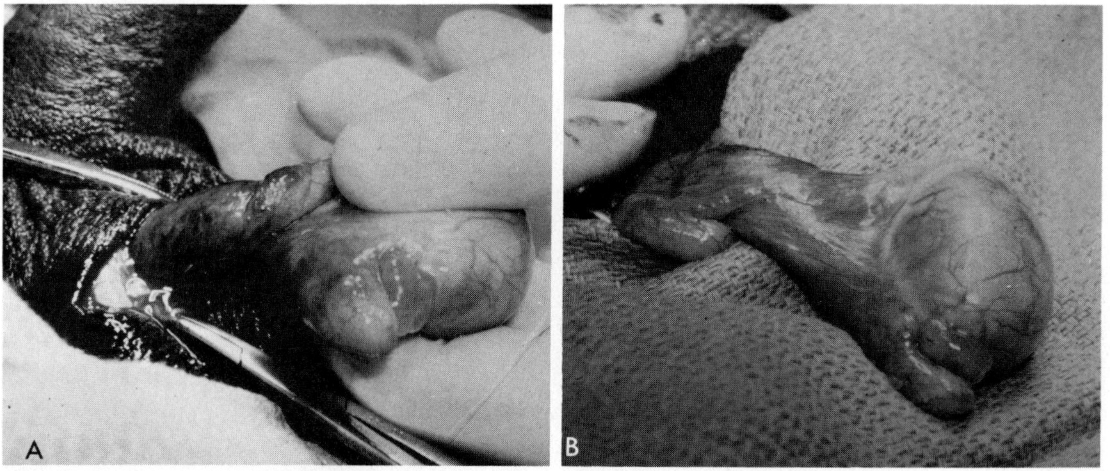

Figure 27–14 Extravaginal torsion *(A)* and detorsion *(B).* Note failure of attachment of tunica vaginalis to the testis.

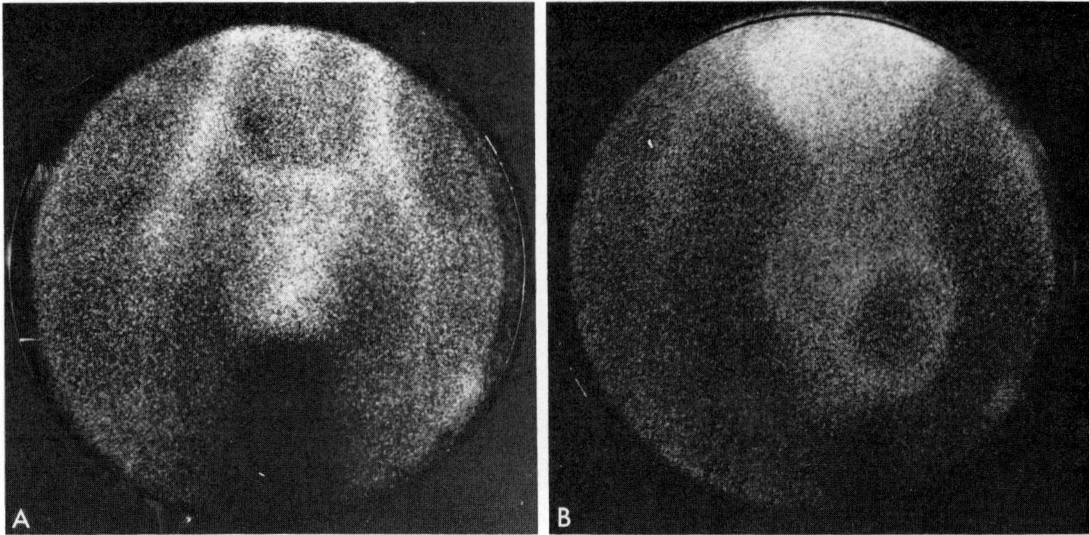

Figure 27–15   *A,* Normal flow pattern with technetium pertechnetate testicular scan. *B,* "Cold" area on testicular scan in boy with proven testicular torsion.

Inflammatory Disease

Inflammatory disease of the scrotum and its contents generally does not require surgical intervention. The exception is scrotal gangrene, fortunately an uncommon problem in children. Epididymitis and epididymo-orchitis may be inadvertently explored when the diagnosis of testicular torsion cannot be ruled out. This cannot be regarded as a complication, however.

Scrotal Swelling

Another entity that does not require surgical exporation is *idiopathic scrotal edema*[9] (Fig. 27–16). The testes must be proved normal. They should be manipulated into the inguinal canals or into the superficial inguinal pouch for accurate palpation. If they are found to be normal, surgical exploration is unnecessary. Children presenting with idiopathic scrotal edema have a swollen, violaceous scrotum or hemiscrotum. The edematous process frequently extends into the perineum and the suprapubic area. Treatment is expectant, with spontaneous resolution occurring within 12 to 36 hours.

Testis and spermatic cord tumors are another cause of scrotal swelling. Failure to recognize the possibility of tumor in a boy who has a hard, nontender scrotal mass is tragic. Transscrotal biopsy of a testis tumor may result in intrascrotal tumor spill. Since the lymphatic drainage of the scrotum is totally separate from that of the testis and spermatic cord, therapy for scrotal contamination by tumors requires excision of the involved

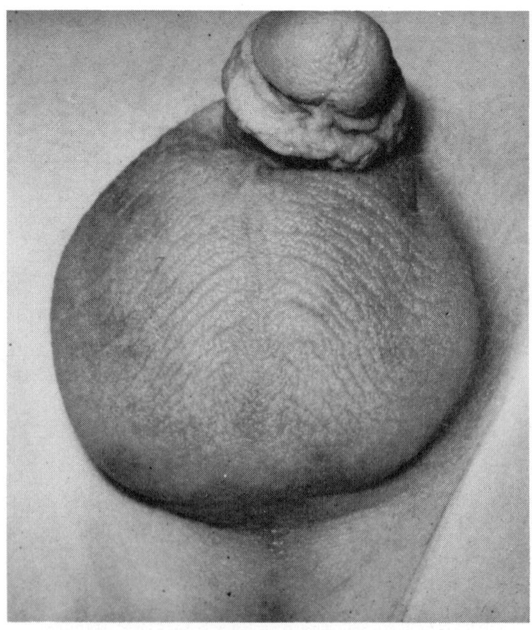

Figure 27–16   Idiopathic scrotal edema.

scrotal wall as well as pathways of inguinal lymphatic spread.

Surgical Trauma

Inadvertent surgical trauma to the scrotum must be quite rare. Hematoma formation within the scrotum following a testicular procedure is not uncommon and may extend to the perineum and inguinal region. Spontaneous absorption is the rule; drainage is rarely necessary.

Scrotal skin devascularization following surgical procedures is also rare. Scrotal skin flaps are often used to cover a variety of defects associated with hypospadias and urethral repairs. Skin necrosis rarely occurs.

References

1. Belman, A. B.: Vascular and related disorders. *In* Kelalis, P. P., King, L. R., and Belman, A. B. (eds.): Clinical Pediatric Urology. Vol. 2. Philadelphia, W. B. Saunders Co., 1976, pp. 850–864.
2. Devine, C. J., Jr., and Horton, C. E.: A one-stage hypospadias repair. J. Urol. 85:166, 1961.
3. Dresner, M.: Torsed appendage: Diagnosis and management: Blue dot sign. Urology 1:63, 1973.
4. Flinn, R. A., and King, L. R.: Experience with the midline transabdominal approach in orchiopexy. Surg. Gynecol. Obstet. 133:285, 1971.
5. Gee, W. F., and Ansell, J. S.: Neonatal circumcision, a ten year overview. Pediatrics 58:824, 1976.
6. Gibbons, D. M., Cromie, W. J., and Duckett, J. W.: Management of the abdominal undescended testicle. J. Urol. 122:76, 1979.
7. Hodgson, N. B.: A one-stage hypospadias repair. J. Urol. 104:281, 1970.
8. Johnston, J. H., and Kogan, S. J.: The exstrophied anomalies and their surgical reconstruction. Curr. Probl. Surg., August 1974, pp. 1–39.
9. Kaplan, G. W.: Acute idiopathic scrotal edema. J. Pediatr. Surg. 12:647, 1977.
10. Kelley, J. H., and Eraklis, A. J.: Procedure for lengthening the phallus in boys with exstrophy of the bladder. J. Pediatr. Surg. 6:645, 1971.
11. Nasrallah, P. F., Manzone, D., and King, L. R.: Falsely negative Doppler examinations in testicular torsion. J. Urol. 118:197, 1977.
12. Puri, P., and Boyd, E.: Torsion of the appendix testis. Clin. Pediatr. 15:949, 1976.
13. Schulman, M. J.: Reanastomosis of the amputated penis. J. Urol. 109:432, 1973.
14. Scorer, C. G., and Farrington, G. H.: Congenital anomalies of the testes. *In* Harrison, J. H., Gittes, R. F., Perlmutter, A. D., et al. (eds.): Campbell's Urology, 4th edition. Vol. 2. Philadelphia, W. B. Saunders Co., 1979, pp. 1549–1565.
15. Smith, E. D.: A de-epithelialized overlap, flap technique in the repair of hypospadias. Br. J. Plast. Surg. 26:106, 1973.
16. Turek, M., and Weir, W. H., Jr.: Successful reimplantation of the traumatically amputated glans penis. Plast. Reconstr. Surg. 48:479, 1971.
17. Winter, C. C.: Care of idiopathic priapism. Urology 8:389, 1976.
18. Zers, M., Walloch, U., and Dentsmen, M.: Staged orchiorrhaphy: Therapeutic procedure in cryptorchid testicles with a short spermatic cord. Arch. Surg. 110:387, 1975.

FEMALE GENITAL TRACT

Donald P. Goldstein, M.D.

28

INTRODUCTION

Gynecologic surgery is rapidly becoming an important subspecialty in the field of pediatric surgery. This trend is evident from the increase in the number of gynecologic procedures performed, the increasing number of gynecologic departments in pediatric institutions, and the increasing number of adolescent females who seek help in emergency rooms and in the offices of pediatricians. In England and Western European nations, well-organized and active pediatric and adolescent gynecologic services have flourished since World War II.

The increased birth rate of the 1960's resulted in an expanded adolescent population today. Changing sexual mores and major advances in the field of gynecology, including diagnostic methods, surgical techniques, and endocrinologic and genetic innovations, have created the need for expertise in dealing with congenital and acquired pelvic pathology. The most frequently performed gynecologic procedure at Children's Hospital Medical Center, Boston, is laparoscopy, a technique developed during the past decade.

This chapter will focus on procedures that are most frequently performed in our institution. Indications for operation, proper technique, and prevention and management of the most important complications will be discussed.

OPERATIONS ON THE PERINEUM AND VULVA

Hymenotomy

Variations in size, thickness, and elasticity of the hymen are common. Anomalies are clinically important and require surgical correction when there is obstruction to vaginal drainage. Imperforate hymen is best corrected when it is discovered, preferably during infancy.[8] The central portion of the membrane is excised in infants and little girls. In older girls, a wedge-shaped portion of the thin posterior part of the hymen is removed. At the time of surgical correction, it is important to evaluate and exclude other abnormalities of the lower genital tract. When the introitus is insufficient to permit adequate examination or sexual activity, it is advisable to perform a perineoplasty by incising the hymen and perineal body in the midline vertically and closing the resultant defect transversely, everting the vaginal epithelium and suturing it to the perineal skin.

Complications. Two major complications of this procedure are postoperative bleeding and persistent stenosis of the introitus. The hymen is served by a network of small vessels, which can bleed vigorously if careful attention is not paid to hemostasis. Packing should not be necessary. Persistent stenosis may occur when there is a rather rigid hymenal ring. If an insufficient introitus persists following simple hymenotomy, a perineoplasty should be performed. An acceptable alternative method is periodic dilations using Young Vaginal Dilators ranging in size from No. 1 to No. 4.

Colpoperineoplasty

Indications. Certain congenital abnormalities, such as congenital adrenal hyperplasia and exstrophy of the bladder, are associated with deformities of the perineum, introitus, and vagina and require correction before normal sexual function can be achieved. It is advisable to postpone

372

operation until after menarche, since the perineum, vulva, and vaginal tissues are underdeveloped.

Operative Technique. Operative technique depends upon the degree of deformity of the perineal body, which is often unusually high, compromising the introitus. The simplest method of repairing this defect is to incise the perineal body down the median raphe externally, continuing the incision into the underlying transverse perineal muscles and into the vagina for a distance of 2 to 3 cm. Dissection is performed with the electrosurgical unit to reduce bleeding. The resulting defect is closed transversely, everting the vaginal epithelium and suturing it to the edge of the perineal skin.

Complications. Three complications may be associated with this procedure — bleeding, perforation of the rectum, and postoperative stenosis. Bleeding requires hemostasis and resuturing. Perforation of the rectum may result from dissection of the vaginal epithelium off the underlying anterior rectum. It is advisable to perform a rectal examination prior to closure of the vaginal epithelium to be sure that the rectal wall is intact. A rectovaginal fistula may result. If a rectal perforation is recognized during dissection, closure can be accomplished quite simply with a finger in the rectum.

Postoperative stenosis can be overcome by the use of dilators unless the patient prefers to undergo a second operation.

Bartholin's Gland Cyst or Abscess

The major vestibular or Bartholin's glands produce a clear, limpid, viscous, mucoid secretion having as its primary function lubrication of the introitus during intercourse. Cysts and abscesses are rare in childhood but can occur. They result from obstruction of Bartholin's gland duct, which is located inside the vestibule just external to the hymenal ring at the base of each labium majus.

SURGICAL TREATMENT

Small Bartholin's gland cysts are commonly found at the time of routine pelvic examination and, if asymptomatic or uninfected, they may not require surgical treatment. Larger cysts usually cause discomfort at coitus, sitting, or walking. Bartholin's gland cysts may be marsupialized or excised. Fluid will reaccumulate if the cyst is merely incised and drained. Excision requires an incision in the epithelium over the cyst, which is then removed by blunt and sharp dissection. Large vessels may be encountered in the region of the cyst; careful hemostasis is required.

An alternative to excision of the cyst is marsupialization, which provides permanent drainage and preserves secretory function for vaginal lubrication. Marsupialization is less involved technically and eliminates most complications resulting from excision. Briefly, a vertical incision is made in the vaginal mucosa over the center of the cyst and outside the hymenal ring. The incision is made as wide as possible to enhance postoperative patency of the stoma. After draining the cysts's contents, the lining of the cyst is everted and sutured to the vaginal mucosa with continuous absorbable sutures.

Complications. Bleeding and hematoma formation are the most common complications following excision of a Bartholin's gland cyst. Treatment consists of bed rest, ice packs, and pressure dressings to the vulva. Attempts to ligate various bleeding points are futile. The hematoma will ultimately resorb. It is sometimes necessary to evacuate blood clot and drain the hematoma cavity.

Complications of marsupialization are rare. There is a 10 to 15 per cent recurrence rate, which results from closure and secondary fibrosis of the cyst orifice. Reoperation is required for such cases.

A short catheter has recently been developed that can be inserted into the Bartholin's gland abscess in the emergency room under local anesthesia. The catheter is inflated and then deflated after several days in the hope that a sinus tract will form. In effect, this is a closed type of marsupialization.

CONGENITAL ABSENCE OF VAGINA

Congenital absence of the vagina is estimated to occur once in every 4000 female live births. Usually there is complete absence of the uterus and cervix, although there are reports of patients in whom the reproductive tract was otherwise normal. Most patients have normal ovaries and fully developed secondary sexual characteristics. The diagnosis of vaginal atresia is made by local examination of the patient, often under general anesthesia. The internal organs are felt by rectoabdominal examination. Ultrasound permits imaging of the internal genitalia. A few women are unconcerned about their condition, but most prefer to have vaginal reconstruction, permitting normal sexual activity. Some patients present to the gynecologist at the age of 14 or 15 years because of primary amenorrhea. It is important to look for associated abnormalities of the urinary tract, most commonly a solitary kidney.

Surgical Treatment

There are four types of repairs recommended for vaginal atresia. First is the nonsurgical method espoused by Frank, using dilators of increasing size.[11] Second is the McIndoe procedure, using a skin graft.[7] Third is the Williams procedure, which utilizes tissues of the external genitalia to create a pouch introitus. Fourth is a procedure involving transfer of an intestinal segment.[9] We believe the McIndoe or skin graft method is the best solution of this difficult problem.[2]

Robert Frank in 1938 reported formation of a vagina by creating local pressure with test tubes.[3] The patient is taught to insert the tube downward and inward and to keep the tube in place every night until an adequate vagina is created. Cooperation is usually not obtainable in a teenager; even with full cooperation, the cavity may fail to form. Complications of this method are rare, though perforation of the bladder and rectum may occur.

McIndoe utilized a split-thickness graft, which is generally obtained from the buttock. It is sutured over an elastic form of the type first described by Councilor. After creation of a vaginal space, the stented graft is inserted and held in place by closure of the labia. The patient is generally kept in bed for 7 to 10 days. The stent is then removed

and the neovagina is carefully irrigated. Graft take is usually excellent. The patient is then discharged and instructed to use the stent continuously for 3 months and nightly for 3 months. Complications of this procedure are perforation of the rectum and the bladder at the time of surgical dissection to create the new vagina. Postoperative hemorrhage and infection may destroy the graft. A frequent late complication is ultimate closure of the neovagina through scarring.

Formation of a neovagina from a transformed segment of ileum or sigmoid is preferred by some surgeons. Complications of this operation are those associated with any anastomosis. In addition, we have seen devascularization of the bowel segment, which leads to contraction that may be difficult to overcome by further internal surgery. Some patients complain of excess mucous discharge. In other respects, the neovagina is satisfactory for sexual intercourse.

In addition to complete vaginal agenesis there may be partial absence of the vagina, which is more common. Vaginal obstruction may be complete, with amenorrhea, or there may be partial obstruction and a sinus tract through which menstruation can occur. With partial obstruction there may be backwash pelvic endometriosis.

Surgical treatment of low or membranous vaginal atresia is relatively easy. An incision is made through the epithelial obstruction, which is removed circumferentially. Complications are rare.

EXCISION OF GARTNER'S DUCT CYST

Gartner's duct cysts develop from müllerian remnants that persist along the anterior and lateral vaginal walls, usually in the upper third of the vagina.

Generally it is recommended that such cysts be removed. The commonest complication is perforation of the bladder, which should be recognized at the time and closed, draining the bladder with a suprapubic catheter for a period of 1 week. Another complication is bleeding or hematoma formation. Generally it is difficult to find the bleeding point. Hematoma formation is treated by incision and drainage. Other cysts must be distinguished from müllerian duct remnants; usually these are lined by squamous epithelium. They should not be excised as a Gartner's duct cyst is; instead they should be incised and marsupialized.

COLPOTOMY/CULDOCENTESIS

Culdocentesis or paracentesis of the posterior cul-de-sac has proved to be an excellent means of differentiating between bleeding and infection in the peritoneal cavity. Culdocentesis is performed with traction on the posterior lip of the cervix, using a 5 inch 18-gauge needle and a 30 to 50 cc. syringe. The commonest complication is perforation of the rectum. The complication is treated with antibiotics; laparotomy is not required. Colpotomy is performed to drain an abscess of the cul-de-sac. Drains are placed through the colpotomy incision.

The main complication of colpotomy is perforation of the rectosigmoid, particularly if there are adhesions between the rectosigmoid and the uterus, which are most common in patients with endometriosis.

CERVICAL CONIZATION AND BIOPSY

The technique of biopsy and cervical conization is performed primarily for the diagnosis of epithelial neoplasia. This is now more common and seen among younger patients because of earlier sexual exposure with multiple partners and increase in infections due to sexually transmitted oncogenic viruses. When an abnormal Papanicolaou smear is reported, the patient should undergo colposcopy. Any surface abnormalities of the transformation zone should be biopsied. In addition, endocervical curettage should be performed. Silver nitrate and ferric subsulfate (Monsel's Solution) have been effective in controlling bleeding from the biopsy sites.

If there is suspicion of carcinoma in situ or invasive cancer, cervical conization should be performed using a cold knife. Conization is carried out under general or regional anesthesia. Schiller's stain should be used in the operating room prior to conization. Cervical conization is not necessary in every patient with abnormal Papanicolaou test results; it is performed when there is suspicion of a serious underlying lesion or when disease extends into the endocervical canal and cannot be treated by cryocauterization.

Complications of conization include immediate postoperative bleeding, which can originate from the highly vascular cervical stroma. The placement of sutures at the 3 and 9 o'clock positions of the cervix may be sufficient. Hot cautery of the conization site after removal of the specimen may be tried. If this fails, the patient must be taken to the operating room. A hemostatic pack is sutured inside and against the conization site.

A late complication of conization may be infertility. Conization occasionally results in cervical stenosis because of scarring. There is decreased production of cervical mucus and poor sperm penetration as well as difficulty with menstruation. Pelvic endometriosis may result.

The procedure may also result in cervical incompetency due to interruption of the fibromuscular integrity of the internal os.

AMPUTATION OF THE CERVIX (MANCHESTER OPERATION)

In certain patients with myelodysplasia and exstrophy, uterine descent may be noted due to weakness of supporting structures in the pelvis. The cervix may protrude through the introitus. When sexual activity is begun, problems with intromission, dyspareunia, and excessive trauma to the cervix occur. The most effective treatment for this condition is the Manchester operation. A portion of the cervix is amputated and the cardinal ligaments are shortened, moving them anterior to the cervix, thus restoring the normal position of the uterus. Cesarean section is required in the event of pregnancy.

Late complications of the Manchester operation include cervical stenosis. Proper placement of the cervical sutures and cervical dilatation for 2 or 3 months will avoid this complication. Because a good portion of the cervical canal has been removed, there may be difficulty in conceiving.

OPERATIONS ON THE UTERUS

Dilatation and Curettage

Indications. Dilatation of the cervix is carried out as a preliminary step to curettage of the uterine cavity, the most frequent gynecologic operation and generally regarded as a simple and harmless procedure. Curettage done under general or conduction anesthesia carries very little risk, but if improperly performed, complications and even death may result. The purpose of curettage of the uterus is the removal of endometrial or endocervical tissue for histologic study and for managing abnormal intrauterine bleeding and unwanted pregnancy. Curettage may be of great value in patients with dysfunctional uterine bleeding, although the exact mechanism by which it produces its effects is not known.

Technique. The technique of uterine curettage is well known to all who perform gynecologic surgery.

Dilatation of the cervix should be performed slowly and carefully, using Pratt dilators commonly used in therapeutic abortion. It is advisable to curette the endocervix prior to dilatation of the internal os in order to determine whether any pathologic tissue is present.

It is important to explore the uterine cavity with a small ureteral stone forceps or uterine packing forceps at the end of the curettage. It may be possible to extract an endometrial polyp which would otherwise be missed.

Perforation of the uterus is the most common complication of curettage. The prepubertal uterus is generally soft and small. The best instrument to use is a Duncan curette, a long, narrow instrument used in performing office endometrial biopsies in older patients. Because the cervix is small, it should not be grasped with a tenaculum. Initially a small Pratt dilator is used. The uterus is usually in a retroverted position rather than anteverted, as in postpubertal patients. Perforation can occur not only during the curettage but also early in the procedure with the insertion of dilators. When perforation occurs, it is best to observe the patient for 24 hours. If hemorrhage occurs, laparotomy with suturing of the site of perforation or laparoscopy with fulguration of the bleeding site may be required. Usually perforation is well tolerated and there is prompt healing. Perforation of the uterus becomes significant when malignancy is present or when there is perforation of a large, boggy, post-abortal uterus. Hemorrhage, endometritis, and peritonitis are common in this situation.

THERAPEUTIC INTERRUPTION OF PREGNANCY

Therapeutic interruption of pregnancy in the first trimester has become a very commonly performed operation. Even though the suction apparatus has greatly simplified the procedure, pediatric surgeons may be faced with a patient who has undergone a therapeutic abortion and has developed one or more complications of this procedure.

Technique. Suction evacuation of the uterus may be performed up to 14 to 16 weeks of gestational age. Beyond that it is advisable to use a large 16-mm. cannula with a special attachment to the suction machine.

Curettage may be carried out under local, conduction, or general anesthesia. Many abortion clinics use intravenous premedication and paracervical blocks. As with curettage of the nonpregnant uterus, care must be taken with dilatation of the cervix to avoid tearing or occult laceration, which may lead to cervical incompetence at some future date. It is particularly important to ascertain the position of the uterine fundus.

Complications. Complications of therapeutic abortions may be immediate or late. One immediate complication is cervical laceration with hemorrhage. This is particularly true in multigravidous patients who have had previous tears of the cervix. The most serious type of laceration is one that extends along the cervix into the base of the broad ligament with injury of the uterine artery. The resulting broad ligament hematoma may be rather extensive, extending along the lateral pelvic side wall to involve the ureter and left adnexal region. This complication requires immediate laparotomy. Hysterectomy is not indicated or required. The peritoneum overlying the lateral pelvic wall should be opened to expose the vessels and the ureter. The ovarian vessels on that side should be ligated and divided and the involved adnexa resected in a retrograde fashion. Sutures should be placed to control the uterine artery, taking care to identify and retract the ureter laterally. Following control of bleeding and repair of the perforation, the lateral wall can be reperitonealized.

Perforation may also be encountered in patients undergoing suction curettage for therapeutic abortion; it usually occurs at the time of dilatation of the cervix and when the uterus is retroverted. When this occurs, it is important to observe the patient in the hospital for 24 hours for evidence of continued bleeding. Perforation should not compromise evacuation of the uterus. If the uterus is not thoroughly evacuated, continuing hemorrhage would ensue. Occasionally on evacuating the uterus in the presence of perforation, small bowel or omentum may be drawn into the uterus. When this occurs, laparotomy should be carried out. The bowel and omentum should be extracted from the uterus and carefully inspected for viability. Bowel resection may be required. Curettage may be completed by use of a simple hysterotomy incision.

Incomplete evacuation of the uterine contents is less common with suction curettage than with sharp technique and can be obviated by performing sharp curettage immediately after suction evacuation of the uterus. With incomplete evacuation of the uterus, there is a higher risk of infection or bleeding. One unusual complication following complete evacuation of the uterus is necrosis of the endometrium and myometrium, with heavy bleeding and ultimate need for hysterectomy. In such cases, curettage apparently suctioned out the endometrial lining.

LATE COMPLICATIONS. The most common complication is persistent irregular bleeding due to retained products of conception, which may be associated with chronic endometritis. Bleeding may be quite heavy and require emergency hospital admission and sharp curettage. Antibiotics are seldom used.

Another complication following suction curettage is the development of intrauterine synechiae (Asherman's syndrome) with partial or complete obliteration of the uterine cavity. This is due to excessive trauma to the endometrium with disruption of the basal layer leading to scar tissue formation. Patients with uterine synechiae may be amenorrheic or oligomenorrheic but have cyclic cramps. Generally, such patients are infertile and require lysis of adhesions and stimulation of the remaining endometrium to promote regeneration. The results of treatment are poor and many such patients are permanently infertile.

A common problem following multiple therapeutic abortions is cervical incompetence due to occult or overt lacerations of the cervix. The use of laminaria stems is becoming more popular in an attempt to achieve a more gradual dilatation of the cervix. Laminaria left in position too long can introduce infection.

No discussion of abortion would be complete without considering postpartum pelvic inflammation. It has become relatively rare following first trimester abortion and is more common with abortion after 10 weeks and following late second trimester procedures. The causative organisms are usually aerobic or anaerobic contaminants from the vagina. In most instances the infection is mild and can be treated on an ambulatory basis with oxytocic agents, such as ergotamine tartrate or maleate and broad-spectrum antibiotics. Hospital admission is required when peritoneal signs develop and when there is evidence of adnexal enlargement. When the infection is severe and does not respond to oxytocics and antibiotics, laparotomy may be required. Either a salpingectomy or, rarely, a hysterectomy is performed as a life-saving procedure.

ABDOMINAL HYSTERECTOMY

Indications. Abdominal hysterectomy is rarely performed in pediatric adolescent gynecology. In all likelihood, the most common indications are the presence of malignant disease and obstructing malformations.[1, 12] Other indications are severe infection due to anaerobic organisms, uncontrollable metrorrhagia, severe cystic and adenomatous hyperplasia, and pelvic inflammatory disease. In rare instances, hysterectomy may be required for pelvic endometriosis. The cervix should be removed unless there is real danger that the ureters may be injured.

Unless ovarian disease is present, it is best to perform a simple, total abdominal hysterectomy with preservation of one or both ovaries. However, when performing hysterectomy for pelvic inflammatory disease, it is best to remove both ovaries and tubes because of the high incidence of residual ovarian syndrome.

INJURIES TO THE BLADDER

When the bladder is injured during the course of hysterectomy, it is not a catastrophe. Indeed, there are occasions when removal of a segment of the bladder with the uterus is indicated. Closure of the bladder in two layers is all that is required. We have not encountered formation of a vesicovaginal fistula after hysterectomy. A Foley catheter should be left in the bladder for 10 days postoperatively.

POSTHYSTERECTOMY HEMORRHAGE

The most common complication following hysterectomy is bleeding. Gray reported a series of 1000 hysterectomies. Bleeding sufficient to require resuturing or transfusion occurred in less than 1 per cent.[6] Most bleeding is due to improper suturing of the vaginal cuff. Bleeding may also occur from the end of the first week to the end of the second week. Once again, the vagina must be resutured. We have always been able to control bleeding by resuturing the edges of the vaginal cuff with figure-of-eight sutures using the vaginal approach. Laparotomy may be required if the hemorrhage originates from the uterine vessels. Transfusions are used as necessary.

Ureteral injury is the most serious complication following abdominal or vaginal hysterectomy. The injury may go unrecognized at the time of operation and become evident because of high fever, costovertebral angle tenderness, signs of urinary tract infection, or reduced urine volume. Total anuria following hysterectomy would suggest bilateral ureteral injury. The most common injury is kinking of the ureter by ligature, although at times the ureter may be divided. The retroperitoneal approach may be utilized if surgery is required. It is wise to identify the location and side of injury by intravenous or retrograde pyelography. On occasion a ureteral catheter may be inserted cystoscopically, allowing time for edema to subside. The surgeon who performs hysterectomy should always be mindful of the relationship between the ureter and uterine vessels and identify the ureter at the time of initial dissection. The ureter should be pushed as far laterally as possible prior to clamping, suturing and dividing the uterine artery on each side.

INFECTION

The most common infection following abdominal hysterectomy is infection of the vaginal cuff. The vagina is opened at the time of hysterectomy, thus permitting spillage of a wide variety of aerobic and anaerobic organisms into the peritoneal cavity. Infection becomes manifest on or about the fifth postoperative day, with fever, ileus and tenderness on vaginal or rectovaginal examination. Administration of prophylactic antibiotics prior to and for 2 days after hysterectomy has reduced the incidence of this complication. Pelvic thrombophlebitis may occur and must be considered a possible source of prolonged and unexplained fever and pelvic pain following hysterectomy. Pulmonary embolization and sudden death may occur. A relatively rare complication of hysterectomy is a hematoma of the pelvic ligament, either with or without ovarian removal.

MYOMECTOMY

Myomata uteri, the commonest tumor of the uterus, is relatively rare but does occur in women under 21 years of age. In black girls the incidence is much higher, accounting for most myomas in the adolescent age group.

Myomas arise in the myometrium and may be subserosal, intramural, or submucosal. They may become pedunculated and obtain some of their blood supply from the omentum and from the uterine pedicle.

Intramural tumors cause more pain, and submucosal myomas cause menorrhagia. All myomas in adolescents should be removed because of symptoms, interference with reproductive function, and the possibility of malignant change. The most common indications for surgery are bleeding, pain, and rapid growth.

When large myomas are removed, a great deal of bleeding may be expected. Bleeding can be minimized by the use of a tourniquet around the cervix and the application of bulldog clamps to the pelvic ligaments. It has been observed that myomectomy is associated with more intestinal ileus than is abdominal hysterectomy. With careful technique and hemostasis, this complication has been reduced. We close the myoma defect in multiple layers, using interrupted and continuous sutures of 3-0 dexon. Then close the serosa with a similar stitch.

METROPLASTY

Metroplasty may be required for uterine duplication or malformations that cause a variety of symptoms and complications.[10] Examples are pregnancy in one horn of a completely septate uterus, pyometra occurring in one or both horns, and habitual abortions. These patients present with incapacitating dysmenorrhea and a tense, cystic mass palpable on one side of the pelvis. Operation generally consists of making an incision through the anterior wall of the cystic portion followed by excision of the septum and reconstruction of two cavities into one.

On occasion, a septum may be present in the endocervical canal as well. Excision should be carried out from below as well as from above. A rubber catheter should be placed through the cervical canal while closing the uterine cavity. Eccentric vaginal pouches may be encountered, often misdiagnosed as a Gartner's duct cyst. These pouches are lined with squamous epithelium and are usually filled with squamous debris. Not infrequently, there is a communication between this pouch and the endocervical canal. The vaginal pouch is treated by simple fenestration of the vaginal wall and excision of the redundant vaginal tissue. Such pouches should not be excised. All

patients who have undergone metroplasty should undergo delivery by caesarean section because of the high incidence of spontaneous rupture of the uterus. The most frequent complication of metroplasty is hemorrhage from the sutured myometrium. One should utilize a cervical band and bulldog clamps, much as has been recommended for the removal of large myomas.

OPERATIONS ON THE ADNEXA

Laparoscopy

During the past decade, laparoscopy has become the most frequently performed gynecologic procedure in both adult and adolescent gynecology. Excellent fiberoptics and induced pneumoperitoneum allow for excellent visualization of the pelvic cavity. A wide variety of surgical procedures are performed during laparoscopy.

Technique. The main indication for laparoscopy in the pediatric and adolescent age group is evaluation of pelvic pain due to pelvic endometriosis and adhesions secondary to previous pelvic surgery.[5] Peritubal and periovarian adhesions often result from previous ovarian cystectomy. The technique has also been utilized in evaluating patients who may have pelvic inflammatory disease but in whom a full clinical picture has not evolved. A third indication is for the differential diagnosis of right lower quadrant pain and to rule out early acute appendicitis. Laparoscopy may also be used as a means of directing needle biopsies of the liver, aspiration of benign ovarian cysts and aspiration of other cystic structures. Laparoscopy has also been used for tubal sterilization, particularly in cardiac patients, patients with severe metabolic disease, and those with cystic fibrosis, in whom pregnancy is contraindicated.

Many procedures are technically possible with laparoscopy; some may not be in the best interest of the patient. Pelvic cavity laparoscopy usually affords a most complete view. Although the view obtained in laparoscopy is similar to that afforded by laparotomy, the comparison ends there. Manipulation of instruments through secondary puncture sites, no matter how great the dexterity of the laparoscopist, will seldom be as informative. Contraindications to the performance of laparoscopy have changed with advancing technology and experience. Prior abdominal surgery is no longer a contraindication. In our experience, roughly 85 per cent of patients who have undergone abdominal operation have no residual adhesions involving the anterior abdominal wall. In others there is only a thin veil of omentum. Very few patients have bowel adhesions to the laparotomy scar. Peritonitis per se is no longer a contraindication. Contraindications to laparoscopy include hiatus hernia, intestinal obstruction, inability to establish pneumoperitoneum, and inability to tolerate general or endotracheal anesthesia.

While laparoscopic technique varies from institution to institution there are a few basic principles involved. These include the following:

Patients undergoing elective laparoscopy are asked to maintain a low-residue diet for 24 hours before entering the hospital. Enemas are not given and patients do not require local shaving. Catheterization is not required if the patient can void just prior to entering the operating room.

The patient is placed in a modified dorsal lithotomy position with the hips in moderate abduction. It is important that the buttocks be moved slightly over the break in the operating room table in order to allow subsequent depression of the tenaculum and cannula. A ground plate for electrocautery is placed under the patient. Light source and gas supply should be checked and the insufflator charged to full capacity with the flow valve off. The skin of the abdomen and the vaginal cavity is cleaned with povidone-iodine (Betadine) solution.

Preinsufflation is the rule, although a highly skilled laparoscopist can direct the main trocar and cannula into the abdominal cavity by tenting up the abdominal cavity and thrusting the instrument to the sacrum. One should be careful not to point the instrument laterally or directly downward because of the danger of lacerating the aorta or the iliac vessels.

The key to low morbidity following laparoscopy is early ambulation, the avoidance of heavy analgesics, and early voiding. Approximately 95 per cent of patients can be discharged home on the day of surgery.

Complications. Most important complications of laparoscopy are due to inexperience of the operator. However, complications can and do occur even in the hands of the most experienced laparoscopist.

Prevention of laparoscopic complications requires thorough understanding of the indications for, the limitations of, and contraindications to the procedure. Once these are understood, there is no substitute for actual experience.

Complications of laparoscopy may be considered under four general categories: (1) complications of pneumoperitoneum; (2) complications of abdominal wall puncture; (3) complications of intra-abdominal manipulation; and (4) minor complications.

COMPLICATIONS OF PNEUMOPERITONEUM. The most common complication is failure to accomplish peritoneal cavity insufflation. Both carbon dioxide and nitrous oxide are rapidly absorbed from bleeding tissues. Introduction of gas intramurally in the abdominal wall is usually of minor significance. In the obese patient, rather large quantities of gas can collect undetected in the subcutaneous tissues. Subcutaneous emphysema can dissect into the vulva or chest wall. In the very thin patient there is danger of introducing the needle through the peritoneal cavity into the retroperitoneal tissues. This is a more serious complication and can result in pneumomediastinum or dissection of gas around the great vessels. If the pneumoperitoneum cannula is introduced or directed away from the midline, the danger of perforating the iliac vessels is great. Failure to recognize the complication immediately could result in pulmonary air embolism. Perforation of the bowel or other pelvic organs can occur if the patient has had previous abdominal surgery or if the insufflating needle is misdirected.

COMPLICATION OF ABDOMINAL WALL PUNCTURE. Perforations made by the small insufflating needle are of less consequence than those due to placement of the larger instrumentation cannula. Lacerations made by a sharply pointed trocar can result in massive intraperitoneal hemorrhage or intestinal contamination of the peritoneal cavity. Laparoscopy should not be performed unless the surgeon and operating room personnel are prepared for immediate laparotomy. Omental perforation and injuries to the uterine fundus may result in bleeding but can be controlled by electrocoagulation. Abdominal wall bleeding may require local incision and vessel ligation. Laparoscopy, except under exceptional circumstances, is a midline procedure. Puncture sites lateral to the midline should be made only under direct vision of the parietal peritoneum.

COMPLICATIONS OF INTRA-ABDOMINAL MANIPULATION. Most complications arising within the peritoneal cavity occur because the laparoscopist attempts to accomplish more than the technique permits. Hemorrhage and hematomas resulting from lysis of adhesions and tumor resection are not uncommon. Biopsies obtained from areas too vascular to be controlled by cautery or from sites in proximity to the bowel, which cause necrosis and subsequent intestinal perforation, are examples of imprudent judgment. Intestinal burns due to electrocautery require laparotomy with resection of the burned area. Only the surgeon should initiate the electric current.

We have encountered an unusual case of prolonged and persistent intraperitoneal bleeding in a cardiac patient on anticoagulation therapy who underwent tubal sterilization by the Falope ring technique. She required two subsequent laparotomies in 24 hours in order to control bleeding because of coagulation problems. Bleeding was due to sloughing of the tube subsequent to placement of the Falope ring. We have changed our technique in anticoagulation patients and now use a Hulka clip, which does not cause necrosis and compresses the tube satisfactorily.

MINOR COMPLICATIONS. Minor complications following laparoscopy include shoulder pain due to diaphragmatic irritation. Perforation of the uterus with a patency cannula has been observed and is easily detected during establishment of the pneumoperitoneum by hearing gas escaping through the cannula or visualizing the tip of the patency cannula through the laparoscope. Inadvertent perforation of a nonpregnant uterus can occur; bleeding is minimal. Skin burns can result from electrical shorting from the coagulation instrument to the metal sleeve of the cannula and is avoided by applying a nonconductive sleeve over the cannula.

ECTOPIC PREGNANCY

The term "ectopic pregnancy" includes any pregnancy in which implantation occurs outside the uterus. Various locations in the fallopian tube account for more than 95 per cent of such gestations. Other sites of implantation include the broad ligament, the peritoneal cavity, and the ovary. The frequency of ectopic pregnancy ranges from 0.3 to 2.2 per cent of pregnancies. There appears to be a higher incidence of tubal pregnancy in patients using intrauterine contraceptive devices and in those in whom there is a prolonged cycle (over 35 days).

Patients in whom an egg is picked up by the contralateral tube are also prone to ectopic pregnancy, presumably because of delay in passage. Patients with a history of pelvic inflammatory disease and who have coexisting adnexal masses are believed to be more susceptible to this problem.

The diagnosis of tubal pregnancy has been considerably advanced by the development of sensitive and specific radioimmunoassay determinations for human chorionic gonadotropins. Pregnancy tests that measure gonadotropin levels over 2000 milliunits (IU) per ml are considered to be too insensitive to detect early cases of ectopic pregnancy. The beta subunit radioimmuoassay is exquisitely sensitive; very low levels of HCG indicate the presence of trophoblastic tissue.

Technique. Over the past few years there has been a shift in emphasis toward earlier detection of ectopic pregnancy, before tubal rupture and hemorrhage occur. This has led to a more conservative approach in the management of this problem — from that of removal of the tube to preservation of the tube by slit salpingostomy. This is the preferred procedure when the tube appears otherwise healthy and normal. Salpingostomy requires optical magnification. An incision should be made in the antimesenteric border and the tubal pregnancy is scraped out bluntly. The tube is closed in one layer using 6-0 prolene sutures. In general, excellent healing occurs and patency is preserved. When the ampullary portion of the fimbriae is destroyed, a cuff fimbrioplasty is employed, with care taken to preserve vessels. If the pregnancy occurs at the distal end of the tube, it may be milked out of the fimbriated portion without actual incision.

Complications. Complications of operation for tubal pregnancy include persistent postoperative bleeding. Late complications include damage to the tube requiring surgical repair at some future date.

traction away from the ureter and dissected away under direct vision. Parovarian masses are located between the leaves of the broad ligament and present as ovarian lesions. They are remnants of the mesonephric duct system and are easily removed by opening the leaves of the broad ligament. The ureter should always be identified and may be abnormally located. Another potential problem is proximity to the pelvic ligaments containing the ovarian vein and artery.

SALPINGO-OOPHORECTOMY

Removal of the tube and ovary may be required for enlarged ovarian or broad ligament cysts or tumors, endometriomas, and tubo-ovarian abscesses that are unresponsive to antibiotic therapy. It is wise to conserve ovarian tissue in the teenage girl or young child, preserving tissue involved in the reproductive process and recognizing that future problems might occur, such as neoplasia. We prefer ovarian resection to ovariectomy. This is possible in dealing with most benign tumors, but it is generally not possible in operations carried out for acute inflammation.

Injudicious and frequently unnecessary incidental ovarian cystectomy performed at the time of appendectomy may lead to development of perioophoritis and salpingitis. Persistent pain may require eventual sacrifice of the tube or ovary, or both. It is best to avoid surgery on the ovary unless this is performed for primary indications. Meticulous technique will avoid trauma to the ovary and tube, diminishing adhesion formation between the tube and ovary and between the ovary and the posterior aspect of the broad ligament or bowel.

Complications. The most important complication of salpingo-oophorectomy is hemorrhage into the infundibulopelvic ligament and damage to the adjacent ureter. It is best to doubly ligate the two infundibulopelvic ligaments because of the large number of veins and a frequently large ovarian artery.

The ureter should be identified, although it is not necessary to open up the posterior peritoneum; the ureter is visible and palpable through it. When the ureter is adherent to the ovary, the ovary should be held in

CONSERVATIVE LAPAROTOMY

This term is generally applied to an operation performed for pelvic endometriosis or adhesions resulting from old inflammatory disease.[4] The tube and ovary are freed, endometrial implants are excised, and the area is reperitonealized. An additional component of the operation is presacral neurectomy and uterine suspension. There is some controversy regarding presacral neurectomy, particularly with the development of some of the newer prostaglandin inhibitors. The operation is designed to preserve reproductive function, to relieve pain, and to promote normal menstruation.

The immediate complications of presacral neurectomy are damage to the ureter, hemorrhage from injury to the middle sacral artery or larger venous structures, and retroperitoneal hematoma. The right ureter is more commonly injured because it is directly in the operative field. It should be freely visible during the operation and retracted out of the way during dissection. If hematoma develops, it is best to let it resolve spontaneously.

Late complications of presacral neurectomy include bladder infection and constipation, which may be a problem for 3 or 4 weeks postoperatively.

UTERINE SUSPENSION

Uterine suspension may be accomplished by plication of the ureterosacral ligaments, round ligament suspension, and by the modified Olshausen technique. Plication of the uterosacral ligaments may compromise the adjacent ureter through kinking or inadvertent suture ligation. Anterior fixation of the uterus can be performed in several ways. Hemorrhage may occur at the site of suture but the main problem is persistent pain in the suspension site, particularly if the anterior fascia is incorporated in the repair. The main indication for suspension is to bring the uterus out of the pelvis during subsidence of a retroperitoneal process and thus avoid excessive adhesions.

References

1. Acosta, A., Kaplan, A. L., and Kaufman, R. H.: Gynecologic cancer in children. Am. J. Obstet. Gynecol. 112:944, 1972.
2. Cali, R. W., and Pratt, J. H.: Congenital absence of vagina: Long-term results of vaginal reconstruction in 175 cases. Am. J. Obstet. Gynecol. 100:752, 1968.
3. Frank, R. T.: The formation of an artificial vagina without operation. Am. J. Obstet. Gynecol. 35:1053, 1938.
4. Goldstein, D. P., DeCholnoky, C., and Emans, S. J.: Adolescent endometriosis. J. Adolescent Health Care 1:37, 1980.
5. Goldstein, D. P., DeCholnoky, C., Emans, S. J., et al.: Laparoscopy in the diagnosis and management of pelvic pain in adolescents. J. Reprod. Med. 24:251, 1980.
6. Gray, L. A.: Indications, techniques, and complications in vaginal hysterectomy. Obstet. Gynecol. 28:714, 1966.
7. McIndoe, A. H.: Reconstruction of the atretic vagina. Proc. R. Soc. Med. 52:952, 1959.
8. Mahoney, P. J., and Chamberlain, J. W.: Hydrometrocolpos in infancy: Congenital atresia of the vagina with abnormally abundant cervical secretions. J. Pediatr. 17:772, 1940.
9. Pratt, J. H.: Vaginal atresia corrected by use of small and large bowel. Clin. Obstet. Gynecol. 15:639, 1972.
10. Raysom, J. H.: Renal agenesis and bicornuate uterus. J. Iowa Med. Soc. 54:6, 1964.
11. Wabrek, A. J., et al.: Creation of a neovagina by the Frank nonoperative method. Obstet. Gynecol. 37:408, 1971.
12. Welch, K. J.: The female genital tract. In Ravitch, M. M., et al. (eds.): Pediatric Surgery, 3rd Ed. Chicago, Year Book Medical Publishers, Inc., 1979.

OTHER SURGICAL CONSIDERATIONS | 6

29

THE ADRENAL GLANDS

Eric W. Fonkalsrud, M.D.

Although the role of surgery in the treatment of adrenal diseases in childhood has been relatively small, there has been a gradual decline in the risk of operations on these glands. The complications almost unique to adrenal surgery are related to the glands' protected anatomic location, which may lead to technical difficulties in addition to the complex metabolic effects of the adrenal hormones when modified either by the pathologic process or by operation.

ANATOMY

The adrenals are dark yellow glands embedded in the perirenal fat along the anteromedial border of the superior poles of the kidneys. The right adrenal is partially covered by the vena cava and the liver and lies on the lower extensions of the diaphragm. The left adrenal is covered by the peritoneum of the lesser omental bursa, the splenic vessels, and the tail of the pancreas. The glands lie beneath Gerota's fascia, supported independently by numerous fibrous bands and vascular attachments, and remain in a relatively fixed position when the kidney is depressed. Although average weight is 3 to 5 gm, it differs with age.

The extensive arterial supply to the adrenals stems from the phrenic artery superiorly, the aorta medially, and the renal artery inferiorly, although variations are frequent (Fig. 29–1). Ovarian or internal spermatic arterial branches on the left and intercostal

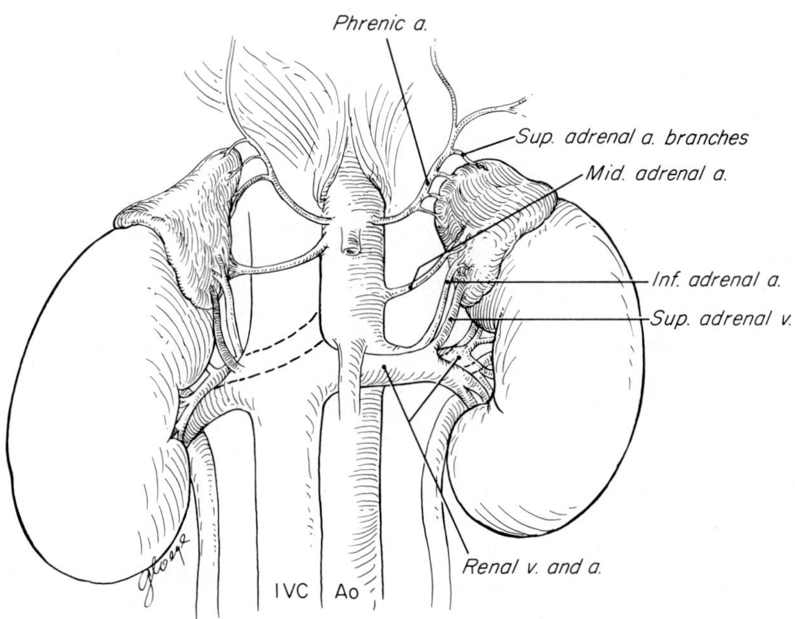

Figure 29–1 Anatomic relationships of the adrenal glands showing major vascular supply.

branches bilaterally may be present. Arterioles in the gland divide into sinusoids extending to the medulla and to the cortex as small capillary loops. Venous drainage returns into the renal vein on the left and directly into the vena cava on the right. Accessory adrenal veins may communicate with the azygous and portal venous systems.

The adrenal nerves are derived from the celiac and renal plexuses and terminate in small ganglia in the medulla. Stimulation of the adrenal nerves produces a prompt release of medullary hormones without influencing cortical activity.[6]

PHYSIOLOGY

Although more than 50 different steroids have been isolated from the adrenal cortex, most are precursors and only a few are actually secreted into the circulation.[8] The corticosteroids are C-21 compounds, including both the glucocorticoids and the mineralocorticoids. The androgens are C-19 steroids and the estrogens are C-18 steroids. The cortex normally contains all enzyme systems necessary for the conversion of cholesterol to cortisol. The zona glomerulosa contains 18-hydroxylase and dehydrogenase, which convert corticosterone to aldosterone. The two most important corticosteroids are cortisol, the major glucocorticoid, and aldosterone, the major mineralocorticoid.[7]

The hypothalamus normally secretes corticotropin-releasing factor (CRF), which releases adrenocorticotropic hormone (ACTH) from the anterior pituitary gland. As blood levels of cortisol rise, a feedback regulatory mechanism inhibits further release of CRF from the hypothalamus except during periods of stress. Androgens are also secreted by ACTH stimulation, although there is no regulatory feedback mechanism. The cortisol regulatory mechanism may be altered by metyrapone (Metopirone), which interferes with 11β-hydroxylation in the cortex. Because cortisol synthesis decreases, there is no feedback to limit continued pituitary secretion of ACTH. The Metopirone test is used to determine whether the pituitary is capable of secreting increased amounts of ACTH.

Secretion of aldosterone depends primarily on stimulation by renin and angiotensin. When renal artery pressure decreases, the renal juxtaglomerular cells release renin. Renin acts on angiotensinogen from the liver to form angiotensin I, which in turn is converted by a circulating enzyme into angiotensin II, which then stimulates the adrenal cortex to release aldosterone. This mechanism is regulated by aldosterone-induced renal retention of sodium that increases the blood volume and reduces the production of renin. Secondary aldosteronism may result from renal artery obstruction, which causes hypersecretion of renin by the juxtaglomerular cells and consequently excess aldosterone with sodium retention, as well as hypertension.

There is considerable overlap of sodium and potassium metabolism between the glucocorticoids and the mineralocorticoids. Cortisol enhances gluconeogenesis, but when it is excessive, protein depletion and diabetes develop. Cortisol also induces a centripetal distribution of fat and hyperlipemia, enhances water diuresis, and assists in maintaining homeostasis of extracellular fluid volume by preventing the shift of water into the cell. Cortisol also sensitizes arterioles to the pressor effects of norepinephrine and related compounds. Glucocorticoids reduce the inflammatory process and the cellular response to injury and inhibit hypersensitivity responses to antigen-antibody complexes.

In contrast, there is no known direct hormonal control of adrenal medullary secretion. Epinephrine, norepinephrine, and dopamine are secreted by at least two types of chromaffin cells in the medulla. The extra-adrenal chromaffin tissues produce norepinephrine and dopamine. Although there is considerable pharmacologic overlap between the catecholamines, epinephrine has greater excitatory, hyperglycemic, and metabolic effects than norepinephrine. The catecholamines are normally metabolized rapidly; about 40 per cent are excreted in the urine as conjugated 3-methoxy-4-hydroxymandelic acid (vanillylmandelic acid, or VMA).

ADRENAL ECTOPIA

The chromaffin tissue masses near the origin of the inferior mesenteric artery are known as the organs of Zuckerkandl and produce only norepinephrine. After birth, the extra-adrenal chromaffin bodies usually involute.

Adrenocortical rests are common and are easily recognized as bright yellow nodules within the kidney or the liver, along the route of descent of the gonads, or within the gonads themselves. Their persistence and hyperplasia in patients with adrenogenital syndrome stems from continued ACTH stimulation. Adrenal insufficiency can occur when ectopic normal adrenal glands are inadvertently removed during nephrectomy or upper abdominal surgery.

COMPLICATIONS RESULTING FROM TECHNICAL DIFFICULTIES

The relatively inaccessible adrenal glands are adjacent to several important organs that are susceptible to operative injury. Good exposure and careful dissection in a dry field are principles that must be followed to avoid injury. Although the majority of operations on the adrenal glands in children can be adequately performed through an abdominal incision, the surgeon should be familiar with other approaches and use them depending upon the type of lesion and the habitus of the patient.

Transabdominal adrenal surgery is particularly useful when the abdominal viscera must be explored and when it is necessary to examine both adrenals before deciding upon the actual procedure to be undertaken. It provides satisfactory exposure for almost all adrenal lesions in thin patients but presents some difficulties in the obese. A bilateral subcostal incision may be extended into the flank, or into the chest for large tumors or in the obese patient.

Transabdominal right adrenalectomy is facilitated by mobilizing the renal fascia from the inferior surface of the diaphragm to bring the adrenal gland closer to the surgical field (Fig. 29–2). The central vein on the right side is short, emptying directly into the vena cava, and mobilization of this structure may injure the vena cava. The hepatic flexure of the colon is retracted downward, and the second portion of the duodenum is mobilized by dividing its later-

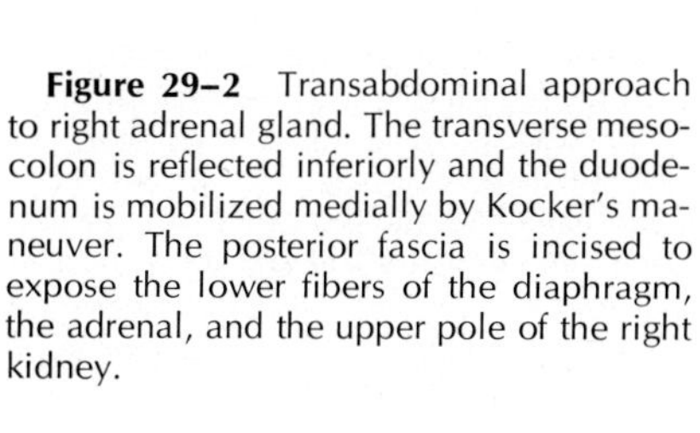

Figure 29–2 Transabdominal approach to right adrenal gland. The transverse mesocolon is reflected inferiorly and the duodenum is mobilized medially by Kocker's maneuver. The posterior fascia is incised to expose the lower fibers of the diaphragm, the adrenal, and the upper pole of the right kidney.

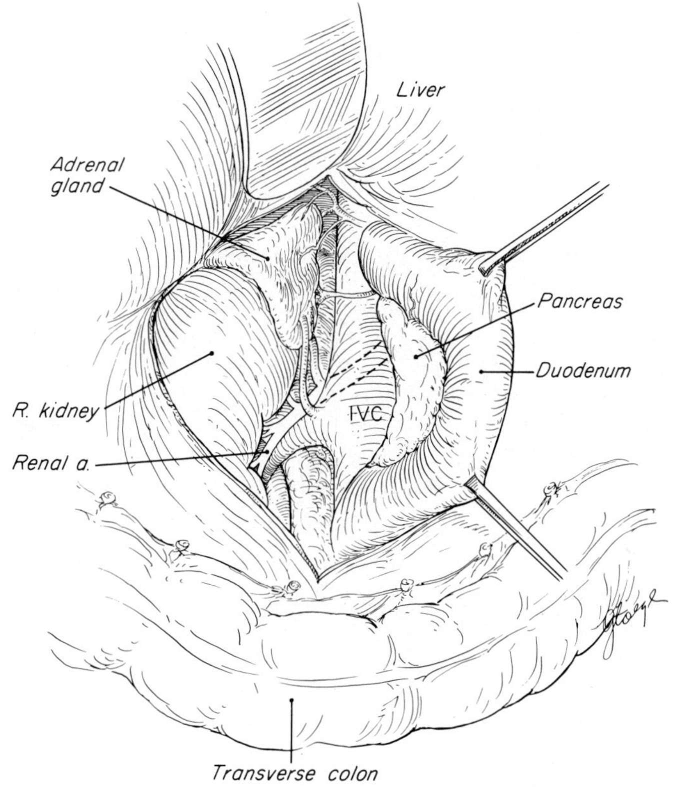

al peritoneal attachments and retracting it medially. Injury to the duodenum may occur during this maneuver but is uncommon.

The left adrenal gland is exposed by reflecting the transverse colon inferiorly, dividing the gastrocolic ligament, and then elevating the stomach (Fig. 29–3). The posterior peritoneum is incised along the lower edge of the pancreas, and the tail of the pancreas is elevated to expose the renal and adrenal veins. An alternative technique is to divide the peritoneum lateral to the splenic flexure of the colon and reflect it medially, exposing the adrenal gland beneath the perirenal fascia. The tail of the pancreas, the splenic vessels, and the spleen must be mobilized carefully to avoid injury. Bleeding from a torn splenic vein can be controlled by digital pressure proximal to the bleeding point to allow repair in a dry field.

The consequences of pancreatic injury are unpredictable; occasional severe damage may heal without difficulty, yet a lesser injury can cause traumatic pancreatitis, abscess, pseudocyst, or pancreatic fistula. Any devascularized portion of the pancreas should be removed. Injury with or without devascularization is an indication for drainage with a Silastic sump.

Laceration of the splenic capsule during adrenalectomy can be avoided by good exposure with minimal blunt dissection. Bleeding from a tear in the splenic capsule can usually be repaired by direct suture, using small pledgets to prevent further laceration of the capsule; by application of microfibrillar collagen (Avitene); and by direct pressure. Total splenectomy is rarely necessary for intraoperative splenic injury in children and should be avoided to obviate the risk of serious sepsis.

A moderate degree of ileus tends to occur after adrenal surgery regardless of the route of exposure. Nasogastric decompression for 24 to 48 hours is recommended.

The lumbar approach provides an entirely extraperitoneal exposure and is used mostly in adults for removal of normal or hyperplastic adrenal glands. It is unsatisfactory for large tumors. To provide bilateral exposure, the patient is placed in the prone position and the twelfth rib is removed. (In obese patients the eleventh rib may be divided posteriorly.) Inasmuch as the pleura ex-

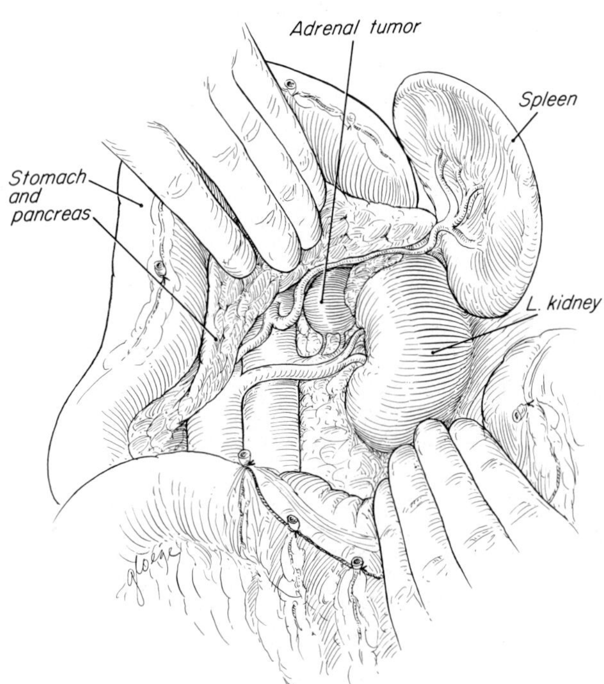

Figure 29–3 The left adrenal gland is readily exposed by dividing the gastrocolic ligament and elevating the stomach. The colon is retracted inferiorly. The peritoneum along the lower border of the pancreas is incised and the pancreas is elevated, exposing the adrenal gland and the renal and adrenal veins.

tends to the level of the twelfth rib posteriorly, care should be taken to avoid entering the pleural space. If the pleura is opened, chest tube drainage must be employed for a short time. Careful auscultation of the chest and a chest roentgenogram are important to identify this problem in the early postoperative period.

The lumbar approach provides less access to the adrenal blood supply than does the abdominal approach. The gland must be mobilized before the vessels are clamped. The risk of hemorrhage is greater on the right side where the adrenal vein is short and easily torn. If a tear extends to the vena cava, rapid bleeding will occur. This can best be treated by placing a gauze pack over the area and applying pressure (Linton maneuver). After 5 minutes, the bleeding will decrease sufficiently to permit identification of the bleeding site, placement of a vascular partial occlusion clamp, and repair of the injury. Transient complete occlusion of the vena cava is rarely necessary, and troublesome bleeding of arterial origin is uncommon.

Transthoracic adrenalectomy is infrequently performed in children even though it provides the wide exposure essential for removing large tumors. The abdominal portion of the incision is made first to confirm the diagnosis, after which the chest is opened by dividing the lower costal cartilages and incising the diaphragm peripherally to avoid injury to the phrenic nerve. Although exposure of the left adrenal gland is excellent, the right adrenal is less accessible because of the intervening liver. Postoperative diaphragmatic hernia may occur. Pulmonary atelectasis, pneumothorax, hemothorax, empyema, and pneumonia are occasional sequelae of thoracoabdominal adrenalectomy. Particular attention should be devoted to managing pulmonary secretions during the postoperative period when the thoracic approach has been employed.

INJURY TO ADRENAL GLANDS DURING NEPHRECTOMY AND RETROPERITONEAL DISSECTION

The adrenal glands are splayed over the surface of the upper pole of the kidneys, although their arterial blood supply is largely independent. Left nephrectomy may lead to inadvertent obstruction of both the arterial and the venous supply to the ipsilateral adrenal gland inasmuch as both artery and vein communicate with the corresponding renal vessels. During nephrectomy, ligation of structures in the renal vascular pedicle should be accomplished distal to the adrenal vessels. Even if the adrenal communications with the renal vessels are interrupted during nephrectomy, there is usually sufficient collateral circulation to permit survival and normal function of the gland. Nephrectomy for Wilms' tumor in most cases may be performed without removing the ipsilateral adrenal gland.

The right adrenal gland is occasionally injured during resection of the right lobe of the liver for tumor or trauma. Phrenic arterial supply is occasionally injured during this dissection. Although the majority of traumatic injuries to the kidney are reparable or can be managed by observation, an occasional severely fractured kidney will require nephrectomy. Under such circumstances it may be difficult to save the ipsilateral adrenal gland.

NEONATAL ADRENAL HEMORRHAGE

Small hemorrhagic cysts of the fetal adrenal cortex are not uncommon; they are frequently bilateral, and are discovered incidentally during laparotomy or postmortem examination. Calcification of the margins is common. Most small cysts are asymptomatic and are absorbed spontaneously. Adrenal hemorrhage in the newborn due to fetal anoxia or difficult labor may produce symptoms of adrenal insufficiency with shock and sepsis, which, if not recognized and treated by adrenocortical hormone replacement, can be fatal.[5] Occasionally there may be an instance of "sudden infant death."[12] The period of required replacement therapy may vary from a few weeks to many months as the hemorrhage is absorbed and function returns. Large cysts, which are rare, may present as an abdominal mass; occasional large adrenal cysts in the newborn result from tumor necrosis, most often neuroblastoma.

ACUTE ADRENAL INSUFFICIENCY

Acute adrenocortical insufficiency is a serious yet avoidable complication of adrenal surgery. It should be anticipated when total or subtotal adrenalectomy is performed. Tumors producing Cushing's syndrome tend to suppress function of the contralateral gland and result in adrenal insufficiency when the tumor is removed. Tumors that primarily produce androgens or estrogens may also be accompanied by atrophy of the contralateral adrenal gland.

Patients with unilateral functioning tumors should be prepared for operation in the same way as those who are to undergo bilateral adrenalectomy, despite the presence of an apparent excess of hydrocortisone, as in Cushing's syndrome. Whereas the patient undergoing total adrenalectomy can be rapidly titrated until his basal adrenal requirements are determined, residual adrenal tissue that is atrophied or injured at operation will require a careful period of "weaning" to promote gradual return of function. The atrophic gland normally resumes function, although the capacity of the residual gland after subtotal adrenalectomy is unpredictable. Many patients who have had bilateral subtotal adrenalectomy must receive permanent substitution therapy.

Children with chronic adrenal insufficiency after bilateral adrenalectomy or as a result of other causes require maintenance steroid replacement with 10 to 40 mg of hydrocortisone daily. Nausea, emesis, and other gastrointestinal symptoms are accurate indicators of the need for increased steroid replacement. Guidelines for corticosteroid replacement in addisonian patients are provided by Frawley.[8]

Acute adrenocortical insufficiency may result from adrenal hemorrhage due to trauma, infection, tumor, or adrenal vascular occlusion. The Waterhouse-Friderichsen syndrome can occur with meningococcal septicemia or may be caused by pneumococcus, staphylococcus, or hemolytic streptococcus and occasionally by other bacterial and viral infections. These patients may experience fever, hypotension, emesis, headache, diarrhea, hypoglycemia, dehydration, weakness, lethargy, and/or abdominal pain. Blood chemical analysis usually shows hyponatremia, hyperkalemia, hypoglycemia, and azotemia. Treatment should begin with prompt hormone replacement, including intravenous infusion of 50 mg of hydrocortisone followed by daily maintenance infusions of 100 to 200 mg. Appropriate antibiotics should be given, and refractory hypotension may require administration of vasopressor drugs.

PREPARATION OF THE PATIENT FOR ADRENALECTOMY

The indications for bilateral adrenalectomy in children are rare. When the procedure is anticipated, the patient is given preoperative hydrocortisone and, for maximal safety, small amounts of a mineralocorticoid such as 0.1 mg of fludrocortisone (Florinef). The dosage of hydrocortisone varies with the size of the patient. During adrenalectomy, an intravenous infusion of 5 per cent dextrose in half-normal saline solution is given, with 100 mg of hydrocortisone per liter added. Although acute intraoperative adrenal insufficiency is rare, the signs are similar to those caused by drugs (hypotension and tachycardia). Acute adrenal insufficiency is most common during the first 72 hours after operation, producing symptoms of apathy, restlessness, weakness, anorexia, emesis, fever, tachycardia, and hypotension. The serum sodium and potassium levels tend to be normal, although the blood urea nitrogen may be elevated under these circumstances. Unless promptly treated with intravenous hydrocortisone (100 mg), the patient may experience progressive shock leading to death. Special precautions must be taken for the adrenalectomized diabetic patient, because insulin requirements often decrease after adrenalectomy. In the presence of infection, both insulin and steroid requirements will increase. Failure to recognize this may lead to adrenal insufficiency and eventually to diabetic coma.

Because of the special risks faced by the adrenalectomized patient, it is recommended that such patients wear an identification card indicating "I am an adrenalectomized patient. In an emergency I will need cortisone."

The period of withdrawal or weaning from corticoids in patients with adrenal insufficiency should be gradual, with the daily dosage being decreased by 5 mg every 1 to 2 weeks. An increase in steroid therapy will be necessary if the patient is exposed to infection or stress.

COMPLICATIONS OF ADRENAL STEROID THERAPY

Continued use of adrenal steroid hormones in excess of physiologic requirements has potentially serious consequences. Although considerable effort has been expended to develop steroid compounds that have potent anti-inflammatory action without the other physiologic effects of cortisone, none of the steroids in current use is entirely free of undesirable effects or complications. Cortisone administration eventually results in atrophy of the adrenal cortex, while ACTH therapy induces pituitary inactivity. The end result of withdrawing either hormone is temporary adrenal insufficiency, causing weakness, fatigability, anorexia, nausea, and diarrhea. When the patient is subjected to stress of sufficient magnitude, such as major infections or surgery, acute adrenal insufficiency may be precipitated. Administration of hydrocortisone during periods of stress may prevent development of the acute symptoms. Our current practice is to administer supplementary hydrocortisone preoperatively, intraoperatively, and throughout the postoperative period to all patients undergoing surgery who received steroid therapy for at least 2 weeks during the preceding year.

The anti-inflammatory properties of steroids reduce resistance to infection and tend to induce a sense of well-being that might mask the symptoms until overwhelming sepsis occurs. Major operative procedures in patients receiving steroid therapy should therefore be accompanied by administration of appropriate antimicrobial agents.

In view of the increased incidence of gastroduodenal ulceration in patients receiving steroid therapy, it is currently our practice to administer cimetidine, a hydrogen ion antagonist, to minimize gastric secretion until the patient is able to tolerate regular oral feedings well.

HYPERFUNCTION OF THE ADRENAL CORTEX

The clinical manifestations of adrenocortical hyperfunction depend upon the age of onset, the nature of the defect, the sex of the patient, the hormones secreted in increased amount, and the underlying pathologic process. Hyperplasia of the adrenal cortex occurring in utero causes male pseudohermaphroditism. After birth, precocious sexual development or heterosexual changes occur either alone or in conjunction with the signs of Cushing's syndrome, predominantly affecting female infants. Moreover, adrenogenital syndrome is far more common than Cushing's syndrome or primary hyperaldosteronism in the pediatric age group. Feminizing changes in men are rare; the cases reported thus far have resulted from malignant cortical tumors. The symptoms of Cushing's syndrome in adolescents include truncal obesity with characteristic fat pads in the upper back, adipose accumulation in the face (moon facies), plethora, hypertension with headaches, peripheral edema, muscular weakness, growth retardation, capillary fragility, ecchymoses, osteoporosis, and pathologic fractures as well as skin fragility with abdominal striae due to protein depletion. In fact, the skin is often so fragile that removal of adhesive tape may de-epithelialize the involved areas. Since cortisol promotes retention of salt and water, electrolyte imbalance tends to develop, along with metabolic alkalosis and hypokalemia, even though aldosterone secretion is normal.[11] Androgen secretion may increase, accounting for the frequent incidence of amenorrhea, hirsutism, and acne in adolescent girls and the virilization often apparent in boys. These patients typically manifest a diabetic glucose tolerance curve with glucosuria and diabetes. The white blood cell count may be elevated. Emotional instability is characteristic.

In patients with Cushing's syndrome secondary to excess pituitary secretion of ACTH and resultant adrenal hyperplasia, bilateral adrenalectomy has been used effectively for many years, although this treatment is directed at the target organ, not at the organ at fault. Less than bilateral total adrenalectomy is usually followed by recurrent symptoms of Cushing's syndrome.[4]

When a benign adenoma is suspected on the basis of preoperative studies, the involved gland should be resected and a biopsy of the contralateral gland done. Adrenocortical carcinoma must be excised widely and a thorough search made of the abdomen for metastases. Prolonged drug treatment is used primarily for patients with Cushing's syndrome due to inoperable carcinoma of the adrenal cortex with metastases. Ectopic ACTH-producing tumors should be resected. If this is not feasible, bilateral adrenalectomy should be performed, depending upon the prognosis for life with the primary tumor.

Although rare in children, primary aldosteronism as described by Conn may be caused by a benign adrenal cortical adenoma or by bilateral adrenal hyperfunction, with or without hyperplasia.[3] Adenomas, which account for almost 90 per cent of cases of primary aldosteronism, are usually small, well encapsulated and solitary. In 1970 a comprehensive review of the many causes of secondary aldosteronism was presented by Kaplan.[10] Bilateral adrenal exploration is indicated for patients with primary aldosteronism in hope of removing an adenoma. However, if an adenoma cannot be identified in the adrenal gland, the course is not clear, since primary aldosteronism may be successfully managed medically. Several surgeons recommend bilateral hemiadrenalectomy with careful sectioning of the gland to search for adenoma or hyperplasia, to be followed by complete adrenalectomy if a tumor is found on the involved side. Although total adrenalectomy is the preferred procedure for definite hyperplasia, unilateral adrenalectomy and 50 to 75 per cent resection of the contralateral gland may be optimal for patients with clear primary aldosteronism in whom neither adenoma nor hyperplasia can be found.

PHEOCHROMOCYTOMAS

Pheochromocytomas produce symptoms by secreting large amounts of epinephrine and norepinephrine in varying proportions, the amount of norepinephrine being greater in children than in most adults.[2] An abdominal exploration encompassing both adrenal glands, the periaortic sympathetic ganglia, the small bowel mesentery, and the pelvis will reveal more than 95 per cent of all pheochromocytomas. The right adrenal gland is affected approximately twice as often as the left. Bilateral tumors have been reported in as many as 25 to 70 per cent of children.[1, 9] Extra-adrenal pheochromocytomas are present in approximately 30 per cent of children, about twice the number found in adults. Malignancy occurs in less than 6 per cent of children with pheochromocytoma. The association of pheochromocytoma with medullary carcinoma of the thyroid (Sipple's syndrome) has been observed occasionally in children. There is a 12 per cent incidence of other anomalies in the families of children with pheochromocytoma (hydrocephalus, neurofibromas, ganglioneuromas, megacolon, megaureter, cryptorchism). The tumor is more likely to occur in children who have congenital heart defects. Approximately 10 per cent of childhood pheochromocytomas are familial, an incidence nearly four times higher than that in adults.

Tumors arising in the adrenal medulla produce both epinephrine and norepinephrine, whereas the majority of extra-adrenal pheochromocytomas yield only norepinephrine. The catecholamines manufactured by pheochromocytomas directly or indirectly activate the alpha- or beta-adrenergic receptors or both, resulting in the adrenergic syndrome (apprehension, hypertension, tachycardia, sweating, manifestations of increased metabolism, constipation, and gastrointestinal bleeding). A functioning tumor usually causes sustained hypertension in children. In contrast, adults tend to experience paroxysmal hypertension. Intravenous pyelography, abdominal ultrasonography, computed axial tomography, and aortography represent the chief diagnostic tools to define the location and size of pheochromocytomas in children. Measurement of catecholamine levels by means of selective adrenal venous catheterization has been helpful in localizing occasional lesions in older children.

Whether it is mandatory to give medical treatment before removing a pheochromocytoma is still undetermined. Epinephrine and norepinephrine from the tumor tend to reduce the blood volume by causing peripheral vasoconstriction. Preoperative vasodilatation with phentolamine or phenoxybenzamine and colloid infusion to restore blood volume before or during surgery will help to obviate the marked swings in blood pressure that characterize tumor excision in the unprepared patient. Patients with high basal metabolic rates and high plasma levels of catecholamines are at high anesthetic risk. Preoperative use of the beta blocker propranolol may be helpful when preparing patients for operation by controlling tachycardia and preventing intraoperative arrhythmias. On the other hand, pretreatment can render the patient unresponsive to norepinephrine after the adrenal tumor is removed.

Anesthetic premedication should consist of meperidine (Demerol) and scopolamine, the combination least likely to produce arrhythmias and tachycardia. The safest anesthetic combination appears to be nitrous oxide, thiopental sodium (Pentothal), Demerol, and succinylcholine. Halothane has been used successfully by many anesthesiologists; if halothane is combined with a beta receptor blocker, arrhythmias are minimized. Beta-adrenergic blockage with lidocaine, 25 to 100 mg, or propranolol, 1 to 5 mg, or both, can be added intravenously for ventricular arrhythmias lasting longer than 20 to 60 seconds if the cardiac output is depressed. Continuous arterial and venous pressure monitoring are helpful guides, and electrocardiographic monitoring is indispensable. Phentolamine or nitroprusside should be used as a continuous drip to control hypertension, which may result from operative manipulation of the tumor. Colloid or blood and norepinephrine or angiotensin II should be used to treat hypotension that occurs precipitously after removal of the tumor. A norepinephrine infusion may be necessary for periods ranging from a few hours to several days. The venous drainage of the involved gland or tumor should be secured promptly, and the tumor should be manipulated as little as possible to minimize the secretion of catecholamines into the circulation. Exploration of the contralateral adrenal gland is mandatory in all children; clear visualization of the entire gland is essential, and even biopsy is recommended by some authors because of the high incidence of bilateral tumors.[1]

In occasional patients the blood pressure may not return to normal levels for several days after removal of the tumor. We have observed that if the blood pressure does not return to normal within 2 to 3 weeks, or if hypertension returns, a second tumor should be suspected. Inasmuch as hypertension due to a second pheochromocytoma is likely to occur within 5 years after removal of the initial tumor, children who undergo resection of a pheochromocytoma should have follow-up examinations at least twice annually, including measurement of blood pressure and urine catecholamine determinations. Moreover, the progeny and siblings of such patients should also be evaluated periodically for hypertension because of the high incidence of familial occurrence.

References

1. Bloom, D. A., and Fonkalsrud, E. W.: Surgical management of pheochromocytoma in children. J. Pediatr. Surg. 9:179, 1974.
2. Cone, T. E., Jr., Allen, M. S., and Pearson, H. A.: Pheochromocytoma in children: Report of three familial cases in two unrelated families. Pediatrics 19:44, 1957.
3. Conn, J. W.: Primary aldosteronism: A new clinical syndrome. J. Lab. Clin. Med. 45:6, 1955.
4. Egdahl, R. H., and Melby, J. C.: Recurrent Cushing's disease and intermittent functional adrenal cortical insufficiency following subtotal adrenalectomy. Ann. Surg. 166:586, 1967.
5. Favara, B. E., Franciosi, R. A., and Miles, W.: Idiopathic adrenal hypoplasia in children. Am. J. Clin. Pathol. 57:287, 1972.
6. Forsham, P. H.: The adrenals. *In* Williams, R. H. (ed.): Textbook of Endocrinology, 3rd edition. Philadelphia, W. B. Saunders Co., 1962, p. 383.
7. Forsham, P. H., and Melmon, K. L.: The adrenals. *In* Williams, R. H. (ed.): Textbook of Endocrinology, 4th edition. Philadelphia, W. B. Saunders Co., 1968, p. 287.
8. Frawley, T. F.: Adrenal cortical insufficiency. *In* Eisenstein, A. B. (ed.): The Adrenal Cortex. Boston, Little, Brown and Co., 1967, p. 439.
9. Hume, D. M.: Pheochromocytoma in the adult and in the child. Am. J. Surg. 99:458, 1960.
10. Kaplan, N. M.: Secondary aldosteronism: With observations on the definition of hypokalemia. Am. J. Clin. Pathol. 54:316, 1970.
11. Migeon, C. J., Green, O. C., and Eckert, J. P.: Study of adrenocortical function in obesity. Metabolism 12:718, 1963.
12. Tsung, S. H., and Loh, W. P.: Sudden infant death and old adrenal hemorrhage. JAMA 241:2507, 1979.

ARTERIES AND VEINS

J. Alex Haller, Jr., M.D.

30

Vascular injuries occur frequently in infants and children and may be increasing with the general increase in blunt trauma and invasive diagnostic studies in this age group.[6] Many vascular injuries are similar to those seen in adults; however, some are unique to the pediatric age group. The sequelae of vascular injuries in children may include claudication with exercise and limb growth disturbances. Growth retardation is due to ischemia; overgrowth is due to increased flow to the involved extremity, commonly seen in patients with traumatic arteriovenous fistulae. Most vascular injuries are preventable through better education of children about home accidents and traffic safety and increased awareness of possible iatrogenic injuries. Better understanding of the mechanisms and range of vascular injuries may make physicians more cautious about recommending invasive intravascular diagnostic studies in children and more aggressive about early diagnosis and operative

intervention when complications of these diagnostic studies occur.[3]

Recent reports of blood vessel injuries due to trauma in children suggest an absolute increase in frequency as well as better collection and collation of data through regional trauma centers. Children share with adults injuries to arteries and veins resulting from cardiac catheterization, arteriography, and other invasive diagnostic studies as well as vascular injuries resulting from blunt and penetrating trauma. A higher incidence of thrombosis occurs in infants and young children undergoing catheterization because of the small size of their vessels. Unusual, if not unique, injuries to blood vessels in small children include damage resulting from injection of therapeutic agents or from falls on sharp objects, such as shards of broken glass, and injury associated with long bone fractures, especially humeral supracondylar and femoral fractures (Fig. 30–1).

In a study of vascular injuries in children

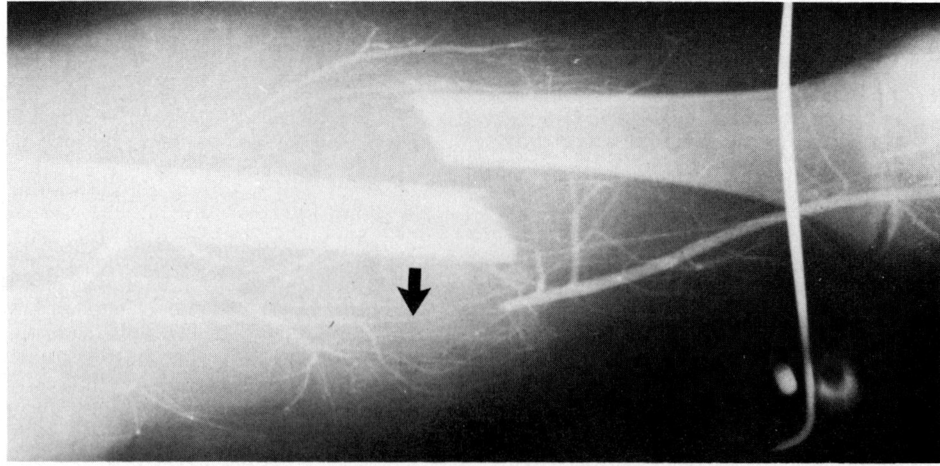

Figure 30–1 Contusion and segmental thrombosis of the superficial femoral artery adjacent to a displaced mid-femoral fracture. The involved segment was resected and replaced with a reversed saphenous vein graft.

TABLE 30–1 ETIOLOGY OF VASCULAR INJURY IN 110 CHILDREN*

Etiology	Number of Patients	Per Cent of Total
Penetrating	39	35
Gunshot	12	11
Knife	4	4
Glass	17	15
Other	6	5
Blunt	13	12
Iatrogenic	55	50
Catheterization	49	45
Other	6	5
Electrical	1	1
Unknown	2	2
TOTAL	110	

*From Haller, J. A., Jr.: Vascular injuries. *In* Touloukian, R. J., ed.: Pediatric Trauma. New York, John Wiley & Sons, 1978.

reported from the Johns Hopkins Hospital and Vanderbilt University Hospital for a 10-year period, 110 patients had major vascular injuries (Table 30–1).[7] More than 50 per cent of these injuries resulted from invasive diagnostic studies, and 47 per cent resulted from trauma (Table 30–2). There is an increasing incidence of vascular as well as other organ injuries in children resulting from handguns, especially on the East Coast of the United States. This is undoubtedly related to the growing number of handguns left unprotected from inquisitive children in private homes.

TABLE 30–2 SITE OF ARTERIAL INJURY IN 110 CHILDREN*

Carotid	3
Vertebral	1
Innominate-subclavian	11
Brachial	24
Radial	13
Ulnar	3
Aorta	4
Iliac	4
Femoral	40
Popliteal	6
Anterior tibial	2
Posterior tibial	1
Peroneal	1

*From Haller, J. A., Jr.: Vascular injuries. *In* Touloukian, R. J., ed.: Pediatric Trauma. New York, John Wiley & Sons, 1978.

Iatrogenic injuries to blood vessels resulting from invasive diagnostic studies are more common in small patients. Many of these infants have severe forms of congenital heart disease. Compromised circulation makes them more liable to stasis thrombosis. In most series, femoral vessel injuries predominate.[3]

SIGNS AND SYMPTOMS OF VASCULAR INJURIES

A vascular injury is easily recognized when there are no distal pulses. However, a vascular injury may be present and can result in ischemia even with weakly palpable pulses. Coolness of an involved extremity on comparison with the opposite one and associated sluggish capillary filling are objective signs of inadequate circulation. Late signs, such as petechial hemorrhage, blister formation, and muscle rigidity, should never occur if the child is under close sequential observation. Occasionally, nerve ischemia will result in paresthesias, anesthesia, or paralysis. More commonly, pain is the chief early symptom associated with tissue ischemia. Symptoms may be difficult to evaluate in the very young child because of the patient's inability to communicate. If a vascular injury is suspected, Doppler pressure measurements are imperative. On occasion, especially with complex multiple-system injuries, arteriography will be necessary. In the Vanderbilt-Hopkins series only 15 per cent of children with major vascular injuries required arteriography to establish the diagnosis.[5]

The question of arteriospasm, which is unlikely, versus thrombosis cannot be resolved without contrast studies. Although spasm may be associated with adjacent soft tissue injury and with hematoma in the vessel wall, it does not result in prolonged absence of distal pulses. A lack of distal pulses beyond 2 to 3 hours is diagnostic of thrombosis.[9] At this point, operative exploration under general anesthesia is mandatory. An extremity that remains ischemic although viable without pulsatile flow should have arterial exploration, because growth retardation or delayed claudication may occur in spite of the development of collateral circulation.

OPERATIVE MANAGEMENT OF VASCULAR INJURIES

Basic principles of operative management of arterial injuries in infants and children are the same as for adults. Local anesthesia is rarely used, because a child cannot cooperate adequately; general anesthesia is almost always required. Occasionally, the site of arterial entry may be re-explored through the operative wound with a local anesthesia supplement if the child is still well sedated from the original procedure. The major considerations are adequate exposure and fine microvascular technique. Because the vessels are small, intraoperative systemic heparinization is usually recommended. Intraoperative arteriography is rarely required and rarely useful. If the arterial injury is an intimal tear or an intramural hematoma, resection of the involved segment with a fresh primary anastomosis is recommended. Occasionally, a diagnostic arteriotomy may be reopened, the edges freshened by excision, and the arteriotomy repaired. Repair and anastomosis should be constructed using 6–0 or 7–0 monofilament vascular suture material under appropriate magnification. The sutures should be interrupted so that growth can occur between them. Fasciectomy, as an adjunct in the management of the ischemic limb, is rarely necessary if the diagnosis is made early and if late ischemic injury to the muscle and soft tissue is avoided. It is occasionally helpful as an adjunctive procedure.

NEEDLE INJECTION INJURIES

Significant vascular complications may result from injections of preoperative and therapeutic medications. A number of reports emphasize errors in technique of injection, especially in neonates and young infants, in whom the injecting needle or solution damaged blood vessels, especially the femoral vessels. Many more such episodes have occurred than have been reported in the literature. In reporting a series of such complications, Talbert et al.[7] discussed the problem and made a number of recom-

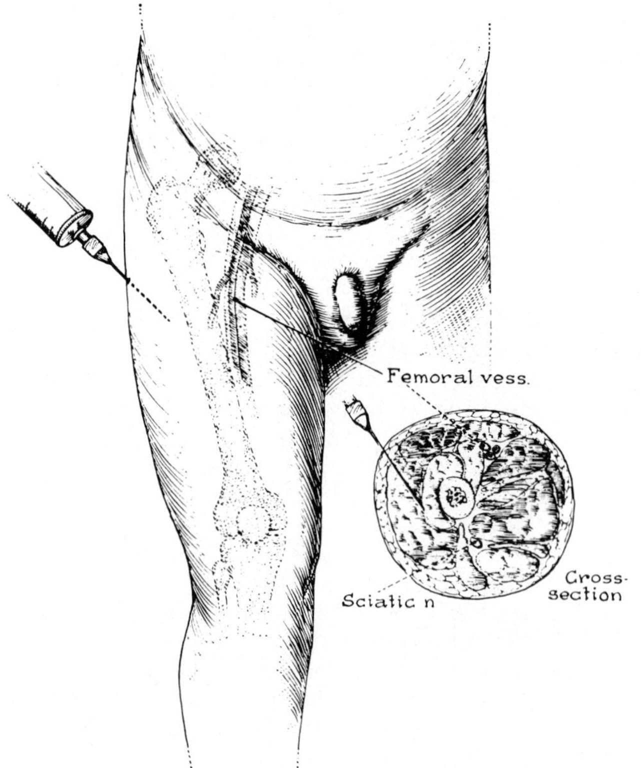

Figure 30–2 Recommended technique of injection to avoid vascular injury: Diagrammatic representation of the optimal site for intramuscular injections in infants. A 1-inch needle should be inserted obliquely into the upper outer quadrant of the thigh at a 45-degree angle with the horizontal and long axes of the leg. The tissues at the injection site are compressed, a maneuver that increases the penetrable mass of the vastus lateralis muscle. (From Talbert, J. L., Haslam, R. J. A., and Haller, J. A., Jr.[7] with permission.)

mendations. Two were modifications of the technique of thigh injection.[1] All 1½-inch 19- and 20-gauge needles have been replaced by 1-inch needles, which are of sufficient length to allow satisfactory intramuscular injection in a child of any age, yet are not so long that transfixion of a major vessel is likely.[2] Instruction of personnel who perform intramuscular injections in infants and small children has also been modified. Increased emphasis is placed on familiarity with the anatomy of the upper thigh, stressing the course of major nerves and vessels. The site of injection has been moved somewhat proximally and is limited to the upper outer quadrant of the thigh. The major muscle mass in this area is utilized, providing buffer between the site of injection and adjacent vital structures. The potential hazard of inserting the needle horizontally is contrasted with the greater safety of more vertical or oblique insertion (Fig. 30–2). The infrequency with which such complications have occurred in the recent past indicates that, with the addition of the safeguards outlined here, the thigh is the safest site for intramuscular injections.

PENETRATING INJURIES

The increased availability of handguns in homes has contributed greatly to increased incidence of penetrating injuries in children. Shards from broken glass doors and windows are particularly dangerous to young children. Brachial and femoral vessel laceration or transection occurs commonly from this type of penetrating injury. Arterial injuries from long bone fractures, especially at the supracondylar level, are common in young people, especially older children and teenagers involved in contact sports. Severe prolonged ischemia to extremities associated with fractures can result in Volkmann's contractures and chronic neurovascular symptoms. Acute and chronic complications can be prevented by early recognition of vascular injury and early arterial repair.

INTRAOPERATIVE INJURIES

The great vessels — aorta and pulmonary artery — are rarely injured during pediatric surgical procedures, but they figure prominently in pediatric cardiac surgical mishaps. Fortunately, many such injuries are repairable because of the availability of a heart-lung machine and means of maintaining the circulation while these life-threatening injuries are corrected.

Arteriovenous fistulae are known complications of pediatric orthopedic procedures, such as rotational osteotomies, and may also result from hurried mass ligation of the renal pedicle for trauma or for resection of large renal tumors and for removal of a ruptured spleen. Secondary arteriovenous fistulae may result when the ligature of arteries and veins cuts through the vascular walls, producing a false aneurysm. Arteriovenous fistulae have also been reported following femoral vein aspiration when the needle penetrates artery and vein, leaving a tract that results in a communication. These accidents are not always detected immediately. A pulsatile mass or loud bruit may present many months after the procedure has been carried out (Fig. 30–3A,B).

The iliac arteries and veins are easily injured during radical iliac lymphadenectomy as a component of treatment of testicular malignancies and other pelvic cancer. The carotid artery has been injured during removal of a large carotid body tumor. In these cases, the saphenous vein has been useful as a bypassing graft. Rarely, the contralateral renal artery has been injured at the time of removal of a large neuroblastoma that crosses over the midline. Although this is uncommon, the injury can usually be repaired if it is recognized.

The inferior vena cava may be injured during resection of large vascular tumors in the upper abdomen, especially lymphangiomas, and has on occasion required ligation at the site of injury. The superior vena cava is less rarely injured, but can be damaged in the removal of large osteosarcomas and other malignancies in the sternal or substernal areas. These large veins can usually be repaired if the operator is competent and exposure is adequate.

In the past, major complications have resulted from use of the brachial artery for catheterization and arteriography. Since the brachial artery is the primary vessel supplying the forearm with very little collateral circulation, cutdowns in the antecubital fossa for brachial artery access should be

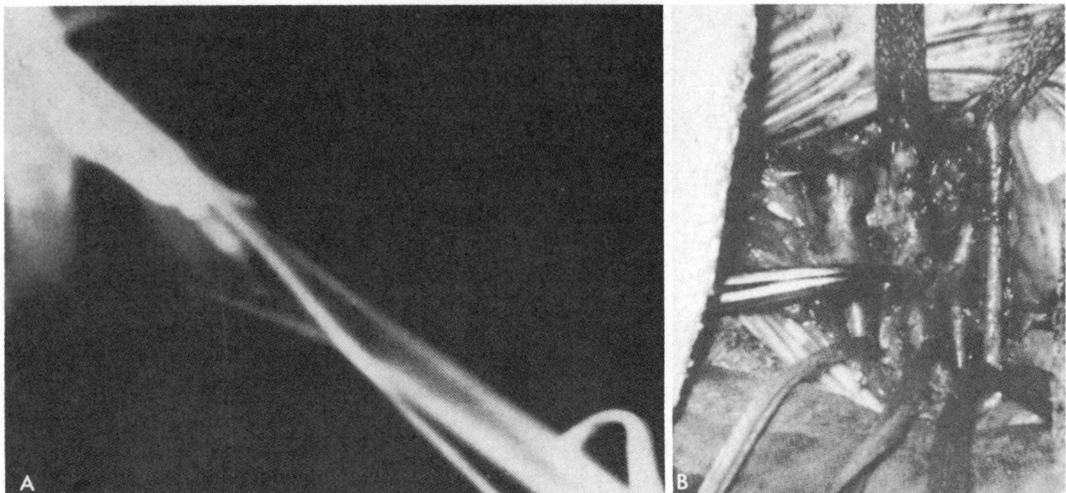

Figure 30–3   *A,* Arteriovenous fistula between profunda femoris artery and deep femoral vein following arterial puncture for blood gas analysis. *B,* The fistulous connection between the profunda femoris and the deep femoral vein is indicated by the instrument tip. (From White, J. J., Talbert, J. L., and Haller, J. A., Jr.,[9] with permission.)

avoided. If the catheter occludes the muscular branch and thrombosis occurs in the primary vessel, loss of peripheral tissue is frequent, including fingers and even the hand. The brachial artery should never be used for catheterization unless it is absolutely mandatory.

The frequent use of central lines, especially percutaneously placed lines, has resulted in perforation of the subclavian vein or the innominate vein with resulting mediastinal hemorrhage and/or pericardial tamponade and massive hemothorax. These known complications can be prevented by careful attention to detail in the placement of percutaneous lines. Awareness of the complication will lead to rapid surgical correction.

Umbilical artery lines, especially if they are left in place for many days, may result in embolic phenomena, which may be responsible for segmental necrotizing enterocolitis on an ischemic basis and for intestinal infarction secondary to occlusion of the superior mesenteric artery. Intraperitoneal hemorrhage has been reported as the result of perforation of the umbilical artery. Aneurysm of the iliac vessels as a result of perforation at that site has also been reported.[4] Although these complications can be managed with appropriate vascular surgical techniques, the diagnosis is often delayed because of the small size of the infants.

The radial artery is popular for the inser-

tion of an arterial monitoring line. Complications include inadvertent disconnection with exsanguination, and gangrene of the fingers due to inadequate volar collateral circulation when the radial artery becomes occluded.

INJURIES DUE TO INVASIVE DIAGNOSTIC STUDIES

Cardiac catheterization and diagnostic arteriography are more and more frequently used in infants and young children to diagnose congenital heart disease, delineate intra-abdominal masses, and determine visceral involvement resulting from blunt abdominal injuries. Complications related to arterial punctures in small children occur quite frequently in spite of improvements in technique and the use of heparin infusions during catheterization.[2] Arterial injuries include intramural hematoma, thrombosis, arteriovenous fistula, false aneurysm, and major bleeding if the arterial line becomes disconnected. The incidence of thrombosis following cardiac catheterization and arteriography in preschool children, formerly reported to be as high as 25 to 30 per cent, more recently has been in the range of 5 to 10 per cent.

The most recent information from the Boston Children's Hospital Medical Center Cardiac Catheterization Unit indicates a marked decrease in complications associated with percutaneous and cutdown arteriography in infants and young children.[2] Of nearly 3700 patients between the ages of 1 and 11 years, only eight sustained thrombosis associated with cardiac catheterization. Circulation was restored in all with operative intervention. There have been no complications in the last 2 years. During that same period, 802 babies under the age of 1 year requiring cardiac catheterization had no thrombosis or none that required operative intervention. This is truly a remarkable record and a testimony to experienced diagnosticians and their awareness of the problem of thrombosis, which can be prevented with attention to detail and use of heparinization during the catheterization procedure.

Arteriography is being used increasingly in the evaluation of children and adults with blunt trauma. Although the site of intra-abdominal bleeding may be determined through diagnostic arteriography, it carries with it the potential for injury to the femoral artery, especially in small children. In addition to small size, factors that predispose to thrombosis in children are congestive heart failure, low cardiac output, polycythemia, dehydration, hypoxia, acidosis, infection, and possibly neoplasia.

Since most iatrogenic injuries from diagnostic procedures occur in preschool children, these invasive tests must be fully justified and carefully evaluated before being recommended. There are potential complications even when the studies are performed by experienced personnel in medical centers where these tests are routine.

A special category of vascular injury is spontaneous thrombosis of major veins and arteries with resulting *gangrene of the extremities*. This dramatic complication has been extensively documented and reported by Welch.[8] It may result from increased coagulability or inflammation of the extremity veins, or it may be iatrogenic. Major problems have been encountered in sick infants under 6 months of age, in whom collapsed veins and low arterial perfusion pressure have been faulted (Fig. 30–4). These babies often have major congenital heart abnormalities. During the prolonged course of diagnostic studies, low perfusion results in venous or arterial occlusion with secondary gangrene. In our own clinic at Johns Hop-

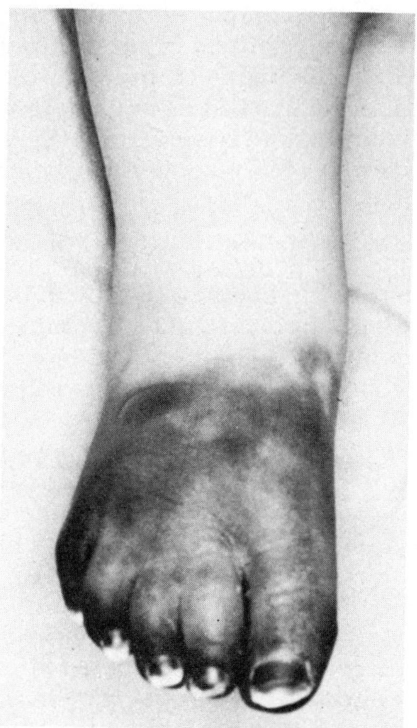

Figure 30–4 Gangrene of forefoot following needle puncture injury to the femoral vessels. The patient, aged 6 months, was hospitalized for diarrheal dehydration with hyperosmolarity and low perfusion.

kins we have encountered a half dozen children with upper extremity gangrene following use of the axillary artery for diagnostic cardiac catheterization; all had complicated congenital heart disease. A transfemoral retrograde study is less likely to result in extremity gangrene. In either instance ischemia is due not to spasm but to thrombosis. These children should have immediate operative intervention as soon as the diagnosis is made. A particular plea for caution should be made about use of a radial artery catheter for injection of drugs or as a feeding line. This should be avoided at all cost! Many drugs, from anesthetic agents to antibiotics to ordinary crystalloids, have been injected. The artery will often go into irreversible spasm with secondary thrombosis. Massive necrosis of the gluteal muscles has been described following the accidental injection of penicillin into the gluteal artery. Many cases of nerve palsy following penicillin injection may have been due not to direct sciatic nerve trauma or chemical neuritis but rather to vascular injury with ischemia.

One of the most important means of

managing the complications of catheterization and arteriography is the administration of heparin during these procedures. Freed et al.[2] noted a marked decrease in complications following the routine use of heparin at the Children's Hospital Medical Center. Immediately after arterial cannulation, heparin (1 mg/kg) or a placebo was administered in an ongoing clinical study. Following catheterization, pulse amplitude in both legs was remeasured and pulse volume index calculated. In patients with evidence of vascular compromise, intravenous infusion of heparin was started. If no improvement was noted within 8 hours, open operation was performed. Seventy-seven children 10 years of age or younger required systemic heparinization after catheterization. The ratio of the placebo group to the heparin group was 2:1. Arteriotomy and thrombectomy was required in seven of 37 children in the placebo group and in none of 40 in the heparin group. No complications related to the use of heparin were noted. It would therefore seem that heparinization at the time of cardiac catheterization should be routine, as has been the practice at Children's Hospital Medical Center in Boston since 1973. During this time only four patients have required surgical intervention for thrombosis. All were treated by thrombectomy with closure. Patency was established in all without a single instance of extremity gangrene.

CONCLUSION

Prevention is extremely important, as in most pediatric diseases, in considering vascular injuries in children. Handguns must be kept in childproof cabinets or drawers.

Careful evaluation of the indications for invasive studies in a young child is required, because most iatrogenic vascular injuries resulting from catheterization and arteriography occur in infants and young children. When clearly indicated, these procedures should be carried out by the most experienced personnel and in centers where invasive studies are frequently performed in small children. Strong suspicion coupled with early recognition of vascular injuries and aggressive operative intervention should prevent limb gangrene or loss of function from ischemic contracture.

References

1. Cahill, J. L., Talbert, J. L., Otteson, O. E., et al.: Arterial complications following cardiac catheterization in infants and children. J. Pediatr. Surg. 2:134, 1967.
2. Freed, M. D., Keane, J. F., and Rosenthal, A.: The use of heparinization to prevent arterial thrombosis after percutaneous cardiac catheterization in children. Circulation 50:565, 1974.
3. Haller, J. A., Jr.: Vascular injuries. *In* Touloukian, R. J. (ed.): Pediatric Trauma. New York, John Wiley & Sons, 1978.
4. Miller, D., Kirkpatrick, B., Kodroff, M., et al.: Pelvic exsanguination following umbilical artery catheterization in neonates. J. Pediatr. Surg. 16:264, 1979.
5. Shaker, I. J., O'Neill, J. A., Foster, J. H., et al.: Vascular injuries in children. J. Pediatr. Surg. (in press).
6. Shaker, I. J., White, J. J., Signer, R. D., et al.: Special problems of vascular injuries in children. J. Trauma 16:863, 1976.
7. Talbert, J. L., Haslam, R. J. A., and Haller, J. A., Jr.: Gangrene of the foot following intramuscular injection in the lateral thigh. A case report with recommendations for prevention. J. Pediatr. 70:110, 1967.
8. Welch, K. J.: Gangrene of the extremities. *In* Ravitch, M. M., Welch, K. J., Benson, C. D., et al. (eds.): Pediatric Surgery. Vol. 2. Chicago, Year Book Medical Publishers, 1979, p. 1508.
9. White, J. J., Talbert, J. L., and Haller, J. A., Jr.: Peripheral arterial injuries in infants and children. Ann. Surg. 167:757, 1968.

31 SURGICAL TREATMENT OF END-STAGE RENAL DISEASE

Raphael H. Levey, M.D.

The dictum that 90 per cent of postoperative care occurs in the operating room unfortunately carries less weight than usual surgical dogma in the case of renal transplantation. Technical perfection does not guarantee a course without complications, for the operation itself is just the first step in what may be a long and difficult period whose course may be totally unrelated to the expertise of the surgical team. However, the corollary of these statements is that without the absolute minimization of surgical complications all the hazards of the ensuing immunologic battle between the host and the grafted organ will be maximized, and an otherwise minor complication can lead to a fatal conclusion. This is all the more true in the pediatric recipient, in whom major technical feats may have to be accomplished in the process of providing vascular access for hemodialysis, urologic reconstruction, and medical management to achieve a steady, if not positive, metabolic state.

The purpose of this chapter is threefold: (1) to summarize those complications that are surgically related, (2) to describe problems arising from immunobiologic considerations, and (3) to point out strategies that may reduce such problems to as low a level as possible. The formulas recommended will be based, to a large extent, on the experience developed at the Children's Hospital Medical Center, Boston, in the course of 155 pediatric renal transplants.

GENERAL CONSIDERATIONS

Renal transplantation cannot be done without extensive planning and requires the commitment of a large multidisciplinary team, each member of which provides a needed expertise for the care of a chronically ill child. Table 31–1 shows the structure of the end-stage renal disease team at our institution. The goal is to bring the recipient to the transplant operation in as good condition as possible by correcting, in advance, as many pre-existing medical, surgical, urological, orthopedic, and psychologic problems as are amenable to treatment.

It is our policy not to perform transplant operations in children without several weeks of prior hemodialysis. During this period, the child can be brought into an anabolic state, the immunologic evaluation of the donor-recipient pair can be carried out, steps may be taken to reduce the level of immunologic reactivity of the recipient, the individual dialysis characteristics and requirements of the patient will be learned, and the entire team will "get to know" better the patient and family. In general, dialysis and transplant patients do not drop from

Supported by a grant from the NIH-NIAID-IAIDP-80-18.

TABLE 31–1   DIALYSIS — TRANSPLANTATION TEAM

1. Director of End-Stage Renal Disease Program
2. Physician (Dialysis)
3. Physician (Chronic Renal Failure Program)
4. Pediatric Surgeon (Recipient)
5. Pediatric Surgeon (Donor)
6. Nursing Coordinator
7. Orthopedic Surgeon
8. Psychiatrist
9. Psychologist
10. Social Worker
11. Nutritionist
12. Play Therapist
13. Physical Therapist
14. Dialysis Nurses
15. Dialysis Technicians

Other Facilities
   Tissue Typing Laboratory
   Immunologic Monitoring Laboratory
   Organ Procurement Facility
   Organ Preservation Facility

the treatment program, and in no area of surgical endeavor, save perhaps oncology, is trust in the team on the part of patient and family more essential.

DONOR SELECTION AND PRE-TRANSPLANT IMMUNOLOGIC MANIPULATION

The kidney donor is selected primarily on the basis of histocompatibility with the recipient. When dealing with a young family, it is unlikely that a histologically identical sibling will be available, and, therefore, a haplotype-identical parent is usually selected, which means that the donor and recipient share one chromosome that codes for transplantation determinants. In addition to conventional typing of the HL-A, HL-B, and HL-C Loci, DR typing is also performed, as well as reactivity in mixed lymphocyte culture (MLC) and cell-mediated lympholysis (CML) assays. If both parents are equally motivated, are ABO blood group compatible with the recipient, and are physiologically fit to be donors, that parent will be selected who is most closely matched to the child in terms of MLC and CML reactivity.

It is our strong belief that a living-related donor is preferable to a cadaveric donor for immunologic reasons, for the chances of long-term immunologic success are greater with the former than with the latter. Complications of many types, to be described later in this chapter, can be obviated or reduced if immunosuppression, especially corticosteroid pulse therapy for rejection episodes, can be avoided. When a living-related donor cannot be identified, the patient is placed on a waiting list for a cadaveric kidney.

Medical evaluation of the living-related donor is carried out by a totally independent team whose judgment is final. It has been our experience[14] that many parents of children whose underlying disease is either dysplasia or a mechanical uropathy may themselves have an anatomic vascular urologic variant, which, while not decreasing renal function, may contraindicate organ donation. Preference is given to removing the left kidney, which has the longer renal vein and which, when placed in a heterotopic location on the right side of the recipient, allows for more facile anastomosis to the laterally lying vena cava or right common iliac vein. If anomalies are present in the donor, that kidney will be selected which will leave the donor with the normal kidney, but a kidney with one renal artery may be picked in preference to the one with two vessels.

The evening prior to the operation the donor is started on intravenous hydration. Intraoperatively, a mannitol-induced diuresis is begun in order to decrease the incidence of early postoperative oliguria in the recipient. Every effort is made to harvest the kidney safely with as long an artery and vein as possible, especially on the right side with the retrocaval renal artery, and to make the warm ischemia time as short as possible. Great care is also essential in preserving hilar and ureteral blood supply, to minimize the chances of ureteral stenosis or fistula formation. Prior careful evaluation of the donor angiogram is useful in determining the need to preserve a polar vessel. In general, if more than 10 per cent of the kidney is supplied by such a vessel it should be saved and either anastomosed to the main renal artery in an end-to-side fashion or anastomosed independently to the iliac vasculature. If such a polar vessel is ligated and a significant portion of the kidney fails to perfuse after revascularization, partial nephrectomy may be required to prevent postoperative hypertension or necrosis and calyceal fistulae.

It is our practice to perfuse and cool all living-related kidneys with a Sacks-Collins solution.[6, 35] Perfusion is performed very gently, using a soft silicon vessel tip so as not to damage the arterial intima, and is continued until the venous washout is grossly clear of red blood cells. The cooling and perfusion allows the recipient operation to be performed at the surgeon's leisure, which has important implications for the avoidance of later complications.

Cadaver nephrectomy should obviously be performed with equal attention to meticulous surgical technique in an effort to ensure the ease and success of the operation in the recipient. Of paramount importance is the prevention of ischemic damage and avoidance of damage to the vasculature that has not been delineated by angiography. If a pediatric donor is used, the kidneys should be removed en bloc with the aorta and vena cava. Both kidneys may then be perfused through the aorta.

RECIPIENT PREPARATION

Immunologic, surgical, and psychologic preparation of the child prior to transplantation is necessary to ensure a good post-transplantation outcome, and to prepare the patient and family to face the situation should the graft fail.

Pretransplant blood transfusions have been shown to improve graft results,[28] although the mechanism for this observation is not firmly established. We undertake planned transfusions in all our patients and give one unit of whole washed cells per week for 3 weeks.

In cases in which a high degree of cytotoxicity has been noted in the CML assay, we have recently begun a program of donor-specific blood transfusions in an effort to decrease the percentage of cell-mediated target killing. Table 31–2 shows the reduction in CML killing against a grandmother donor following specific blood transfusions.

Parathyroidectomy for secondary hyperparathyroidism is now rarely indicated before transplantation because of improved medical management. However, in those intractable patients in whom persistently high parathormone levels occur and who have severe bone lesions, subtotal parathyroidectomy should be performed to facilitate bone healing. The results may be dramtic; in one case we have seen the disappearance of calcium deposits in arterial walls following such an operation.

It is our policy now to perform native nephrectomies in virtually all patients prior to engraftment. The rationale for this rests on our observations that the incidence of post-transplant hypertension is less following nephrectomy, even in those patients who were not hypertensive before, and also that the hypertension that does occur is easier to manage. Clearly, in those patients who have reflux nephropathy or infection, or both, native nephroureterectomies are mandatory. Unless there is significant reflux with ureteral dilation, the native ureters are left in situ in case they should be needed for future use. Clinically important reflux into the unused ureters following successful transplantation has not been noted in our series.

Urologic evaluation consists primarily of a voiding cystourethrogram. It has been possible to utilize small, long-unused bladders

TABLE 31–2   RESULTS OF CELL-MEDIATED LYMPHOLYSIS* ASSAY BETWEEN A RECIPIENT AND HER DONOR GRANDMOTHER

	Patient	Grandmother	Control
Before Blood Transfusions			
Patient + Grandmother	3.5 ± 0.2†	79.1 ± 0.97	12.7 ± 3.7
Patient + Control	10.4 ± 0.5	26.6 ± 1.6	15.0 ± 1.2
After Donor Specific Blood Transfusions			
Patient + Grandmother	3.0 ± 0.2	12.5 ± 0.86	10

*Cell-mediated lympholysis (CML) measures the ability of lymphocytes to kill target lymphocytes, as opposed to simply proliferating, as happens in mixed lymphocyte culture (MLC).

†Results are shown as per cent of specific ^{51}Cr release.

in patients who have been previously diverted, provided the voiding cystourethrogram (VCUG) demonstrates minimal residual urine in the bladder. Only one patient in our series has required diversion after use of a bladder that was normal urodynamically. If a diversion has been necessary, we have chosen to perform an ileal conduit at the time of transplantation.

RECIPIENT OPERATION

There is a generally held belief, albeit poorly documented, that the transplantation operation should be carried out rapidly in order to avoid a long warm ischemia time and subsequent acute tubular necrosis and oliguria. This has too often meant sacrificing precision for unnecessary speed, for with a cooled and perfused kidney it is possible to proceed judiciously and carefully and thus to be certain that every stitch is placed exactly where it should be.

It is usually possible to transplant an adult kidney into the right retroperitoneal space in children, even in infants weighing as little as 5.0 kg and measuring 73 cm in length.

Prior to the start of the transplant operation, a formal central Silastic line is placed through either the external or internal jugular vein. The line is brought out through a tunnel on the anterior chest wall. This line is used intraoperatively to measure central venous pressure and post-operatively for drawing blood, giving fluids, and administering antilymphocyte serum, when indicated. The line will stay in for at least 2½ to 3 months, unless there are specific contraindications. We have not experienced clinically significant episodes of sepsis with these lines.

In small children and infants, adequate exposure of the abdominal great vessels and iliac vasculature is mandatory. Therefore, the standard adult transplant incision has been modified to achieve this goal. The retroperitoneum is entered by means of long incision, which divides both rectus muscles approximately one fingerbreadth above the pubis and then turns laterally along the border of the right rectus muscle and extends to the midcostal margin. Prior to dividing the rectus muscles, sutures are used to anchor the muscles to the anterior fascia to prevent their retraction, which occurs more readily below the umbilicus than above, because below the posterior sheath is absent. This precaution not only facilitates later closure but also helps to eliminate a potential dead space and area of hematoma and seroma formation.

The lateral abdominal musculature is divided with the electrocautery. Great pains are taken to achieve excellent hemostasis. The inferior epigastric vessels are ligated and divided. In the male the spermatic cord is spared; in the female the round ligament is clamped, divided, and ligated. The entire operation is carried out with the use of magnifying aids which help in the identification of small bleeding points and lymphatic channels and in performing the meticulous vascular anastomoses and ureteral reimplantation.

The lymphatic channels overlying the vasculature are very carefully ligated in continuity and divided. Using this technique, only one patient in our series has developed a lymphocele, and two patients have had prolonged lymph drainage, which spontaneously subsided.

When control has been gained of the major vessels, the kidney is either removed from the donor or the cadaveric kidney is taken off the portable perfusion apparatus. An important technical consideration at this juncture is the proper positioning of the kidney in the recipient. It is our practice to place the organ in the paravertebral gutter from its inferior pole resting in the iliac fossa, so that the kidney assumes a vertical orientation.

With the kidney thus positioned, we are able to accurately determine where the venous and arterial anastomoses will best lie to prevent any vascular kinking that may lead to subsequent low-flow states and thrombosis or stenosis.

Control of the vena cava or iliac vein is achieved by means of a large side-biting vascular clamp. The venotomy in the recipient is of a length that is sufficient to provide adequate flow but not to lead to tenting or tearing of the vessel when an end-to-side anastomosis is carried out between the donor renal vein and the recipient vein. Often, in small children, the recipient vein is extremely thin, and the anastomosis must be performed with very fine vascular sutures. In practice, this means that the recipient venotomy should be smaller than either the orifice of the donor renal vein or its attached caval patch and that 6-0 monofilament suture is used. The venous anastomosis is performed with a running stitch, which is carried on the medial and lateral sides from each corner after placing a mattress suture at the superior and inferior corners. No venous obstruction has occurred in any of our patients using this technique.

The arterial anastomosis is usually performed in an end-to-side fashion either to the distal aorta or to the common iliac artery. After carefully positioning the arterotomy, a small window of recipient vessel is removed and an end-to-side anastomosis performed using interrupted horizontal mattress sutures of 7-0 monofilament suture. We prefer this end-to-side technique to an end-to-end anastomosis between the donor renal artery and the recipient hypogastric artery. Often the recipient hypogastric artery is either too short or too narrow to allow for an adequate-sized orifice between the two vessels or else it tethers the vessels in such a way that there is kinking at the take-off of the hypogastric artery. There is a far greater degree of freedom when the end-to-side technique is used.

The ureteroneocystostomy is carried out by the technique first described by Leadbetter.[31] The ureter is trimmed to a point at which adequate bleeding occurs after the vascular clamps are released and is brought beneath the spermatic cord, through a capacious opening in the bladder and through a large submucosal tunnel to be fixed in place with interrupted sutures of 5-0 chromic catgut. The bladder is closed in two layers and an indwelling catheter is left for 1 week following the surgery. The operative field is extensively irrigated with antibiotic solution. The rectus muscles are reapproximated with interrupted figure-eight sutures of nonabsorbable suture material and the lateral abdominal musculature with running sutures of nonabsorbable material. Small drains are left in the right paravesical space and suction catheters are placed in front of and behind the kidney in an effort to reduce seroma formation.

The intraoperative fluid and pharmaco-logic management of the patient is important to ensure the establishment of a good diuresis and adequate immunosuppression. It has been our practice to raise the central venous pressure to the 12 cm level and to administer 5 per cent albumin solution as well as a solution containing 25 gm of mannitol in 400 ml of 5 per cent dextrose in normal saline. The appropriate dose of azathioprine (Imuran), usually 2 mg/kg body weight, is given slowly at the outset of the operation. Prior to the opening of the vascular clamps, a methylprednisolone pulse dose of 10 mg/kg is administered intravenously, as well as a furosemide bolus at a dose of 3 mg/kg. In over 100 living-related transplant operations, only one patient has required immediate postoperative hemodialysis and only 10 per cent of the recipients of cadaveric kidneys have required immediate post-transplant hemodialysis.

COURSE FOLLOWING TRANSPLANTATION

Maneuvers to avoid the major surgical and urologic complications of renal transplantation have been described in the preceding sections. A description of the natural history of both a successful and unsuccessful allograft will encompass a discussion of diagnostic techniques used to follow their fate in an effort to differentiate an overt correctable problem (conventional complication) from a routine or not so routine difficulty that is peculiar to this type of surgery.

Physiologic Aspects

In the immediate postoperative period, with both a living-related and cadaveric kidney, urine will start to flow. This urine has a higher sodium content (70 to 140 mEq/L), which is typical of the polyuric phase of high-output renal failure. Most transplanted kidneys will show evidence of tubular damage even from the cold ischemia period, which will self-correct over a period of days.[10, 13, 37] The diuresis is exacerbated by a possible high urea load in the recipient as well as by the intraoperative priming and rehydration of the patient. The urine may also contain a significant amount of potassium (10 to 20 mEq/l).

During this time, it is our practice to follow the diuresis milliliter for milliliter as well as to replace insensible and other fluid losses. The electrolytes of intravenous solutions are adjusted to replace the measured urinary losses and to maintain a serum electrolyte homeostasis. Therefore, it is imperative to closely monitor these values. In addition, since large volumes of fluid are given, the serum blood sugar levels will rise to unacceptable heights (greater than 400 mg/dl) unless the replacement solutions are dextrose-poor (2.5 per cent or less).

It is our preference to manage the patient in this polyuric state for several days. However, if the output exceeds 30 ml/kg/hour, we make every effort to diminish it by giving 50 per cent or 80 per cent replacement of losses. However, if the polyuria persists unabated, it is necessary to pursue it to equivalence so that dehydration and the oliguric or anuric phase of acute tubular necrosis does not supervene.

In the small child, especially, high-output acute tubular necrosis (ATN) may lead to serious disequilibria, which are difficult to measure but are presumed to exist. These disequilibria can cause central nervous system seizures. Therefore, we treat such patients prophylactically with appropriate anticonvulsant therapy, even if there is no history of a previous seizure disorder.

Within 72 hours of the transplant, the polyuria and urinary sodium values decrease and a steady state will have been reached. Prior to this time we routinely obtain, usually during the first 24 hours postoperatively, a radionuclide renal scan to measure blood flow and function. If a graft forms no urine in the first 3 hours following revascularization, the scan will be performed in the recovery room to assess the status of renal blood flow. Failure to demonstrate perfusion would be sufficient cause for re-exploration, since seeking angiographic confirmation of renal artery thrombosis, an event which has been described in 1 to 2 per cent of allografts,[26, 44] would cause undue delay. Thrombosis may be a sequel of a mechanical problem, hyperacute rejection, or nonrecognized damage from pulsatile perfusion.[23]

Venous thrombosis may be partial or complete.[38] If two major renal veins are present in the donor kidney, both must be reanastomosed in the recipient or signs and symptoms of renal vein thrombosis will ensue, such as swelling of the graft, sluggish arterial flow, and significant proteinuria. Just as in the case of arterial problems, the allograft can only be salvaged by prompt re-exploration, cooling, and washout of the kidney and correction of the underlying pathology.

Vascular Aspects and Hypertension

It is our view that angiography should not be performed routinely in the transplant recipient, but it should be done only for specific indications, such as persistent severe hypertension that is still present after corticosteroid therapy has reached maintenance levels. In children, post-transplant hypertension is common in the immediate postoperative period[2, 9, 17, 20, 25, 45] and may be related to a number of factors. In general, the causes of hypertension are multifactorial, but there is a correlation between the severity and frequency and the original disease, the presence of hypertension per se pre-transplant while on adequate hemodialysis, the occurrence of rejection episodes, and the reappearance of the original disease. In our patients, we define normal blood pressure as one that is below the 95th percentile for age and sex, mild hypertension as blood pressure that is persistently at or above the 95th percentile, moderate hypertension as 3 to 4 standard deviations above the 95th percentile, and severe hypertension as 3 to 4 standard deviations above the 95th percentile plus encephalopathy.

Despite the absence of renal artery anastomotic stenosis in our series, we strongly believe that every case of moderate to severe hypertension should be investigated thoroughly and treated vigorously because it carries with it the risk of serious morbidity.[16]

Renal artery stenosis is the most frequent vascular complication involving the renal vessels.[13, 18] Its location may be variable, and, if amenable to surgical repair, correction should be attempted. Distal renal artery stenosis may be discovered late after transplantation and has been attributed to intimal damage or to chronic rejection. In one of our patients, such a narrowing was corrected by a saphenous vein interposition graft. The vessels should be approached by a transperitoneal route so that the kidney itself will not be disturbed. In a second patient, a distal stenosis was significantly modified by transluminal balloon angioplasty, with subsequent return of normal blood pressure for 6 months. A repeated effort 8 months after the first was unsuccessful and the kidney was lost because of chronic rejection.

Urologic Aspects

The literature is replete with a litany of urologic complications of renal transplantation. Wherever uroepithelium is present and whenever an attempt is made to join a conduit of urine to another tube or anatomic reservoir — especially when there is a decreased blood supply, disuse atrophy of an organ, a history of multiple previous operations, and a past history of infection — a fistula may develop, stenosis and obstruction may ensue, or reflux may be found.

Fistulae occur in 4 to 25 per cent of cases[8, 29, 36, 43] and are life-threatening complications. The diagnosis is established by a falling urine output and extravasation of urine from a drain site. It is confirmed by radionuclide scanning, ultrasonography, cystourethrography, and intravenous pyelography, the last to localize the site of leak if not known.

In one patient, a leak from the renal pelvis secondary to damage to a small branch of the renal artery that occurred during harvest of a cadaveric kidney was successfully treated by tube pyelostomy. No patient in our series has had either a ureterovesical fistula or a stenosis at the site of ureteral reimplantation.

Extravasation of urine from the bladder occurred in four patients who previously had had extensive bladder surgery. In three, the leakage was managed by an indwelling catheter for 2 to 3 weeks. The fourth case required surgical repair.

Three patients have developed late (3 to 5 years post transplant) long segment distal ureteral obstruction, which required exploration and treatment by ureteroureteros-

tomy between the proximal donor ureter and distal recipient ureter. It has been our practice to protect this anastomosis by proximal tube diversion and not to use stents.

We strongly believe that leakage and fistulae are sequelae principally of technical problems, which can by and large be prevented by judicious anticipation and are not assignable to entities such as a rejection process uniquely directed against the ureter.[11]

Infectious Complications and Mortality

The causes of death in 11 patients who received kidney transplants and in two who were maintained on chronic hemodialysis are shown in Table 31–3. Six of the 11 deaths were related to infection. In our series, there was no change in patient mortality following the incorporation of rabbit antihuman thymocyte serum[21, 22] into the standard post-transplant immunosuppressive regimen.

The transplant and chronic hemodialysis patients are immunodepressed of necessity and, therefore, are at greatly increased risk for conventional and opportunistic invasion by bacterial, viral, fungal, and parasitic pathogens. Cytomegalovirus (CMV) infection can occur as either a primary infection in the recipient, perhaps transmitted from the donor, or as reactivation of latent virus in the host. The primary infection with CMV is the more serious disorder and is characterized by progressive deterioration of hepatic function, fever, and interstitial pneumonitis. The CMV may itself cause a direct glomerulitis, and the syndrome then is compounded by rising serum creatinine levels. Reduction or withdrawal of immunosuppression is the most rational approach to therapy, and before the fever and worsening renal function are ascribed to rejection and steroid pulse therapy administered, it is mandatory to rule out infection. With CMV disease, renal function will improve as the viral assault comes under control.

Over the past 8½ years at the Children's Hospital Medical Center, an analysis of 216 transplantation or dialysis courses in 120 patients, with no exclusions from treatment or review, showed an overall actuarial survival of 92 per cent at 6 months, 90 per cent

TABLE 31–3   PATIENT DEATHS FOLLOWING RENAL TRANSPLANTATION

Treatment	Diagnosis	Cause of Death*	Time on Current Treatment	Previous Treatment and Duration
LRD Tx	Chronic GN	Anaphylaxis	1 day	
LRD Tx	Hypoplasia-dysplasia	Bacterial sepsis	1 month	
LRD Tx	Hypoplasia-dysplasia	Hypertension	2 months	CH, 6 months
LRD Tx	Wilms' tumor	Hypertension	1 day	CH, 4 months
LRD Tx	Obstructive uropathy	Pancreatitis	6 months	CH, 8 months
LRD Tx	Chronic interstitial nephritis	Viral sepsis	2 months	CH, 5 months
CAD Tx	Membranoproliferative GN	Bacterial sepsis	2 months	STH, 2 months
CAD Tx	Membranoproliferative GN	Bacterial sepsis	3 months	CH, 10 months
CAD Tx	Chronic GN	Hypertension	6 months	
CAD Tx	Polyarteritis nodosa	Fungal sepsis	3 months	CH, 9 months
CAD Tx	Obstructive uropathy	Viral sepsis	3 months	STH, 4 months; LRD Tx, 21 months
CH	Hypoplasia-dysplasia	Hepatic failure	17 months	
CH	Me-CCNU Toxicity	Brain tumor	8 months	

*Causes of death in patients with living-related transplants (LRD Tx), with cadaveric transplants (CAD Tx), and on chronic hemodialysis (CH). Noted is any previous therapy, including short-term hemodialysis (STH).

GN, Glomerulonephritis; Me-CCNU, trans-1-(2-chloroethyl)-3-(4-methylcyclohexyl)-1-nitrosourea.

(From Avner, E. D., Harmon, W. E., Grupe, W. E., et al.: Mortality of chronic hemodialysis and renal transplantation in pediatric end-stage renal disease. Pediatrics 67:412, 1981. Copyright American Academy of Pediatrics 1981.)

at 12 months, and 89 per cent at 5 years. The data demonstrated a 5-year cumulative patient survival of 92 per cent with living-related donor transplants, 85 per cent with cadaver transplants, and 95 per cent with chronic hemodialysis.[1]

Since the major cause of mortality in our series and in other centers was infection during periods of maximal immunosuppression — namely, during the first 12 months following transplantation — it has made great sense to always act very cautiously before increasing drug therapy[41] and to accept graft loss as calmly as possible, remembering that children with end-stage renal disease can be kept alive quite well with chronic hemodialysis, even if a successful allograft provides a better life.

Aseptic Necrosis of Bone

Aseptic osteonecrosis, especially in the adolescent, is a major problem, which has been observed by most transplantation groups.[24, 39, 46] In our series, the incidence has been 12 per cent and has been correlated with the total dose of administered prednisone. If conservative therapy fails to halt the development of symptoms or x-ray progression of the disease, surgical treatment

has been used, and 4 per cent of the patients have required joint replacement.

IMMUNOLOGIC COMPLICATIONS OF RENAL TRANSPLANTATION

Rejection of the allograft is the bête noire of the patient, family, surgeon, and transplant team. It is our practice always to inform the patient and family that immunologic success cannot be guaranteed, even in cases of apparent histologic identity, but we do not think it wise to quote actuarial graft survival figures except to express our belief, founded on fact, that a living-related kidney is preferable to a cadaveric organ. Rejection may occur at any time following revascularization, but three main types are recognizable: (1) hyperacute or accelerated rejection; (2) acute reversible rejection; and (3) chronic rejection.

Hyperacute rejection is due to presensitization of the donor against HL-A antigens present on the donor cells.[3, 30] Its incidence has been decreased first by routine cross-matching of the most current recipient serum against donor lymphoid cells and second by concomitant use of the serum that expressed the greatest percentage of reactivity in complement-mediated cytotoxic assays against panels of lymphoid cells expressing most of the known HL-A determinants. Furthermore, augmented assays have been developed to elicit low levels of reactivity in the recipient, which may lead to accelerated rejection when the offending antigens are presented. Computer analysis of past and present reactivity can now make possible an analysis of those specificities against which the recipient reacts and which, therefore, must be excluded from the donor kidney.

In cases of hyperacute rejection, minutes after blood flow is re-established, the kidney will lose its pink color and turgor and become livid and flaccid. The histopathologic lesions are well described[4, 5] and lead to severe vascular damage, hemorrhagic necrosis, and the deposition of platelets, fibrin, and immunoglobulins.

The course following such rejections may dictate immediate removal of the transplant, with the development of a toxic syndrome that may even include disseminated intravascular coagulation. However, in one recent episode, we have apparently been able to reverse this type of rejection, which was biopsy proved, with a prolonged and multiple course of plasmapheresis and concomitant heavy immunosuppression.

Acute rejection is usually reversible and typically manifests itself on or about the fifth postoperative day or within the first 2 weeks after transplantation. It is characterized by a falling urine output, fever that may reach 41° C, tenderness over the allograft, a rising serum creatinine level, and a deteriorating renal scan. The fever may or may not be associated with systemic symptoms. Oliguria may progress to anuria, and although this classic "crise du transplant" is more often than not effectively treatable by methylprednisolone pulse therapy, it can take weeks to months for the kidney to rectify the sequelae.

The explanation of this observation would seem to lie in the renal histopathology, which shows marked interstitial edema and cellular depositions of lymphocytes, plasma cells, and macrophages.[7, 40] The swelling, in turn, combined with peritubular capillary damage, leads to a picture consistent with ATN. Therefore, despite instant defervescence, normal renal function returns only slowly. On the other hand, the entire pic-

ture may be extremely short-lived and not necessitate prolongation of the patient's hospital stay.

No single test short of biopsy establishes the diagnosis of rejection. We rely on the clinical picture, the renal scan, which shows delayed transit of[131]I hippuric acid, and time of onset to aid in making the diagnosis. If doubt persists, an open biopsy will be done, since with the operative technique we use the right colon comes to overlie the graft, precluding the need for a percutaneous needle biopsy. If normal renal function does not return by 2 weeks after the onset of acute rejection, we then also proceed with open biopsy in order to assess the extent of renal damage and both the short-term and long-term prognosis of the graft.

The mechanism of action of steroid pulse therapy remains obscure and may be related more to an anti-inflammatory action than to augmented immunosuppression.[19] It has been our experience that rabbit antihuman thymocyte serum significantly reduces the incidence of early or acute rejection[22] and, thus, the need for high-dose glucocorticoids, with their associated morbidity.

An acute rejection episode may manifest itself as a de novo phenomenon any time after transplantation, from weeks to months to years, in a previously perfectly well tolerated graft. Such an occurrence can be triggered by an intercurrent viral illness, by noncompliance with drug therapy, by too rapid tapering of steroid dosage, or by events unknown. It is called "acute" because of the associated clinical picture, which is then confirmed by open biopsy and the symptoms treated appropriately.

Once the hyperacute and acute periods are passed, danger still lurks in the form of chronic rejection, which progresses as a manifestation of the failure of the host to accept the graft as "self." The ongoing conflict may produce no immediate overt symptoms, and the first signs may be the reappearance of an anemia, which is then followed by a slow, inexorable rise in serum creatinine level. This may remit for a time, rise to a new plateau, and then ascend again. Ultrasonography is an aid in diagnosis and shows a loss of the homogeneous pattern of renal tissues and an increase in echogenicity of the kidney parenchyma.

Biopsy will show progressive destruction

of the kidney, with arterial narrowing, intimal hyperplasia, and medial fibrosis.[32-34] Interstitial fibrosis also progresses, with thickened tubular basement membrane and Bowman's capsule. Rejection glomerulonephritis has also been described[12] and is characterized by ischemic glomeruli, which shows lesions similar to those of thrombotic microangiopathy, with clear deposits in the subendothelial region.

The treatment of chronic rejection consists in a short-term increase in oral steroid dosage, usually at a level of 3 mg/kg/day of prednisone for 3 days. We are reluctant to give major intravenous pulse therapy at this time. If there is an associated heavy interstitial cellular infiltrate, it has been our policy to add a 5-day course of antihuman thymocyte serum to the immunosuppressive regimen. The results are encouraging.

RECURRENT DISEASE

In our series, hereditary nephropathy constitutes the single most frequent indication for placing patients in the end-stage renal disease program, as shown in Table 31–4. Fortunately, these conditions do not lead to recurrence of the underlying pathology in the transplant. However, the reappearance of glomerulonephritis is a well-described entity and may lead to destruction of the new kidney, as it did the old.

Focal segmental glomerulosclerosis with the nephrotic syndrome and membranoproliferative glomerulonephritis are the two major entities characterized by recurrence,[15, 42] with recurrence rates as high as 25 per cent and 10 per cent, respectively. These diagnoses may be of more interest to the pathologist than to the clinician, for associated clinical manifestations are not always seen. Furthermore, they do not constitute a contraindication to transplantation, because even if graft failure should eventuate, it may be 5 to 15 years after allografting, during which time the child can lead a normal life and grow and mature.

TABLE 31–4 PRIMARY DIAGNOSIS LEADING TO CHRONIC RENAL FAILURE*

Disease Category	Number	Per cent Total
Congenital/hereditary	57	(48%)
Hypoplasia-dysplasia	25	
Obstructive uropathy	18	
Nephronophthisis	4	
Alport's syndrome	3	
Cystinosis	3	
Prune-belly syndrome	2	
Polycystic kidney disease	1	
Tuberous sclerosis	1	
Glomerulonephritis	43	(36%)
Chronic GN (unclassified)	13	
Membranoproliferative GN	11	
Focal segmental sclerosing GN	10	
Rapidly progressive GN	4	
Mesangioproliferative GN	3	
Anaphylactoid purpura GN	1	
Systemic lupus GN	1	
Chronic tubulointerstitial	8	(6%)
Chronic interstitial nephritis	8	
Vascular	6	(5%)
Hypertensive glomerulosclerosis	2	
Renal vein thrombosis	2	
Polyarteritis nodosa	1	
Hemolytic uremic syndrome	1	
Other	6	(5%)
Wilms' tumor	2	
Me-CCNU toxicity	2	
Unknown	1	
Diabetes	1	
Total	120	

*GN, Glomerulonephritis; Me-CCNU, trans-1-(2-chloroethyl)-3-(4-methylcyclohexyl)-1-nitrosourea.

(From Avner, E. D., Harmon, W. E., Grupe, W. E., et al.: Mortality of chronic hemodialysis and renal transplantation in pediatric end-stage renal disease. Pediatrics, 67:412, 1981. Copyright American Academy of Pediatrics 1981.)

References

1. Avner, E. D., Harmon, W. E., Grupe, W. E., et al.: Mortality of chronic hemodialysis and renal transplantation in pediatric end-stage renal disease. Pediatrics 67:412, 1981.

2. Belzer, F. O., Schweitzer, R. T., and Holliday, M.: Renal homotransplantation in children. Am. K. Surg. 124:270, 1972.

3. Boehmig, H. J., Giles, G. R., Amemiya, H., et al.: Hyperacute rejection of renal homografts with particular reference to coagulation changes, humoral antibodies and formed blood elements. Transplant. Proc. 3:1105, 1971.

4. Busch, G. J., Reynolds, E. S., Galvanek, E. G., et al.: Human renal allografts. The role of vascular injury in early graft failure. Medicine 50:29, 1971.

5. Callard, P., Bedrossian, J., Idatte, J. M., et al.: The arterial lesions in the course of renal allograft rejection phenomena. *In* Hamburger, J., Crosnier, J., and Maxwell, M. H. (eds.): Advances in Nephrology, Vol. 5. Chicago, Year Book Medical Publishers, 1975, p. 333.

6. Collins, G. M., Bravo-Shugarman, M., and Terasa-

ki, P. I.: Kidney preservation for transportation. Lancet 2:1219, 1969.

7. Damin, G. J.: The pathology of human renal transplantation. *In* Rapaport, F. T., and Dausset, J. (eds.): Human Transplantation. New York, Grune and Stratton, 1968.

8. Gil-Vernet, J. M.: Le remplacement du rein: Technique chirurgicale. 63e Session, Association Francaise d'Urologie. Paris, Masson, 1969, p. 221.

9. Gonzales, L. L., Martin, L., West, C .D.: Renal homotransplantation in children. Arch. Surg. 101:232, 1970.

10. Gyorgy, A. Z., Stewart, J. H., George, C. R. P., et al.: Renal tubular acidosis, acidosis due to hyperkalemia, hypercalcemia, disordered citrate metabolism and other tubular dysfunctions following human renal transplantation. Q. J. Med. 38:231, 1969.

11. Haber, M. H., and Putong, P. B.: Ureteral vascular rejection in human renal transplants. J.A.M.A. 192:417, 1965.

12. Hamburger, J., Crosnier, J., and Dormont, J.: Observations in patients with a well tolerated homotransplanted kidney. Ann. N.Y. Acad. Sci. 120:558, 1964.

13. Hamburger, J., Crosnier, J., Dormont, J., et al.: Homotransplantation renale humaine. Resultats personnels chez 52 malades. II. Histoire naturelle du greffon dans les cas de tolerance prolongée. Presse Med. 73:2873, 1965.

14. Hollenberg, N., and Levey, R.H.: Unpublished observations.

15. Hoyer, J. R., Raij, L., Vernier, R. L., et al.: Recurrence of idiopathic nephrotic syndrome after renal transplantation. Lancet 2:343, 1972.

16. Ingelfinger, J. R., Grupe, W. E., and Levy, R. H.: Post-transplant hypertension in the absence of rejection of recurrent disease. Clin. Nephrol. 15:236, 1979.

17. Ingelfinger, J. R., Lazarus, J. M., Levey, R. H., et al.: Hypertension in pediatric renal transplant patients. Pediatr. Res. 9:376, 1975.

18. Kincaid-Smith, P., Hare, W. S. C., Morris, P. J., et al.: Renal artery stenosis due to the vascular lesions of rejection in cadaveric allografts. Proc. Eur. Dial. Transplant. Assoc. 6:235, 1969.

19. Kreis, H., Lacombe, M., Noel, L. H., et al.: Kidney graft rejection: Has the need for steroids to be reevaluated? Lancet 2:1169, 1978.

20. LaPlante, M. P., Kaufman, J. J., and Goldman, R.: Kidney transplantation in children. Pediatrics 46:665, 1970.

21. Levey, R. H., Ingelfinger, J., Grupe, W. E., et al.: Unique surgical and immunologic features of renal transplantation in children. J. Pediatr. Surg. 13:576, 1978.

22. Levey, R. H., and Parkman, R.: Whole antilymphocyte serum: A potent safe immunosuppressive agent for intravenous use in man. Transplant. Proc. 9:1019, 1977.

23. Merkel, F. A., Seim, S. K., Armbruster, K., et al.: Thrombosis of perfused cadaver kidney. Urology 4:709, 1974.

24. Murray, W. R.: Hip problems associated with organ transplants. Clin. Orthop. 90:57, 1973.

25. Najarian, J. S., Simmons, R. L., and Tallent, M. B.: Renal transplantation in infants and children. Ann. Surg. 174:583, 1971.

26. Nerstrom, B., Ladefoged, J., and Lung, F. L.: Vascular complications in 155 consecutive kidney transplantations. Scand. J. Urol. Nephrol. *15*(Suppl. 6):65A, 1972.

27. Ogden, D. A., Sitprija, V., and Holmes, J. H.: Function of the renal homograft in man immediately after transplantation. Am. J. Med. 38:873, 1965.

28. Opelz, G., and Terasaki, P. I.: Improvement of kidney graft survival with increased numbers of blood transfusions. N. Engl. J. Med. 299:799, 1978.

29. Pfeffermann, R., Vidne, B., Leapman, S., et al.: Urologic complications in renal primary and retransplantation. Experience with 202 consecutive transplants. Am. J. Surg. 131:242, 1976.

30. Pierce, J. C., Cobb, G. W., and Hume, D. M.: Relevance of HLA antigens to acute humoral rejection of multiple renal allotransplants. N. Engl. J. Med. 285:142, 1971.

31. Politano, V. A., and Leadbetter, W. F.: An operative technique for the correction of vesicoureteral reflux. J. Urol. 79:932, 1958.

32. Porter, K. A.: Renal transplantation. *In* Heptinstall, R. H. (ed.): Pathology of the Kidney, Vol. 2. Waltham, MA, Little, Brown, 1974, p. 977 2nd ed. Vol. 2.

33. Porter, K. A., Thomson, W. B., Owen, K. et al.: Obliterative vascular changes in four human kidney homotransplants. Br. Med. J.,2:639, 1963.

34. Rowlands, D. T., Hill, G. S., and Zmijewski, C. M.: The pathology of renal homograft rejection. A review. Am. J. Pathol. 85:774, 1976.

35. Sacks, S. A., Petritsch, P. H., Leong, C. H., et al.: Experiments in renal preservation: 48- and 72-hour canine kidney preservation by initial perfusion and hypothermic storage. J. Urol. 111:434, 1974.

36. Schiff, M. J., McGuire, E. J., Weiss, R. M., and Lytton, B.: Management of urinary fistulas after renal transplantation. J. Urol. 115:251, 1976.

37. Skov, P. E., and Hansen, H. E.: The functional pattern of the cadaveric kidney in early post transplant period. Acta Med. Scand. 196:285, 1974.

38. Sorenson, B. L., Hald, T., and Nissen, H. M.: Silent iliac compression syndrome as a cause of renal vein thrombosis after transplantation. Scand. J. Urol. Nephrol. 6 (Suppl. 15):75, 1972.

39. Starzl, T. E., Marchioro, T L., Porter, K. A., et al.: Renal homotransplantation. Late function and complications. Ann. Intern. Med. 61:470, 1961.

40. Starzl, T. E., Marchioro, T. L,. and Waddell, W. R.: The reversal of rejection in human renal homografts with subsequent development of homograft tolerance. Surg. Gynecol. Obstet. 117:385, 1963.

41. Tilney, N. L., Strom, T. B., Vineyard, G..C., et al.: Factors contributing to the declining mortality

rate in renal transplantation. N. Engl. J. Med. 299:1321, 1978.

42. Turner, D. R., Cameron, J. S., Rewick, M., et al.: Transplantation in mesangiocapillary glomerulonephritis with intramembranous dense "deposits." Recurrence of disease. Kidney Int. 9:439, 1976.

43. Walsh, A.: Some practical problems in kidney transplantation. Transplant. Proc. 1:170, 1969.

44. White, R. I., Najarian, J., Loken, M., et al.: Arteriovenous complications associated with renal transplantation. Radiology 102:29, 1972.

45. Williams, G. M., Lee, H. M., and Hume, D. M.: Renal transplants in children. Transplant. Proc. 1:262, 1969.

46. Woods, J. E., de Weerd, J. H., Johnson, W. J., et al.: Experience in human renal allotransplantation. Surg. Gynecol. Obstet. 134:934, 1972.

32 | RADIATION THERAPY

J. R. Cassady, M.D.

With the advent of newer and more sophisticated equipment permitting much larger tumor doses with an equivalent reduction in damage to normal tissues, radiation therapy has assumed an increasingly prominent role in the treatment of most pediatric neoplasms. Major improvements in successful treatment, in terms of both cure and, in several instances, improved function, have accompanied the introduction of radiation therapy for patients with Wilms' tumor,[20] rhabdomyosarcoma,[38] leukemia,[37, 62] Ewing's tumor,[50] retinoblastoma,[23] and numerous other tumors of childhood.

With the introduction of more aggressive multidisciplinary treatment regimens, both the number of children exposed to irradiation and the varieties of normal tissue reactions observed have increased.

It is important to separate radiation reactions into acute, intermediate, and chronic effects. Acute effects most often result from irradiation of rapidly proliferating normal tissues (i.e., skin, mucosa, bone marrow, gastrointestinal tract). Their intensity is a function of dose rate and fractionation schedule and is rapidly modified by relatively minor changes in dose schedules. Subacute, or intermediate, effects result from injury to more slowly proliferating cells such as vascular endothelium and are manifest late in the course of treatment or, more commonly, 1 or more months after completion of irradiation. Clinically significant subacute effects are dose-, volume-, and organ-related and, when related to endothelial effects, are often rapidly relieved by steroids. Chronic effects are primarily related to total radiation dose and to size of the daily radiation fraction.[12] Often postulated to be related to vascular endothelial effects,[95] the true mechanism(s) of the chronic changes is unknown.[111] The severity of acute effects has no bearing on the likelihood or nature of late effects, which are usually more important clinically.

In addition to classification on the basis of time of onset, toxic reactions to irradiation in children undergoing treatment for malignancy can be further subdivided into several categories. These include the following:

1. Conventional organ toxicity to irradiation, unrelated to unique characteristics of children or to the interrelationship of radiation and any chemotherapeutic agent.

2. Organ or organ system toxicity primarily related to the child's lack of adult maturation or development.

3. Multidisciplinary toxicity related to the interaction of several agents and/or classes of therapy, perhaps aggravated by the child's immature state.

4. Radiation neoplasia and the influence of Categories 1 and 2 on its course.

Many excellent reference works and symposia exist on the subject of radiation toxicity.[74, 111, 123, 131, 133]

Although acute effects of irradiation with or without surgery or chemotherapy frequently present troublesome temporary problems of medical management, they rarely assume the overall importance of the more insidious subacute and chronic damage. It is our general impression that children tolerate the acute consequences of radiation therapy at least as well as and probably significantly better than their adult counterparts. As an example of this, children with non-Hodgkin's lymphoma or Wilms' tumor who require irradiation of all peritoneal surfaces ("whole abdomen") regularly tolerate daily radiation fractions of 150 to 175 rad to this volume with significantly less nausea and vomiting and hematologic depression than adults receiving similar radiation volumes and doses, e.g., for ovarian cancer.[24, 101]

Complications requiring stem cell proliferation for restoration of normal tissue integrity (i.e., mucositis, gastrointestinal toxicity, or bone marrow suppression) appear to resolve more rapidly in the child than in the older adult. For these reasons, as well as for considerations of treatment efficacy, we do *not* think that the very conservative daily radiation parameters espoused by some when dealing with children are either necessary or appropriate.[138] Daily radiation fraction size and volumes noted to be safe and effective in adult practice may be used for children with at least equal acute safety and tolerance, assuming that other factors such as surgery and chemotherapy are equivalent.

Prescription of the total tumor dose delivered to a patient depends on a complex relationship between the tumor involved, the volume and nature of the tissue to be irradiated, the importance of local failure to possibility of survival, and any other agent(s) to be utilized in the overall management of the child. When a clear need for treatment exists, the dose of radiation deemed necessary to ensure a reasonable likelihood of tumor control should be the goal of the therapist. With rare exception, this will vary only minimally with the age of the patient. We therefore disagree with published schemas that suggest a sliding scale of radiation doses for children, depending on age and tumor type.[31] Such schedules have in the past recommended unnecessarily high doses for a number of older children and have almost certainly been responsible for underdosage in a number of younger individuals.[33] Pediatric malignancies are often relatively radiocontrollable and may not necessarily require the total radiation dose needed to achieve a high level of local control of most adult epithelial malignancies. In one unique instance (neuroblastoma), modest radiation doses almost always produce local control in infants less than 13 months of age. Such doses are clearly not suitable for older children with this tumor. No other examples are known.

Should the consequences of adequate radiation treatment be deemed unacceptable, radiation therapy should be either deferred (i.e., by use of chemotherapy) or replaced (i.e., by surgery, perhaps inappropriate in a more fully developed individual) rather than utilized at a dose level that is probably ineffective. Such partial efforts almost always produce more ultimate morbidity for the child.

Some injury to normal tissues as a consequence of radiation treatment is inevitable. However, it is usually possible to markedly reduce the frequency and severity of such injury by innovative treatment planning, technically expert delivery of radiation, and use of appropriate radiation beam modifiers and shielding devices.

MUSCULOSKELETAL SYSTEM

Skeletal and muscular tissue growth are clearly essential in the transition from childhood to adulthood. One of the earliest recognized adverse consequences of irradiation was the production of scoliosis, kyphosis, or lordosis as a result of inhomogeneous irradiation of immature bony[102] or muscular[112] tissue (Fig. 32–1). Currently, megavoltage techniques with significantly lessened skin dose and bone absorption and im-

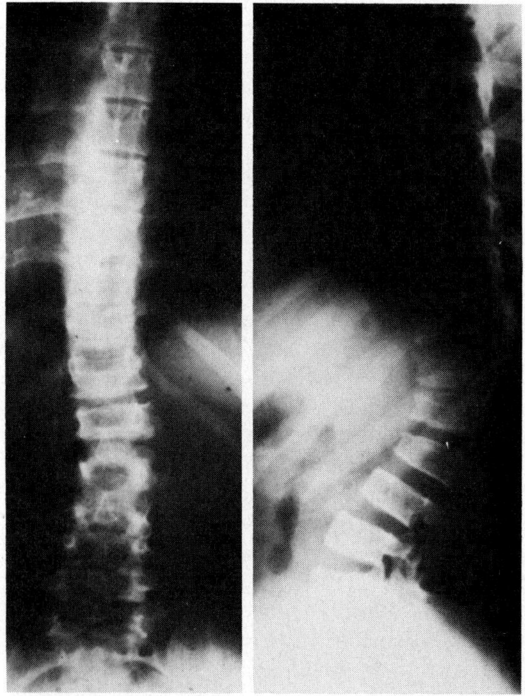

Figure 32–1 Kyphoscoliosis following unknown dose and field orthovoltage treatment for Wilms' tumor.

proved depth dose characteristics for a given tumor have markedly reduced the incidence of these conditions, provided that treatment volumes sufficient to irradiate growing bone homogeneously and symmetrically are used.[109] As both tumor control and normal tissue complications follow a steep dose-response curve with irradiation, seemingly small differences in dose across a bony structure (i.e., the vertebral column) can produce major differences in ultimate effect.[12]

Neuhauser et al., reviewing bone changes of orthovoltage treatment in 34 children, found that exposures of 2000 R or more produced increasingly prominent effects on irradiated bone during growth.[102] Experiments in laboratory animals show that a variety of types of deformity can be produced, depending on the portion of bone treated, the dose used, and the age of the patient.[32] Probert and coworkers have demonstrated that radiation delivered during the two periods of rapid growth (before age 6 years and during the adolescent growth spurt) produced greater relative deformities.[109]

Experimental studies have demonstrated that certain chemotherapeutic agents such as actinomycin D can considerably augment ultimate radiation effect on bone.[86]

Irradiation of muscle and soft tissue, by creating muscle imbalance and by muscle maldevelopment and fibrosis, may indirectly cause clinically progressive bony abnormalities. Clearly, any pre-existing muscle imbalance such as surgical- or tumor-related nerve or muscle weakness or von Recklinghausen's disease may predispose the patient to resulting indirect structural abnormalities (Fig. 32–2).

Circumferential irradiation of an extremity leads to constrictive fibrosis with lymphatic obstruction and subsequent intractable edema and is clearly to be avoided in irradiation of bone or soft tissue sarcomas involving extremities.[125] Approximately 6 to 8 weeks following more appropriate extremity irradiation, we have observed transient erythema, warmth, slight local discom-

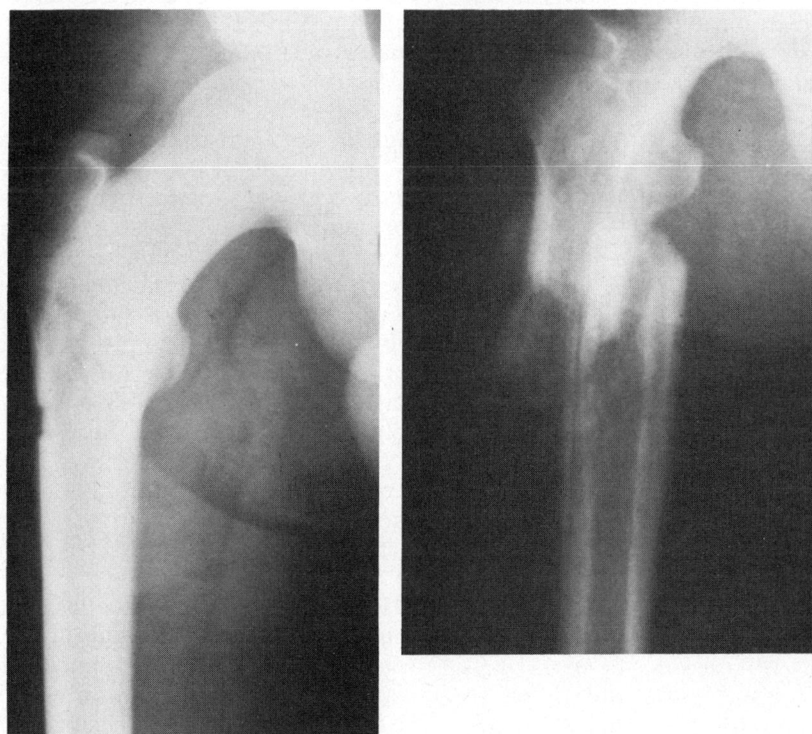

Figure 32–2 Pathologic fracture at biopsy site during treatment of child with round cell tumor by both irradiation and intensive multiagent chemotherapy.

fort, and edema in the irradiated field lasting 2 to 3 weeks. The cause of this subacute reaction is not known, but it does not appear to herald late complications. We suspect that it represents a subacute transient vasculitis.[18]

Acute symptoms immediately following bone or muscle irradiation are almost unheard of and, with the exception of the treatment-associated subacute myositis and the syndrome previously noted, do not pose clinical problems. Almost all significant musculoskeletal effects are chronic in nature and often are related to the incompletely developed state of the child. An excellent example of this is the development of a slipped caput femoral epiphysis many years after high-dose irradiation.[141]

CARDIOVASCULAR SYSTEM

Acute Complications

As vascular endothelium and other structural tissues of the cardiovascular system are either slowly proliferating (e.g., endothelium) or nonproliferating (e.g., heart), acute cardiovascular complications of irradiation are equally rare with conventional techniques, fractionation, and usual total dose ranges.

Chronic Complications

Subacute, or chronic, endothelial vasculitis is currently thought by many to account for the clinical entities of radiation pneumonitis, nephritis, pericarditis, and hepatitis.[19, 46, 48, 53, 98] In the absence of drugs that augment radiation reactions, these clinical abnormalities are total dose– and dose-fraction size–dependent, are partially treatment volume–dependent, and most commonly occur 4 to 12 weeks after completion of a planned course of irradiation. Although a considerable individual range exists, approximately 1800 rad/12 fractions/16 days to both lungs (uncorrected), 2000 to 2500 R/10 to 13 fractions/14 to 17 days to both kidneys, and 3000 rad/15 to 18 fractions/21+ days to the entire liver are usually thought to represent threshold doses beyond which a steeply rising incidence of complications begins to be seen.[64, 89, 107]

Clinically apparent acute pericardial reactions occurring 6 weeks to 6 months following irradiation are observed in fewer than 2 per cent of patients receiving cardiac radiation totaling 4000 rad, delivered in 200-rad daily fractions by equally weighted anterior and posterior fields over 4 weeks. Small increases in either total dose or daily fraction size rapidly increase the incidence of pericarditis, as with other radiation complications.[120] Increasing volumes of heart irradiated and pre-existing pericardial tumor involvement both increase the incidence of this complication. Animal experiments suggest that this subacute pericardial reaction is also related to endothelial vasculitis of the pericardium.[46, 47, 120] None of the described endothelial vascular problems is unique to childhood, nor do they seem to occur with greater frequency or with lower total doses of irradiation.

Clinically apparent damage to cardiac muscle requires significantly higher doses of radiation and occurs over a longer period.[121] Enhancement of atherosclerotic plaque development following irradiation has been suggested by collected case reports and animal experiments.[10, 45]

A chronic complication unique to pediatrics may be encountered after relatively high-dose (3500 to 5000 rad) treatment of infants usually less than 13 months of age. Many years following irradiation, usually for neuroblastoma or a neoplasm of the central nervous system, there is a marked narrowing of arterial caliber that is geographically related to the irradiation portal(s) (Fig. 32–3). Symptoms suggestive of arterial coarctation or an arteritis such as Takayasu's disease occur. An etiologically complicating feature in these patients is the occasional coexistence of von Recklinghausen's disease, a condition known to cause such abnormalities in some persons (especially in the cerebral vessels) in the absence of irradiation.[105]

Concurrent or temporally associated administration of chemotherapy, especially with actinomycin D or doxorubicin (Adriamycin), significantly enhances the visceral changes described, especially pneumonitis and hepatitis.[19, 42, 78, 106] Actinomycin D, in the absence of irradiation but in association

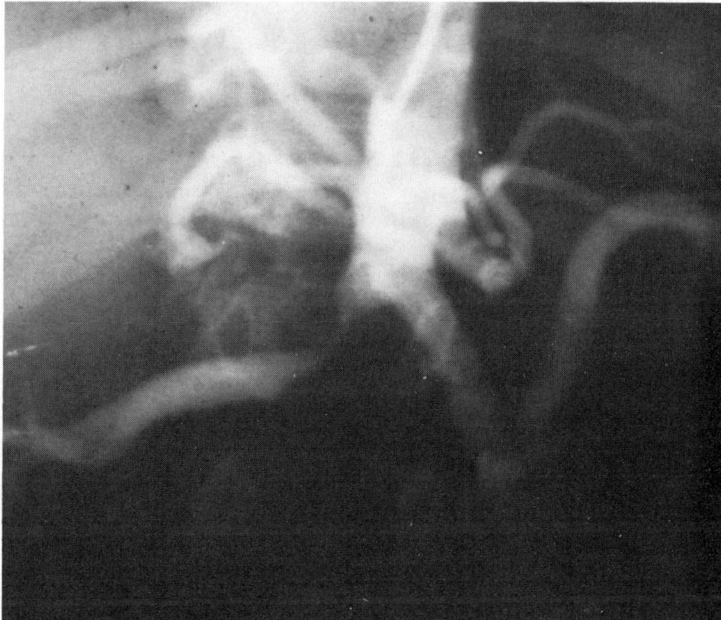

Figure 32–3 Arterial hypoplasia (abdominal aorta) following unknown dose of orthovoltage irradiation for treatment of neuroblastoma in an infant.

with surgical injury or trauma, produces a similar endothelial reaction. In most clinical reports and when tested experimentally, a reduction in radiation dose of 20 to 25 per cent is required to produce a given incidence of complication when irradiation is combined with actinomycin D.[106]

A different type of interaction between Adriamycin, known to be potentially cardiotoxic, and irradiation has been suggested by Gilladoga et al., who describe an increased incidence of cardiac failure when a given cumulative dose of Adriamycin is administered in combination with cardiac irradia-

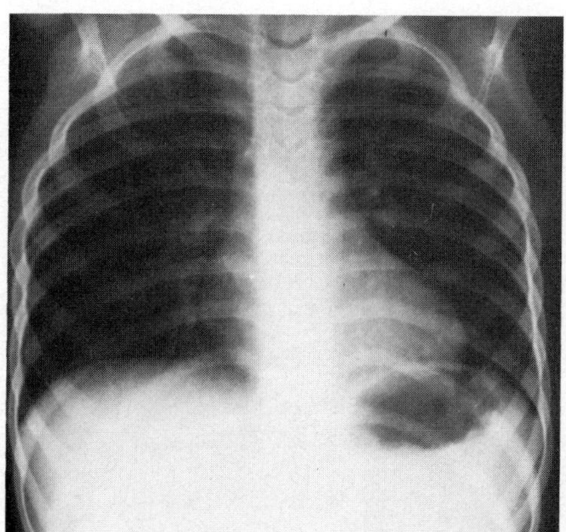
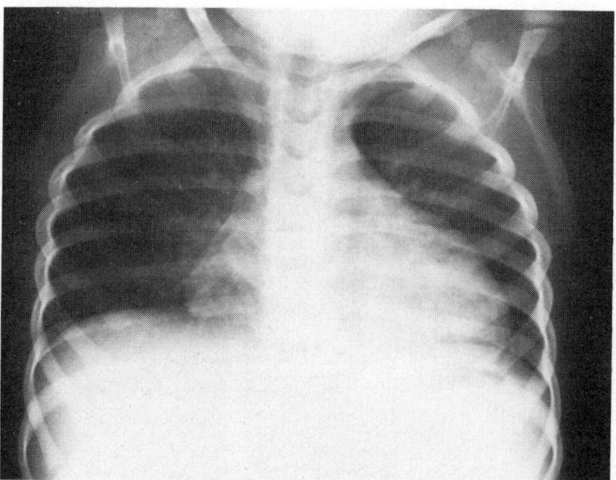

Figure 32–4 Cardiac enlargement and congestive heart failure in child treated for metastatic (from lung) Wilms' tumor with 4 MV whole-lung irradiation (1650 rad/11 fractions/2+ wk) and Adriamycin. Digitalization completely reversed clinical failure. Roentgenogram on left was made before treatment (and before development of metastases).

tion.[52] Experimental work by Eltringham and coworkers supports this contention[44] (Fig. 32–4).

GASTROINTESTINAL SYSTEM

Unlike the cardiovascular and musculoskeletal systems, the gastrointestinal system is subject to acute as well as subacute and chronic complications after irradiation.

Nausea and emesis following abdominal irradiation are not uncommon. The incidence and severity are related to daily radiation fraction size, dose rate, radiation volume, and region treated as well as to a number of other factors such as concurrent administration of a variety of chemotherapeutic agents, recent surgery, and so forth. Treatment fields including the stomach or small bowel or both are more likely to produce acute symptoms than are lower abdominal or pelvic fields. A variety of antiemetics are often effective, and, as noted previously, a decrease in daily radiation dose often alleviates these acute symptoms. Radiation-related diarrhea occurring somewhat later in a treatment course is similarly amenable to symptomatic treatment combined with treatment delays, decreased daily radiation fractions, or both.

When concurrent or closely interposed administration of Adriamycin and esophageal irradiation occurs, a marked increase in the incidence and severity of acute esophagitis is seen. This occasionally leads to stric-

ture formation, especially if Adriamycin administration is repeated.[103] Radiation doses necessary to produce this complication appear to be lower in the child than in the adult.[61, 103]

Subacute hepatic changes were briefly discussed earlier. Hepatic cells, usually in a mitotically resting state, are induced into cycle by destruction or surgical removal of a portion of the liver. The liver, under these circumstances, has been shown to be much more sensitive to irradiation.[51] When agents such as actinomycin D or vincristine are administered concurrently, hepatic injury is further augmented.[19] A precipitous decrease in platelets and other formed elements of the blood is often noted in association with hepatitis and may be responsible for a variety of clinical findings, including hepatic tenderness, ascites, jaundice, and hepatic enzyme abnormalities.

Gastrointestinal mucosal stem cells have been shown to possess a striking capacity to absorb and repair sublethal radiation injury when compared with other stem cell populations.[140] Actinomycin D and Adriamycin have both been shown to interfere with this capacity.[9, 42] It might be expected, therefore, that moderate to high doses of abdominal irradiation combined with actinomycin D or Adriamycin would cause a variety of subacute and chronic bowel complaints. This has in fact been noted in a review of patients treated for Wilms' tumor.[24] Gastrointestinal complaints predominated, and there was a significant incidence of bowel

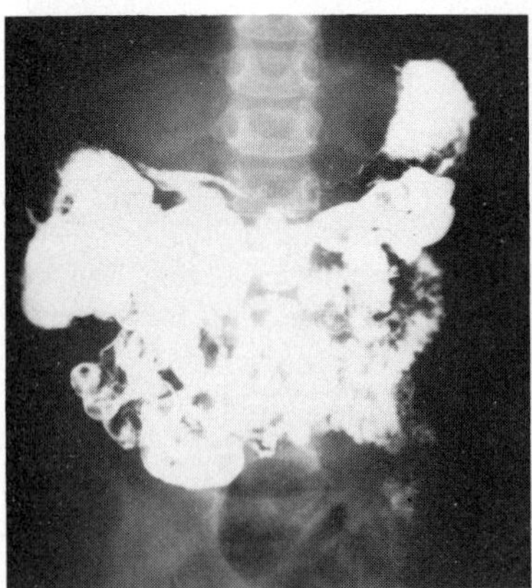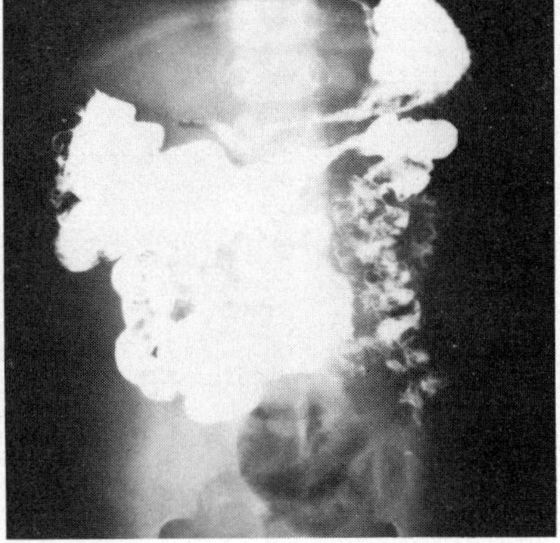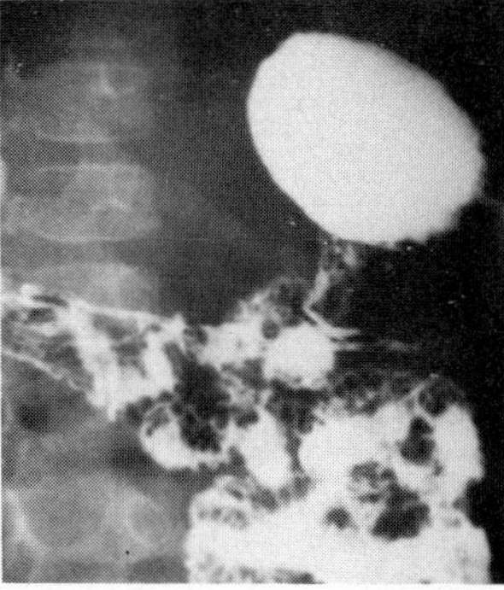

Figure 32–5   Chronic and severe enteritis following 4400 rad midplane orthovoltage abdominal treatment combined with administration of actinomycin D in child with Wilms' tumor. Note thickening of mucosal pattern.

obstruction. Fistula formation, chronic enteritis, and malabsorption have also been described[36, 55, 122] (Fig. 32–5).

Prior surgery, presumably by fixing bowel loops that might otherwise move in and out of limited radiation fields by peristalsis, appears to increase the risk of subsequent injury for a given dose of radiation.[66, 126]

Other chronic changes range from dental abnormalities to small bowel and colonic disturbances.[29, 100, 118, 137] Failure of teeth to erupt and a variety of assorted dental abnormalities have been described following irradiation of head and neck tumors.[29, 34, 85, 137] The salivary gland is also irradiated in the course of such treatment. Depending on the total dose administered and the volume of salivary tissue treated, this may produce chronic xerostomia with a resultant increase in dental caries. Prophylactic fluoride treatments before or after irradiation are effective in diminishing dental complications.[29, 57, 137] Children appear to recover a greater degree of salivary gland function than do adults after moderate-dose irradiation. Long-term studies of salivary gland function in children who have received moderate levels of irradiation have not been done.

A complication analogous to that described in the cardiovascular section may occur many years after moderate- to high-dose abdominal irradiation of an infant. Abrupt narrowing of the caliber of bowel, especially the colon, may be noted and is geographically related to the irradiation portal. Such abnormalities may be responsible for chronic bowel complaints, including constipation.

RESPIRATORY SYSTEM

Acute effects immediately following pulmonary irradiation have not been clinically troublesome. Radiation pneumonitis manifested by cough, dyspnea, fever, and varying degrees of shortness of breath is the most common respiratory complication, occurring 4 to 6 weeks or more after irradiation of the lung.[12, 46, 98, 106, 107] Its clinical severity is volume- and dose-dependent and may be considerably augmented by actinomycin D, Adriamycin, or high-dose methotrexate[68, 106, 107] (Fig. 32–6). Prednisone is usually quite effective in relieving or improving symptoms and signs of treatment-associated pneumonitis.[14, 135] Sudden with-

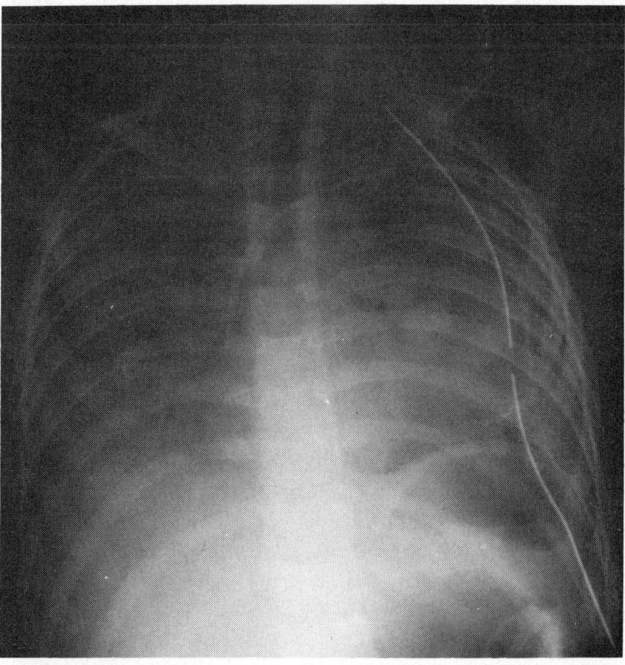

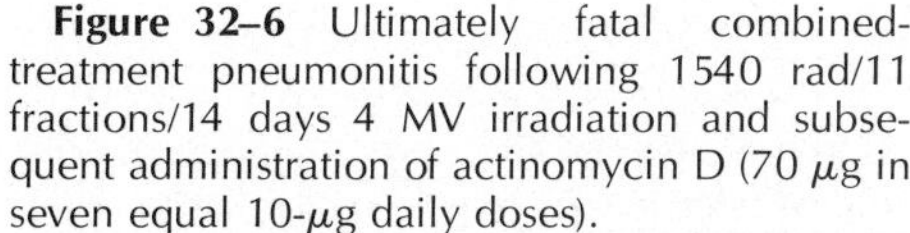

Figure 32–6 Ultimately fatal combined-treatment pneumonitis following 1540 rad/11 fractions/14 days 4 MV irradiation and subsequent administration of actinomycin D (70 μg in seven equal 10-μg daily doses).

drawal or cessation of prednisone has been recognized as activating radiation pneumonitis.[25]

Following moderate- to high-dose irradiation, shunting of blood through poorly aerated lung occasionally occurs, resulting in significant desaturation of blood and cardiorespiratory symptoms.[108] When possible, resection of this abnormal lung often results in clinical improvement, occasionally to a striking degree.

Bullae and pneumatoceles resulting in pneumothorax are also known to occur after lung irradiation. Severely injured lung tissue following treatment may also pose a risk as a site of chronic recurring infection.

GENITOURINARY SYSTEM

Radiation nephritis has previously been noted as a subacute, probably endothelially based response to irradiation.[53, 89] Sudden renal shutdown may occur following irradiation and/or chemotherapy of an extremely resposive neoplasm such as Burkitt's lymphoma or leukemia owing to renal tubular occlusion with precipitated urates. Good hydration and alkalinization of the patient and use of allopurinol to increase solubility will minimize this problem.

Unilateral renal irradiation may result in hypertension by a Goldblatt-type mechanism. Nephrectomy, if indicated and clinically feasible, may be necessary and curative.[28]

Loss of renal cortical substance has been noted following moderate-dose irradiation of a portion or all of a kidney.[81, 113] Compensatory renal hypertrophy following nephrectomy may be modified by irradiation of the remaining kidney when combined with administration of certain chemotherapeutic agents.[21, 99]

Ureteral obstruction following irradiation usually suggests recurrence of the neoplasm. However, on rare occasions it may occur, usually when tumor encircling the ureter has been irradiated, with resultant scarring and stenosis.[116, 122, 130]

A moderately frequent pediatric complication, seen most often in treatment of genitourinary rhabdomyosarcomas and pelvic bone tumors such as Ewing's sarcoma, is an augmentation by irradiation of hemorrhagic cystitis occurring after administration of cyclophosphamide. This agent is excreted in an active form in the urine. Prolonged contact with the bladder mucosa causes marked irritation and is aggravated by significant prior irradiation.[69] Attention to appropriate hydration is helpful, but substitution of another alkylating agent such as nitrogen mustard, which is not excreted in active form in the urine, may be necessary.

REPRODUCTIVE AND ENDOCRINE SYSTEMS

With rare exceptions, sterility regularly follows fractionated treatment totaling approximately 2000 rad given over 1 to 2 weeks in both sexes.[8, 16, 54, 67, 88] Fractionation with even smaller doses causes prolonged periods of aspermia.[119] The relative effect of age and pubertal development on radiation sensitivity of germ cells is not certain. Presumably, the full complement of ova are present at birth; therefore, ovarian sensitivity should not change with increasing age. The status of spermatogonia is less clear.

It is known that radiation sterilization in the young girl will also cause failure of development of secondary sexual characteristics; however, interstitial cells in the boy are much more resistant, and testicular sterilization does not preclude normal male secondary sexual development.

Irradiation of breast tissue in infancy and early childhood to more than 1500 to 2000 rad will cause decrease or failure or development at adolescence despite normal endocrine stimulation.

Thyroid irradiation to more than 3000 to 3500 rad may cause subsequent hypofunction or frank hypothyroidism.[40] A 5 per cent incidence of clinically evident hypothyroidism has been reported after delivery of 4400 rad/19 fractions/4½ weeks to a mantle field for Hodgkin's disease in adults.[110] Both young age and prior lymphangiography appear to increase the risk of this complication.[40] Careful assessment in follow-up care permits early diagnosis and appropriate treatment of this complication. Clinical symptoms may be rather mild. Tumor induction following head and neck irradiation will be discussed separately.

Pituitary hypofunction with decreased growth hormone production and reduction in the output of other pituitary hormones may occur after very high doses of irradiation, as in the treatment of rhabdomyosarcoma affecting the nasopharynx, middle ear, or paranasal sinuses.[13, 40, 127] Treatment of craniopharyngioma may also result in pituitary deficient states; however, determination of cause may be difficult in such patients in view of possible preirradiation tumor effects or sequelae of surgery.

CENTRAL NERVOUS SYSTEM

Acute effects following irradiation of the central nervous system are rare. In the presence of significant intracranial or intraspinal tumor, especially with borderline compensation, acute swelling following irradiation is occasionally seen, with resultant rapid and marked worsening of neurologic signs and symptoms. This situation represents a clinical emergency, and rapid administration of very high doses of steroids, possibly with concurrent mannitol therapy, is essential. Unless performed prior to irradiation, surgical decompression, especially with intraspinal lesions, may provide the most rapid and effective therapy.

With the exception of these acute reactions, most central nervous system complications are delayed or chronic in nature.

Brain necrosis following irradiation is quite rare in the absence of other contributing causes.[77, 139] Myelinization of the child's brain continues for the first 3 to 4 years of life. It has been thought that the brain is more sensitive to the effects of irradiation during this period. A subsequent learning disability has been noted in children irradiated to more than 2000 to 2400 rad with concurrent intrathecal and systemic methotrexate combined with other agents.[41] Other evidence of increased sensitivity of the young child's brain is scanty or absent. Several authors have documented leukoencephalopathy following irradiation in childhood, almost always in the presence of administration of both systemic and intrathecal or intraventricular methotrexate.[5, 104] On occasion, a clinically inseparable abnor-

mality has followed either very high systemic doses or intrathecal administration of methotrexate, usually in the presence of overt central nervous system tumor or leukemia.[1] In one study, a nearly 50 per cent incidence of clinically significant leukoencephalopathy occurred in children treated for leukemia following cranial irradiation (2400 rad) with concurrent intrathecal, and moderate-dose systemic, Methotrexate. However, when similar irradiation and intrathecal methotrexate have been administered in the absence of central nervous system tumor or systemic methotrexate, this complication has not been seen.[5, 37]

Radiation myelitis is one of the most serious of all complications. This chronic injury is thought to occur as a result of progressive vascular compromise following irradiation. It is extremely rare in children or adults when less than 4500 rad delivered in 150-rad fractions have been administered. However, the incidence increases significantly, especially with radiation doses greater than 5000 to 5500 rad.[6, 92, 136] Possible potentiation by actinomycin D has recently been reported.[87] Most commonly, a technical error in delivery of radiation is responsible, with overlap occurring between two irradiated fields in a region of the spinal cord (i.e., between mantle and para-aortic fields in treatment of Hodgkin's disease).

Peripheral nerve injury as a result of irradiation is uncommon.[7] As with radiation-related cranial nerve damage, high doses of radiation are required.[11, 27, 43]

Keratoconjunctivitis is commonly seen as an acute complication of treatment of tumor near the eye and may be considerably worsened by concurrent or subsequent chemotherapy, especially with agents such as actinomycin D or Adriamycin.

Irradiation of the lens in childhood, necessary in the treatment of orbital rhabdomyosarcoma, invariably produces cataract formation when fractionated doses greater than 1000 rad are administered.[26, 82, 96] Cataracts usually do not form until at least 12 to 14 months have elapsed and are often progressive in severity until at least 18 to 24 months have passed. Depending on the total dose delivered, such cataracts may never become visually significant and may stabilize at this level. It is usually possible in most clinical settings to provide sufficient lens shielding to minimize or eliminate this problem. Other eye complications such as retinal vascular degeneration and production of a phthisic, dry, or painful eye require substantially larger radiation doses.[43]

SKIN AND MUCOUS MEMBRANES

With the advent of megavoltage equipment, chronic skin abnormalities, formerly among the most frequent of long-term radiation effects, have become quite uncommon.[3, 39, 129, 134] Acute skin reactions continue to be seen after high-dose irradiation, especially when tangential skin treatment has been necessary or when sensitive areas such as the perineum must be treated.

A clinically inapparent or minimal skin reaction may be rapidly transformed into a striking erythema with areas of moist desquamation by administration of radiopotentiators such as actinomycin D, Adriamycin, or high-dose methotrexate. When these agents are given after completion of irradiation, they may produce a phenomenon whereby prior radiation reactions are "recalled."[22, 30, 35] This recall phenomenon usually becomes progressively less severe with each subsequent administration of chemotherapy. Recall by actinomycin D administration, however, has been noted to occur more than 1 year following irradiation (Fig. 32–7).

Acute mucosal reactions are common during the course of therapy. In general, they respond quickly to a short break in treatment or a decrease in daily radiation fraction size. Mucosal reactions may be worsened by significant leukopenia from systemic chemotherapy and clearly may be substantially worsened by additive or synergistic chemotherapy administration. The severity of acute skin or mucosal reactions is not of predictive value for development of late complications.

A potentially unanticipated sequela of intensive, wide-field irradiation for children with Hodgkin's disease may be the development of herpes zoster. A number of factors, including irradiation and prior splenectomy, appear to influence the incidence of this finding.[56]

Although there is experimental evidence demonstrating some delay in wound healing following irradiation of a surgical incision,[79] many pediatric patients have been treated with radiation including the surgical incision without increased risk of wound dehiscence or breakdown.

INDUCED TUMORS

Second tumors occurring many years after treatment for malignant childhood tumor are one of the most disturbing complications of radiation therapy. Accumulating data suggest that tumor incidence is

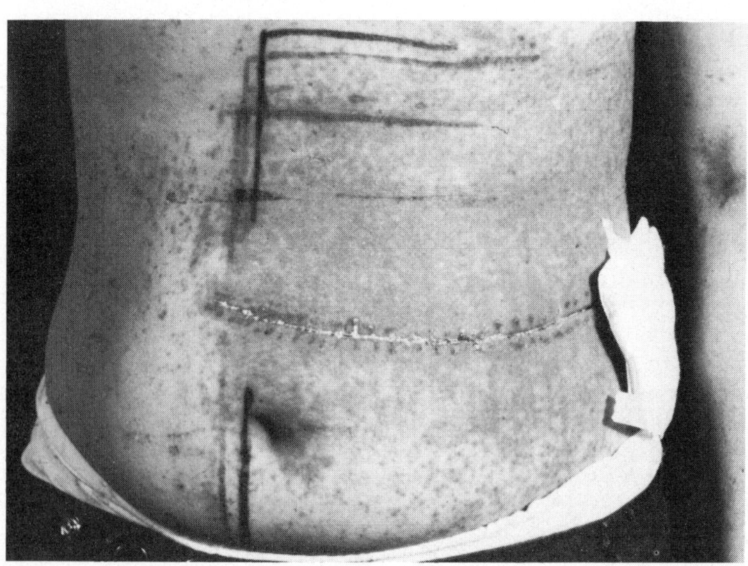

Figure 32–7 Actinomycin D recall of radiation dermatitis following irradiation for Wilms' tumor. Child had no evident skin reaction before intravenous administration of actinomycin D. Note should also be made of accentuation and reaction at prior tape sites (unirradiated) and at intravenous sites of left arm, indicating that actinomycin D recall may occur at the site of any prior injury, regardless of cause.

related to age; site of treatment; therapy with radiation, chemotherapy, or combinations; and duration of follow-up, as well as to the intensity and technique of treatment.* In addition to these variables, the long latent period between exposure and development of a possible second tumor further complicates evaluation of treated populations.[84, 93] Genetic predisposition has been observed and confirmed by Jensen and Miller[70] and, more recently, has been extended to other conditions by Knudson and others.[17, 73, 75, 80] From these observations, it would appear that children with certain genetic structures carry a heightened risk of developing tumors of many varieties independent of their therapy (Fig. 32–8).

Radiation technique, including both total dose and equipment used, appears to strongly influence the incidence of radiation-associated neoplasms.[58, 114] A direct relationship between dose and incidence was noted in survivors of retinoblastoma and other treated tumors as well as in survivors of the atomic bomb.[2, 65, 114]

With the exception of the atomic bomb experience, virtually all available data represent series of patients treated only with orthovoltage equipment, with its higher relative bone and subcutaneous tissue doses.[58] Only two series are available detailing the radiation-associated tumor incidence in

---

*See references 4, 15, 17, 48, 59, 60, 63, 74, 84, 90, 91, 94, 97, 114, and 142.

megavoltage-treated patients followed up for more than five years[58, 114] Sagerman et al. reported a less than 2 per cent incidence of second tumors in patients receiving 4500 rad or less.[114] Virtually all of these patients were treated with megavoltage techniques using a 22.5 MV betatron. Haselow et al. reported a similarly low incidence in children treated with cobalt 60 (^{60}Co).[58] The incidence in orthovoltage-treated patients has been considerably greater, even when lower doses have been used.[84, 114] The duration of follow-up has been significantly longer in the orthovoltage-treated patients. Of interest is the absence of an excess of second tumors occurring in the radiation field in adult women treated with high doses for carcinoma of the cervix.[76, 142] A significant incidence of in-field tumors has been noted in women treated with lower radiation doses for benign conditions.[117] These observations suggest a possible region in the tumor incidence vs. radiation dose curve where increasing dose actually produces a lower incidence of associated tumors.[63] Experimental animal systems also suggest that this phenomenon can occur.[132]

The importance of age at time of treatment in predicting both the incidence and, in certain cases, the type of tumor is clearly evidenced by an examination of series of children and adults receiving thyroid irradiation. A substantial incidence of thyroid tumors has been noted in irradiated children.[49, 59] Adults treated for both Hodgkin's

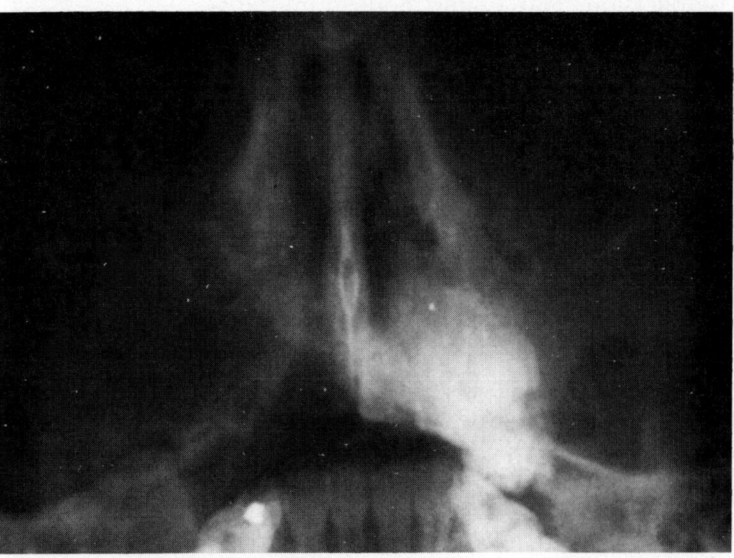

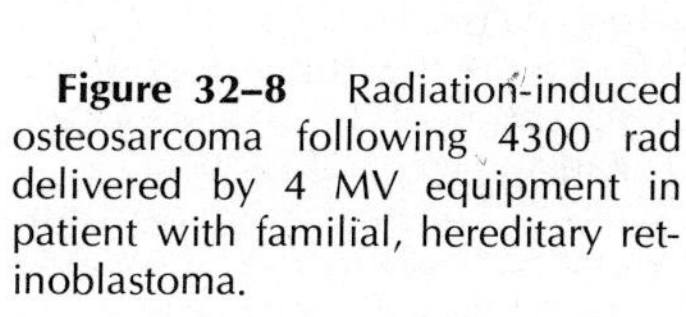

Figure 32–8 Radiation-induced osteosarcoma following 4300 rad delivered by 4 MV equipment in patient with familial, hereditary retinoblastoma.

disease and other lymphomas, as well as for a variety of head and neck tumors, appear to be affected much less frequently.[72, 80]

Irradiation in utero, even with very low doses delivered for diagnostic purposes, appears to carry a substantially increased risk of tumor development.[91] The heightened risk of subsequent adenocarcinoma of the breast following significant radiation exposure appears to largely disappear by age 35 years; however, sarcoma may still develop in the irradiated older patient.[90, 115, 128]

Combinations of chemotherapy with irradiation may substantially increase the likelihood of certain tumors such as acute myelogenous leukemia or lymphoma. Patients treated for Hodgkin's disease with either radiation or MOPP chemotherapy (combination of mechlorethamine, vincristine, procarbazine, and prednisone) have a very low likelihood of leukemia development. However, when these therapies are combined, a many-fold increase in incidence of myelogenous leukemia and non-Hodgkin's lymphoma has been observed.[4, 17]

The study of Li et al. indicates the importance of duration of follow-up in establishing the "true" incidence of second tumors. A steadily increasing risk of tumors has been observed with increasing length of follow-up.[84, 93]

CONCLUSION

Clearly, an extensive array of potential complications may follow modern multidisciplinary treatment. Accurate knowledge of the nature, incidence, and, when possible, prevention or successful treatment of these complications is important in making therapeutic management decisions.

It must be stressed that many reported complications of irradiation are related to technique and could be prevented by more satisfactory radiation practice.[83, 124] Second-tumor incidence and bone, skin, and subcutaneous complications related to the use of orthovoltage equipment are clear examples. Brief analysis of two reports on radiation pericarditis provides another. When equally weighted anterior and posterior mediastinal portals are used to deliver a midmediastinal dose of 4000 rad in 200-rad fractions over 4 weeks, a 2 per cent incidence of pericarditis

is observed. However, when essentially the same midmediastinal dose is delivered using solely an anterior field, the incidence rises to nearly 25 per cent.[71, 121] It must also be noted that no improvement in tumor control accompanied this increased morbidity.

Signal improvements in treatment of children with cancer have strikingly increased the number of children cured of malignancy. Only by a clear understanding of radiation-associated morbidity and use of optimal technique to minimize its occurrence will the radiation therapist be able to ensure that this increased survival is as normal as possible.

References

1. Allen, J. C., Thaler, H. T., Deck, M. D., and Rottenberg, D. A.: Leukoencephalopathy following high-dose intravenous methotrexate chemotherapy: Quantitative assessment of white matter attenuation using computed tomography. Neuroradiology 16:44, 1978.
2. Anderson, R. E., Nishiyama, H., Ishida, K., et al.: Pathogenesis of radiation-related leukemia and lymphoma. Lancet, 1:1060, 1972.
3. Arcangeli, G., Friedman, M., and Paoluzi, R.: A quantitative study of late radiation effect on normal skin and subcutaneous tissue in human beings. Br. J. Radiol. 47:44, 1974.
4. Arseneau, J. C., Sponzo, R. W., Levin, D. L., et al.: Nonlymphomatous malignant tumors complicating Hodgkin's disease. N. Engl. J. Med. 287:1119, 1972.
5. Aur, R., Hustu, H. O., and Simone, J.: Leukoencephalopathy in children with acute lymphocytic leukemia receiving preventive central nervous system therapy. Proc. Am. Soc. Clin. Oncol. 17:97, 1976.
6. Backmark U. B.: Neurologic complications after irradiation of the cervical spinal cord for malignant tumor of the head and neck. Acta Radiol. (Ther.) 14:33, 1975.
7. Bagley, F. H., Walsh, J. W., Cady, B., et al.: Carcinomatous versus radiation-induced brachial plexus neuropathy in breast cancer. Cancer 41:2154, 1978.
8. Beaumont, H. M.: The radiosensitivity of germ cells at various stages of ovarian development. Int. J. Radiat. Biol. 4:581, 1966.
9. Belli, J., and Piro, A. J.: The interaction between radiation and Adriamycin damage in mammalian cells. Cancer Res. 37:1624, 1977.
10. Berdjis, C. C.: The cardiovascular system. *In* Berdjis, C. C. (ed.): Pathology of Irradiation. Baltimore, Williams & Wilkins Co., 1971, pp. 377–407.
11. Berger, P. S., and Bataini, J. P.: Radiation-induced cranial nerve palsy. Cancer 40:152, 1977.
12. Bloomer, W. D., and Hellman, S.: Normal tissue

responses to radiation therapy. N. Engl. J. Med. 293:80, 1975.

13. Bradley, J. M.: Radiotherapy of pituitary tumors. J. Coll. Radiol. Aust. 9:36, 1965.

14. Braun, S., Dopico, G. A., Olsen, C. G., and Caldwell, W.: Low-dose radiation pneumonitis. Cancer 35:1322, 1975.

15. Brown, J. M.: Linearity vs. non-linearity of dose response for radiation carcinogenesis. Health Phys. 31:231, 1976.

16. Callaway, J. L., Moseley, V., and Barefoot, S. W.: Effects of roentgen ray irradiation on testes of rabbits; possible harmful effects on human testes from low voltage roentgen ray therapy. Arch. Dermatol. Syph. (Berlin) 56:471, 1947.

17. Canellos, G. P., Arseneau, J. C., DeVita, V. T., et al.: Second malignancies complicating Hodgkin's disease in remission. Lancet 1:947, 1975.

18. Cassady, J. R.: Radiation therapy in Ewing's sarcoma. *In* Jaffe, N. (ed.): Bone Tumors in Children. Littleton, Mass., PSG Publishing Co., 1979.

19. Cassady, J. R., Carabell, S., and Jaffe, N.: Chemotherapy-irradiation related hepatic dysfunction in patients with Wilms' tumor. Front. Rad. Ther. Oncol. 13:147, 1979.

20. Cassady, J. R., Jaffe, N., and Filler, R. M.: The increasing importance of radiation therapy in the treatment of Wilms' tumor. Cancer 39:825, 1977.

21. Cassady, J. R., Lebowitz, R., Jaffe, N.: Effect of low-dose irradiation on renal enlargement in children following nephrectomy for Wilms' tumor (in press).

22. Cassady, J. R., Richter, M. P., Piro, A. J., et al.: Radiation-Adriamycin interactions: Preliminary clinical observations. Cancer 36:946, 1975.

23. Cassady, J. R., Sagerman, R. H., Tretter, P., and Ellsworth, R. M.: Radiation therapy in retinoblastoma. Radiology, 93:405, 1969.

24. Cassady, J. R., Tefft, M., Filler, R. M., et al.: Considerations in the radiation therapy of Wilms' tumor. Cancer 32:598, 1973.

25. Castellino, R. A., Glatstein, E., Turbow, M. M., et al.: Latent radiation injury of lungs or heart activated by steroid withdrawal. Ann. Intern. Med. 80:593, 1974.

26. Chan, R. C., and Shukovsky, L. J.: Effects of irradiation on the eye. Radiology 120:673, 1976.

27. Cheng, V. S. T., and Schulz, M. D.: Unilateral hypoglossal nerve atrophy as a late complication of radiation therapy of head and neck carcinoma: A report of four cases and a review of the literature on peripheral and cranial nerve damages after radiation therapy. Cancer 35:1537, 1975.

28. Crummy, A. B., Hellman, S., Stansel, H. C., and Hukill, P. B.: Renal hypertension secondary to unilateral radiation damage relived by nephrectomy. Radiology 84:108, 1965.

29. Daly, T. E., and Drane, J. B.: Management of teeth related to the treatment of oral cancer. Proceedings of the Seventh National Cancer Conference, Los Angeles, Sept. 27–29, 1972. pp. 147–154.

30. D'Angio, G. J.: Clinical and biologic studies of actinomycin D and roentgen irradiation. Am. J. Roentgenol. 87:106, 1962.

31. D'Angio, G. J., Evans, A. E., and Breslow, N.: The treatment of Wilms' tumor. Results of the National Wilms' Tumor Study. Cancer 38:633, 1976.

32. D'Angio, G. J., Jung, J., Wright, K., and Cohen, J.: Disturbance in bone growth produced by 3.5 MeV electron irradiation of young rabbit limbs. Am. J. Roentgenol. 91:1132, 1964.

33. D'Angio, G. J., Tefft, M., Breslow, N., et al.: Radiation therapy of Wilms' tumor. Results according to dose, field, postoperative timing, and histology. Int. J. Radiat. Oncol. Biol. Phys. 4:769, 1978.

34. Doline, S., Needleman, H. L., Petersen, R. A., and Cassady, J. R.: The effect of radiotherapy in the treatment of retinoblastoma upon the developing dentition. J. Pediatr. Ophthalmol. 17:109, 1980.

35. Donaldson, S. S., Glick, J. M., and Wilbur, J. R.: Adriamycin activating a recall phenomenon after radiation therapy. Ann. Intern. Med. 81:407, 1974.

36. Donaldson, S. S., Jundt, S., Ricour, C. L., et al.: Radiation enteritis in children: A retrospective review, clinicopathologic correlation and dietary management. Cancer 35:1167, 1975.

37. Dritschilo, A., Cassady, J. R., Camitta, B., et al.: The role of irradiation in central nervous system treatment and prophylaxis for acute lymphoblastic leukemia. Cancer 37:2729, 1976.

38. Dritschilo, A., Weichselbaum, R. W., Cassady, J. R., et al.: The role of radiation therapy in the treatment of soft tissue sarcomas of childhood. Cancer 42:1192, 1978.

39. Dutriex, J., Wambersie, A., and Bonhik, C.: Cellular recovery in human skin reactions: Application to dose fraction number, overall time relationship in radiotherapy. Eur. J. Cancer 9:159, 1973.

40. Einhorn, J., and Einhorn, N.: Effects of irradiation on the endocrine glands. Front. Rad. Ther. Oncol. 6:386, 1972.

41. Eiser, C., and Lansdown, R.: Retrospective study of intellectual development in children treated for acute lymphoblastic leukaemia. Arch. Dis. Child. 52:525, 1977.

42. Elkind, M. M., and Sakamoto, K.: Combined effects of x-irradiation and chemotherapeutic drugs (nitrogen mustard and actinomycin D). Front, Rad. Ther. Oncol. 4:53, 1969.

43. Ellingwood, K. E., and Million, R.: Cancer of the nasal cavity and ethmoid/sphenoid sinuses. Cancer 43:1517, 1979.

44. Eltringham, J. R., Fajardo, L. F., Stewart, J. R., and Klauber, M. R.: Investigation of cardiotoxicity in rabbits from Adriamycin and fractionated cardiac irradiation: Preliminary results. Front. Rad. Ther. Oncol. 13:21, 1979.

45. Fajardo, L. F.: Radiation induced coronary artery disease (editorial). Chest 71:563, 1977.

46. Fajardo, L. F., and Berthrong, M.: Radiation injury in surgical pathology. Am. J. Surg. Pathol. June 1978, p. 159.

47. Fajardo, L. F., and Stewart, J. R.: Experimental radiation induced heart disease. I. Light microscopic studies. Am. J. Pathol. 59:299, 1970.

48. Fajardo, L. F., and Stewart, J. R.: Capillary injury preceding radiation-induced myocardial fibrosis. Radiology 101:429, 1971.

49. Favus, M. J., Schneider, A. B., Stachura, M. E., et al.: Thyroid cancer occurring as a late consequence of head-and-neck irradiation. N. Engl. J. Med. 294:1019, 1976.

50. Fernandez, C. H., Lindberg, R. D., Sutow, W. W., et al.: Localized Ewing's sarcoma: Treatment and results. Cancer 34:143, 1974.

51. Filler, R. M., Tefft, M., Vawter, G. F., et al.: Hepatic lobectomy in childhood: Effects of x-rays and chemotherapy. J. Pediatr. Surg. 4:31, 1969.

52. Gilladoga, A. C., Manuel, C., Tan, C. T. C., et al.: The cardiotoxicity of Adriamycin and daunorubicin in children. Cancer 37:1070, 1976.

53. Glatstein, E., Fajardo, L. F., and Brown, J. M.: Radiation injury in the mouse kidney. I. Sequential light microscopic study. Int. J. Radiat. Oncol. Biol. Phys. 2:933, 1977.

54. Glucksman, A.: The effects of radiation on reproductive organs. Br. J. Radiol. 1(suppl.):101, 1947.

55. Goldstein, H. M., Rodgers, L. F., Fletcher, G. H., and Dodd, G.: Radiologic manifestations of radiation induced injury to the normal upper gastrointestinal tract. Radiology 117:135, 1975.

56. Goodman, R., Jaffe, N., Filler, R., and Cassady, J. R.: Herpes zoster in children with stages I–III Hodgkin's disease. Radiology 118:429, 1976.

57. Guggenheimer, J., Fischer, W. G., and Pechersky, J. L.: Anticipation of dental anomalies induced by radiation. Radiology 117:405, 1975.

58. Haselow, R. E., Nesbit, M., Kehner, L. P., et al.: Second neoplasms following megavoltage radiation in a pediatric population. Cancer 42:1185, 1978.

59. Hempelmann, L. H.: Risk of thyroid neoplasms after irradiation in childhood. Science, 160:159, 1968.

60. Hirohata, T.: Radiation carcinogenesis. Semin. Oncol. 3:25, 1976.

61. Horwick, A., Lokich, J. J., and Bloomer, W. D.: Doxorubicin, radiotherapy and oesophageal stricture. Lancet 2:561, 1975.

62. Hustu, H. O., Aur, R. J. A., Verzosa, M. S., et al.: Prevention of central nervous system leukemia by irradiation. Cancer 32:585, 1973.

63. Hutchison, G. B.: Late neoplastic changes following medical irradiation. Radiology 105:645, 1972.

64. Ingold, J. A., Reed, G. B., Kaplan, H. S., and Bagshaw, M. A.: Radiation hepatitis. Am. J. Roentgenol., 93:200, 1965.

65. Ishimaru, T., Hoshino, J., Ichimaru, M., et al.: Leukemia in atomic bomb survivors, Hiroshima and Nagasaki, 1 Oct. 1950–30 Sept. 1966. Radiat. Res. 45:216, 1971.

66. Jackson, B. T.: Bowel damage from radiation. Proc. R. Soc. Med. 69:683, 1976.

67. Jacox, H. W.: Recovery following human ovarian irradiation. Radiology 32:538, 1939.

68. Jaffe, N., Farber, S., Traggis, D., et al.: Favorable response of metastatic osteogenic sarcoma to pulse high-dose methotrexate with citrovorum rescue and radiation therapy. Cancer 31:1367, 1973.

69. Jayalakshmamma, B., and Pinkel D.: Urinary bladder toxicity following pelvis irradiation and simultaneous cyclophosphamide therapy. Cancer 38:701, 1976.

70. Jensen, R. D., and Miller, R. W.: Retinoblastoma: Epidemiologic characteristics. N. Engl. J. Med. 285:307, 1971.

71. Kagan, A. R., Hafermann, M., Hamilton, M., et al.: Etiology, diagnosis and management of pericardial effusion after irradiation. Radiol. Clin. Biol. 41:171, 1971.

72. Kaplan, H. S.: Hodgkin's Disease. Cambridge, Harvard University Press, 1972.

73. Kitchin, F. D., and Ellsworth, R. M.: Pleiotropic effects of the gene for retinoblastoma. J. Med. Genet. 11:244, 1974.

74. Kligerman, M. M.: Principles of radiation therapy. *In* Holland, J., and Frei, E., III (eds.): Cancer Medicine. Philadelphia, Lea & Febiger, 1973, pp. 541–565.

75. Knudson, A. G., Jr.: Mutation and cancer: Statistical study of retinoblastoma. Proc. Nat. Acad. Sci. 68:529, 1971.

76. Kohn, H. I., Bailar, J. C., and Zippin, C.: Radiation therapy for cancer of the cervix: Its late effect on the lifespan as a function of regional dose. J. Natl. Cancer Inst. 34:345, 1965.

77. Kramer, S., Southard, M. E., and Mansfield, C. M.: Radiation effects of tolerance of the central nervous system. Front. Rad. Ther. Oncol. 6:332, 1972.

78. Kun, L. E., and Camitta, B. M.: Hepatopathy following irradiation and Adriamycin. Cancer 42:81, 1978.

79. Lawrence, W., Nickson, J. J., and Wajshaw, L. M.: Roentgen rays and wound healing. Surgery 33:376, 1953.

80. Lawson, W., and Som, M.: Second primary cancer after irradiation of laryngeal cancer. Ann. Otol. Rhinol. Laryngol. 84:771, 1975.

81. Lebowitz, R.: Personal communication.

82. Leinfelder, P. J., Evans, T. C., and Riley, E.: Production of cataracts in animals by x-rays and fast neutrons. Radiology 65:433, 1965.

83. Levene, M. B., Kijewski, P. K., Chin, L. M., et al.: Computer-controlled radiation therapy. Radiology 129:769, 1978.

84. Li, F. P., Cassady, J. R., and Jaffe, N.: Risk of second tumors in survivors of childhood cancer. Cancer 35:1230, 1975.

85. Lines, L. G., Hazra, T. A., Howells, R., and Shipman, B.: Altered growth and development of lower teeth in children receiving mantle therapy. Radiology 132:447, 1979.

86. Littman, P. S., and D'Angio, G. J.: Growth considerations in the radiation therapy of children with cancer. Ann. Rev. Med. 30:405, 1979.

87. Littman, P., Rosenstuck, J. G., and Bailey, C.: Radiation myelitis following craniospinal irradiation with concurrent actinomycin-D therapy. Med. Pediatr. Oncol. 5:145, 1978.

88. Lushbaugh, C. C., and Ricks, R. C.: Some cytokinetic and histopathology considerations of irradiated male and female gonadal tissues. Front. Rad. Ther. Oncol. 6:228, 1972.

89. Luxton, R. W., and Kunkler, P. B.: Radiation nephritis. Acta Radiol. 2:169, 1964.

90. Mackenzie, I.: Breast cancer following multiple fluoroscopies. Br. J. Cancer 19:1, 1965.

91. MacMahon, B.: Prenatal x-ray exposure and childhood cancer. J. Natl. Cancer Inst. 28:1173, 1962.

92. Maier, J. G., Perry, R. H., Saylor, W., and Sulak, M.: Radiation myelitis of the dorsolumbar spinal cord. Radiology, 93:153, 1969.

93. Makuch, R., and Simon, R.: Recommendations for the analysis of the effect of treatment on the development of second malignancy. Cancer 44:250, 1979.

94. Mayneord, W. V.: Radiation carcinogenesis. Br. J. Radiol 41:241, 1968.

95. Mendelsohn, M. L.: Radiotherapy and tolerance. *In* Vaeth, J. (ed.): Frontiers of Radiation Therapy and Oncology. Vol. 6: Radiation Effect and Tolerance, Normal Tissue. Basel, S. Karger, 1972, pp. 512–523.

96. Merriam, G. R., Szechter, A., and Fucht, E. F.: The effects of ionizing radiations on the eye. Front. Rad. Ther. Oncol., 6:346, 1972.

97. Mole, R. H.: Ionizing radiation as a carcinogen: Practical questions and academic pursuits. Br. J. Radiol. 48:157, 1975.

98. Moosavi, H., McDonald, S., Rubin, P., et al.: Early radiation dose-response in the lung, and ultrastructural study. Int. J. Radiat. Oncol. Biol. Phys. 2:921, 1977.

99. Moskowitz, P. S., and Donaldson, S. S.: Chemotherapy-induced inhibition of compensatory renal growth in the immature mouse. 21st Annual Meeting of Society for Pediatric Radiology, 1978. Abstract in Am. J. Roentgenol. 132:306, 1979.

100. Mossman, K. L., and Henkin, R. I.: Radiation-induced changes in taste acuity in cancer patients. Int. J. Radiat. Oncol. Biol. Phys. 4:663, 1978.

101. Nelson, D. F., Cassady, J. R., Traggis, D., et al.: The role of radiation therapy in localized resectable intestinal non-Hodgkin's lymphoma in children. Cancer 39:89, 1977.

102. Neuhauser, E. B. D., Wittenborg, M. H., Berman, C. Z., and Cohen, J.: Irradiation effects of roentgen therapy on the growing spine. Radiology 59:637, 1952.

103. Newburger, P. E., Cassady, J. R., and Jaffe, N.: Esophagitis due to Adriamycin and radiation therapy for childhood malignancy. Cancer 42:417, 1978.

104. Norrell, H., Wilson, C. B., Slage, D. E., and Clark, D. B.: Leucoencephalopathy following the administration of methotrexate into the cerebrospinal fluid in the treatment of primary brain tumors. Cancer 33:923, 1974.

105. Painter, M. J., Chutorian, A. M., and Hilal, S. K.: Cerebrovasculopathy following irradiation in childhood. Neurology 25:189, 1975.

106. Phillips, T. L.: Effects on lung of combined chemotherapy and radiotherapy. Front. Rad. Ther. Oncol. 13:133, 1979.

107. Phillips, T. L., and Fu, K. K.: Acute and late effects of multimodal therapy on normal tissues. Cancer 40:489, 1977.

108. Prato, F. S., Kurdyak, R., Saibil, E. A., et al.: Physiological and radiographic assessment during the development of pulmonary radiation fibrosis. Radiology 122:389, 1977.

109. Probert, J. C., Parker, B. R., and Kaplan, H. S.: Growth retardation in children after megavoltage irradiation of the spine. Cancer 32:634, 1973.

110. Rogoway, W. M., Finkelstein, S., Rosenberg, S. A., and Kriss, J. P.: Myxedema development after lymphangiography and neck irradiation. Clin. Res. 14:133, 1966.

111. Rubin, P., and Casarett, G. W.: Clinical Radiation Pathology, Vols. 1 and 2. Philadelphia, W. B. Saunders Co., 1968.

112. Rubin, P., Duthie, R. B., and Young, L. W.: Significance of scoliosis in post irradiated Wilms' tumor and neuroblastoma. Radiology 79:539, 1962.

113. Sagerman, R. H., Berdon, W. E., and Baker, D.: Renal atrophy without hypertension following irradiation in infants and children. Ann. Radiol 12:278, 1969.

114. Sagerman, R. H., Cassady, J. R., Tretter, P., et al.: Radiation induced neoplasia following external beam therapy for children with retinoblastoma. Am. J. Roentgenol. 105:529, 1969.

115. Simon, N.: Breast cancer induced by irradiation. JAMA 237:789, 1977.

116. Sklaroff, D. M., Gnaneswaran, P., and Sklaroff, R. B.: Post irradiation ureteric structure. Gynecol. Oncol. 6:538, 1978.

117. Smith, P. G., and Doll, R.: Late effects of x-irradiation in patients treated for metropathia haemorrhagica. Br. J. Radiol. 49:224, 1976.

118. Smith, J. S., and Milford, H. E.: Management of colitis caused by irradiation. Surg. Gynecol. Obstet. 142:519, 1976.

119. Speiser, B., Rubin, P., and Casarett, G.: Aspermia following lower truncal irradiation in Hodgkin's disease. Cancer 32:692, 1973.

120. Stewart, J. R., and Fajardo, L. F.: Dose response in human and experimental radiation-induced heart disease. Application of the nominal standard dose (NSD) concept. Radiology 99:403, 1971.

121. Stewart, J. R., and Fajardo, L. F.: Radiation induced heart disease. Clinical and experimental aspects. Radiol. Clin. North Am. 9:511, 1971.

122. Strockbine, M. F., Nahcock, J. E., and Fletcher, G. F.: Complications in 831 patients with squamous cell carcinoma of an intact uterine

cervix treated with 3000 rads or more pelvis irradiation. Am. J. Roentgenol. 108:293, 1970.

123. Suit, H. D.: Radiation biology: A basis for radiotherapy. *In* Fletcher, G. H. (ed.): Textbook of Radiotherapy. Philadelphia, Lea & Febiger, 1966, pp. 65–97.

124. Suit, H. D., and Goitein, M.: Dose-limiting tissues in relation to types and location of tumours: Implications for efforts to improve radiation dose distributions. Eur. J. Cancer 10:217, 1974.

125. Suit, H. D., and Russell, W. O.: Radiation therapy of soft tissue sarcomas. Cancer 36:759, 1975.

126. Swan, R. W., Fowler, W. C., and Bornow, R. C.: Surgical management of radiation injury to the small intestine. Surg. Gynecol. Obstet. 142:325, 1976.

127. Tan, B. C., and Kunaratnam, N.: Hypopituitary dwarfism following radiotherapy for nasopharyngeal carcinoma. Clin. Radiol. 17:302, 1966.

128. Tokynaga, M., Norman, J., Asano, M., et al.: Malignant breast tumors among atomic bomb survivors, Hiroshima and Nagasaki, 1950–1974. J. Natl. Cancer Inst. 62:1347, 1979.

129. Traenkle, H. L., and Mulay, D.: Further observations on late radiation necrosis following therapy of skin cancer. Arch. Dermatol. 81:908, 1960.

130. Underwood, P. B., Lutz, M. H., and Smoak, D. L.: Ureteral injury following irradiation therapy for carcinoma of the cervix. Obstet. Gynecol. 49:663, 1977.

131. Upton, A. (ed.): Time and Dose Relationships in Radiation Biology as Applied to Radiotherapy (BNL50203 C-57). New York, Brookhaven National Laboratory, 1970.

132. Upton, A. C.: The dose response relation in radiation-induced cancer. Cancer Res. 21:717, 1961.

133. Vaeth, J. (ed.): Radiation Effect and Tolerance, Normal Tissue. Vol. 6 of Radiotherapy and Tolerance. Basel, S. Karger, 1972.

134. Von Essen, C. F.: Radiation tolerance of the skin. Acta Radiol. (Ther.) 8:311, 1969.

135. Wara, W. M., Phillips, T., Margolis, L. W., and Smith, V.: Radiation pneumonitis: A new approach to the derivation of time-dose factors. Cancer 32:547, 1973.

136. Wara, W. M., Phillips, T. L., Sheline, G. E., and Schwade, J. G.: Radiation tolerance of the spinal cord. Cancer 35:1558, 1975.

137. Wescott, W. B., Starcke, E. N., and Shannon, I. L.: Chemical protection against postirradiation dental caries. Oral Surg. 40:709, 1975.

138. Williams, I. G., and Price, B. S.: Tumours of Childhood. New York, Appleton-Century-Crofts, 1973.

139. Wilson, G. H., Byfield, J., and Hanafee, W. M.: Atrophy following radiation therapy for central nervous system neoplasms. Acta Radiol. 11:361, 1972.

140. Withers, H. R., and Elkind, M. M.: Microcolony survival assay for cells of mouse intestinal mucosa exposed to irradiation. Int. J. Radiat. Bio. 17:261, 1970.

141. Wolf, E., Berdon, W. E., Cassady, J. R., et al.: Slipped caput femoral epiphysis as a sequela to childhood irradiation for malignant tumors. Radiology 125:781, 1977.

142. Zippin, C., Bailar, J. C., Kohn, H. I., et al.: Radiation therapy for cervical cancer: Late effects on lifespan and on leukemia incidence. Cancer 28:937, 1971.

33 | CANCER CHEMOTHERAPY

Norman Jaffe, M.D.

Optimum treatment for cancer involves a multimodal approach, including surgery, radiation therapy, and chemotherapy. Prior to initiation of treatment, a plan of management should be formulated. This should consider the histologic nature of the tumor, anatomic site, local extent, areas of dissemination, and the patient's physiologic status. The utility and interdependence of each therapeutic discipline should also be acknowledged. This will permit their integrated use to best advantage. Surgery and occasionally radiation therapy are generally employed as primary treatment. Postopera-

tively, chemotherapy or radiation therapy or both may be administered to eradicate residual disease. Occasionally, however, a preoperative chemotherapy-radiation strategy may be employed to reduce the size of a tumor or render an inoperable tumor operable. Rarely, such treatment without surgery may also prove curative.

Results of multimodal therapy also reveal that chemotherapy has improved the survival of patients with localized and disseminated disease. This is due primarily to its administration as adjuvant therapy after eradication of the primary tumor. In most

TABLE 33–1 CHEMOTHERAPY FOR CHILDHOOD UROLOGIC CANCER

Tumor	Chemotherapeutic Agent	Comments
Wilms' tumor	Actinomycin D Vincristine Adriamycin Cyclophosphamide	Conventional protocols comprise combinations of actinomycin D and vincristine (Adriamycin under investigation)
Renal cell carcinoma	Actinomycin D Vincristine Androgens	

Rhabdomyosarcoma
  Paratesticular
  Prostatic
  Bladder
	Vincristine
	Actinomycin D
	Cyclophosphamide
	Adriamycin
		Commonly used protocols comprise combinations of actinomycin D, vincristine, and cyclophosphamide

Testis
  Teratoma
  Germ cell cancer
	Vincristine
	Actinomycin D
	Cyclophosphamide
	Adriamycin
	Methotrexate
	Chlorambucil
	Mithramycin
		Methotrexate and actinomycin D generally incorporated in nongestational choriocarcinoma regimens

	Cis-dichlorodiammineplatinum II	Cis-dichlorodiammineplatinum II used to treat testicular cancer
	Velban Bleomycin	
Leukemia Lymphoma	Methotrexate 6-Mercaptopurine Arabinosyl cytosine L-Asparaginase Corticosteroids Cyclophosphamide	Leukemia/lymphoma infiltration of testes

malignant diseases, microscopic foci of tumor are disseminated at presentation. Chemotherapy is designed to destroy such metastases. The rationale underlying this approach was initially investigated in experimental animals.[23, 32, 34] It produced increase in survival time and a high percentage of cures. It may aptly be designated microablative treatment. Chemotherapy is currently administered to most children with cancer.[8, 14, 16, 17, 39]

Modifications of treatment may occur as a result of interactions between the different therapeutic modalities and their anticipated complications. In this context, chemotherapeutic agents tend to cause acute and chronic side effects.[15] Most agents are also immunosuppressive and may cause additional problems. A knowledge of these side effects and the special precautions essential in administering the drugs is crucial. Chemotherapeutic agents generally used to treat childhood urologic cancer are listed in Table 33–1.

GENERAL PRINCIPLES

All anticancer drugs are potentially harmful. The decision to administer these agents should not be made without careful consideration. Clinicians should be fully aware of potential side effects, and measures to combat or prevent complications should be available. The selection of drugs is based upon a knowledge of their probable effect on cancer. In general, chemotherapy is administered for three major purposes: curative, adjunctive, and palliative. The goals of treatment should be clearly defined. Occasionally, it may be possible to convert palliation to potential cure.

Chemotherapeutic agents interfere with the vital functions of cells by interrupting complex biochemical pathways. These generally involve DNA-RNA mechanisms, which may be affected by alkylating agents, antibiotics, antimetabolites, and miscellaneous compounds. Alkylating agents bind to DNA, producing fragmentation and clumping of chromosomes. This can lead to incorrect reduplication of the code or dissociation from the regulator genes. The antibiotics form relatively stable complexes with DNA, thereby inhibiting synthesis of DNA and RNA. Antimetabolites may affect pyrimidine and purine biosynthesis, which in turn affects DNA formation. Protein synthesis may be affected by damage to RNA or by prevention of synthesis of specific amino acids, as occurs with L-asparaginase treatment. The mechanisms for action for each class of agents are outlined later in greater detail.

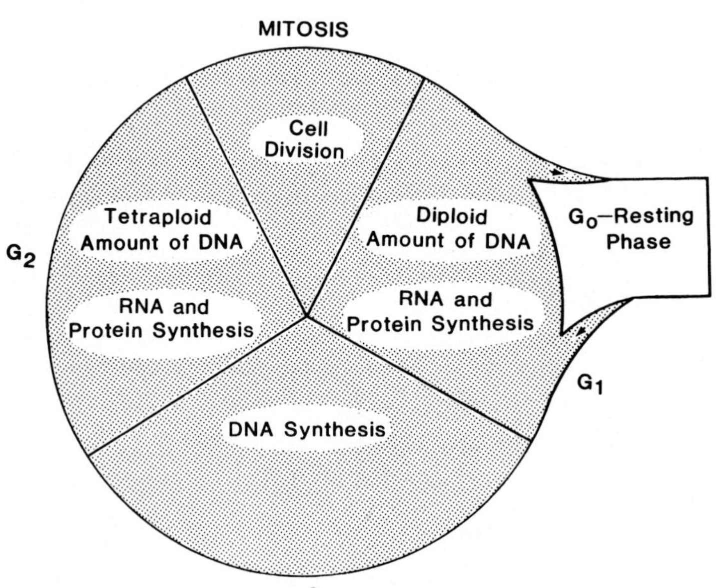

Figure 33–1   The cell cycle.

The selection and sequence of administration of chemotherapuetic agents are also dependent upon a knowledge of their activity in the cell cycle. Classically, the life history of a proliferating cell is divided into mitosis and interphase. Currently, replication time of the genetic material is called the DNA synthetic period (S) (Figure 33–1). During this phase, the dividing cells double their complement of DNA prior to cell division. The latter occurs at mitosis (M). The periods between these two events are designated the presynthetic gap (G_1) and the postsynthetic gap (G_2). The resting phase of the cell is designated G_0. During the G_0 phase, the cell is minimally susceptible to the action of chemotherapeutic agents. Drugs are characterized as cell cycle–specific and cell cycle–nonspecific according to their effect on specific phases of the cell cycle.

Not all cells proliferate at the same time. There may be a large pool of nonproliferating cells that, during this phase, are unresponsive to chemotherapeutic agents. This is particularly characteristic of the solid tumors. Chemotherapeutic agents also are not equally effective throughout the cell cycle; several are active only during cell division. This is the rationale for the administration of combination chemotherapy, in which agents with different mechanisms of action and minimal overlapping toxicity are employed.

Maximum chemotherapeutic effect may also be attempted by administering agents to manipulate the phases of the cell cycle. Thus, one agent may be utilized to synchronize cells into a particular phase. This is followed by a second agent immediately before entry of the cell into the next phase, during which the second agent is most effective. This phenomenon is designated "recruitment." Other factors influencing cytotoxic activity of drugs include absorption, conversion of the drug to its active form, distribution in the blood stream, and penetration into specific sites.

SIDE EFFECTS OF DRUGS

All chemotherapeutic agents have the potential to cause side effects. Details are outlined in the sections dealing with each agent. In general, side effects influence growing tissues to a greater or lesser degree and may be summarized as follows.

Hemopoietic Tissues

All elements of the hemopoietic system may be affected by chemotherapeutic agents. Depression of the peripheral leukocyte and platelet count is usually adopted as a means of monitoring the need for dose adjustments. It is customary to discontinue an agent when the total leukocyte count falls below 1500 cells/mm³ and when the platelet count falls below 100,000/mm³. The effect on the red cell series, manifested as a fall in hemoglobin level, is usually delayed in comparison with the effect on other formed elements. Severe depressions in the hemopoietic system are treated by transfusions of blood, platelets, and white blood cells. These should not be administered indiscriminately, since frequent transfusions may stimulate antibody formation in the recipients.

Gastrointestinal Toxicity

Early signs of toxicity are lesions involving the mucous membranes of the mouth. The patient may complain of soreness when drinking acidic beverages, and on physical examination there is generalized erythema. The entire gastrointestinal tract may be involved, producing diarrhea. Chemotherapy should be interrupted under these circumstances. A mouthwash with a local anesthetic is sometimes helpful. Occasionally, an oral antibiotic preparation containing polymyxin B, neomycin, and bacitracin may prevent secondary infection of the mucous membranes. Citrovorum factor may be added to the antibiotic preparation if the ulcers are methotrexate-induced.

Severe episodes of gastrointestinal toxicity may be followed by cachexia. To avoid or treat this complication, total parenteral nutrition is being employed with increasing frequency.[9] When effectively applied, it has permitted delivery of planned courses of treatment. Nutritional repletion also assists in restoration of an anabolic state, healing of wounds, and correction of metabolic derangements.

Liver Toxicity

Occasional elevations of liver enzymes may be detected after the administration of chemotherapy. These are usually not significant. However, gross elevations and abnormal serum bilirubin levels call for temporary discontinuation of treatment. Some drugs are excreted through the liver and should be withheld or the doses reduced in the presence of severe hepatic dysfunction. Radiation therapy administered to the liver, particularly in association with actinomycin D, may produce selective thrombocytopenia.[36] This is probably due to congestive splenomegaly.

Renal Toxicity

Several agents are excreted through the kidney. Some may cause renal dysfunction. If renal function is poor, a normally tolerated dose will have to be decreased because of prolonged retention of the drug. Chemotherapy may occasionally cause excessive tumor destruction with elevation of the serum uric acid level and uric acid nephropathy. Prophylactic use of allopurinol, alkalinization, and a large intake of fluid may prevent this complication.

SPECIFIC CLASSES OF AGENTS

Alkylating Agents

Alkylating agents probably act by replacing a hydrogen atom in the DNA molecule with an alkyl group. This interferes with DNA replication or RNA transcription and subsequent protein synthesis. Similar effects are produced by ionizing irradiation. There are several varieties of alkylating agents. Differences in their activity are related to site and rate of metabolism and tissue affinity rather than mode of action. They are active against most childhood urologic cancers.

Nitrogen Mustard. Nitrogen mustard was the first anticancer agent to undergo clinical investigation. It retains its role as progenitor because of its rapidity of action. It must be administered intravenously; extravasation causes local ulceration. The drug also causes nausea, vomiting, leukopenia, and thrombocytopenia. The dose-limiting toxicity is myelosuppression, with the nadir occurring 2 to 3 weeks after each administration. Recovery usually occurs 2 weeks later, when the drug may again be administered. The drug may also be given intrapleurally for recalcitrant effusions. Systemic effects may follow absorption from this site. The drug is used in the treatment of the lymphomas and as a substitute for cyclophosphamide.[5]

Cyclophosphamide. This is a cyclic nitrogen mustard compound that must be metabolized to an active form by the liver. It is excreted through the kidney and may irritate the bladder mucosa. This becomes manifest as hematuria, dysuria, or both and may eventually result in irreversible bladder fibrosis. The latter is more likely to occur when the bladder is exposed to radiation therapy.[20] With continued cystitis, an intravenous pyelogram should be obtained, and cyclophosphamide should be permanently discontinued if bladder fibrosis or other abnormalities are detected. Prior to each course of treatment, it is advisable to examine the urine for microscopic hematuria. The main dose-limiting toxicity of cyclophosphamide is myelosuppression. Other common side effects include nausea, vomiting, and alopecia.

A variety of doses and schedules are in use. The drug may be administered intravenously, intramuscularly, or by the oral route. With very large intravenous doses, it is advisable to dissolve the drug in 250 to 1000 ml of 5 per cent dextrose in water and follow with liberal amounts of fluids to prevent hemorrhagic cystitis. This technique is particularly useful when single large doses (of the order of 40 mg/kg/day) are administered. Another commonly used schedule is 10 mg/kg for 5 to 10 days, repeated at 6-week intervals. Long-term maintenance treatment usually consists of 2 to 3 mg/kg/day administered orally. Dose modifications should be introduced as dictated by the hemogram.

A form of inappropriate antidiuretic secretion has been described when massive doses of cyclophosphamide are given.[4] This manifests as oliguria or anuria and may take several days to resolve. During this period, fluids should be withheld or administered judiciously. Massive doses of cyclophosphamide have recently been reported to cause heart failure and death.[27] Diffuse pulmonary fibrosis, similar to that reported with bleomycin, has also been observed.[30]

Cyclophosphamide is used in the treatment of sarcomas, testicular tumors, lymphomas, leukemias, and resistant or recurrent cases of Wilms' tumor.

Chlorambucil. Chlorambucil is a nitrogen mustard compound. It may be utilized if the patient's tolerance of cyclophosphamide or nitrogen mustard is poor, and it can be administered orally. The principal dose-limiting toxicity is myelosuppression; blood counts should be obtained frequently. Hepatic toxicity and occasionally diarrhea, dermatitis, nausea, and vomiting have been observed. Chlorambucil is generally used in the treatment of lymphomas.

CHRONIC EFFECTS OF ALKYLATING AGENTS

Sterility and ovarian dysfunction have been reported following administration of most of the alkylating agents.[7, 22, 37] The effect on the ovary may be a consequence of oocyte destruction. In the testis the consequences are more pronounced after the pubertal period and may manifest as aspermia. These complications are not inevitable and may not be permanent. Normal reproductive function in patients exposed to alkylating agents has been documented.[24]

Recent publications have described an increasing number of second malignant neoplasms occurring in patients exposed to alkylating agents and radiation therapy. In several instances, the alkylating agent has been incriminated.[29, 31] The reports particularly concern older patients. A chemotherapeutic agent that is a distinct cause of oncogenesis in the pediatric age group has not been reported.[26] Continued surveillance of long-term survivors of pediatric cancer to detect abnormalities is currently in progress. This includes examination of the prog-

eny, which to date has failed to reveal any increased incidence of teratogenesis or congenital abnormalities.[24]

Antibiotics

A number of antibiotics have been found to be effective against malignant diseases in man. Those employed in pediatric patients with urologic cancer include actinomycin D, the anthracyclines (doxorubicin and daunorubicin), bleomycin, and mithramycin.

Actinomycin D. The actinomycins were discovered by Waksman in 1940. In 1952, Hackman reported on their carcinolytic effects. Of these, actinomycin D has been utilized most extensively. The drug intercalates with the minor groove of the DNA helix and inhibits RNA transcription. It has three major clinical anticancer properties: It is tumoricidal, enhances radiation effects, and occasionally reactivates latent radiation activity in previously irradiated sites.[3] When administered concurrently with radiation therapy, it requires skillful and judicious application.

The major side effects are nausea, vomiting, and myelosuppression. The drug is excreted primarily by the liver. Simultaneous administration of actinomycin D and radiation therapy to the liver should therefore be undertaken with caution. Similarly, if there is any evidence of liver damage, a reduction in actinomycin D dosage may be indicated. Finally, if hepatic resection has been performed (as for example, in metastatic Wilms' tumor), administration of actinomycin D or radiation therapy or both should be delayed until hepatic regeneration is complete.[10] The drug is administered intravenously; extravasation results in ulceration. Actinomycin D is used in the treatment of Wilms' tumor, sarcomas, and testicular tumors.

Doxorubicin (Adriamycin) and Daunorubicin. These agents belong to the class of antibiotics known as the anthracyclines. They are derived from *Streptomyces peucetius* and have similar properties and toxicities. They probably intercalate with the major groove of the DNA helix, preventing DNA transcription and replication. They are administered intravenously; extravasation results in ulceration. The major dose-limiting toxicity is myelosuppression, which occurs 10 to 14 days after administration. Stomatitis and alopecia are common. Adriamycin also interacts with radiation therapy and may cause complications similar to those described with actinomycin D.

The long-term limiting toxicity of the anthracyclines is cardiomyopathy.[11] This is prone to occur with doses in excess of 450 mg/M^2. Prior irradiation of the mediastinum also exacerbates the complication; therefore, doses in such patients should probably not exceed 300 mg/M^2.[12] The drugs are excreted principally by the liver, and dose adjustments should be made for hepatic dysfunction. They are also excreted through the kidneys, causing a reddish discoloration of the urine. Severe hyperpigmentation of the nails may occur with Adriamycin.

The anthracyclines are used in treatment of sarcomas and leukemias and as investigational drugs in patients with Wilms' tumor.

Bleomycin. This is a mixture of several polypeptide antibiotics derived from *Streptomyces verticillus*. The drug probably causes lethal effects by binding to DNA, producing scission and fragmentation of the helix. It has minimal myelosuppressive activity and is therefore useful in combination chemotherapy.

Animal studies demonstrate that the drug reaches its highest concentration in the lungs and skin. The major dose-limiting toxicity is pulmonary fibrosis, which occasionally may be fatal.[33] Pulmonary complications are characterized by an insidious onset of dyspnea 4 to 10 weeks after initiation of therapy. Early indications of toxicity include crepitations and rhonchi. Radiographic examination of the lungs may reveal diffuse infiltrates, found in 5 to 10 per cent of patients. Pulmonary function tests have not been helpful in predicting toxicity. In some patients, discontinuation of the drug leads to reversal of pulmonary side effects; in others, progression is inexorable and leads to death. Pulmonary toxicity may not be related to total dose, but in children the maximum allowable cumulative dose is 300 mg/M^2.

Cutaneous complications have also been observed. They appear as induration and erythema of the fingers and hands, which may proceed to desquamation and ulceration. Other toxicities include a low-grade fever and fatigue. Bleomycin is used particularly in treatment of testicular tumors and the lymphomas.

Mithramycin. Mithramycin is derived from *Streptomyces argillaceus.* It complexes with DNA, preventing RNA transcription. The principal dose-limiting toxicity is a hemorrhagic diathesis. This occurs as a result of damage to the vascular walls and platelets, decreased coagulation factors, and enhancement of fibrinolytic activity. Mithramycin may also cause hypocalcemia and is therefore useful in the treatment of hypercalcemia of malignancies. Gastrointestinal toxicity, skin necrosis, and fever have also been reported. The drug is used to treat metastatic testicular cancer.

Antimetabolites

Antimetabolites are used principally in treatment of leukemias and lymphomas. Testicular infiltration by these diseases is being recognized with increasing frequency. Orchiectomy may occasionally be requested as a mode of therapy. Such patients may also receive leukemia-lymphoma therapy. A discussion of the properties and side effects of antimetabolites is therefore provided.

Methotrexate. Methotrexate is a folic acid antagonist. It acts by inhibiting the dihydrofolic reductase enzyme that converts folic acid to reduced folate cofactors. These are essential for the synthesis of purine nucleic acid bases and the pyrimidine DNA base thymidine. Depletion of reduced folates leads directly to inhibition of DNA synthesis in the S phase of the cell cycle.

Methotrexate is administered by the oral, intravenous, intrathecal, and intramuscular routes. Toxicity includes myelosuppression, stomatitis, diarrhea, and hepatic and renal dysfunction. Pneumonitis has also been observed, but it is uncertain whether this is directly related to the drug. Severe osteopenia and fractures and hepatic fibrosis have been reported with prolonged administration. The antidote to methotrexate is citrovorum factor. Methotrexate is also administered to patients with teratocarcinoma of the testes.

6-Mercaptopurine. This is a purine analogue and acts as a purine antagonist. It is used principally in treatment of leukemia and lymphoma. The major side effects are nausea, vomiting, and myelosuppression. Prolonged administration may result in hepatic fibrosis.

Arabinosyl Cytosine. This inhibits DNA polymerase. The drug is administered intravenously or intramuscularly. Its principal side effects are nausea and vomiting. Mild hepatic dysfunction may also be observed.

Plant Alkaloids

The vinca alkaloids are derived from the periwinkle plant, *Vinca rosea.* They exert a striking cytotoxic effect by damaging protein microtubule subunits. This prevents normal spindle cell formation and eventually results in metaphase mitotic arrest. Following administration of a vinca alkaloid, the cells exhibit bizarre mitotic appearances. These drugs also interfere with normal DNA and RNA mechanisms.

Vincristine. This vinca alkaloid has relatively little myelosuppressive effect and is generally used in combination with other agents. It has a wide range of anticancer activity and is used in the treatment of most pediatric urologic cancers. The major side effects involve the nervous system and are manifested as peripheral neuropathy, severe jaw pain, obstipation, and decreased deep tendon reflexes. If obstipation lasts more than 3 to 4 days, subsequent doses of vincristine should be reduced or withheld. Loss of deep tendon reflexes is not necessarily an indication for discontinuation of the drug. If, however, there is weakness and difficulty in walking or in picking up fine objects, resumption of therapy should await return of neurologic function. Severe hyponatremia and convulsions have been observed when excessive doses have been inadvertently administered. Alopecia is a frequently observed complication.

The drug is used extensively in treatment of the sarcomas, Wilms' tumor, leukemias, and lymphomas.

Vinblastine. Vinblastine has a more limited spectrum of activity than vincristine. It is used more frequently in the treatment of the lymphomas. Toxicity is similar to that of vincristine. However, the nervous system is usually less severely affected, and, unfortunately, myelosuppression is more frequent.

Both alkaloids are excreted primarily by the liver and therefore should be administered cautiously to patients who have hepatic dysfunction.

MISCELLANEOUS AGENTS

L-*Asparaginase.* This is an enzyme that depletes asparagine in tumor cells. It is administered intravenously or subcutaneously, usually to patients with leukemia. The side effects include hypersensitivity with occasional anaphylactic reactions. Hepatoxicity and pancreatitis have also been reported. Myelosuppression is not prominent.

Procarbazine. Procarbazine is a methyl hydrazine compound. Its exact mechanism of action is unknown, although many of its biologic reactions resemble those of alkylating agents. It is used principally in patients with lymphoma. Side effects include nausea, myelosuppression, central nervous system depression, and a synergism with monoamine oxidase inhibitors.

Dimethyl Triazino Imidazole Carboxamide (DTIC). This is an analogue to an aminoimidazole carboxamide originally thought to exert its toxic effect by inhibiting nucleic acid synthesis. The mechanism of action is unknown, but DTIC probably acts as an alkylating agent. It is administered intravenously to patients with soft tissue sarcomas. It is usually employed to potentiate the action of Adriamycin.

Nitrosoureas. These are compounds that probably react by means of alkylating properties. They also have an isocyanate metabolite that inhibits DNA repair. There are several varieties. BCNU is an intravenous preparation, and CCNU and methyl-CCNU are administered orally. They are utilized principally in the treatment of lymphomas and brain tumors. The principal dose-limiting toxicity is bone marrow suppression, with the nadir occurring as long as 4 to 6 weeks after administration. Other toxicities include nausea, vomiting, and hepatic dysfunction.

Rapid intravenous administration of BCNU may cause pain along the site of the injection and phlebitis. Chronic renal dysfunction has recently been reported in long-term survivors.[13] This is probably related to the total cumulative disease. A prolonged form of hypoplastic anemia and occasionally leukemia have also been noted.[28]

Cis-dichlorodiammineplatinum II(Cis-platinum). This is a heavy metal coordination compound with a unique antitumor property. The exact mode of action is unclear. Certain similarities to the bifunctional alkylating agents suggest that it may act by cross-linking NDA. Cis-platinum also seems to be a cell cycle–nonspecific agent. There is preliminary evidence that it may enhance tumor immunogenicity. The drug is administered intravenously.

The major dose-limiting toxicity is renal damage. The mechanism is unclear but presumably is similar to that seen with other heavy metals such as mercury. Mannitol is frequently used as a diuretic to prevent this complication. Saline hydration may possibly be just as effective.[6] Aminoglycoside antibiotics should probably be avoided if possible when cis-platinum is administered.

Cis-platinum is only modestly myelosup-pressive and is thus an ideal agent for combination chemotherapy. Neurotoxicity evidenced by paresthesias and, rarely, seizures has been reported.[21] Hearing loss is an important side effect. Anaphylaxis may also occur, but successful treatment of the allergic reactions has been reported.[38] Nausea and vomiting are almost universal. Hyponatremia, hypomagnesemia, hypocalcemia, and hyperuricemia occur but may not necessarily be of clinical importance. This drug is used in the treatment of testicular cancer. Pretreatment studies include an evaluation of the patient's creatinine clearance.

PROTOCOLS

Wilms' Tumor

Investigations have shown that the combination of vincristine and actinomycin D produces optimum results as adjuvant therapy. Survival of patients with localized and regional disease (Stage I and II) receiving such adjuvant therapy is in excess of 80 per cent.[1, 2] Wilms' tumor protocols utilized in several of the major centers are outlined in Figure 33–2 and Table 33–2. Chemothera-

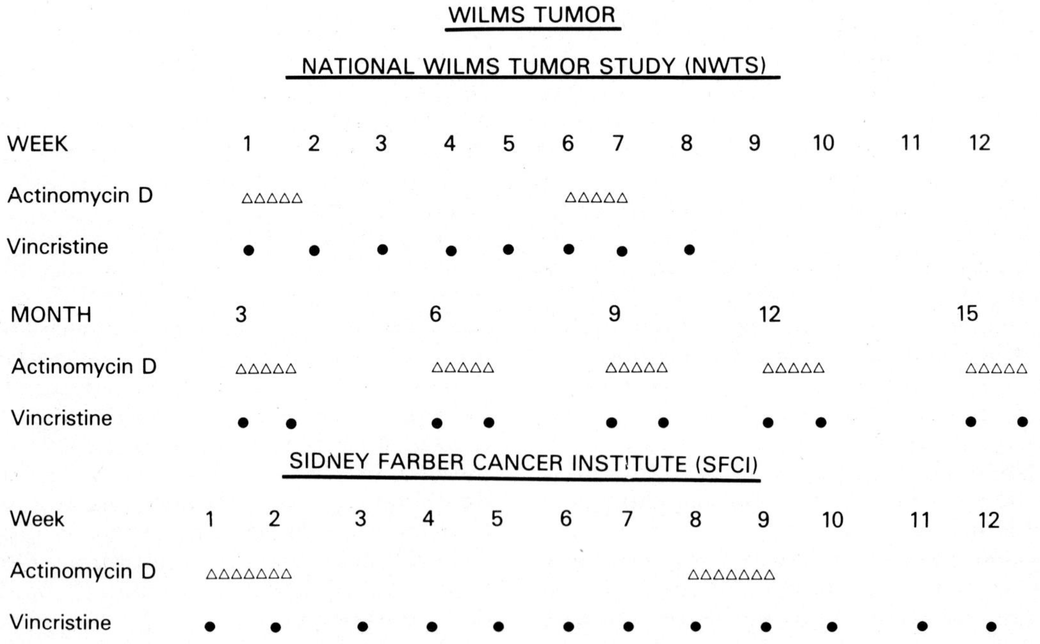

WILMS TUMOR

NATIONAL WILMS TUMOR STUDY (NWTS)

WEEK	1	2	3	4	5	6	7	8	9	10	11	12
Actinomycin D	△△△△△					△△△△△						
Vincristine	●	●	●	●	●	●	●	●				

MONTH	3		6		9		12		15
Actinomycin D	△△△△△		△△△△△		△△△△△		△△△△△		△△△△△
Vincristine	● ●		● ●		● ●		● ●		● ●

SIDNEY FARBER CANCER INSTITUTE (SFCI)

Week	1	2	3	4	5	6	7	8	9	10	11	12
Actinomycin D	△△△△△△△							△△△△△△△				
Vincristine	●	●	●	●	●	●	●	●	●	●	●	●

Figure 33–2 Schematic presentation of selected Wilms' tumor protocols. Consult individual protocols for details.

TABLE 33–2   CHEMOTHERAPY FOR WILMS' TUMOR AND RHABDOMYOSARCOMA—DOSES AND SCHEDULES

Agent	Protocol	Dose	Schedule
Vincristine	NWTS*	1.5 mg/M²	Weekly × 8, then at 3, 6, 9, 12, and 15 mo
	SFCI†(Wilms')	2 mg/M²	Weekly × 12 or more if tolerated
	IRS‡	1.5 mg/M²	Weekly as per protocol
	SFCI(Rhabdo)	2 mg/M²	Weekly × 12 or more if tolerated
Actinomycin D	NWTS	15 µg/kg/day × 5	q 6 wk × 2, then at 3, 7, 9, 12, and 15 mo
	SFCI(Wilms')	10 µg/kg/day × 7	q 8 wk × 18 mo
	IRS	15 µg/kg/day × 5	q 4 wk × 12
	SFCI(Rhabdo)	225 µg/M²/day × 7	q 12 wk × 8
Cyclophosphamide	IRS	10 mg/kg/day × 3	q 4 wk × 12
	SFCI(Rhabdo)	300 µg/M²/day × 7	q 6 wk × 16

Note: 1. Vincristine administered weekly only if tolerated.
2. Cyclophosphamide omitted during bladder irradiation.
3. Actinomycin D omitted during bowel or oral irradiation.
4. Doses adjusted to hematologic tolerance.
5. Consult specific protocols for full details.
*National Wilms' Tumor Study.
†Sidney Farber Cancer Institute.
‡Intergroup Rhabdomyosarcoma Study.

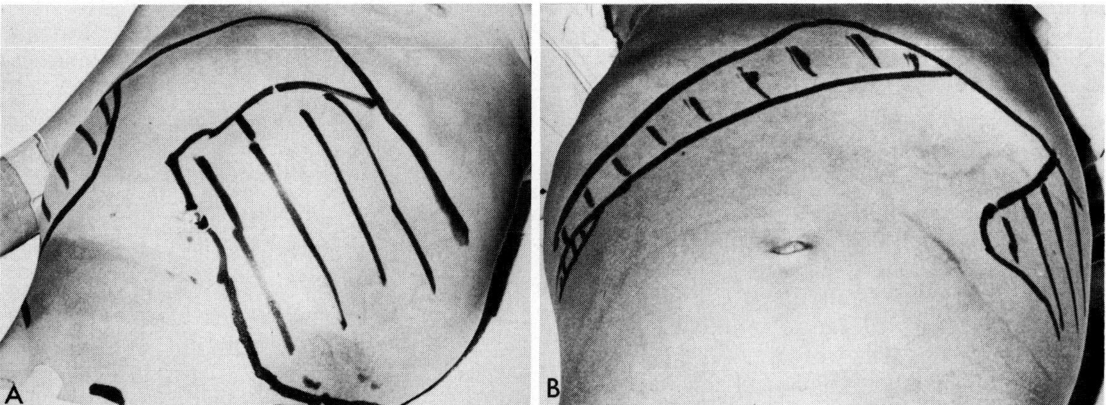

Figure 33–3   *A,* Abdominal distension in a 3-year-old child with bilateral Wilms' tumor. The size of the tumor masses is outlined. *B,* Photograph of patient 3 weeks after a course of actinomycin D and three injections of vincristine. Reduction in abdominal distension and tumor masses permitted palpation of the liver, which was not possible previously. The liver was found to be free of tumor at operation.

RHABDOMYOSARCOMA

INTERGROUP STUDY (IRS)

WEEK	1	2	3	4	5	6	7	8	9	10	11	12
Actinomycin D	△△△△△			△△△△△				△△△△△				△△△△△
Vincristine	●	●	●	●	●	●	●	●	●	●	●	●
Cyclophosphamide	XXX			XXX				XXX				XXX

SIDNEY FARBER CANCER INSTITUTE (SFCI)

Week	1	2	3	4	5	6	7	8	9	10	11	12
Actinomycin D	△△△△△△△											△△△△△△△
Vincristine	●	●	●	●	●	●	●	●	●	●	●	●
Cyclophosphamide	XXXXXXX					XXXXXXX						XXXXXXX

Figure 33–4   Schematic presentation of selected rhabdomyosarcoma protocols. Consult individual protocols for details.

py, particularly as vincristine, may occasionally be administered preoperatively to render a large tumor operable.[35] A favorable response in a patient with bilateral Wilms' tumor is illustrated in Figure 33–3.

Rhabdomyosarcoma

Vincristine, cyclophosphamide, actinomycin D, and adriamycin are all effective in the treatment of rhabdomyosarcoma. Combinations of these agents are therefore employed.[19, 25] The basis for this approach is primarily the heterogeneity of the neoplastic cells. Cyclophosphamide should be omitted while large areas of the bladder are being irradiated. Protocols utilized in various major centers are outlined in Figure 33–4 and Table 33–2.

Leukemia-Lymphoma

Invasion of the testes should be treated initially with antileukemic therapy. Occasionally, radiation therapy may be administered. Orchiectomy may be indicated for resistant disease confined to one or both testes.

Priapism may occasionally be encountered in patients with acute leukemia. Such patients should be treated initially with intensive antileukemic therapy.[18] Surgical intervention with irrigation of the corpora cavernosa may occasionally be helpful.

References

1. Cassady, J. R., Jaffe, N., and Filler, R. M.: Multimodality therapy for Wilms' tumor. Applied Radiology 7:71, 1978.
2. D'Angio, G. J., Evans, A. E., Breslow, N., et al.: The treatment of Wilms' tumor. Results of the National Wilms' Tumor Study. Cancer 38:633, 1976.
3. D'Angio, G. J., Maddock, C. L., Farber, S., et al.: The enhanced response of Ridway osteogenic sarcoma to roentgen radiation combined with actinomycin D. Cancer Res. 25:1002, 1965.
4. De Fronzo, R. A., Braine, H., Coloin, M., and Davis, P. J.: Water intoxication in man after cyclophosphamide therapy. Ann. Intern. Med. 78:861, 1973.
5. DeVita, V. T., Jr., Serpick, A., and Carbone, P. P.: Combination chemotherapy in the treatment of advanced Hodgkin's disease. Ann. Intern. Med. 73:881, 1970.
6. Einhorn, L. H., and Williams, S. D.: The role of

cis-platinum in solid-tumor therapy. N. Engl. J. Med. 300:289, 1979.

7. Fairley, K. F., Barrie, J. U., and Johnson, W.: Sterility and testicular atrophy related to cyclophosphamide therapy. Lancet 1:568, 1972.

8. Farber, S.: Chemotherapy in the treatment of leukemia and Wilms' tumor. JAMA 198:826, 1966.

9. Filler, R. M., Jaffe, N., Cassady, J. R., et al.: Parenteral nutritional support in children with cancer. Cancer 39:2665, 1977.

10. Filler, R. M., Tefft, M., Vawter, F., et al.: Hepatic lobectomy in childhood: Effects of x-ray and chemotherapy. J. Pediatr. Surg. 4:31, 1969.

11. Gillidoga, A. C., Tan, C., et al.: Adriamycin cardiomyopathy: Diagnosis and management. Case reports. Proc. Am. Assoc. Cancer Res. 14:95, 1973.

12. Greenwood, R. D., Rosenthal, A., et al.: Constrictive pericarditis in childhood due to mediastinal irradiation. Circulation 50:1033, 1974.

13. Harmon, W. E., Cohen, H. J., Schneeberger, E. E., et al.: Chronic renal failure in children treated with methyl CCNU. N. Engl. J. Med. 300:1200, 1979.

14. Heyn, R. M., Holland, R., Newton, W. A., Jr., et al.: The role of combined chemotherapy in the treatment of rhabdomyosarcoma in children. Cancer 34:2128, 1974.

15. Jaffe, N.: Pediatric cancer—delayed sequelae of treatment. Care of the child with cancer. Am. Cancer Soc. 179:118, 1979.

16. Jaffe, N., Filler, R. J., Farber, S., et al.: Rhabdomyosarcoma in children. Improved outlook with a multidisciplinary approach. Am. J. Surg. 125:482, 1973.

17. Jaffe, N., Frei, E., III, Traggis, D., et al.: Adjuvant methotrexate and citrovorum-factor treatment of osteogenic sarcoma. N. Engl. J. Med. 291:994, 1974.

18. Jaffe, N., and Kim, B. S.: Priapism in acute granulocytic leukemia. Am. J. Dis. Child 118:619, 1969.

19. Jaffe, N., Murray, J., Traggis, D., et al.: Multidisciplinary treatment for childhood sarcoma. Am. J. Surg. 133:405, 1977.

20. Jayalakshmamma, B., and Pinkel, D.: Urinary-bladder toxicity following pelvic irradiation and simultaneous cyclophosphamide therapy. Cancer 38:701, 1976.

21. Kedar, A., Cohen, M. E., and Freeman, A. I.: Peripheral neuropathy as a complication of cis-dichlorodiammineplatinum(II) treatment: A case report. Cancer Treat. Rep. 62(5):819, 1978.

22. Koyama, H., Wada, T., et al.: Cyclophosphamide-induced ovarian failure and its therapeutic significance in patients with breast cancer. Cancer 39:1403, 1977.

23. Laster, W. R., Jr., Mayo, J. G., Simpson-Herren, L., et al.: Success and failure in the treatment of solid tumor. H. Kinetic parameters and "cell cure" of moderately advanced carcinoma 755. Cancer Chemother. Rep. 53:169, 1966.

24. Li, F. P., and Jaffe, N.: Progeny of childhood cancer survivors. Lancet 2:707, 1974.

25. Maurer, H. M., Moon, T., Donaldson, M. H., et al.: The Intergroup Rhabdomyosarcoma Study: A preliminary report. Cancer 40:2015, 1977.

26. Meadows, A. T., D'Angio, G. J., Miké, V., et al.: Patterns of second malignant neoplasms in children. Cancer 40(suppl 4):1903, 1977.

27. Mills, B. A., and Robert, R. W.: Cyclophosphamide-induced cardiomyopathy. A report of two cases and review of the English literature. Cancer 43:2223, 1979.

28. Osband, M., Cohen, H. J., Cassady, J. R., et al.: Severe and protracted bone marrow dysfunction following long-term treatment with methyl CCNU. Proc. Am. Assoc. Cancer Res. 18:303, 1978.

29. Reimer, R. R., Hoover, R., Fraumeni, J. F., Jr., et al.: Acute leukemia after alkylating-agent therapy of ovarian cancer. N. Engl. J. Med. 297:177, 1977.

30. Rodin, A. E., Haggard, M. E., and Travis, L. B.: Lung changes and chemotherapeutic agents in childhood: Report of a case associated with cyclophosphamide therapy. Am. J. Dis. Child 120:337, 1970.

31. Rosner, F.: Acute leukemia as a delayed consequence of cancer chemotherapy. Cancer 37:1033, 1976.

32. Schabel, F. M., Jr.: Concepts for systemic treatment of micrometastases. Cancer 35:15, 1975.

33. Shastri, S., Slayton, R. E., et al.: Clinical study with bleomycin. Cancer 28:1142, 1971.

34. Skipper, H. E., Schabel, F. M., Jr., and Wilcox, W. S.: Experimental evaluation of potential anticancer agents. XIII. On the criteria and kinetics associated with "curability" of experimental leukemia. Cancer Chemother. Rep. 35:1, 1964.

35. Sullivan, M. P., Sutow, W. W., Cangir, A., et al.: Vincristine sulfate in management of Wilms' tumor. Replacement of preoperative irradiation by chemotherapy. JAMA 202:381, 1967.

36. Tefft, M., Mitus, A., Das, L., et al.: Irradiation of the liver in children: Review of experience in the acute and chronic phases, and in the intact normal and partially resected. Am. J. Roentgenol. 108:365, 1970.

37. Warne, G. L., Fairley, K. F., Hobbs, J. B., et al.: Cyclophosphamide-induced ovarian failure. N. Engl. J. Med. 289:1159, 1973.

38. Wiesenfeld, M., Reinders, E., Corder, M., et al.: Successful re-treatment with cis-dichlorodiammineplatinum(II) after apparent allergic reactions. Cancer Treat. Rep. 63(2):219, 1979.

39. Wolff, J. A., D'Angio, G. J., Hartmann, J., et al.: Long-term evaluation of single versus multiple courses of actinomycin D therapy of Wilms' tumor. N. Engl. J. Med. 290:84, 1974.

SOLID NEOPLASMS

Philip R. Exelby, M.D.

34

Current multidisciplinary treatment of childhood cancers requires good surgery integrated carefully with chemotherapy and radiation therapy. The role of surgery has changed, and newer procedures are often more difficult technically. Surgery is performed on children who have received large doses of radiation and whose physiologic status and healing powers have been altered by multidrug chemotherapy. The surgeon operating on a child with cancer must be aware of the toxicity of chemotherapeutic agents and appreciate the tissue changes caused by radiation therapy. Complications of surgery can be reduced in frequency and severity by correct planning and timing of the surgical procedure.

GENERAL PROBLEMS

Cancer may cause disturbances in blood clotting that must be corrected preoperatively. Tumors such as neuroblastoma and non-Hodgkin's lymphoma invade and replace normal bone marrow cells, causing reduced platelet levels. Liver involvement with tumor may lower fibrinogen levels or other coagulation factors. Even with normal bone marrow and liver function, disseminated intravascular clotting may occur, which may be incipient at the time of diagnosis but develop fully during operation. A coagulation profile and bone marrow examination are required in all children with cancer before any surgical procedure is performed. Coagulation defects should be corrected preoperatively, which will prevent bleeding complications during or after operation.

Septic complications are more common in children with cancer for several reasons. The white blood cell count may be low because of marrow replacement by tumor or previous radiation therapy or chemotherapy. Some tumors such as lymphoma and advanced neuroblastoma may produce depression of the child's immune defenses. In addition, the surgical procedure may lower resistance to infection, as in the postsplenectomy syndrome seen after staging laparotomy for Hodgkin's disease.

INCREASED RISK OF SURGICAL COMPLICATIONS FOLLOWING CHEMOTHERAPY AND RADIATION THERAPY

Toxic reactions to some chemotherapeutic agents cause problems of particular interest to the surgeon. Cyclophosphamide may produce acute or chronic delayed hemorrhagic cystitis, increasing the hazards of pelvic surgery.[7, 11] Bleomycin has caused nonspecific interstitial changes in lung parenchyma that result in acute postoperative respiratory failure.[14] Reduction of oxygen concentration to less than 25 per cent and careful fluid replacement with colloids rather than excessive loads of crystalloids during anesthesia lessen the risk of these respiratory problems. Adriamycin and daunomycin are cardiotoxic at certain cumulative doses[13] (Fig. 34–1). Careful cardiac monitoring during and after surgery, with maintenance of normal P_{O_2} and fluid balance, will help reduce cardiac problems. Vincristine is neurotoxic and may produce a particularly troublesome paralytic ileus 4 to 10 days after administration. Abdominal surgery should be avoided during this period because of the prolonged ileus. Delayed wound healing or disruption in patients receiving chemotherapy appears not to be as great as originally thought. Methotrexate given in high doses seems to be the only agent that significantly delays wound heal-

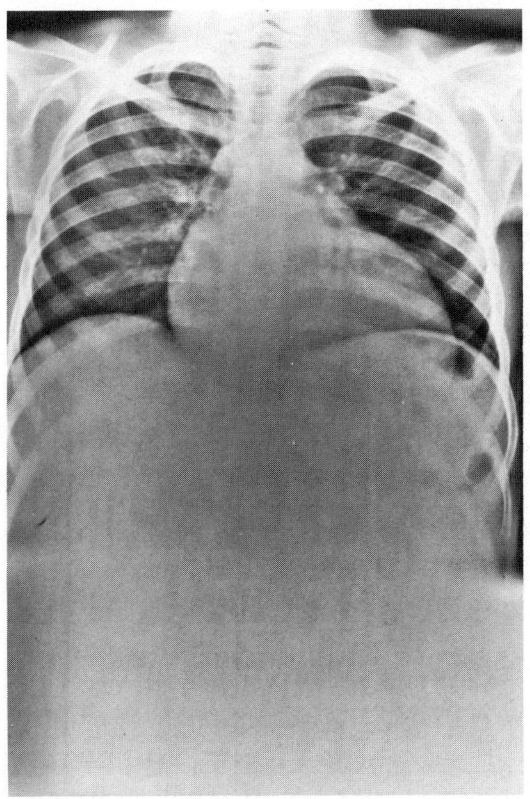

Figure 34–1 Cardiomegaly due to Adriamycin toxicity. The cardiothoracic ratio is 66 per cent; a normal ratio is less than 50 per cent.

ing. Major surgery should be postponed more than 1 week after treatment with this drug.

Irradiation effects on tissues, particularly when combined with chemotherapy, increase surgical complications, including poor tissue healing of wounds and anastomoses, fistula formation, and disruption of conduits. The higher the radiation dose, the greater the surgical risks; less than 3000 rads may produce little additional risk. Surgery performed in areas of the body that have received more than 3000 rads, however, is associated with a significant increase in surgical complications.[10] Some chemotherapeutic agents, particularly actinomycin D, appear to be synergistic and increase the toxic effects of radiation therapy. The surgeon should be aware of the type, accumulated dose, and date of the most recent chemotherapy and radiation therapy. Ideally, the type and timing of surgical procedures should be discussed with the radiation therapist and chemotherapist before operation.

NEUROBLASTOMA

Several years ago, extensive radical resections of large upper abdominal neuroblastomas were commonly carried out, with loss of large amounts of blood, uncontrolled hemorrhage, and even intraoperative deaths. Our policy today is to perform much more conservative surgery at the initial operation. Small primary adrenal neuroblastomas, pelvic neuroblastomas, or tumors of the organ of Zuckerkandl are usually excised as a primary procedure. Large hemorrhagic tumors filling the upper abdomen, enveloping the vena cava and aorta, and extending into the porta hepatis and around the pancreas and spleen are now only biopsied. Chemotherapy with or without radiation therapy is then given. After several months, formal resection is attempted as a second-look procedure. Following chemotherapy, the tumors are usually smaller, are more mature, and bleed less than during the first procedure. Nevertheless, the main intraoperative complications of surgery remain hemorrhage and injury to surrounding structures.

Excision of an adrenal tumor may be difficult, particularly on the right side, when the tumor extends high under the liver. A tear of the right adrenal vein, which is very short and enters directly into the vena cava, may cause severe hemorrhage that is difficult to control because of poor exposure. Resection of a left-sided adrenal neuroblastoma is usually easier because the left adrenal vein drains into the renal vein. Tear of the renal vein may occur but is usually easily controlled, and the kidney can be saved. The spleen and pancreas are subject to injury during resection of these tumors. Such injuries are less likely if the spleen and pancreas are mobilized and reflected medially before large left adrenal neuroblastomas are resected. High midline lesions are technically difficult to remove even after being made smaller by chemotherapy. Injury to the liver, vena cava, aorta, celiac axis, and superior mesenteric artery may occur in these dissections. Structures at the portal triad, the pancreas, and even the transverse colon are also commonly injured.

A rare but troublesome problem is management of the small neuroblastoma with massive metastatic liver involvement, producing a large, distended abdomen. Laparotomy in such infants should consist of the minimum procedure required to establish a diagnosis, usually biopsy of a liver nodule. Any further attempt to resect the adrenal or celiac axis primary tumor is unwarranted. Closure of the abdominal incision, even a small one, can be very difficult, and wound dehiscence may occur. Even without surgery the massive enlargement of the abdomen may so interfere with intestinal or renal blood flow that decompression is necessary. Opening the fascia and inserting a prosthetic mesh, as described by Schnaufer and Koop, expands the abdominal cavity until specific antitumor treatment can be given.[21] In most cases, radiation and chemotherapy rapidly shrink these tumors, avoiding the need for insertion of mesh.

Intrathoracic neuroblastomas have a tendency to extend in dumbbell fashion through the intervertebral foramina and into the extradural space, compressing the spinal cord. Severe compression of the cord may occur without any symptoms or signs of long spinal tract involvement (Figs. 34–2 and 34–3). Intraspinal extension must be defined preoperatively so that combined

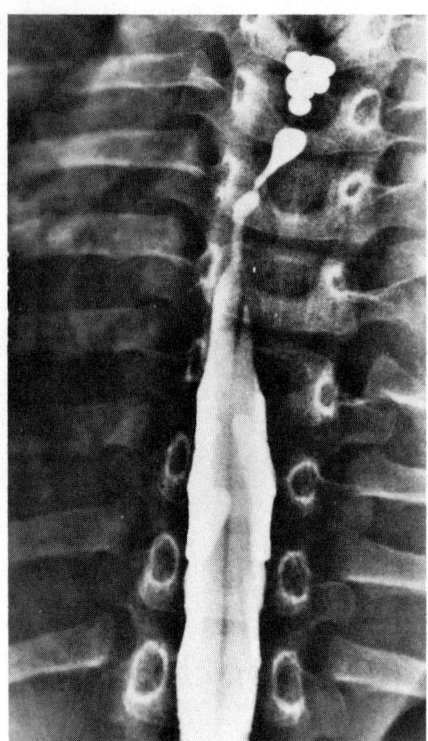

Figure 34–3 Asymptomatic cord compression caused by mediastinal neuroblastoma.

thoracic resection and laminectomy may be carried out appropriately and safely. An intrathoracic neuroblastoma occasionally extends beyond the midline into the mediastinum. Such tumors may be extremely difficult to excise. Injury to the esophagus, aorta, or trachea may occur during removal of left-sided lesions, while injury to the vena cava occurs with right-sided lesions. A common location of thoracic neuroblastoma is in the superior sulcus region, often compressing the subclavian vessels. Surgical injury to the subclavian vessels is difficult to avoid but rarely serious, since these vessels have been chronically compressed, and collateral circulation is adequate to supply the upper extremity. Tumors in this location may involve the stellate ganglion, and surgical removal will produce Horner's syndrome even if this is not present preoperatively. A particular danger in removing high left mediastinal lesions is injury to the recurrent laryngeal nerve, as it lies in close proximity to the back of the aortic arch.

Postoperative complications of abdominal

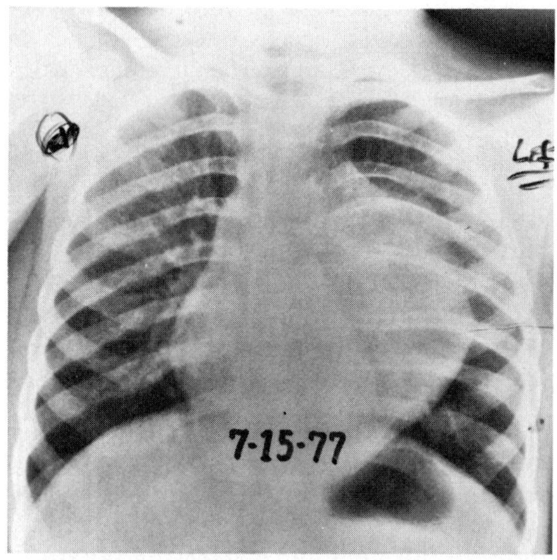

Figure 34–2 Mediastinal neuroblastoma. The large tumor is seen merging with the left cardiac border. The patient was asymptomatic.

surgery for neuroblastoma are infrequent. Wound dehiscence is rare when a transverse incision is used. Wound infections are uncommon except in patients with advanced disease and severe immune depression or neutropenia due to bone marrow involvement. Postoperative intestinal obstruction is not common, because the tumors are retroperitoneal and bowel surgery is usually not performed in the resection. The peritoneal surfaces should be closed as carefully as possible and rents in the mesentery repaired to avoid internal hernias, volvulus, or obstruction due to adhesions. The greatest danger during the postoperative period is still hemorrhage, usually from an unrecognized laceration of the spleen or major vessels. Postoperative pancreatitis may occur if there is excessive manipulation of the pancreas during surgery for large midline lesions. Pancreatitis must be differentiated from a pancreatic laceration with chemical peritonitis, which requires urgent surgical drainage. Complications may be kept to a minimum by careful inspection of the spleen and pancreas at the end of each procedure to make sure that there are no small tears in these organs.

WILMS' TUMOR

The most common complication of surgery for Wilms' tumor is rupture of the tumor during nephrectomy.[17] This can best be avoided by careful dissection and limited manipulation of the tumor until it is freed from the renal bed. If spill is unavoidable or if rupture has occurred preoperatively and remains localized, it should be walled off from the rest of the abdomen during dissection. Localized spill of tumor does not change the prognosis provided that tumor cells are not spilled into the general peritoneal cavity. The renal vessels should be isolated at a convenient and safe time during surgery.[16] Attempting to isolate these vessels too early may cause excessive manipulation of the tumor and unnecessary rupture. Other major complications of the surgery of Wilms' tumor are associated with the renal vessels. Tumor in the renal vein or vena cava may be dislodged accidentally and cause fatal embolism into the right atrium and lungs. Schullinger et al. described a

Wilms' tumor extending into the renal vein, inferior vena cava, and right atrium.[22] It is extremely important to recognize these cases preoperatively by cavagram and sonography. Otherwise, death from tumor embolization can occur on the operating table. Any child with evidence of vena caval obstruction and a cardiac murmur should have cavagrams and cardiac evaluation, and a cardiac bypass team should be available. In most instances, tumor in the renal vein or extension into the vena cava can be removed by cavotomy and suction, with the vena cava isolated by vascular clamps either above or below the liver. Occasionally, tumor thrombus will extend into the opposite renal vein, a problem that should be suspected with bilateral nonfunction of the kidneys on intravenous pyelograms. If there is tumor in the vena cava or renal vein, it is important that the opposite renal vein be suctioned clear of tumor during cavotomy. Failure to clear the renal vein on the opposite side may lead to tumor embolus postoperatively. Hemorrhage from a tear in the renal vein or from avulsion of the renal artery is a risk when handling a large tumor. Careful surgery and freeing up of the tumor before attempting to isolate the vessels will usually avoid this complication.

A further problem associated with large tumors is tenting up of the aorta and vena cava and possible rotation of these vessels due to the size and extent of the tumor. On occasion the opposite renal vein and artery will be pulled over into the operative field. Clamping or dividing the opposite renal vein or artery can occur if this distortion is not recognized. It is important to identify both renal arteries and both renal veins before dividing any of the major vessels. In excising right-sided tumors, inadvertent damage to the duodenum or even the structures of the portal triad may occur. Careful reflection of the hepatic flexure of the colon and a Kocher maneuver mobilizing the duodenum will facilitate exposure and help avoid injury to the duodenum and portal triad. Injury to the spleen and pancreas may occur during dissection of left-sided tumors. After the colon is dissected off left-sided tumors, the pancreas may be seen splayed out over the tumor and thinned by pressure. The tail of the pancreas may be inadvertently divided, and leakage of pancreatic juice may go unrecognized. Dissection superiorly may injure the spleen, usually causing a capsular tear near the hilum. These complications may be reduced by dividing the posterior peritoneal attachments of the spleen and reflecting the spleen and pancreas upward and medially. This procedure also facilitates exposure of the upper pole of the kidney. Small lacerations of the pancreas should be closed with either metal clips or nonabsorbable sutures to prevent leakage of pancreatic juice. Injury to the colon during removal of Wilms' tumor is uncommon. The tumor in its growth usually lifts the transverse colon mesentery. The left or right colon is usually draped over the tumor and can be easily separated from its anterior surface. It is rare for the tumor to invade the mesentery or the colon itself. The colon mesentery may, however, be thinned, and tears in the mesentery or vessels are common. It is important that any tears or defects in the mesentery, however small, be closed carefully. At the end of the procedure it is wise to again check the colon mesentery, which may have been further thinned by dissection. Division of one or more of the major vessels in the colon mesentery will not usually cause any serious problem in a child. However, careful inspection of the entire mesentery and the colon for satisfactory blood supply and viability should be done at the end of the procedure.

Complications following surgery for Wilms' tumor are relatively uncommon. The reasons are that these children are usually in good general health and that the surgery for removal of even large tumors is relatively straightforward if simple precautions are taken. Postoperatively, it is important to monitor urine output, which may provide an early indication of operative damage to the contralateral renal vessels. Unrecognized damage to the pancreas or spleen may lead to pancreatitis, chemical peritonitis, or postoperative hemorrhage from the spleen. Intestinal obstruction due to postoperative adhesions is more common following multidisciplinary treatment than previously. In the past 10 years we have noted a 6 per cent incidence of intestinal obstruction, due mostly to adhesions but including one case of volvulus secondary to a hernia through a rent in the mesentery.

Two other children were operated on for intestinal obstruction produced by radiation ileitis. Both received total abdominal irradiation and actinomycin D for Stage III tumors. Wound infections as well as subphrenic or other intra-abdominal abscesses are extremely rare following surgery. Good hemostasis and careful wound closure are important prophylactic measures, since these children will be given intensive chemotherapy immediately postoperatively and many will also receive radiation therapy.

SACROCOCCYGEAL TERATOMAS

Operative complications in removing the benign sacrococcygeal teratoma are rare.[1] Despite the fact that the tumor may be very large, it often outgrows its blood supply. Ligation of the lateral sacral vessels early in the operation minimizes blood loss, and hemorrhage is usually not a problem. Since the dissection is done between the sacrum and the rectum, injury to the rectal wall is possible if this structure is not carefully identified. It is a good idea to have the bowel mechanically clean at the time of surgery in case the rectum is inadvertently entered. A small hole in the posterior wall of the rectum can be easily repaired and does not affect the outcome adversely if the bowel is clean. Fluid may collect in the space between the rectum and the sacrum if the soft tissues are not sutured back in place or if a large dead space is left under the skin flaps. If a large space cannot be obliterated, drainage by Hemovac suction catheters is advisable. Otherwise, two small subcutaneous rubber drains, one at each side of the transverse incision, will suffice. Since the coccyx is always removed, the posterior attachment of the levator sling is divided. It is important that the two halves of the levator muscle be resutured in the midline to preserve normal anal function. The baby is nursed face down during the immediate postoperative period, thus avoiding soiling of the wound by urine or feces. The postoperative course of these children is usually benign.

Complications associated with the surgery of malignant sacrococcygeal teratomas are usually more serious.[2] The tumor itself may have caused the loss of bladder or anal sphincter control by neurologic involvement before surgery. It is important to accurately assess neurologic function in patients with malignant presacral teratomas before any surgery is performed. There may be neurologic changes in the lower extremities as a result of extension and involvement of parts of the lumbosacral plexus. Postoperative neurologic deficits are difficult to interpret unless careful evaluation has preceded surgery. Whereas benign tumors have a pseudocapsule and can be shelled out from between the presacral fascia and the rectum, malignant tumors are infiltrative and extend beyond the presacral fascia into the very vascular region of the presacral plexus. Resection of a malignant teratoma must be carried out by either an abdominoperineal or a two-stage procedure. Hemorrhage may be extremely troublesome unless the blood supply from the abdominal vessels is controlled. Ligation of the lateral and middle sacral vessels from above through the laparotomy incision helps to avoid excessive bleeding while the tumor is mobilized from above. During this procedure it is easy to damage the base of the bladder or the rectum. The perineal part of the dissection of these malignant tumors may be difficult owing to extension of the tumor laterally into the ischiorectal region. Attempts to separate the tumor from the anterior wall of the rectum may result in severe hemorrhage even though the tumor has been mobilized from above. Blind clamping during such hemorrhage may result in injury to the rectum.

Postoperative complications of surgery for benign tumors are unusual provided that there is adequate drainage of the wound. Fluid collection and postoperative infection are uncommon. Healing of skin flaps is usually prompt, and there is rarely any problem with urination or defecation. In contrast, postoperative complications of surgery for malignant presacral teratomas are common. Postoperative hemorrhage is the most serious complication and most commonly emanates from the presacral veins, which are difficult to control either through the abdominal approach or through the perineum. Postoperatively there may be urinary retention necessitating prolonged catheter drainage with risk of urinary infection. Anal sphincter control may be impaired postoperatively. Only after time can results of surgery be determined. There is usually a large surgical defect after resection of a malignant tumor, and it is important, as with benign tumors, to attempt some sort of reconstruction of the perineal floor. It may be difficult to approximate the levator ani muscles, but this should be tried. If dead spaces are left, they must be adequately drained or packed open. Late complications following this surgery are usually due to recurrence of tumor or are the result of added radiation therapy or chemotherapy. Worsening of neurologic deficits, particularly the loss of bladder or rectal sphincter mechanisms, usually means recurrent tumor but may represent progressive side effects of treatment.

EMBRYONAL RHABDOMYOSARCOMA

The complications of surgery for embryonal rhabdomyosarcoma vary with the site of origin of the primary tumor. Most tumors of the extremities are excised by wide local excision, resecting gross tumor with a good margin of normal tissue. This often means encroaching on bone, nerves, or vessels. In some cases the correct operative procedure entails sacrificing vessels and nerves. With modern multidisciplinary treatment, however, major vessels and nerves in the extremity can be preserved and dissected free of tumor, since microscopic residual disease can be treated successfully by radiation and chemotherapy. Inadvertent damage to a large extremity vessel may occur. However, in limb surgery, the vessels are rather easily controlled and can be repaired or reanastomosed if necessary. Complications associated with lymph node dissections in the groin or axilla are largely related to lymph collection and damage to skin flaps. Excessive loss of lymph may occur during and after regional lymph node dissection. It is important to ligate every small lymphatic vessel that can be identified to prevent loss or collection of lymph postoperatively. The most common complication of wide excision and regional lymph node dissection in an extremity is the loss of skin flaps. Approximately 80 per cent of thigh lesions having incontinuity groin dissections will be associated with loss of a portion of the skin flap. Usually the loss of skin is small and will heal without secondary closure. A complication of skin loss is secondary infection extending to the major vessels beneath the flap. Suture of the vessel is rarely possible if blowout occurs in the presence of infection. More likely, excision of the vessel and arterial graft will have to be carried out. This complication is rare and can be prevented by moving muscle flaps over the major vessels at the end of the procedure before closing the skin. In the thigh the sartorius muscle makes a convenient covering for the femoral artery and vein before skin flaps are closed. In the axilla, the pectoral muscles form a natural covering over the vessels after completion of dissection. Lymph collections under the skin flaps are relatively common following inguinal and axillary node dissection. These are best avoided by careful ligation of lymphatic channels during surgery and good drainage using Hemovac catheters for 5 to 7 days.

A late complication of regional node dissection in the extremities is edema due to interruption of lymph flow. Significant edema occurs after approximately 20 per cent of regional node dissections of the groin and axilla and is accentuated in cases requiring postoperative irradiation. Edema of the extremity usually follows complications such as necrosis of skin flap, infection, or excessive fluid collection in the immediate postoperative period. Excellent care during the immediate postoperative period will help avoid late complications. During the period of immobilization following an inguinal or axillary node dissection, Venodyne boots are placed on the extremities to maintain good venous flow.

Surgery of embryonal rhabdomyosarcoma of the genitourinary tract, including bladder, prostatic, vaginal, and paratesticular lesions, is difficult, and morbidity is high.[8, 10, 12] Radical cystectomy including prostatectomy with pelvic node dissection and urinary diversion creates major anatomic and physiologic changes in the child. The immediate postoperative complications are bleeding, pelvic collection, and leakage from the urinary conduit. The complication rate is increased when preoperative radiation therapy or chemotherapy is given. The most difficult surgery is radical excision

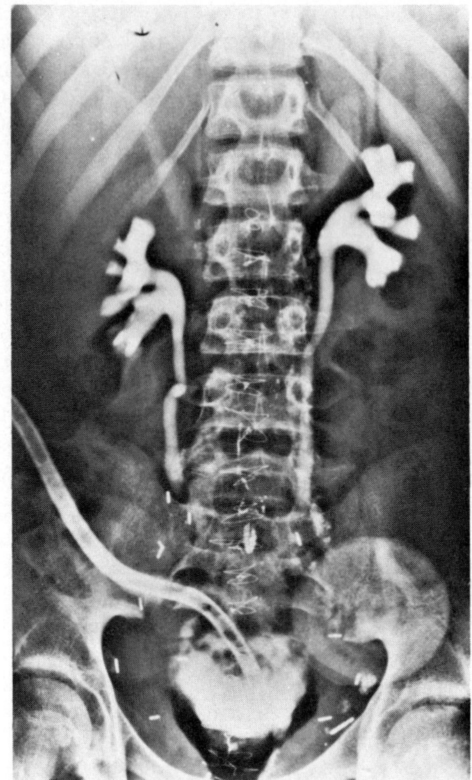

Figure 34–4 Disruption of a sigmoid conduit occurred following postoperative chemotherapy and irradiation. Extravasation of contrast material is demonstrated by intravenous pyelogram.

after failure of primary chemotherapy and radiation therapy. Slough of the conduit with urinary leakage into the pelvis was seen in one of our patients with a bladder lesion who failed to respond to 3000 rads and chemotherapy (Fig. 34–4). Drainage of a pelvic abscess and construction of a second conduit was necessary (Fig. 34–5). This boy has had chronic problems, including intermittent small bowel obstruction and chronic pelvic abscess in a fibrotic pelvis. Despite these complications he completed college while receiving total parenteral nutrition at home. In another child treated initially with radiation and chemotherapy, small bowel obstruction developed after cystectomy, necessitating resection of part of the ileum. Subsequently, a small bowel fistula developed, necessitating further surgery. The long-term problems with urinary diversion have been well documented[5, 24]; they include stricture, chronic infection, hydrone-

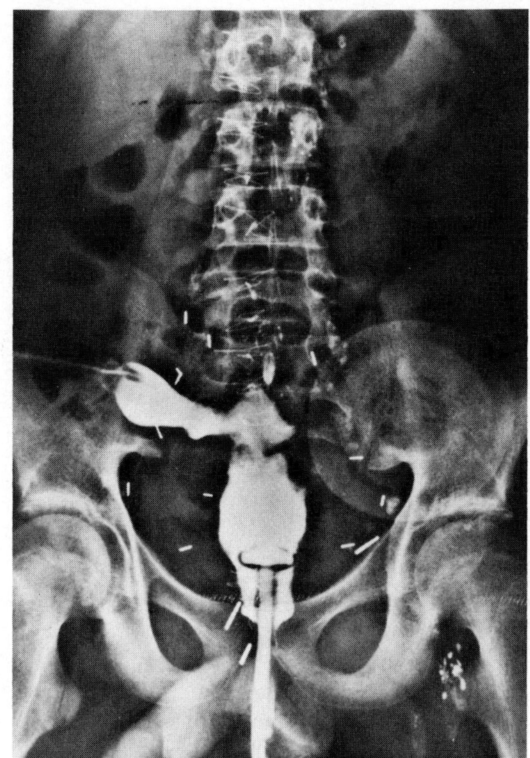

Figure 34–5 Drainage of pelvic abscess resulting from disrupted conduit.

toneal and pelvic irradiation is required, complications may be severe. In one adolescent who had resection of bulky nodes followed by radiation therapy and chemotherapy, chronic small bowel obstruction and malabsorption developed (Fig. 34–7). This boy requires intermittent total parenteral nutrition to maintain his weight. Impotence and failure of ejaculation may follow extensive bilateral retroperitoneal node dissections. These problems can be minimized by limited node dissection as described by Whitmore.[26] Pelvic vein thrombosis is a hazard in all pelvic procedures, less so in children than in adults. One of our adolescent patients developed pelvic vein thrombosis and a subsequent fatal pulmonary embolus after pelvic and retroperitoneal node dissection. Early activity, including ambulation, is the best prophylaxis. We use Venodyne boots extensively in older children and adolescents who have undergone major pelvic surgery.

phrosis, and renal failure (Fig. 34–6). The choice between radical surgery and an attempt at less radical surgery by preoperative chemotherapy and radiation therapy remains difficult.[19] Failure of conservative treatment means more difficult radical surgery later with more complications.

Pelvic exenteration is now rarely performed for vaginal and uterine rhabdomyosarcoma.[16] If exenteration is necessary, the complications are similar to those of cystectomy. The most common procedure for these tumors is now radical hysterectomy and pelvic node dissection. The main complication of this procedure is devascularization of a ureter with fistula formation. Although frequently seen in adults, urinary fistulae rarely form in children unless the ureters or the bladder is injured during surgery. Retroperitoneal and pelvic node dissections are carried out for perineal and paratesticular embryonal rhabdomyosarcoma. When bulky retroperitoneal lymph node metastases are removed and retroperi-

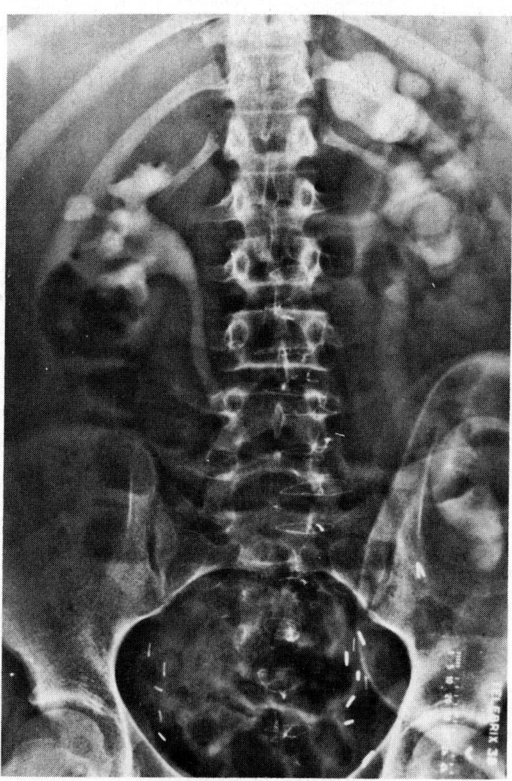

Figure 34–6 Left hydronephrosis following anastomotic stricture at the level of the ureterosigmoid conduit.

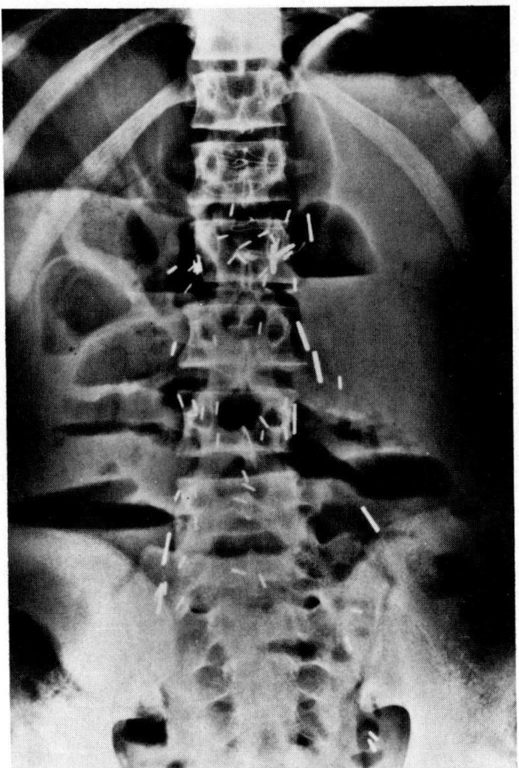

Figure 34–7   Severe chronic small bowel obstruction following retroperitoneal node dissection and irradiation.

LYMPHOMA

Children with lymphoma are operated on more frequently now than previously for specific indications: (1) staging laparotomy for Hodgkin's disease, (2) surgical resection of primary non-Hodgkin's lymphoma in the abdomen, and (3) complications of the treatment of these diseases.

The immediate postoperative problems with Hodgkin's disease staging laparotomy are unexplained fever, prolonged ileus from the retroperitoneal dissection, third-space fluid sequestration, and bleeding. High temperatures are frequent during the first few days after staging laparotomy. Chest x-ray studies, blood cultures, and urinalysis usually show no abnormality, and the fever abates without special treatment or specific identifiable cause. Adynamic ileus following staging laparotomy is often troublesome and may last 5 to 7 days. It is important to continue nasogastric tube drainage and in-travenous alimentation for this period. Forcing of oral feeding led to acute abdominal distention and wound disruption in one of our patients. Lymph collection in the retroperitoneal space or splenic bed requires active replacement during the first 1 or 2 days postoperatively. Postoperative hemorrhage is uncommon if careful attention is paid to hemostasis during surgery, particularly in the splenic bed and short gastric vessels. Delayed hemorrhage in the subdiaphragmatic region is usually responsible for subphrenic collections and abscess formation, though these are extremely rare in our experience.

The best known late complication of staging laparotomy is a particularly virulent and rapidly fatal pneumococcal infection attributed to loss of the spleen.[3, 4] However, children with Hodgkin's disease have disturbed immune defenses that are further depressed by radiation therapy and chemotherapy.[9, 15, 20] A variety of causes in addition to splenectomy may contribute to septic episodes in these patients.[25] All children at our institution are given prophylactic penicillin or erythromycin after splenectomy and are further protected by polyvalent pneumococcal vaccine.[6] We have encountered no deaths from pneumococcal sepsis in more than 100 staging laparotomies for Hodgkin's disease. The most common late surgical complication has been intestinal obstruction due to adhesive bands. Six children were seen with small bowel obstruction 6 months to 8 years after staging laparotomy. Four required laparotomy for release of adhesions; one required bowel resection.

Children with abdominal non-Hodgkin's lymphoma are sicker than children with other lymphomas and are often operated on while undergoing intensive chemotherapy.[9, 27, 28] Multidrug chemotherapy will sometimes cause a rapid necrosis of lymphoma and produce perforation of lymphomatous deposits in the small bowel. Three of our patients who had initial laparotomy elsewhere sustained perforations of the small intestine while in the induction phase of intensive chemotherapy. Each had fewer than 500 white blood cells and 40,000 platelets per ml at the time of surgery. All three patients sustained massive necrosis of a loop or loops of small bowel with gross fecal contamination of the peritoneal cavity.

Treatment consisted of povidone-iodine (Betadine) irrigation, resection of the necrotic bowel, and exteriorization of the bowel ends as ileostomy and mucous fistula. Multiple sump drains were left in the abdomen and irrigated daily with dilute Betadine solution. The patients all had a stormy course and required total parenteral nutrition, multiple antibiotics, and irrigation of sump tubes for several weeks. All survived and eventually had bowel continuity restored by further surgical procedures. Primary resection of bowel lesions is well tolerated and postoperative complications are uncommon even though intensive chemotherapy is given immediately in the postoperative period. The most difficult complications occurred when primary surgery was inadequate and chemotherapy was delayed, as in the three patients just described. Another child had bowel resection elsewhere and no other treatment for 2 months. This child developed intussusception from tumor and required a second small bowel resection before receiving chemotherapy and eventually entering remission. No patients require more careful evaluation by all members of the multidisciplinary team than children with non-Hodgkin's lymphoma.[9] Correct surgery and properly timed chemotherapy are imperative for cure and avoidance of complications.[28]

OSTEOGENIC SARCOMA

The surgeon treats the primary long-bone lesion and the common pulmonary metastases in children with osteogenic sarcoma. Primary surgery is often amputation or, increasingly, some kind of limb-saving procedure following preoperative chemotherapy. Amputations are performed as simple procedures and have fewer complications. Apart from minor wound separations, low grade stump infections, and later neuromas, amputations distal to the mid-humerus and midthigh are relatively straightforward. When proximal disarticulations or forequarter or hindquarter amputations are necessary, complications are more frequent. Hindquarter amputations have a high incidence of skin flap loss and wound problems as a result of devascularization. An attempt should be made to save the superior gluteal artery and thus preserve the posterior flap blood supply. The most distressing complication of ablative surgery for osteogenic sarcoma is recurrence of tumor in the amputation stump due to inadequate margins of resection. Amputations removing the joint proximal to the tumor or leaving a margin of at least 8 cm proximal to any area shown to be positive on bone scan will help avoid this problem. Tumor recurrence in the stump is usually associated with metastatic spread either locally or to the lung. It makes overall management more difficult and the chance of cure much less.

Modern limb surgery for osteogenic sarcoma involves an attempt to save the extremity and replace the resected bone with a metal prosthesis or bone grafts.[18] These procedures are complex and prone to early and late complications. Preserving the vascular supply requires careful dissection. Even so, blood supply to skin flaps, and rarely to major portions of the distal part of the extremity, may be lost. Preoperative arteriography and careful evaluation of the patient help select those children in whom limb salvage procedures can be carried out safely. In 14 Tikhoff-Linberg procedures performed for osteogenic sarcoma of the humerus at our institution, no limbs were lost. The radial nerve was injured in two patients and wound healing was delayed in two others. Three patients had chronic wound infections, one requiring removal of the metal prosthesis because of osteomyelitis of the distal humerus. Prolonged use of antibiotics may control minor infections and prevent progression to osteomyelitis. Edema of the distal part of the extremity after limb-sparing surgery is often seen initially. In most patients it will subside with elevation and active exercising of the extremity. Breakage of the internal prosthesis has been seen in lower extremity procedures. Because weight-bearing is the main function of the lower extremity, development of stronger metals and more physiologic prostheses is necessary. Ischial weight-bearing braces are currently used in many active children to prevent breakage of the prosthesis. Despite these problems, more children have a painless, functional extremity after these procedures for osteogenic sarcoma than survived the disease 10 years ago.

Metastatic osteogenic sarcoma in the lungs is becoming less common with improved chemotherapy. Surgical resection of metastatic lung nodules and surgical treatment of pneumothorax caused by chemotherapy necrosis of lung nodules (Fig. 34–8) still play an important role in total management of osteogenic sarcoma. Unrecognized lung disease will sometimes first be manifested by a pneumothorax while the patient is receiving chemotherapy. This is usually treated by tube thoracotomy and conservative management, with subsequent expansion of the lung. Occasionally thoracotomy is necessary for prolonged air leak. At surgery a necrotic tumor nodule will usually be found, with a persistent bronchial leak through the necrotic area.

In our experience, excision of pulmonary metastases in osteogenic sarcoma has had very few complications provided that the patients were well selected. After more than 100 thoracotomies for osteogenic sarcoma

we have had one death, which was related to unresectable disease that progressed after surgery. This patient's course was complicated by failure of the lung to expand, empyema, and prolonged tube drainage. One of the patients developed a wound infection and a small, persistent fluid collection in the chest; the low-grade empyema responded to antibiotics and conservative management. When multiple peripheral nodules were excised and a large amount of pleura denuded, a prolonged air leak following surgery was not uncommon but finally responded to conservative management. Even though great care is taken in positioning children on the operating table, one patient had a transient radial nerve palsy that disappeared completely within 6 weeks. The type of surgery carried out for metastatic osteogenic sarcoma was usually multiple wedge excisions using the mechanical stapling machine. Since using the stapler, air leaks have been fewer and recovery from surgery more rapid. Even those children who required multiple thoracotomies tolerated the procedures well and had few complications.[23] When multiple thoracotomies are required, careful preoperative evaluation of pulmonary function is necessary to be sure the child can tolerate at least lobectomy should this become necessary. If care is taken to remove only metastatic disease with a minimal surrounding area of lung tissue, pulmonary function will remain good despite multiple resections.

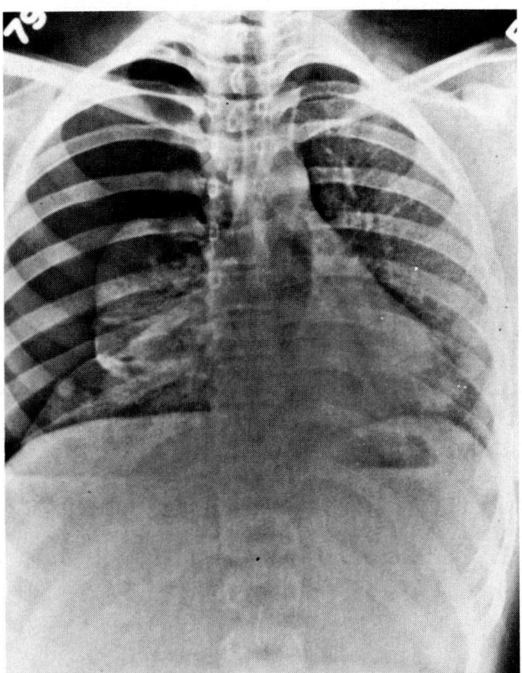

Figure 34–8 Right pneumothorax secondary to necrosis of osteogenic nodule during chemotherapy in a patient with metastatic osteosarcoma.

References

1. Altman, R. P., Randolph, J. G., and Lilly, J. R.: Sacrococcygeal teratoma, American Academy of Pediatrics, Surgical Section Survey 1973. J. Pediatr. Surg. 9:389, 1974.
2. Applebaum, H., Exelby, P. R., and Wollner, N.: Malignant presacral teratoma in children. J. Pediatr. Surg. 14:352, 1979.
3. Boles, E. T., Haase, G. M., and Hamoudi, A. B.: Partial splenectomy in staging laparotomy for Hodgkin's disease. An alternative approach. J. Pediatr. Surg. 13:581, 1978.
4. Chilcote, R. R., Baehner, R. L., and Hammond, D.: Septicemia and meningitis in children splenectomized for Hodgkin's disease. N. Engl. J. Med. 295:798, 1976.
5. Delgado, G. E., and Muecke, E. C.: Evaluation of 80 cases of ileal conduits in children: Indication, complications and results. J. Urol. 109:311, 1973.

6. Donaldson, S. S., Vosti, K., Berberich, F. R., et al.: A comparison of responses to pneumococcal vaccine among children with Hodgkin's disease. Proc. Am. Assoc. Cancer Res. 2:393, 1980.

7. Duckett, J. W., Peters, P. C., and Donaldson, M. H.: Severe cyclophosphamide hemorrhagic cystitis controlled with phenol. J. Pediatr. Surg. 8:55, 1973.

8. Exelby, P. R.: Management of embryonal rhabdomyosarcoma in children. Surg. Clin. North Am. 54:849, 1974.

9. Exelby, P. R.: Malignant lymphomas in children. World J. Surg. 4:49, 1980.

10. Exelby, P. R., Ghavimi, F., and Jereb, B.: Genitourinary rhabdomyosarcoma in children. J. Pediatr. Surg. 13:746, 1978.

11. Gellman, E., Kissane, J., Frech, R., et al.: Cyclophosphamide cystitis. J. Can. Assoc. Radiol. 22:99, 1969.

12. Ghavimi, F., Exelby, P. R., D'Angio, G. J., et al.: Multidisciplinary treatment of embryonal rhabdomyosarcoma in children. Cancer 35:677, 1975.

13. Gilladoga, A. C., Manuel, C., Tan, C. T. C., et al.: The cardiotoxicity of Adriamycin and Daunomycin in children. Cancer 37:1070, 1976.

14. Goldiner, P. L., and Scheizer, O.: The hazards of anesthesia and surgery in bleomycin treated patients. Semin. Oncol. 6:121, 1979.

15. Jenkin, D., Freeman, M., McClure, P., et al.: Hodgkin's disease in children: Treatment with low dose radiation and MOPP without staging laparotomy. A preliminary report. Cancer 44:80, 1979.

16. Kumar, A. P. M., Wrenn, E. L., Jr., Fleming, I. D., et al.: Combined therapy to prevent complete pelvic exenteration for rhabdomyosarcoma of the vagina or uterus. Cancer 37:118, 1976.

17. Leape, L. L., Breslow, N. E., and Bishop, H. C.: The surgical treatment of Wilms' tumor — results of the National Wilms' Tumor Study. Ann. Surg. 187:351, 1978.

18. Marcove, R. C., and Rosen, G.: En bloc resections for osteogenic sarcoma. Cancer 45:3040, 1980.

19. Rivard, G., Ortega, J., Hittle, R., et al.: Intensive chemotherapy as primary treatment for rhabdomyosarcoma of the pelvis. Cancer 36:1593, 1975.

20. Rosenstock, J. C., D'Angio, G. J., and Keisewetter, W. B.: The incidence of complications following staging laparotomy for Hodgkin's disease in children. Am. J. Roentgenol. Radium Ther. Nucl. Med. 120:531, 1974.

21. Schnaufer, L., and Koop, C. E.: Silastic abdominal patch for temporary hepatomegaly in stage IV-S neuroblastoma. J. Pediatr. Surg. 10:73, 1975.

22. Schullinger, J. N., Santulli, T. V., Casarella, W. J., and MacMillan, R. W.: Wilms' tumor: The role of right heart angiography in the management of selected cases. Ann. Surg. 185:451, 1977.

23. Shah, A., Exelby, P. R., Rao, B., et al.: Thoracotomy as adjuvant to chemotherapy in metastatic osteogenic sarcoma. J. Pediatr. Surg. 12:983, 1977.

24. Smith, E. D.: Follow-up of 150 ileal conduits in children. J. Pediatr. Surg. 7:1, 1972.

25. Walzer, P. D., Armstrong, D., and Tan, C.: Serum immunoglobulin levels in childhood Hodgkin's disease: Effect of splenectomy and long term follow-up. Cancer 45:2084, 1980.

26. Whitmore, W. F., Jr.: Germinal tumors of the testis. Sixth National Cancer Conference Proceedings. Philadelphia, J. B. Lippincott Co., 1970, p. 219.

27. Wollner, N., Exelby, P. R., and Lieberman, P. H.: Non-Hodgkin's lymphoma in children. A progress report on the original patients treated with the LSA(2)L2 protocol. Cancer 44:1990, 1979.

28. Zea, J. M., Exelby, P. R., and Wollner, N.: Abdominal non-Hodgkin's lymphoma in childhood. J. Pediatr. Surg. 11:363, 1976.

INDEX

Numbers in *italics* refer to illustrations; (t) denotes tabular material.